Your Health Today
Choices in a Changing Society

FIFTH EDITION

Michael L. Teague
University of Iowa

Sara L. C. Mackenzie
University of Washington

David M. Rosenthal
Columbia University

Mc
Graw
Hill
Education

YOUR HEALTH TODAY: CHOICES IN A CHANGING SOCIETY, FIFTH EDITION

2 3 4 5 6 7 8 9 0 RMN/RMN 1 0 9 8 7 6 5

ISBN   978-0-07-802859-5
MHID   0-07-802859-0

Senior Vice President, Products & Markets: *Kurt L. Strand*
Vice President, General Manager, Products & Markets: *Michael Ryan*
Vice President, Content Design & Delivery: *Kimberly Meriwether David*
Managing Director: *Gina Boedeker*
Brand Manager: *Courtney Austermehle*
Director, Product Development: *Meghan Campbell*
Product Developer: *Rhona Robbin*
Product Developer: *Kirstan Price*
Marketing Manager: *Phil Weaver*
Digital Product Analyst: *John Brady*

Director, Content Design & Delivery: *Linda Avenarius*
Program Manager: *Mark Christianson*
Content Project Managers: *Kathryn D. Wright and Emily Kline*
Buyer: *Michael R. McCormick*
Design: *Debra Kubiak*
Content Licensing Specialists: *Lori Hancock and Ann Jannette*
Cover Image: © *13/Tony Anderson/Ocean/ Corbis*
Compositor: *Laserwords Private Limited*
Printer: *R. R. Donnelley*

Library of Congress Cataloging-in-Publication Data

Teague, Michael L., 1946–
    Your health today : choices in a changing society loose leaf edition /
Michael Teague, University of Iowa-Iowa City, Sara Mackenzie, University of Washington, David Rosenthal, Columbia University—Fifth edition.
        pages cm
    Includes bibliographical references and index.
    ISBN 978-0-07-802859-5
    1. Health education. 2. Health promotion. I. Mackenzie, Sara L. C.
II. Rosenthal, David M. III. Title.
    RA440.T43 2015
    613—dc23
                                                            2014026738

www.mhhe.com

Dear Readers,

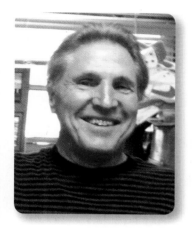

The story of this book began 12 years ago when three friends—a health educator, a family physician, and a family therapist—had a conversation about their beliefs about teaching health. While our clinical and academic paths differed, we found that we shared a fundamental belief that, while the individual plays a role in the wellness process, society has a responsibility to promote the well-being of all individuals. Many personal health books at the time focused on personal responsibility for health. While it is indeed a major part of health, we wanted to emphasize a model where individuals make health decisions within the context of their relationships, cultures, communities, policies, and physical surroundings. What eventually came of that conversation was the decision to create a book that emphasizes putting personal health in context.

Since we started working on the first edition of what became *Your Health Today*, we have visited health educators across the county and learned from their many different approaches to teaching personal health. We have tried to incorporate a range of those strategies and resources into our revisions and our own personal health courses.

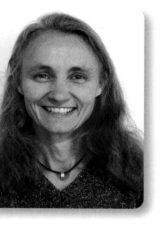

Like instructors who use our book, we too have been challenged through the years by the dynamic nature of health. The world is changing—interpersonally, financially, politically, and environmentally—so, what does that mean to personal health? How do students of the 21st century learn best, and where does their current understanding of personal health come from? What will be the health priorities of the future? What skills will today's students need 20 years from now to maintain a healthy lifestyle? Examining history and our own beliefs about those questions encouraged us to incorporate several health topics that are not traditionally covered (or covered only briefly) in other personal health books. As learners, we also believe that today's students generally do not need to memorize facts so much as learn how to access and assess health information, critically consider implications, and respond. In essence, our program fills the need for an approach to personal health that balances individual and cultural responsibility.

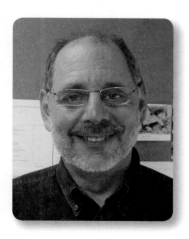

Our mission and passion for this endeavor has remained true years later. We continue to learn how to create small change in personal, professional, and community lives in an attempt to improve the health outcomes for all future generations. We hope that the fifth edition will challenge students to think of themselves as agents of change. Students can make personal changes in lifestyle behaviors that affect their own health, and they can also influence communities to make changes in response to social, political, and economic factors that affect the health of broader segments of the population.

Michael Teague
Sara Mackenzie
David Rosenthal

Brief Contents

p. 2
What does health mean to you?

Contents

p. 3

Who knew so many things influence the choices you make?

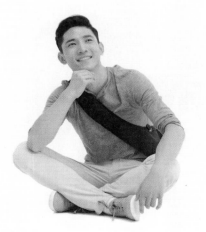

p. 55

Friendship matters
to your health.

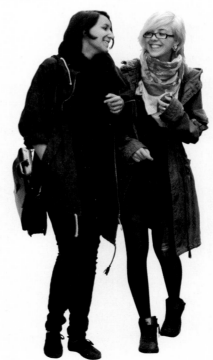

p. 124

Physical activity benefits your physical, cognitive, and emotional health.

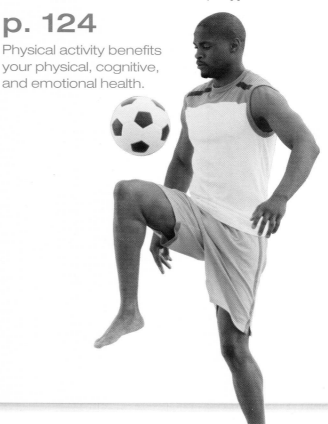

p. 180
Many body types and sizes can be associated with good health.

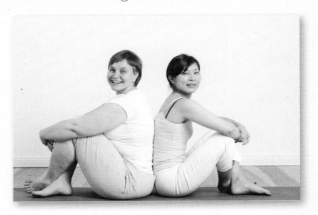

p. 235

Should recreational use of marijuana be legal?

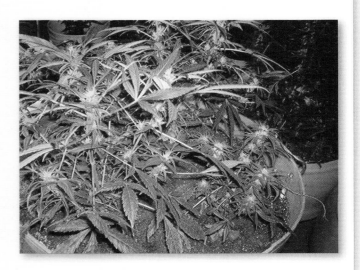

p. 288

What vaccines are recommended?

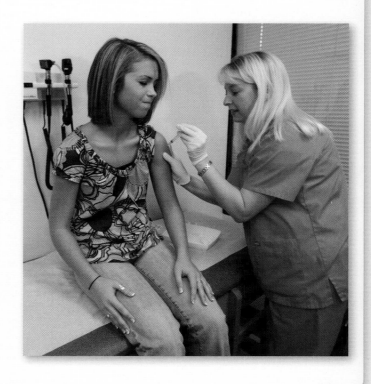

p. 325
What foods are part of a heart-healthy diet?

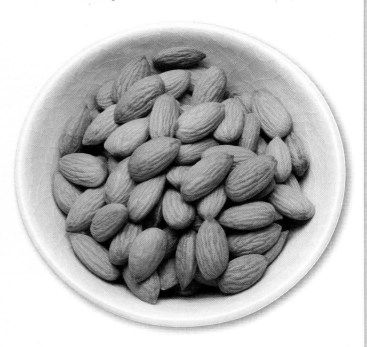

p. 371

How loud is too loud?

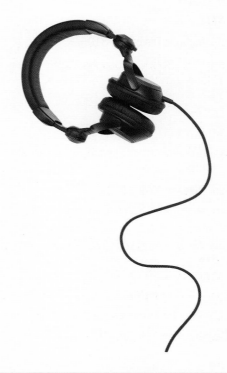

p. 426

What can and can't be recycled?

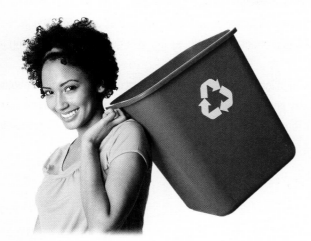

Features of *Your Health Today*

Your Health Today teaches personal health from a truly inclusive and socially responsible perspective. While each of us has a unique set of individual characteristics that shape our health, other environmental factors have an impact on our well being too. *Your Health Today* incorporates the individual, interpersonal, and broader social factors that affect our health, acting as a guide for healthy living in college and beyond.

The student-focused features in the fifth edition of *Your Health Today* highlight current topics, illustrate concepts with new photos and graphs, and invite dialogues among personal health students. For every chapter, these features serve as entry points to classroom discussion, critical thought, and practical application of health concepts to students' lives. Many also have accompanying assignable online activities within Connect.

Action Skill-Builders present manageable first steps in making meaningful behavior changes that relate to chapter topics. These include strategies for overcoming barriers to physical activity, improving body image, and getting a better night's sleep, as well as steps to healthier eating and how to deal with alcohol poisoning or perform routine self-exams for cancer. They show how even a small change can make a big difference.

Consumer Clipboards show students how to weigh information, evaluate product claims, and make savvier, healthier choices in a world full of misinformation and gimmicks. Topics include what to look for in an over-the-counter drug label, how to evaluate claims about e-cigarettes, and how to select a pair of running shoes.

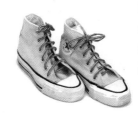

Public Health Is Personal boxes highlight the institutions of health and how issues that might otherwise seem remote—governmental limits on cigarette packaging, community-sponsored needle-exchange programs, or FDA regulation of antibiotic use in animal agriculture—can have a profound impact on students' individual health choices and priorities.

Who's at Risk? boxes highlight data that show health outcomes and trends among diverse groups of people: drinking problems by gender, sugar consumption by income level, illicit drug use by geographical region, and stress symptoms and strategies by age and gender. With graphs and visuals for students to examine, these boxes invite students to think about and discuss the reasons for these trends in an informed way.

Life Stories boxes feature lively and relatable stories that personalize chapter concepts and show how topics play out in real life. Among the topics covered are cohabitation, family planning pressures, exercise addition, eating disorders, and sexual assault.

Starting the Conversation boxes are designed to invite meaningful classroom discussion. Each box poses a question about a relevant news item or current event related to the chapter, followed by information to inform the discussion, and ending with two critical thinking questions. Topics in the fifth edition include social media and health-related apps, "sex tech" and the quality of sexual interactions, and whether cell phone use causes cancer.

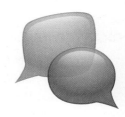

You Make the Call features present the facts behind a contentious social issue related to the chapter topic, followed by the pros and cons of each side of the issue. Designed to foster in-class discussion and/or personal reflection by the student, topics include marijuana legalization, vaccination requirements for college students, the legality of revenge porn websites, taxation of unhealthy foods, and the pros and cons of digital connectivity.

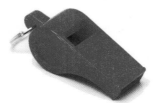

Personal Health Portfolio self-assessment activities that can be completed on paper or online guide students in exploring their personal health strengths and challenges. Activities include assessments of heart health and body image, creation of a family health tree, and evaluation of current physical activity, diet, and sleep habits. Students are able to see how their own family history, community, and culture affect their personal health decisions.

Chapter-by-Chapter Changes

Changes to the fifth edition reflect new research findings, updated statistics, and current hot topics that affect students' health choices and challenges. Revisions to the fifth edition were also guided by student performance data anonymously collected from the thousands of students who have used LearnSmart with *Your Health Today.* LearnSmart is an adaptive learning system that provides students with an individualized assessment of their own progress. Because virtually every text paragraph is tied to several questions that students answer while using LearnSmart, the specific concepts with which students are having the most difficulty can be pinpointed through empirical data.

Chapter 1: Self, Family, and Community

- New coverage of epigenetics.
- Updates to the ecological model of health and expanded discussion of health inequities, including the role of poverty.
- Updated material on Healthy People 2020.

Chapter 2: Mental Health and Stress

- Material on mental health updated to reflect DSM-5; stress statistics updated from the annual "Stress in America" survey.
- New "You Make the Call" feature focused on the stress and mental health impacts of digital connectivity.

Chapter 3: Social Connections

- Updated "Consumer Clipboard" feature on online dating, including new material on dating apps such as Lulu and Tinder.
- Updated discussion of same-sex marriage and related issues.

- Updated statistics and information on cohabitation and divorce, including new material on divorce patterns and ethnicity.

Chapter 4: Sleep

- Updated information provided on sleep quality, including the impact of technology (television, cell phones, computers) and caffeinated energy drinks.
- New "Who's at Risk?" box reviews how the amount and type of exercise an individual engages in affects sleep quality.
- Updated information on Adderall use by college students; "You Make The Call" feature focuses on whether colleges should conduct random drug testing for Adderall.

Chapter 5: Nutrition

- New coverage of gluten-free diets; celiac disease; the dangers of combining alcohol with energy drinks; probiotics, prebiotics, and symbiotics; and proposed FDA changes to the Nutrition Facts label for packaged foods.
- Updated coverage of sugar and artificial sweeteners, including information on whether sugar is addictive; recent findings on potential health risks of artificial sugars; and a new "Who's at Risk?" box with statistics on sugar consumption by age, gender, and income.
- New "Public Health Is Personal" box focuses on the Preservation of Antibiotics for Medical Treatment Act, designed to address concerns over the link between use of antibiotics for farm animals and the development of "superbugs."

Chapter 6: Fitness

- New coverage of high-intensity interval training, resistance cords for strength training, fitness apps, and the benefits of exergaming.

- Updated and expanded coverage of the dangers of sitting and the benefits of exercise for the immune system.
- The Human Capital Model is presented as a way to effectively argue the societal benefits of physical activity.

Chapter 7: Body Weight and Body Composition

- Updated coverage of U.S. obesity trends and medications for weight loss.
- Addition of the life course perspective for weight management.
- New "You Make the Call " feature considers reality television *Biggest Loser* competitions.

Chapter 8: Body Image

- New and updated coverage of social media and tracking tools and their impact on body image; also, the role of media in body image, including warning labels for digitally enhanced photographs.
- Updated coverage of eating disorder diagnosis criteria from DSM-5.

Chapter 9: Alcohol and Tobacco

- New boxed features: "Starting the Conversation" focuses on Driver Alcohol Intoxication Systems, and "You Make the Call" looks at proposals to lower the legal limit for alcohol to 0.05 percent.
- New coverage of ingestion fads for alcohol consumption (for example, alcohol enemas, vaporizing alcohol), dissolvable tobacco products, and the impact of DSM-5 changes on the classification of students as mild alcoholics.
- Updated and expanded coverage of the risks of e-cigarettes and hookah parlors, the dangers of pre-gaming and spring break excursions, biopsychosocial pathways to alcohol-related problems, and nonsmoker rights on college campuses.
- Updated statistics and discussion of health risks of drinking problems among college students and binge drinking as an underreported problem for college women.
- Updated material on the debate over graphic tobacco product labels.

Chapter 10: Drugs

- Updated statistics throughout on drug use prevalence and patterns.
- Material added on new drugs of abuse, including krokidil, N-Bomb, Syrup, and Devils Breath.

Chapter 11: Sexual Health

- New box features: "Public Health Is Personal" focuses on sex trafficking, "Who's At Risk?" examines condom use and sexual activity among college students, "Starting the Conversation" raises the question of whether sex tech reduces the human quality of sexual interactions, and "You Make the Call" examines the question of whether revenge porn should be illegal.

- New and updated information included on choosing condoms, sexting, and telidildonics.
- Updated information provided on hooking up among college students ("party and play" using drugs like crystal meth) and on college organizations promoting abstinence and working counter to the hook-up culture (for example, the Love and Fidelity Network and Anscombe Society).

Chapter 12: Reproductive Choices

- New "You Make the Call" feature on the role of paid family leave in health outcomes of children and families.
- New and expanded coverage of the role of long-acting contraceptives in pregnancy planning for young adults and the role of early childhood education in health.

Chapter 13: Infectious Diseases

- Expanded and updated material on climate change and infectious disease patterns, pertussis outbreaks, and Tdap and flu vaccination recommendations.
- New "Public Health Is Personal" box on reducing antibiotic resistance.

Chapter 14: Cardiovascular Disease, Diabetes, and Chronic Lung Diseases

- Newly released American Heart Association cholesterol guidelines, with key changes to recommendations.
- New "Who's at Risk?" box focuses on geographical variation in noncommunicable disease patterns.

Chapter 15: Cancer

- New "Starting the Conversation" box considers the potential role of cell phones in cancer development.
- Updated cancer screening guidelines, including new Pap recommendations and lung cancer screening.
- Updated statistics throughout on cancer prevalence and patterns.

Chapter 16: Injury and Violence

- New boxed features: "Who's at Risk?" box provides a profile of sexual harassment on college campuses, "Public Health Is Personal" focuses on curbing gun violence and recent mass shootings, and "You Make the Call" examines the question of whether stop-and-frisk laws are legal.
- New material included on Stand Your Ground laws, the Heimlich maneuver, and the association between smart phone use and neck problems.
- Expanded coverage of concussions from sports and recent studies citing long-term health problems.
- Updated information on use of 3-D printers for constructing guns and updated statistics and information on safety and sexual assaults on college campuses.

Digital Tools for Today's Instructors and Students

liveWell: A Healthy Foundation for Life

liveWell is an innovative online, multimedia program designed to help college students improve their exercise, eating, and stress management habits. liveWell, created by Dr. James Prochaska, is a two-part, self-administered program that includes the following:

- An online, personalized assessment of current health-related behaviors and readiness to make meaningful behavior change.

- A Personal Activity Center containing activities, such as exercise videos and stress management tools, matched to each individual's behavior change goals and readiness to change.

The program leverages state-of-the-science best practices to tailor behavior change messages and activities to promote student well-being and behavior change.

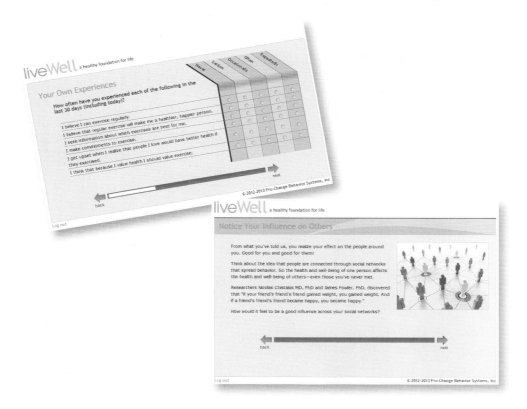

Get Connected and Make It Count

McGraw Hill Education **connect** | PERSONAL HEALTH

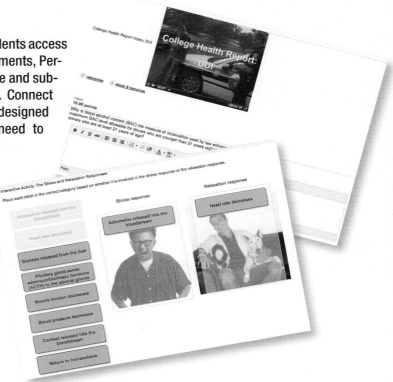

Connect for *Your Health Today* gives students access to a wealth of online interactive activities and assignments, Personal Health Portfolio activities that they can complete and submit, and practice quizzes with immediate feedback. Connect provides a highly interactive learning environment designed to help students connect to the resources they need to achieve success in the course.

With the *Connect* e-book, students can access *Your Health Today* anywhere, any time. And, they have access to an additional two chapters, "Complementary and Alternative Medicine" and "Environmental Issues." Through the *Connect* e-book, they can also manage notes, highlights, and bookmarks in one place for simple, comprehensive review.

McGraw Hill Education **connect** INSIGHT

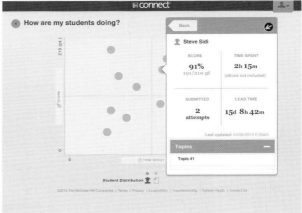

New to *Connect* is Connect Insight™, the first and only analytics tool of its kind. Connect Insight™ is a series of visual data displays—each framed by an intuitive question—to provide at-a-glance information for instructors regarding how a class is doing. Instructors can easily view student performance matched with student activity, and the real-time analytics allows instructors to take action early to keep struggling students from falling behind. Instructors can leverage aggregated information about their courses and students to provide a more personalized teaching and learning experience.

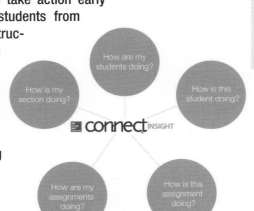

Adaptive Learning to Improve Student Performance

Adaptive technology uses continual assessment and artificial intelligence to personalize the learning experience for each individual student. By identifying a student's strengths and weaknesses, you can ensure that every minute a student spends studying has the highest possible impact. With users experiencing an average of a letter grade improvement, adaptive learning is a proven way to increase student success and confidence.

LEARNSMART

LearnSmart is an adaptive study tool designed to strengthen memory recall, increase class retention, and boost grades. Students are able to study more efficiently because they are made aware of what they know and don't know. Real-time reports quickly identify the concepts that require more attention from individual students—or the entire class.

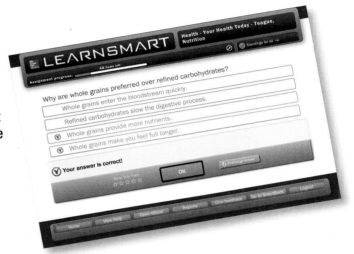

SMARTBOOK

SmartBook is the first and only adaptive reading experience designed to change the way students read and learn—it adds value to every minute a student spends studying *Your Health Today.* SmartBook creates a personalized reading experience by highlighting the most impactful concepts a student needs to learn at that moment in time. As a student engages with SmartBook, the reading experience continuously adapts by highlighting content based on what the student knows and doesn't know. This ensures that the focus is on the content he or she needs to learn, while simultaneously promoting long-term retention of material. Use SmartBook's real-time reports to quickly identify the concepts that require more attention from individual students—or the entire class. The end result? Students are more engaged with course content, can better prioritize their time, and come to class ready to participate.

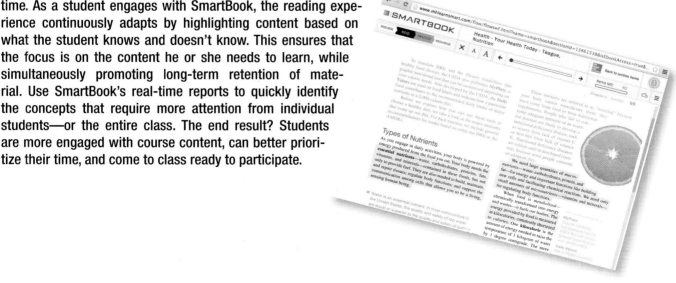

Customize Your Course Materials

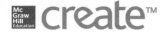 Craft your teaching resources to match the way you teach! With McGraw-Hill Create™, www.mcgrawhillcreate.com, you can easily rearrange chapters, combine material from other content sources, and quickly upload content you have written like your course syllabus or teaching notes. Find the content you need in Create by searching through thousands of leading McGraw-Hill textbooks. Arrange your book to fit your teaching style. Create even allows you to personalize your book's appearance by selecting the cover and adding your name, school, and course information. Order a Create book and you'll receive a complimentary print review copy in 3 to 5 business days or a complimentary electronic review copy (eComp) via email in minutes. Go to www.mcgrawhillcreate.com today and register to experience how **McGraw-Hill Create**™ empowers you to teach *your* students *your way.*

Instructor Teaching Resources

Instructor teaching resources that will help you get your course up and running include:

- The *Course Integrator Guide* includes chapter learning objectives, lists of outside resources, and an integrator guide to help you make the most of Connect Personal Health.

- A *Test Bank* features more than 2,000 multiple-choice, true/false, matching, and short-answer questions. McGraw-Hill's computerized EZTest allows instructors to create customized exams using these test items or instructors' own questions. A version of the test bank is also provided in Microsoft Word files for instructors who prefer that format.

- *PowerPoint presentations* for each chapter of the text can be used as-is or modified to meet the needs of individual instructors.

CourseSmart CourseSmart offers thousands of the most commonly adopted textbooks across hundreds of courses from a variety of higher education publishers. It is the only place for faculty to review and compare the full text of a textbook online, providing immediate access without the environmental impact of requesting a printed exam copy. At **CourseSmart**, students can save up to 50 percent off the cost of a printed book; reduce their impact on the environment; and gain access to powerful Web tools for learning, including full text search, notes and highlighting, and email tools for sharing notes among classmates. Learn more at *www.coursesmart.com*.

Campus McGraw-Hill Campus is the first of its kind—an institutional service providing faculty with true single sign-on access to all of McGraw-Hill's course content, digital tools, and other high-quality learning resources from any learning management system (LMS). This innovative offering allows for secure and deep integration and seamless access to any of our course solutions, such as McGraw-Hill Connect, McGraw-Hill Create, McGraw-Hill LearnSmart, or the Tegrity lecture capture tool. McGraw-Hill Campus includes access to our entire content library, including e-books, assessment tools, presentation slides, and multimedia content, among other resources, providing faculty open and unlimited access to prepare for class, create tests/quizzes, develop lecture material, integrate interactive content, and much more.

ACKNOWLEDGEMENTS

Thanks to the reviewers who provided feedback and suggestions for enhancing the fifth edition of *Your Health Today.*

Rachelle Franz, University of Central Oklahoma

Kathi Fuller, Western Michigan University

Linda-Marie Hamill, The Citadel

Ray Lomax, Kean University

Steve Owens, Tallahassee Community College

Kelly Schoonaert, University of Wisconsin—Stevens Point

Dana Sherman, Ozarks Technical Community College

Debra Tavasso, East Carolina University

Sharon K. Woodard, Wake Forest University

Matt Wright, Folsom Lake College

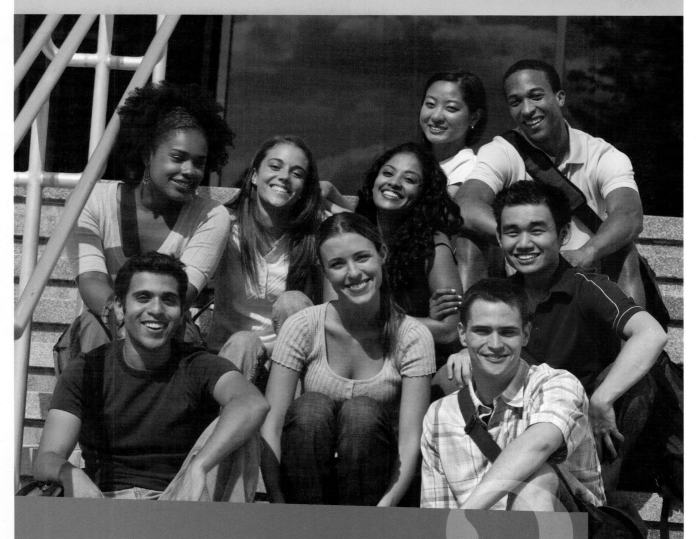

Ever Wonder...

- why it's so hard to break a bad habit?
- how much your parents' health predicts your own?
- what you are most likely to die of?

As individuals, we are all responsible for our own health. Each of us makes choices about how we live—about whether to be physically active, whether to eat a healthy diet, whether to get enough sleep, whether to see a doctor when we need to. And yet to talk about health only as a matter of individual choice assumes that we are always aware of the choices we are making and that we are always "free" to make them. The truth is that there are differences in how we live and the contexts in which we make decisions.

In this book, we explore personal health within the context of our social, cultural, and physical environment. We recognize that individuals are ultimately responsible for their own health, but we also know that people make healthier choices when their environment supports those choices, especially when it provides a nudge in more positive directions.[1]

PERSONAL HEALTH IN CONTEXT

To begin, we consider the difference between the terms *health* and *wellness,* and then we explore the personal and environmental factors that shape and influence our personal health.

Health and Wellness

---

health
State of complete physical, mental, social, and spiritual well-being.

wellness
Process of adopting patterns of behavior that can lead to improved health and heightened life satisfaction; wellness has several domains and can be conceptualized as a continuum.

Traditionally, people were considered "healthy" if they did not have symptoms of disease. In 1947, the World Health Organization (WHO) broke new ground with its positive definition of **health** as a state of complete physical, mental, and social well-being, not merely the absence of disease and infirmity. Physical health refers to the biological integrity of the individual. Mental health includes emotional and intellectual capabilities, or the individual's subjective sense of well-being. Social health means the

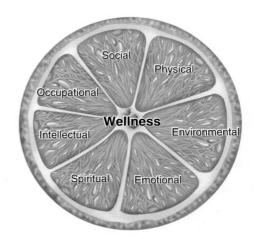

figure 1.1   **Dimensions of wellness.**
Sources: Adapted from *The World Health Report 2006: Working Together for Health,* by World Health Organization, 2006, Geneva, Switzerland; *Wellness Index: A Self-Assessment for Health and Vitality,* by J. W. Travis and S. R. Ryan, 2004, Berkeley, CA: Ten Speed Press (Celestial Arts).

ability of the individual to interact effectively with other people and the social environment.[2]

More recently, a spiritual domain has been added to the WHO definition, reflecting the idea that people's value systems or beliefs can have an impact on their overall health. Spiritual health does not require participation in a particular organized religion but suggests a belief in (or a search for) some type of greater or higher power that gives meaning and purpose to life. Spiritual health involves a connectedness to self, to significant others, and to the community.

Wellness is a slightly different concept from health. It is generally defined as an active process of adopting patterns of behavior that can lead to improved health and heightened life satisfaction. Like health, wellness is seen as encompassing multiple dimensions: physical, emotional, intellectual, spiritual, interpersonal or social, environmental, and occupational (see Figure 1.1).

Wellness may also be conceptualized as a continuum. One end of the continuum represents extreme illness and premature death; the other end represents wellness and optimal health (see Figure 1.2). Historically, Western medicine has focused primarily on the illness side of the continuum,

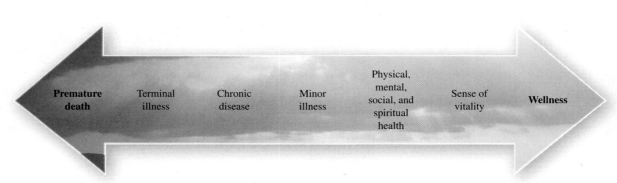

| Premature death | Terminal illness | Chronic disease | Minor illness | Physical, mental, social, and spiritual health | Sense of vitality | Wellness |

figure 1.2   **The wellness continuum.**
Source: Adapted from "Definition of Health Promotion" by M. P. O'Donnell in *American Journal of Health Promotion, 1* (5), Premier Issue, 1986.

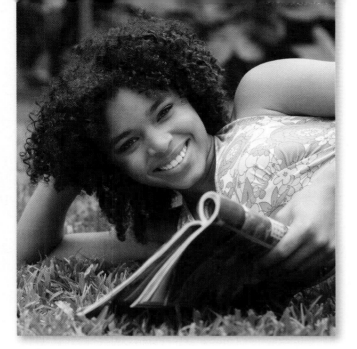

■ Qualities associated with wellness include self-confidence, optimism, a sense of humor, an active mind, vitality, and joy in life, among many others.

treating people with symptoms of disease. More recently, approaches to health have focused on the wellness side of the continuum, seeking ways to help people live their lives fully, as whole people, with vitality and meaning. For example, in the approach called *salutogenesis,* individuals (or communities) are encouraged to assess and understand their current situation, find reasons to move in a health-promoting direction, and then develop the capacity to do it.[3]

Although most people want to have good health, it typically is not an ultimate goal in itself. Usually, people desire good health in order to reach other goals—to be more productive, more attractive, more comfortable, more independent—in other words, to have a higher quality of life. In the next section, we'll look at how our environment can promote or deter our capacity for good health.

The Ecological Model of Health and Wellness

Although there are many theories about health behavior and decision making, we focus here on the **ecological model of health and wellness**. As shown in Figure 1.3, the model is a framework that addresses the interrelationships between individuals and their environment, taking into account all the factors that influence individuals' choices. It recognizes that we each have a unique set of characteristics—our genetics, age, and sex, along with our knowledge, beliefs, values, and skills that guide the decisions we make about how to live our life. We also live within an environment, which in this model is defined very broadly

ecological model of health and wellness A framework that recognizes the interrelationship between individuals and their environment; emphasizes the multiple social determinants that influence health.

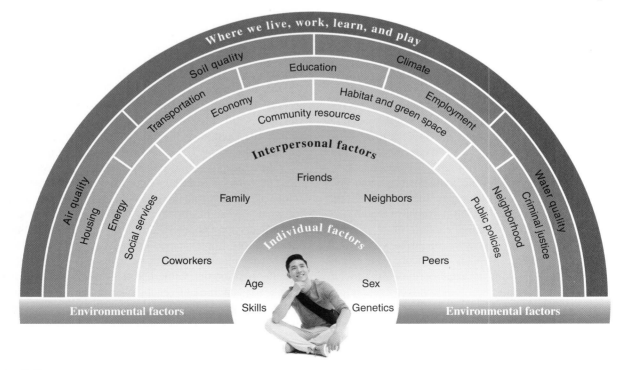

figure 1.3   The ecological model of health and wellness.
Our health is shaped both by our unique set of individual characteristics and by environmental factors, also called the social determinants of health.
Source: Adapted from *Health in All Policies: A Guide for State and Local Governments* by L. Rudolph, J. Caplan, K. Ben-Moshe, and L. Dillon, 2013, Washington, DC and Oakland, CA: American Public Health Association and Public Health Institute.

as anything external to us. The environment encompasses our relationships with other people, our interactions with social institutions, our community affiliations, and public policies that impact each of these.

According to the ecological model, friends, family, community norms, economic, social, and public policy, and even global events affect your health opportunities. In addition, societies' practices can influence your health by shaping your environment in ways that increase or decrease your opportunities for making healthy or unhealthy choices. For example, in most supermarkets candy is placed near the checkout counter, where you (or your child) can grab it impulsively as you're getting ready to pay. The practice increases sales but discourages healthy choices.

social determinants of health
Societal conditions that affect health and can potentially be altered by social and health policies and programs.

These external environmental factors are also known as the **social determinants of health**. This term highlights the fact that the conditions in which you are born, grow, live, work, and age influence the options you have available and the choices you make. Social determinants of health include such factors as income, socioeconomic status, educational attainment, literacy, employment status, working conditions, housing, transportation, social support networks, and access to health care services.[4,5] Your health is also affected by your physical environment. Factors in the *built* physical environment—such as kinds of housing, streets, schools, and sanitation and transportation systems—and factors in the *natural* physical environment—such as air and water quality, proximity to environmental hazards, and access to parks and natural settings—all affect your health.

How does the ecological model play out in your life? As an example, let's say you decide you want to have a healthier diet. What influences your ability to achieve this goal, according to the ecological model? First, consider your personal history: your knowledge, attitudes, and skills—ideas about what constitutes a healthy diet, attitudes toward different foods and diets, and skills that enable you to prepare certain foods. In addition, depending on your genetic predispositions, age, and health conditions, you may need to pay attention to certain components of your diet, such as salt if you have high blood pressure or red meat if you have high cholesterol.

Next, consider how the people closest to you—your family, friends, coworkers, and peers—influence your eating patterns. As you were growing up, you became familiar with the foods your family ate. In turn, your family's food preferences were influenced by their cultural background and geographic location. You may still prefer those foods, seek them out, and eat them when you go home. Your friends may like to eat out at fast-food restaurants and you may go with them. Or your friends may be vegetarian, so you find yourself eating more vegetarian foods. If your friends are overweight or if they gain weight, it's likely that you will find weight gain more acceptable for yourself.[6,7]

Your decisions about what to eat also take place in the context of where you live, work, learn, and play. Your dining hall may have unlimited soda refills and fried foods, or your church may serve donuts after services. In your community, you may have opportunities to buy fresh fruits and vegetables, or the corner store may have only candy and liquor. Your income can also significantly affect the foods you purchase. Finally, local, state, and national laws influence the safety of the food you eat, the nutritional labeling it features, and its cost. When all these environmental factors are taken into account, it is clear that choosing a healthier diet is not just a matter of your individual choices—though the choices you make within the context of your environment are critical. One way to make your diet healthier is to promote healthful eating options in your community.

Both in the United States and worldwide, worse health outcomes are associated with poverty, unemployment, poor housing, low educational attainment, environmental pollution, and other negative social, economic, and physical factors. Addressing these factors to reduce inequities is one of the goals of national and international health policies; health policy in the United States will be discussed in more detail later in the chapter.

SELF AND FAMILY: HEREDITY AND FAMILY HEALTH HISTORY

Are you the way you are because of your genetic endowment or because of your experiences? This is the classic question of "nature versus nurture," and the answer isn't black and white. Who we are as individuals is the result of a complex, ongoing interaction among (1) our genetic inheritance, (2) our lifestyle choices, and (3) environmental factors of many kinds (including our first environment—in utero)[8]. Even though these influences are woven together in life, in this chapter we treat them separately—genetic inheritance first, then lifestyle choices, and finally environmental factors.

At conception, you received what is perhaps your biggest inheritance, your genetic makeup. Your genetic inheritance plays a key role in establishing some of the parameters of what you can be and do in your life, but it does not determine everything about you. It gives you the potential to be tall or short; apple-shaped or pear-shaped; brown-eyed or blue-eyed; blonde, brunette, or bald. It gives you a unique bundle of strengths, vulnerabilities, and physical characteristics. You can think of genetic inheritance as your blueprint, or starting point. The blueprint is filled in and actualized over the course of your entire life.

Genetics used to be confined to the realm of scientists. Now, however, due to significant advances, the language of genetics has entered the realm of everyday conversation. You will need to understand some basic genetic concepts to engage in personal health decisions, public debates, and policy decisions.

DNA and Genes: The Basis of Heredity

Our bodies are made up of about 260 different types of cells, each performing different, specific tasks. Except for red blood cells, every cell in the body contains one nucleus that acts as the control center. Within the nucleus, the entire set of genetic instructions is stored in the form of tightly coiled, threadlike molecules called **deoxyribonucleic acid**, or **DNA**. If we were to uncoil the DNA and magnify it thousands of times, we would find it consists of two long strands arranged in a double helix—a kind of spiraling ladder (Figure 1.4). DNA has four building blocks, or bases, called adenine (A), guanine (G), cytosine (C), and thymine (T). The two strands of DNA are held together with bonds between the building blocks; an A on one strand always connects to a T on the opposite strand, and a G on one strand connects to a C on the opposite strand. The consistent pairing is important—each strand is an image of the other (see Figure 1.4).

The complete set of DNA is called a person's **genome**. Within the nucleus, DNA is divided into 23 pairs of **chromosomes** (one set of each pair comes from each parent). One pair of chromosomes—the sex chromosomes—is slightly different and is labeled with an X or a Y rather than a number. Females have two X chromosomes; males have an X and a Y chromosome.

DNA is the body's instruction book. The four bases are like a four-letter alphabet. Just as the letters in our 26-letter alphabet can be arranged to make thousands of words with different meanings, a series of thousands or millions of A-T-G-C combinations can be arranged to form a distinct message; this message is a gene. Each chromosome contains hundreds or thousands of genes located at precise points along the chromosome. Approximately 21,000 of these genes serve as protein-coding templates, meaning they are transcribed into *RNA*, which carries the template out of the nucleus to the cell sites where proteins are made. The sequence of RNA is translated into a precise sequence of amino acids, creating a protein with a specific composition, shape, and role. Different proteins make up structural components of the body and help direct the activities of cells and body processes. Much of the rest of the genome had been thought to contain "junk" DNA, also known as noncoding DNA because it's not involved in coding for proteins. But it is now known that many genes are transcribed into noncoding types of RNA, which in turn are believed to play vital roles in cell function and regulation.[9]

deoxyribonucleic acid (DNA)
Nucleic acid molecule that contains the encoded, heritable instructions for all of a cell's activities; DNA is the genetic material passed from one generation to the next.

genome
The total set of an organism's DNA.

chromosome
Gene-carrying structure found in the nucleus of a cell, composed of tightly wound molecules of DNA.

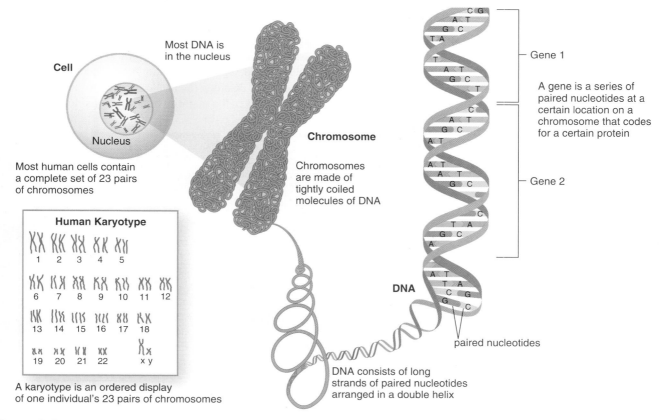

Most DNA is in the nucleus

Cell

Nucleus

Most human cells contain a complete set of 23 pairs of chromosomes

Chromosome

Chromosomes are made of tightly coiled molecules of DNA

Gene 1

A gene is a series of paired nucleotides at a certain location on a chromosome that codes for a certain protein

Gene 2

DNA

paired nucleotides

DNA consists of long strands of paired nucleotides arranged in a double helix

Human Karyotype

1	2	3	4	5

6	7	8	9	10	11	12

13	14	15	16	17	18

19	20	21	22	x y

A karyotype is an ordered display of one individual's 23 pairs of chromosomes

figure 1.4 **Chromosomes, genes, and DNA.**

Although our cells contain the same full set of genes, most of the cells in our body become specialized—that is, they take on characteristic shapes or functions, such as skin, bone, nerve, or muscle. Genes turn on or off to regulate this activity in a process called **differentiation**. Once a cell is differentiated, it can no longer become other cell types (it is as if certain "chapters" of the DNA instruction book are locked shut). Unspecialized cells, called **stem cells**, are present in an embryo (embryonic stem cells) and are retained within tissues (adult stem cells).

differentiation
The process by which an unspecialized cell divides and gives rise to a specialized cell.

stem cell
An undifferentiated cell that is capable of giving rise to different types of specialized cells.

mutation
Alteration in the DNA sequence of a gene.

Genetic Inheritance

You inherited one set of chromosomes from each of your parents and thus have two copies of each gene (excluding genes on the sex chromosome). The position of each gene is in a corresponding location on the same chromosome of every human. However, your two copies may be slightly different because every so often, changes occur in a gene; such a change is called a **mutation**. The change may involve a letter being left out (e.g., a series A-T-G becomes A-G), an incorrect letter being inserted (e.g., a series A-T-G becomes A-A-G), or an entire series of letters being left out, duplicated, or reversed. The location of the mutation determines the effect. If we go back to the analogy of the alphabet, consider what happens to the following sentence when a single letter change is made:

"When my brother came home, he lied."

If we change one letter to a "d," it can turn the sentence into nonsense:

"When my drother came home, he lied."

Or it can change the meaning entirely:

"When my brother came home, he died."

Something similar happens with a mutation in a gene. The change can cause different "meanings" or instructions to be sent to cells. Many mutations are neither harmful nor beneficial (such as changes that lead to blue eyes or brown eyes). Other mutations may be harmful and cause disease. For example, in sickle cell disease, an adenine (A) is replaced by a thymine (T) in the gene for hemoglobin (a protein that carries oxygen in red blood cells). This single change at a crucial spot changes the gene's instructions and causes it to produce an altered form of hemoglobin that makes red blood cells stiff and misshapen. This leads to an increased risk of red cells blocking arteries and causing pain, infection, and damage to organs.

Two important facts about mutations are that (1) they are passed on from generation to generation, and (2) they allow for human diversity. You share 99.9 percent of the same DNA with your classmates. Slight differences in the remaining 0.1 percent account for all your genetic variations in appearance, functioning, and health.[8,10]

Most characteristics (like height or skin color) are determined by the interaction of multiple genes at multiple sites on different chromosomes. However, some traits are determined by a single gene, such as whether earlobes are attached or detached (Figure 1.5). To explain the relationship between genes and appearance, we will use this trait. An individual inherits two alleles (alternative forms) of the gene for earlobe structure (one copy from each parent). The two alleles can be the same version of the gene or they may be different versions, and one version is likely to be dominant over the other. In our example, the detached-earlobe allele is the *dominant allele,* and it will be expressed and will determine appearance. The other version, the attached-earlobe allele, is a *recessive allele*—it will be hidden by the dominant allele and will not be expressed. A recessive allele is expressed only if both copies of the gene are the recessive version. Other relationships are possible between alleles as well: some alleles have incomplete dominance or codominance, meaning that both alleles affect appearance in varying degrees.

How does genetic inheritance affect your health? As previously noted, a genetic mutation in just one gene can cause a disease or disorder (as in the example of sickle cell disease). However, the majority of health conditions are caused

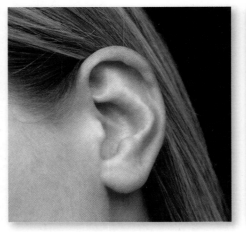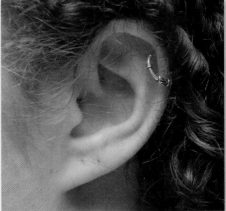

figure 1.5   Dominant and recessive alleles.
A single gene appears to determine whether earlobes are detached (left) or attached (right). We all have two copies (alleles) of the "earlobe" gene. The detached allele is dominant, meaning a single copy will make the earlobes appear detached (remember, if a dominant allele is present, it determines appearance). The attached allele is recessive, meaning two copies are required for the earlobes to appear attached. Think about your parents and siblings; can you figure out which alleles you have?

Starting the Conversation

Genetic Testing Online

Q: If you could find out if you have a gene that increases your risk for breast cancer or depression by ordering a home test kit on the Internet, would you do it?

A growing number of companies are now advertising genetic testing directly to the public over the Internet. For a few hundred dollars or less, you can order a testing kit online, submit a sample of saliva or blood, and receive information about your individual genome within a few weeks. The companies assert that the tests assess your genetic risk for a wide range of health conditions, including heart disease, stroke, various types of cancer, type 2 diabetes, allergies, migraine, osteoporosis, Alzheimer's disease, Parkinson's disease, rheumatoid arthritis, and multiple sclerosis. Some companies offer advice about diet and nutritional supplements based on your results.

For most of the 20th century, genetic disorders were diagnosed primarily by noting the presence of the disorder in a family tree across multiple generations. In the past 20 years, however, advances in genetic research have allowed scientists to identify the genes responsible for many inherited single-gene diseases, such as sickle cell disease, Tay-Sachs disease, Huntington's disease, and cystic fibrosis. At first, genetic testing was done to determine whether someone who showed symptoms of a genetic disease was a carrier of a genetic disorder, to predict the adult onset of a genetic disorder, or to screen newborns for genetic defects. Testing was done in a clinical laboratory by order of a physician, and genetic counseling was available to help the patient understand the results.

Now, with the rapid expansion of expertise and technology, genetic testing has moved into the commercial realm of for-profit business. Direct-to-consumer marketing bypasses physicians, clinics, and insurance companies to appeal directly to healthy people who may or may not have a family history of a genetic disorder. The vast majority of the diseases they test for are multi-factorial—that is, several or many genes interact with each other and the environment to affect risk.

The advantages of personal genetic testing appear evident at first glance—convenience, time savings, cost savings, privacy. You may also feel a sense of empowerment by gathering your own health information, and you may be motivated by this information to make healthy lifestyle choices or follow screening recommendations if you know you have a genetic risk for a condition.

There are also disadvantages. Often the claims made about how much information the testing can provide are not adequately backed by evidence and thus may be misleading. There is currently no federal regulation of direct-to-consumer genetic testing, although the U.S. Food and Drug Administration (FDA) has informed several home testing companies that they need to submit tests to the FDA for approval. Home testing may also have less quality control over the collection, transport, and testing of your DNA sample than in a medical setting.

Perhaps most importantly, interpreting the results of genetic testing is complicated, and most consumers report they want guidance by a professional. Except in rare circumstances, genetic profiling can only suggest a risk of disease but does not diagnose disease or predict disease with certainty. Because most diseases with a genetic component are multifactorial, information about genetic risk factors may not be any more meaningful than information about other risk factors, such as poor diet or smoking.

If you are thinking about ordering your genetic profile, consider how the results could affect you and how you would use them. If you already know from your family health tree that you are at risk for heart disease, cancer, or other multifactorial diseases, would genetic testing provide any additional information or be more likely to cause you to pursue the lifestyle behaviors that would reduce your risk?

Q: Under what circumstances do you think you would consider ordering a genetic testing kit? What would you hope to find out?

Q: Genetic testing is available for diseases that as yet have no cures, such as some degenerative neurological disorders. If your family history suggested you might have a gene for such a disease, would you want to know? Why or why not?

Sources: "Direct to Consumer Genetic Testing: A Systematic Review of Position Statements, Policies and Recommendations," by H. Skirton, L. Goldsmith, L. Jackson, and A. O'Connor, 2013, *Clinical Genetics, 82,* pp. 210–218.

---

by interactions among one or more genes, the environment, and health behaviors; these are called **multifactorial disorders**. Examples of multifactorial disorders include heart disease, cancer, diabetes, obesity, and schizophrenia. Many personal characteristics, predispositions, and behaviors are also the results of interactions among genes and multiple environmental factors.

To further complicate this story, gene–environment interactions can actually be passed on from generation to generation. In a new area of study called *epigenetics,* researchers are identifying how health risks, such as stress or poor nutrition, can be passed from generation to generation independent of actual DNA sequence changes. What they have found is that the environment can modify the structure of DNA without changing the sequencing of nucleotides, the DNA building blocks (A-T-G-C), through a process called methylation—small methyl (carbon and hydrogen) particles that attach to the DNA. Methylation changes how DNA is used within cells. To use the book analogy again, methylation is like glue between some of the pages, making it more difficult to read sections. [11]

multifactorial disorder
Disease caused by the interaction of genetic and environmental factors.

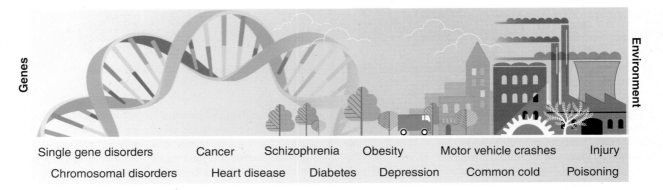

figure 1.6   **Relative contribution of environment and genetics.**
Source: Adapted from Figure 12.1: Relative contribution of environment and genetic factors in some common disorders, in *ABC of Clinical Genetics* by Helen Kingston, 3rd edition, 2002, London: BMJ Publishing Group.

Because so many diseases with a genetic component are multifactorial, paying attention to the lifestyle and environmental factors that contribute to them is crucial. Figure 1.6 shows the continuum of genetic and environmental contributions for some common diseases and incidents. Notice that there is no clear distinguishing line between environment and genetics because the precise roles of each are not always clear. For instance, poisoning may seem to have purely environmental causes, but some children may be genetically more predisposed to take risks and thus more prone to eat or drink unknown substances.

You have probably already noticed within your own family that some traits are passed from one generation to the next (see the box, "Genetic Testing Online"). You have inherited not only the color of your skin, hair, and eyes but also other traits and predispositions. Your grandmother's history of colon cancer may mean you have inherited an increased risk for colon cancer. Your uncle's heart attack at age 40 may mean you have received an increased risk of heart disease from his side of the family. A family health tree is a useful way to organize this information.

Creating a Family Health Tree

A **family health tree**, also called a *genogram* or *genetic pedigree,* is a visual representation of your family's genetic history. Creating a health tree can help you see your family's patterns of health and illness and pinpoint any areas of special concern or risk for you.

family health tree
Diagram illustrating the patterns of health and illness within a family; also called a genogram or genetic pedigree.

To construct your family health tree, you need to assemble information concerning as many family members as you can. (A sample tree is shown in Figure 1.7.) The more detailed and extensive the tree, the easier it will be for you to see patterns. Your tree should include parents, siblings, grandparents, cousins, aunts, and uncles. Basic information for each family member should include date of birth, major diseases, and, for deceased relatives,

age and cause of death. You might include additional data such as the age of family members when their diseases were diagnosed as well as disabilities, major operations, allergies, reproductive problems, mental health disorders, and behavioral problems. Because we are learning more about genetic responses to medications, you may want to include information about what medications worked well to treat your uncle's depression or your father's high cholesterol. The Personal Health Portfolio activity for this chapter at the end of this book provides detailed instructions on how to put together your own family health tree. As the tree reveals patterns in your family's health, you can think about the roles that lifestyle habits, community factors, and even public policies may play.

Gathering family health information to construct a tree may not be easy. In some cultures, it is taboo to discuss the dead or certain diseases, such as cancer, depression, or HIV. Such cultural views may influence the information you are able to collect. In addition, if you were adopted, you may not have the same access to your biological family's health history. Only one-third of Americans report that they have tried to gather information for a family health tree. In recognition of the importance of the task, the U.S. surgeon general has launched a national public health campaign called the U.S. Surgeon General's Family History Initiative. The initiative encourages families to use opportunities when they are gathered together to discuss and record health problems that seem to run in the family.[12]

What Can You Learn From Your Health Tree?

Certain patterns of illness or disease suggest a genetic link, as in the following instances:

- An early onset of disease is more likely to have a genetic component.

- The appearance of a disease in multiple individuals on the same side of the family is more likely to have a genetic correlation.

Life Stories

Janet: A Family History of Breast Cancer

Janet, a college sophomore, lost her mother to breast cancer when she was 10 years old and her mother was just 34. Since then, Janet had felt sure that she too was destined to get breast cancer. In high school, she struggled with decisions about whether to go to college and pursue a career or to start a family as early as she could so she would have at least some time with her children. She chose to go to college, but her ambivalence about that decision was reflected in her often risky approach to contraception. On those occasions when she had sex with her boyfriend without using birth control, she knew that on some level, she hoped she would get pregnant.

A turning point came when Janet learned in one of her classes that some cases of breast cancer are associated with specific genes, referred to as BRCA1 and BRCA2. Genetic tests can be performed to determine if a person has a mutated copy of either of these genes. Learning this empowered Janet to find out more. Using her college library and online sources, she learned about options available to high-risk people like herself. They included starting mammograms (breast screenings) at an earlier age than recommended for the general population, taking certain medications, and even mastectomy (breast removal) to prevent cancer.

For the first time since her mom died, Janet felt she had some control over her future. She couldn't change her genes, but there were actions she could take to reduce her risk. She had never really talked to her dad about her mom's health history because she didn't want to upset him by stirring up sad memories. Now she realized it was important to her own health to get as much information as possible about her mom's cancer. She decided to talk to him about it the next time she was home. She also decided to make an appointment with a genetic counselor to find out more about testing for the BRCA1 and BRCA2 genes.

- What obstacles—psychological as well as logistical—do you think make it hard for people to find out more about their family health histories?

- What conditions or diseases seem to run in your family? What behavioral choices or environmental factors might increase or decrease the likelihood that these conditions will actually occur?

connect
ACTIVITY

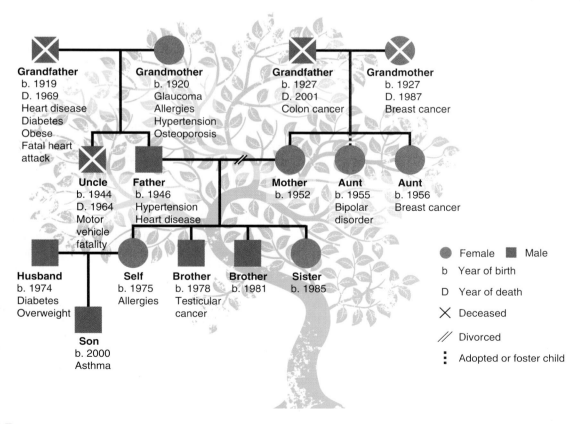

figure 1.7 A family health tree.

What conclusions can you draw from this tree? Perhaps the grandfather's obesity played a role in his heart attack at age 50. Perhaps the uncle would have survived the motor vehicle injury if seat belt laws had been in place in 1964.

- A family member with multiple cancers represents a greater likelihood of a genetic association.

- The presence of disease in family members who have good health habits is more suggestive of a genetic cause than is disease in family members with poor health habits.

If you discover a pattern of illness or disease in your health tree, you may want to consult with your physician or a genetic counselor about its meaning and implications (see the box, "Janet: A Family History of Breast Cancer"). You may want to implement lifestyle changes, have particular screening tests, or watch for early warning signs. Again, a pattern of illness in your family does not automatically mean that you will be affected. The main use of a health tree is to highlight your personal health risks and strengths so you can make informed lifestyle choices.

SELF AND LIFESTYLE CHOICES

Now that you understand something about how your genes influence your health, we turn to the lifestyle choices you can make that affect how your genetic inheritance will play out in your life. Genes and lifestyle choices are not the only factors contributing to your health, as the ecological model makes clear, but they are critical components. In this section, we look at how your behavior choices affect your health and how people change unhealthy behaviors.

Health-Related Behavior Choices

Your health-related behavior choices (or lifestyle choices) are actions you take and decisions you make that affect your individual health (and, possibly, the health of your immediate family members). They include choices concerning your physical, mental, emotional, spiritual, and social well-being—what you eat, how much you exercise, whether you spend time developing meaningful relationships, and so on. For example, having an apple instead of a bag of chips is a healthy behavior choice, as is quitting smoking. Other examples are getting enough sleep, practicing safe sex, wearing a seatbelt in a car, finding effective ways to manage stress, drinking alcohol in moderation if at all, and getting regular health checkups. Lifestyle choices are what individuals have the most control over in managing their health.

Interesting questions arise when we consider why people make choices that don't enhance their health and why they don't change behaviors they know are hurting them.

Health Belief Model
Model of behavior change that uses the constructs of perceived susceptibility, seriousness of consequences, benefits of action, and barriers to action.

Stages of Change Model
Model of behavior change that focuses on stages of change.

Psychologists have proposed many theories about health behavior choice and change. The Health Belief Model and the Stages of Change Model are especially useful.

The Health Belief Model

The **Health Belief Model** was developed in the 1950s as a framework for understanding why people make the health choices they do. According to the model, health behaviors are influenced by four perceptions:

- *Perceived susceptibility.* Do you believe you are at risk for a problem?

- *Perceived seriousness of consequences.* Do you perceive the problem as serious if it were to occur?

- *Perceived benefits of specific action.* If you change behavior, do you believe it will reduce the threat?

- *Perceived barriers to taking action.* What factors will get in the way of your making a change, such as time, money, or beliefs?

To illustrate how this works, imagine that you are a smoker in a family where people are prone to heart disease. Your uncle and grandfather both died from heart disease at relatively young ages, and you know that you too are susceptible to the same fate. You also know that your smoking habit increases your risk for this disease and that the consequence for your continuing the habit could be death. If you quit, the benefits are a reduced risk for heart disease within a few years and a potentially longer life. You also recognize a huge barrier: most of your friends smoke, and it would be hard to go out with them and resist a cigarette. According to the Health Belief Model, all of these considerations enter into your decision-making process when you think about quitting smoking.

In the chapters to come, you will come across information and ideas that may prompt you to consider changing your health behavior in one way or another. You will examine a variety of factors that affect your health, such as the nutritional content of your favorite foods, the amount of exercise you get, and your choices around alcohol and drugs. One way to organize your decision-making process is by using the concepts offered by the Health Belief Model.

The Stages of Change Model

Developed in the 1990s by psychologists James Prochaska and Carlo DiClemente, the **Stages of Change Model**, or Transtheoretical Model (TTM), is another widely accepted framework for understanding individual health behavior change. The model acknowledges that people are often ambivalent about making significant changes in their lives, and it recognizes that change happens as a process, not a one-time event. It also takes into account not just a person's knowledge but also her feelings, behaviors, relationships, and perceived **self-efficacy** (belief that one can perform a certain task). The stages of change are as follows:

- *Precontemplation.* In this stage, you have no motivation to change a behavior. In fact, you may not even realize or acknowledge that you have a problem. You just want people to quit bothering you about your behavior. You may be helped to see a problem by events that highlight discrepancies between your behaviors and your goals.

- *Contemplation.* You realize you may have a problem behavior. You are thinking that you should make a change in the near future (usually within six months). You are trying to understand the problem and may search for solutions. Often you are weighing the pros and cons of making a change. Self-efficacy becomes important, as you are more likely to prepare for change if you believe in yourself and the fact that you can make a change.

- *Preparation.* The pros have won and you are making a plan for change. You are setting goals and have a start date. You are looking for tools to help support the change. You are building your skill set and supporting your self-efficacy.

- *Action.* You are implementing behavior change. You are committing time and energy to make it work. From this point forward, you can support your efforts to change by rewarding yourself for change, avoiding environments that trigger the unhealthy behavior, and enlisting the help of friends and family.

- *Maintenance.* You have been maintaining the new behavior for at least six months. You are working to prevent yourself from falling back into old habits. You are well on your way! This can be a long, ongoing stage—for some behaviors, lasting a lifetime.

- *Termination.* The new behavior has become such a part of your life that you have no temptation to return to the old behavior, and you have 100 percent confidence in your ability to maintain the behavior.[13,14]

Understanding that change is a process with different stages is important because you may need different information or different types of support, depending on where you are in the process (some are included in the list of stages). It's also important to realize that change is more like a spiral than a linear progression. You can enter and exit the process at any point, and you often cycle back through some or all of the steps (Figure 1.8). Most of us try several times to make changes before they really stick. **Relapse** is the rule rather than the exception. It should be seen not as failure but as a normal part of the process.[13,14,15] The important thing is to keep trying and not get discouraged.

Let's consider an example of the stages of change. Say you are determined to get better grades this term, especially in psychology, your major. To improve, you've been studying a lot in the afternoons and drinking coffee and energy

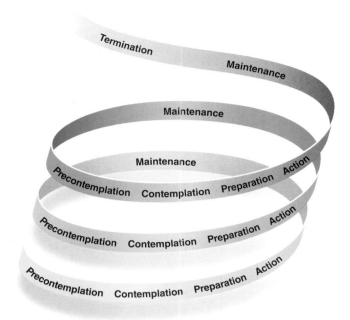

figure 1.8 **The stages of change: A spiral model.**
Source: Adapted from "In Search of How People Change," by J. O. Prochaska, C. C. DiClemente, and J. C. Norcross, 1992, *American Psychologist, 47* (9), pp. 1102–1114.

drinks to stay focused. Unfortunately, you keep oversleeping and missing your 8 a.m. psych class, where surprise quizzes are often given. Because you've missed several quizzes, your grade is suffering. The reason you're oversleeping is that you're having trouble falling asleep at night, which you've been attributing to stress. You don't make the connection between the caffeine you're consuming in the afternoon and your insomnia. This sort of behavior marks the precontemplation stage, in which you do not recognize that your caffeine consumption may be causing you a problem.

When a friend mentions that you might sleep better if you cut out the caffeine, your first thought is that you really enjoy those drinks in the afternoon and might not be able to study without them. But then you start to weigh the benefits of caffeine (you feel sharper, you can concentrate more easily) against the problem of insomnia (you oversleep and miss class). This thought process marks the contemplation stage, in which you weigh the pros and cons of behavior change.

You decide to try decaffeinated coffee and see what happens. You buy some decaf at the grocery store (preparation) and make a switch the following week, at the same time cutting out energy drinks (action). Although you feel fuzzier and less focused at first, and you have a pounding headache for a day, you are able to get to sleep more easily

self-efficacy
Internal state in which you feel competent to perform a specific task.

relapse
Backslide into a former health state.

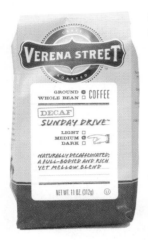

and start making it to class. You ace some of the quizzes, so you know your grade will be going up. You also notice how much better you feel, and how much sharper your mind is, when you get enough sleep.

A few weeks later, you're at a friend's house and she offers you regular coffee. Your sleep problems seem to be over, so you drink it. You lie awake till 3 a.m. that night and have to force yourself out of bed in the morning. Though not a full-blown relapse, this slip reminds you of why you wanted to make this behavior change. It's not as hard to get back on track, skipping the caffeine, as it was to give it up in the first place. You are on your way to the maintenance stage.

Have you ever had an experience like this one? If so, were you able to make the necessary connections and stick with the behavior change you made?

Creating a Behavior Change Plan

Research has given us a great deal of information about how behavior change occurs. How can you use this information to change your own behavior? The first step is accepting responsibility for your health and making a commitment to change. Ask yourself these questions:

■ *Is there a health behavior I would like to change?* It could be smoking, overeating, procrastinating, being sedentary, eating too much sugar, or a host of other behaviors.

■ *Why do I want to change this behavior?* There can be many reasons and motivations, but it's best if you want to change for yourself.

■ *What barriers am I likely to encounter?* Having a plan to deal with barriers will increase your chances of success.

■ *Am I ready to change the behavior?* Beginning a behavior change plan when you haven't fully committed to it will likely result in relapse.

Although making an initial commitment is an important step, it isn't enough to carry you through the process of change. For enduring change, you need a systematic behavior change plan. Once you have identified a behavior you would like to change, assessed your readiness to change, and made a commitment to change, follow the steps in the box, "Change to a New Behavior."

Although behavior change theories offer valuable insights into the change process, they also have limitations. The major limitation of the behavior change approach is that

Action Skill-Builder

Change to a New Behavior

1. Set goals. Make them Specific, Measurable, Attainable, Realistic, and Time-bound (SMART goals). An example of a SMART goal might be "I will increase my consumption of vegetables, especially dark green and orange vegetables, to three cups per day over the next four weeks, reaching my goal by October 30."

2. Develop action steps for attaining goals within a set time frame. For example, "I will include baby carrots in my lunch starting October 1."

3. Identify benefits associated with the behavior change. For example, "Eating more vegetables will help me lose weight, improve my complexion, and be healthier overall."

4. Identify positive enablers (skills, physical and emotional capabilities, resources) that will help you overcome barriers. An important capability is a sense of self-efficacy. Another capability might be the confidence that comes from having succeeded at behavior change in the past, along with skills that were used at that time. For example, "I was able to cut out caffeine last semester. I think I'll be able to improve my diet now."

5. Sign a behavior change contract to put your commitment in writing. Ask a friend or family member to witness your contract to increase your commitment. Signing a behavior change contract is one of the most effective strategies for change. An example of a behavior change contract is provided in the Personal Health Portfolio activity for Chapter 1 at the end of the book.

6. Create benchmarks to recognize and reward interim goals. Particularly when a goal is long term, it is useful to have rewards for short term goals reached along the way. Reward yourself with something that particularly appeals to you (e.g., buying a new iPhone app, going to a movie).

7. Assess your accomplishment of goals and, if necessary, revise the plan.

it does not take into account health factors beyond the control of the individual, primarily the kinds of social environmental factors in the outer layers of the ecological model illustrated earlier in Figure 1.3. Another complicating factor is the glut of health-related information that inundates our daily lives and environments, especially on television and the Internet. Some of this information is confusing, some is contradictory, and some is even misleading or wrong. To make good choices, you need skills that allow you to access accurate health information, to understand the evidence underlying health recommendations, and to evaluate important health issues in society.

Being an Informed Consumer of Health Information

Part of taking responsibility for your health is learning how to evaluate health information, sorting the reputable and credible from the disreputable and unsubstantiated—in other words, becoming an informed consumer of health information.

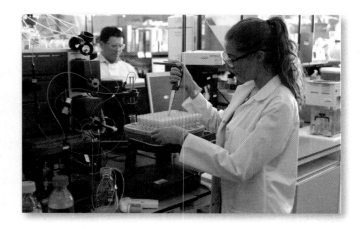

Developing Health Literacy Do you read and understand the labels on foods you buy? Do you know which clinics are covered by your health insurance plan? If you learn that your dad is taking Lipitor, do you know how to find out more about it and its associated risks? These are all questions that relate to **health literacy**—the ability to read, understand, and act on health information. Health literacy includes the ability to critically evaluate health information, to understand medical instructions and directions, and to navigate the health care system. Eighty million American adults are said to have limited health literacy skills.[16,17] Without these skills, they are at risk for poor health outcomes, especially as they receive more conflicting health information from a variety of sources such as websites and television.

Evaluating health information is complicated by the fact that we process information not just logically but also emotionally, and our emotional responses can affect how we interpret and react to that information. Interpreting our **health risk**, defined as the probability of exposure to a hazard that can result in negative consequences, can be especially difficult. Many factors contribute to our health risk for a particular condition, including age, gender, family history, income, education, geographical location, and other factors that make us unique. So, for example, if you have a family history of breast cancer and you learn that 13 percent of women will develop breast cancer in their lifetime, you may feel alarmed and anxious about your risk, based on that information. If you don't have a family history of breast cancer and learn the same information, you may feel relieved and reassured about your risk. Recognizing the part played by your emotions can help you assess your risk in more balanced ways.[18]

As with other skills, health literacy can be developed, and this book will help you develop your own health literacy. Each chapter will introduce you to basic health and medical language related to the topic, coach you on how to find accurate information, and encourage you to apply your critical thinking skills. For some general guidelines related to health literacy, see the box, "Evaluating Health Information on the Internet."

Understanding Medical Research Studies Being an informed consumer also involves understanding research studies, which inform most of the health recommendations that you hear about on the news or in health journals or magazines. Most sources will cite the study, the researcher, and the journal in which the study appeared, and very often you can look up the study online and read the original article or a summary of it.

A formal research study follows a specific design and tests a specific hypothesis. The research process is clearly enough described in the study that other researchers can replicate it and confirm the results themselves. There are many possible ways to categorize research studies. Formal studies can generally be of three types, with different methods and different goals:

health literacy
The ability to read, understand, and act on health information.

health risk
Probability of an exposure to a hazard that can result in negative consequences.

- *Basic medical research.* This type of research typically involves work on a cellular level or in animals. It contributes to a baseline of scientific knowledge, which then can be applied to humans in clinical or epidemiological research.

- *Epidemiological studies.* In this type of research, scientists study large groups of people (cohorts), using interviews, surveys, and measurements to identify and explore the relationships between risk factors and disease (or health) over time.

- *Clinical studies.* This type of research involves human participants, typically individuals who have received screenings, diagnostic tests, treatments, or other interventions. Clinical research usually identifies whether or not an intervention—such as a drug, a product, or a behavior—produces a particular effect. Randomized, double-blind studies are considered the gold standard, meaning that study participants are randomly assigned to either the group that receives the intervention or the group that receives a placebo and that neither the participants nor the researchers know until the end of the study who got what.

Any of these types of medical research studies can serve as credible supporting sources for news stories, product endorsements, and your own personal health decisions, as long as you know the limitations and goals of each type.

Consumer Clipboard

Evaluating Health Information on the Internet

You can find accurate health information on the Internet—but you can also find information that's misleading or just plain wrong. Ask yourself these questions to evaluate and deconstruct health messages you find on websites.

What techniques are used to catch your attention?

Dramatic images and language are frequently used to make you pay attention. How are the creators trying to influence you, either overtly or covertly?

What evidence is cited?

Reliable information is based on scientific research, not opinion. Be cautious if the "evidence" consists of personal stories or testimonials, and be wary about "miracle cures." A healthy dose of skepticism is helpful when assessing health information.

Is the information current?

Information about health and medicine is always changing. Use sources of information that are current and frequently updated. Remember that websites can stay on the Internet unchanged for years.

Who sponsors the website or advertises on it?

Ads give you another clue about the possible bias of the information and its providers.

Who created the website?

Look for the organization or individuals providing the information and consider whether there is an agenda, bias, or hidden message. The most reliable sources of health information are government organizations, educational institutions, and nonprofit (URLs ending in gov, edu, or org).

What values, lifestyles, or points of view are represented (or omitted) in the message?

Look for clues about the site's targeted audience in terms of gender, age, ethnicity, educational level, income, and political persuasion. If you identify with the audience, you may be more likely to overlook bias.

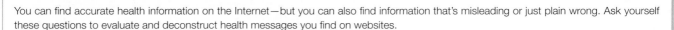

| Home | Health News | Drugs | Healthy Living | Eating & Diet | Parenting/Pregnancy | Health Facts |

MedConnect™
Medical information for everyone

Search criteria | Sign in | New User | Search

Doctors Symptoms Medical terms

How to get the most from the MedConnect community, where to go when you need answers, and how to talk to your doctor, are just a few of the topics currently running in our online forums.

Featured forums:
Ask a nurse
Heart disease facts
Hypertension
Diet and exercise
STDs
Cold and flu remedies
Migranes

Featured videos:

Baby Q&A   Sleep disorders

Stress relief   Relationship tips

Video   Diet and Diabetes

Sources: "Health Literacy," by the National Network of Libraries of Medicine, retrieved from www.nnlm.gov/outreach/consumer/hlthlit.html; *Literacy for the 21st Century* (5th ed.), by G. L. Tompkins, 2010, Boston: Allyn & Bacon.

When you are considering a health recommendation and the study that supports it, ask these questions:

- *Is the recommendation based on a formal research study, or is it simply an expert opinion?* Sources often cite experts when no clinical research is available to guide recommendations or when current research results are conflicting. Keep in mind that an expert's opinion hasn't necessarily been subjected to any formal testing.

- *If it was a formal clinical study, was it randomized and double-blind?* If the study was randomized, you can be more confident that the results were not influenced by factors outside of the treatment, such as differences between participants at the outset of the study. If it was a double-blind study, you can be more confident that the results weren't unduly influenced by the placebo effect or researcher bias.

- *Were the people in the study similar to you?* If the participants were different from you in some significant way—for example, if they were all over the age of 65 and you are 20—the results are less likely to apply to you than if the participants were similar to you.

- *How many participants were involved?* Larger studies, involving many participants, are generally more reliable than studies involving a small number of participants.

- *Who sponsored or funded the study?* Some sponsors stand to benefit from certain results, such as drug companies. The most impartial sponsors are research institutes and government agencies.

- *Was the study published in a reputable, peer-reviewed medical or health journal?* Such a study has been evaluated by other researchers in the field, who are in a position to judge the strength of the methods and the accuracy of the results.

The answers to these questions affect how much credence you can put in the research results. Keep in mind that scientists typically consider individual studies stepping-stones in the ongoing search for answers to complex questions.

SELF AND COMMUNITY

The ecological model shows us that personal health is influenced by factors well beyond the control of the individual. Accordingly, responsibility for health and wellness extends beyond the individual to public health and community health.

Public Health

Public health is a discipline that focuses on the health of populations of people (whereas the discipline of medicine focuses on the health of individuals). Public health efforts include both health promotion and disease prevention. **Health promotion** focuses on actions designed to maintain a current health state or encourage a more desirable state of health (such as campaigns to promote physical activity). **Disease prevention** focuses on defensive actions taken to ward off specific diseases and their consequences (such as food and water safety standards or flu shot campaigns). Public health measures can improve the health of populations through education, engineering, and enforcement. Public health initiatives balance the needs and rights of individuals against the needs and rights of other members of the population. It is important to keep in mind that your health is inherently linked to the health of the people around you!

Specific public health agencies and organizations are responsible for public health. Many such agencies are parts of the federal or state governments (one responsibility of government is to ensure safety of society). In the United States, nationwide government-sponsored public health initiatives are conducted by the Public Health Service, led by the surgeon general and the Centers for Disease Control and Prevention in Atlanta, Georgia. State, county, and city health departments are involved at the state and local levels, and many public health actions take place at the local, or community, level (see the box, "What Is Public Health?").

Nongovernmental organizations also promote population health through work in politics, education, and research advocating for a range of health-related issues, including environmental rights, women's health, economic development, health care, and cancer research. An increasing need for work by agencies and organizations not traditionally considered "health" related has arisen due to the vital role of social determinants in health.[5] For example, city planners may not consider themselves in a health-related field, but parks and community walkability directly influence citizens' health and are determined by zoning and planning.

public health
The study and practice of health promotion and disease prevention at the population level.

health promotion
Public-health-related actions designed to maintain a current healthy state or advance to a more desirable state.

disease prevention
Public-health-related actions designed to ward off or protect against specific diseases.

community health
Issues, events, and activities related to the health of a whole community, as well as activities directed toward bettering the health of the public and/or activities employing resources available in common to members of the community.

Community Health

Community implies an interdependence of people and organizations within a defined region. **Community health** refers to activities directed toward improving the health of those people or activities employing resources shared by the members of the community. It is similar to public health, but the population is defined as a geographic community rather than people with shared characteristics, and it specifically recognizes ties and connections within the community. For example, the health department in a town (the community) with a large immigrant population may decide as part of its emergency preparedness planning that it needs to design messages in different languages in order to reach all members of the community. Ideally, the health department would create partnerships with members of the various groups within the town to ensure cultural sensitivity, relevance, and engagement. Research

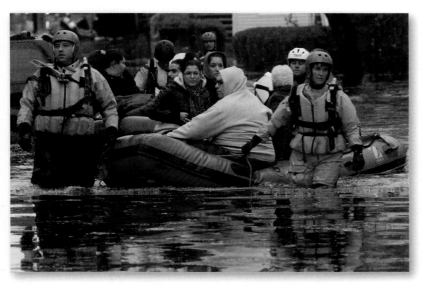

■ Heavy rains and floods periodically necessitate the evacuation of communities. Extreme weather, natural disasters, and other events that affect whole populations fall into the domain of public health.

Public Health Is Personal

What Is Public Health?

The benefits of public health are all around you, reducing your risk for disease and injury and helping you live a healthier life.

When you get up in the morning, you brush your teeth with the water from your tap. You don't have to worry about contracting an infectious disease because tap water in the United States is safe to drink and presents a minimal risk of infectious disease. You have had fewer cavities and dental problems than people did a century ago, because the tap water you drink contains fluoride, which strengthened your teeth when you were younger.

If you drive to campus, you buckle your seatbelt out of habit. Your state has seatbelt laws in place to reduce traffic fatalities, and even if you would prefer not to buckle up, you do not want to get a ticket. If you bike to campus, you can avoid dodging cars by taking the bike lane, which has been put in place to protect bicyclists. You meet a friend for a bagel and cream cheese before class. You don't worry about eating the food from a coffee shop because sanitation inspectors ensure that all restaurants follow regulations that reduce incidences of foodborne illness.

After breakfast, you continue your commute to school, past "clean buses" that run on emissions-controlled diesel as part of your city's green energy campaign. A road worker directs you around a lane closure, where construction workers are wearing helmets and hearing protection, following occupational safety and health laws.

You enter your class building, where the air you breathe is fresh and smoke-free. Because tobacco smoke has been recognized as a health hazard, your campus follows regulations that prohibit smoking within 25 feet of public buildings.

After class, you head to the campus health center to pick up a month's worth of contraceptive supplies. You and your partner are not ready for pregnancy; you're planning to delay starting a family until after you finish school. While at the center, you pass signs promoting HIV/AIDS awareness and a supply of free condoms. Free vaccinations are available as part of a campaign to reduce students' risk of illness during the approaching flu season.

Later in the day, you go for a run on a trail in a city park near your home. People are out walking their dogs and obeying the signs to clean up after them in compliance with local ordinances. On your way home, you stop at a local grocery store to pick up some fruit and packaged foods for dinner. You assume the ingredients list printed on the packaged foods accurately reflects what is in them, because food-labeling laws have been in place your whole life. When you get home, you know you need to wash the fruit you bought, just as you know you should wash your hands frequently. The wealth of information you have about keeping yourself well and safe comes from the health education you have received in your schools and community.

Ten great public health achievements in the past century include vaccination, motor vehicle safety, safer workplaces, control of infectious diseases, safer and healthier foods, healthier mothers and babies, family planning, fluoridation of drinking water, the recognition of tobacco as a health hazard, and reduced deaths from heart attacks and stroke. Beyond these achievements, innumerable other developments and advances have contributed to your health, including health education initiatives and campaigns. In this book, you can learn more about public health from the "Public Health Is Personal" boxes that appear in each chapter and draw your attention to the different ways that your personal health depends on public health.

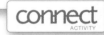

Sources: "Ten Great Public Health Achievements—United States, 1900–1999," 1999, *Morbidity and Mortality Weekly Reports, 48* (12), pp. 241–243; "Healthiest Nation in One Generation," by the American Public Health Association, retrieved from www.generationpublichealth.org.

---

demographics
The statistical characteristics of a population in terms of such categories as age, gender, ethnicity and race, income, disability, geographical location, migration patterns, and many others.

suggests that a healthy community is one that meets the basic needs of all its citizens, offering adequate housing, transportation, access to quality schools, health care, healthy foods, and parks, job opportunities and living wages, and opportunities for civic engagement and social cohesion free from violence.[5]

To develop public health policies, officials have to know the demographics of the population and its subgroups. **Demographics** are the statistical characteristics of a population in terms of such categories as age, gender, ethnicity and race, income, disability, geographical location, and migration patterns. Information about these characteristics, and about changes in them, informs planning and policy. For example, the general trend of population migration in the United States has been away from rural areas and into cities. Of the entire U.S. population of 317 million, approximately 82 percent now live in urban centers. But since 2000, the

Hispanic population has grown in nonmetropolitan areas, and immigrants in general are dispersing more widely across rural areas. Understanding population trends enables improved planning for services—for example, the increased Hispanic population growth in nonmetropolitan areas suggests that services in rural areas increasingly need to be bilingual or multilingual.[19,20]

Similarly, the overall makeup of the U.S. population is changing in terms of age. With the baby boomer generation (those born between 1946 and 1964) reaching retirement age, the nation is aging. This profile places complex new pressures on society and the economy, as the number of people in retirement facilities increases quickly while the number of people in the workforce decreases. Knowing the composition of communities helps policy makers address the needs of all segments of the population.

The Healthy People Initiative

Another example of government interest in the health of the population is the Healthy People Initiative, an effort among federal, state, and territorial governments and community partners (private and public) to set health objectives for the nation. The objectives identify the significant preventable threats to health and establish goals for improving the quality of life for all Americans.[21] The U.S. government issued the first *Healthy People* report in 1980 and has issued revised reports every 10 years since.

The initiative's most recent version, *Healthy People 2020,* envisions "a society in which all people live long, healthy lives" and sets the following broad national health goals:[21]

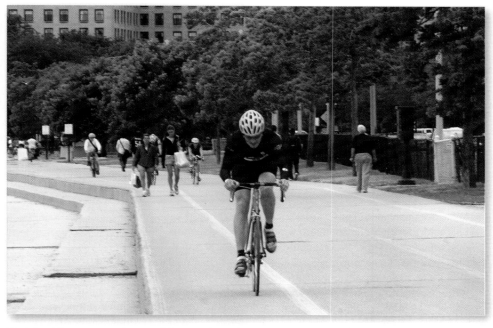

■ A healthy community provides services that support the health and wellness of community members. As an example, community pedestrian and bike trails encourage physical activity and decrease the need for automobiles.

■ Attain high-quality, longer lives free of preventable disease, disability, injury, and premature death.

■ Achieve health equity, eliminate disparities, and improve the health of all groups.

■ Create social and physical environments that promote good health for all.

■ Promote quality of life, healthy development and healthy behaviors across every stage of life.

In a shift from the previous versions, *Healthy People 2020* increases emphasis on "health determinants"—factors that affect the health of individuals, communities, or entire populations. Using the same concepts as the ecological model, the report focuses on the range of personal, social, economic, and environmental factors that affect health. It also takes a life stages focus—recognizing that risk factors are different at different life stages, so interventions are most effective at different critical moments. The report emphasizes the importance of reducing health inequities—differences in health outcomes between populations. Race or ethnicity, socioeconomic status, gender, sexual identity, age, and geographic location can all contribute to differences in health outcomes, as we will discuss in detail shortly.

The Healthy People Initiative further identifies the nation's "leading health indicators"—a set of priority public health issues that can be targeted and measured. In *Healthy People 2020,* the initiative reported the leading health indicators as follows:

■ Nutrition, Physical Activity and Obesity

■ Maternal, Infant, and Child Health

■ Tobacco

■ Substance Abuse

■ Reproductive and Sexual Health

■ Mental Health

■ Injury and Violence

■ Environmental Quality

■ Clinical Preventive Services (such as immunizations)

■ Access to Health Care

■ Oral Health

■ Social Determinants of Health

The indicators are intended to motivate individuals and communities to action by helping to determine where action is necessary.

INDIVIDUAL CHOICE VERSUS SOCIETAL RESPONSIBILITY

The ecological model shows us how individual and societal factors are involved in creating outcomes in everyday life. Within this context, some thorny ethical questions arise:

■ To what extent are individuals responsible for their choices, given the powerful influence of environment? Does someone who drinks excessively to suppress memories of childhood poverty and trauma have the same right to a liver transplant as a child with liver cancer?

- On the other hand, to what extent should individuals be held accountable if their choices pose a cost to society, such as the cost of fighting a fire caused by someone smoking in bed, the cost of EMTs at the scene of a motorcycle crash where the rider wasn't wearing a helmet, or the cost of medical care for a heart attack patient who ignored advice to lose weight and exercise?

- To what extent is government justified in enacting laws, regulations, and policies to "nudge" individuals toward what society considers better choices, such as taxes on tobacco and alcohol or CDC recommendations that girls and boys as young as 11 be vaccinated against HPV infection?

- What are the responsibilities of society to protect individuals and those around them from poor choices, such as drinking and driving? When should society take action to prevent individuals from participating in risky behaviors? When are violations of confidentiality or restrictions on individual rights justified for the sake of the "greater good," such as reporting sexually transmitted infections and quarantine for cases of multiple-drug-resistant tuberculosis?

Your life is influenced by policies related to questions like these. Your choices are constrained by certain policies—think of seat belt laws, speed limits, drinking age laws, gun control laws—because your choices have effects on others and on society. When you are making decisions, whether choosing a personal behavior or supporting or opposing a public policy, consider this complex web of relationships and interactions. In particular, ask yourself, How great a risk does this behavior pose for the individual and for the community? How strongly do individuals oppose restrictions on their ability to participate in the behavior? How much evidence is there that imposing a restriction will affect the behavior? Are there social or environmental factors that limit the options available for an individual's "choice"? Use these questions to inform your thinking and guide you in making reasoned, responsible decisions.

ethnicity
The sense of identity an individual draws from a common ancestry and/ or a common national, religious, tribal, language, or cultural origin.

race
Term used in the social sciences to describe ethnic groups based on physical characteristics, such as skin color or facial features; race does not exist as a biological reality.

HEALTH IN A DIVERSE SOCIETY

As a nation of immigrants, the United States has always been a melting pot of different races and ethnic groups, and it will become even more diverse as the 21st century unfolds. Immigration currently accounts for approximately 50 percent of growth in the United States. According to the U.S. Census Bureau, the primary racial/ethnic groups in the country are Black or African American, American Indian or Alaska Native, Asian, Native Hawaiian or Other Pacific Islander, and White. Hispanic origin is treated as a separate category, because people of Hispanic origin may be of any race or ethnic group. Within each group, there is tremendous diversity: Asian Americans, for example, include people from China, Japan, Korea, Vietnam, Laos, Cambodia, the Philippines, and many other countries. In 2010, approximately 28 percent of the population consisted of members of racial or ethnic minority groups. In some states and cities, minorities are the new majority—that is, Whites now make up less than 50 percent of the population.[22] This is the case, for example, in Hawaii, California, New Mexico, and Texas.

Culture, Ethnicity, and Race

Although diversity includes many kinds of differences among individuals—including gender, age, sexual orientation, ability or disability, educational attainment, socioeconomic status, and geographical location—three important dimensions of diversity that impact groups of people are culture, ethnicity, and race. There are many different meanings of the term *culture,* but we are using the term here to mean a shared pattern of values, beliefs, language, and customs within a group. You may have a sense of belonging to a particular culture or to different subcultures, based on such factors as geographical location, socioeconomic status, religious affiliation, and so on. Your culture helps shape what you view as acceptable and unacceptable (including health-related behaviors) and may even influence how you define or view illness and wellness.[23]

Ethnicity refers to the sense of identity individuals draw from a common ancestry, as well as from a common national, religious, tribal, language, or cultural origin. This identity nurtures a sense of social belonging and loyalty for people of common ethnicity, helping to shape how they think, relate, feel, and behave both within and outside their group. Ethnicity is often confused with **race**, a term used to describe ethnic groups based on physical characteristics, such as skin color or facial features. Although classifying people by race has been a common practice, the fact is that biologically distinct and separate races do not exist within the human species. Genetic traits are inherited individually, not in clumps, groups, or "races." Thus, it is more accurate to view race as a social category rather than a biological one and to think of similarities or differences among people as a matter of culture or ethnicity.

Health Inequities

Over the past 100 years, advances in medical technology, lifestyle improvements, and environmental protections have produced significant health gains for the general U.S. population. These advances, however, have not produced equal health benefits for all. Health inequities are differences in health outcomes that result from systemic, avoidable, and unjust social and economic practices and policies that create barriers to opportunity.

Health inequities are an ongoing issue for the country's ethnic or racial minority populations. Morbidity and mortality (rates of illness and death, respectively) for ethnic and racial minority populations are disheartening. Many have higher rates of cancer, diabetes, cardiovascular disease, infant mortality, alcoholism, drug abuse, unintentional injury, and premature death than the general population does (see the box, "Variations in Leading Causes of Death Among Americans"). Most also have significantly higher lifestyle risk factors, such as high-fat diets, lack of exercise, and more exposure to carcinogens and other environmental toxins.[24,25,26,27]

Why might this be occurring? In the United States, rates of residential segregation by race remain high. Racial minority neighborhoods are more likely to have higher rates of poverty and thus be areas of limited opportunity and limited infrastructure (limited access to the health-promoting social determinants). Community poverty appears to be more important than racial or ethnic group in determining health outcome. Race may determine where people live, and where people live plays a major role in health outcomes! Of concern is the fact that despite decreasing rates of racial segregation in the past 30 years, residential segregation by income is on the rise in the United States.[25,26]

We are also experiencing a time of increasing income disparity—the rich are getting richer and the poor are getting poorer. Multiple factors contribute to the income segregation, including zoning laws, historical settlement patterns, discrimination, real estate practices, and transportation and job opportunities. Much of the disparity in health outcomes

■ *Race* exists only as a social construct, not as a biological reality. People with biracial backgrounds—like Blake Griffin, whose father is African American and whose mother is White—inherit a random mix of individual traits from each parent.

can be attributed to social and economic conditions, including poverty, discrimination, and limited access to health information and other resources. Reducing or eliminating health disparities is a critical challenge of the 21st century and a specific national health goal and will require looking closely at practices and policies that support (intentionally or unintentionally) segregation and thus restrict access to equal opportunities.[21,24,25,26,27]

Health outcomes also vary by factors other than race or ethnicity and income,

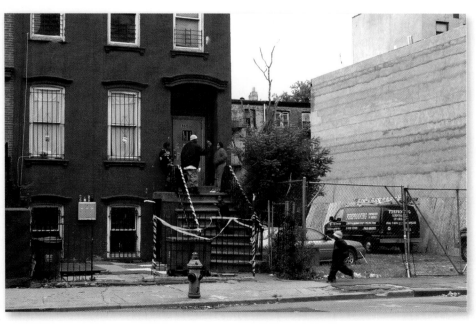

■ Health inequities between racial and ethnic groups are largely attributable to social and economic conditions. A poor neighborhood does not provide the same opportunities for a healthy life as a more affluent neighborhood.

such as age, sexual orientation, educational attainment, and geographical location. For example, the leading cause of death for those between ages 15 and 24 is unintentional injuries (accidents) (see Figure 1.9). For those age 60 and over, the leading causes of death are heart disease and cancer. If we look at the overall leading causes of death for all ages, we see that the major health concerns are chronic diseases—heart disease, cancer, stroke, diabetes, chronic respiratory diseases—and the lifestyle behaviors that contribute to them. They are the focus of both individual behavior change plans and broad public health initiatives.

Who's at Risk?

Compare differences in the overall leading causes of death for Americans across racial/ethnic groups. For example, diabetes is the fourth leading cause of death for African Americans but seventh leading cause overall. Chronic lower respiratory disease is the third leading cause of death for Caucasians but the seventh leading cause for African Americans. Can you hypothesize factors that may be contributing to these differences? What social, economic, or cultural components may be involved?

10 Leading Causes of Death, 2011, by Race and Hispanic Origin

Rank	All	White	Black/African American	American Indian/ Alaska Native	Asian/Pacific Islander	Hispanic/Latino
1	Heart disease	Heart disease	Heart disease	Cancer	Cancer	Cancer
2	Cancer	Cancer	Cancer	Heart disease	Heart disease	Heart disease
3	Chronic lower respiratory disease	Chronic lower respiratory disease	Stroke	Unintentional injury	Stroke	Unintentional injury
4	Stroke	Stroke	Diabetes mellitus	Diabetes mellitus	Unintentional injury	Stroke
5	Unintentional injury	Unintentional injury	Unintentional injury	Chronic liver disease/cirrhosis	Diabetes mellitus	Diabetes mellitus
6	Alzheimer's	Alzheimer's	Kidney disease	Chronic lower respiratory disease	Influenza/ pneumonia	Chronic liver disease/cirrhosis
7	Diabetes mellitus	Diabetes mellitus	Chronic lower respiratory disease	Stroke	Chronic lower respiratory disease	Chronic lower respiratory disease
8	Kidney disease	Influenza/ pneumonia	Homicide	Suicide	Kidney disease	Alzheimer's
9	Influenza/ pneumonia	Kidney disease	Septicemia (overwhelming bacterial infection)	Kidney disease	Alzheimer's	Kidney disease
10	Suicide	Suicide	Alzheimer's	Influenza/pneumonia	Suicide	Influenza/ pneumonia

Source: Health, United States, 2012, by National Center for Health Statistics, 2013, Hyattsville, MD: Author.

connect
ACTIVITY

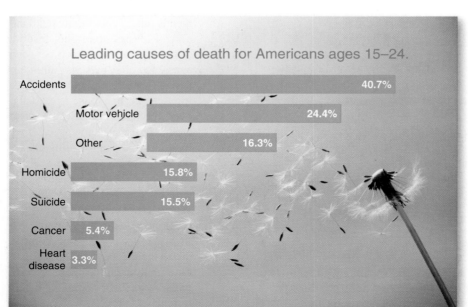

Leading causes of death for Americans ages 15–24.

Accidents — 40.7%
Motor vehicle — 24.4%
Other — 16.3%
Homicide — 15.8%
Suicide — 15.5%
Cancer — 5.4%
Heart disease — 3.3%

figure 1.9 **Leading causes of death for Americans ages 15–24.**
Source: "Deaths: Preliminary Data for 2010," by the National Center for Health Statistics, 2013, *National Vital Statistics Report 60* (4).

LOOKING AHEAD

When compared with other high-income countries, the United States spends more on health care but has a shorter average life span and worse health outcomes. The United States has higher rates of infant mortality, injury and homicide, sexually transmitted infections and pregnancy among youth, chronic disease, obesity, and drug- and alcohol-related mortality.[28] Clearly we have many challenges on both the personal and the community/societal level. Throughout this book, we will ask you to consider your personal health and health choices within the context of your environment. As you read each chapter, reflect on your current level of health in that area. What are your predispositions based upon family history? Which of your behaviors is affecting your health in that area? If there is a behavior you would like to change, assess your readiness to change; then develop a behavior change plan based on the guidelines in this chapter and throughout the rest of the book.

At the same time, think about the influences that shape your decisions. What factors restrict your choices or support them? Consider your family and friends, your classmates and peers, your school and instructors, the community you live in, government policies, and the prevailing socioeconomic and political climate. What do you have to take into account to be successful at behavior change? To help you think more deeply about these issues, we have provided a Personal Health Portfolio section at the end of the book. It includes assessments and critical thinking activities for every chapter.

Even if you decide not to make a personal change right now, perhaps you can share health information with a family member or encourage a friend to change a worrisome habit. Maybe you can do something to make a difference in your community, such as participating in a community garden or a recycling drive or advocating for schools. Or maybe you will become involved in the health care debate or in activities aimed at improving quality of life for underserved segments of the population. The ecological model of health is not just about how your environment influences you—it's also about how your efforts shape your environment.

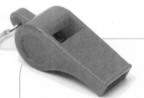

You Make the Call

Access to Health Care: For Everyone, or Just for Some?

Access to health care accounts for an estimated 15 to 20 percent of health and longevity. In March 2010, Congress passed the Affordable Care Act (ACA, or "Obamacare"), and President Obama signed it into law. This landmark legislation made sweeping changes to the current system of health care insurance in the United States. A primary goal of the bill was to extend health insurance to the millions of uninsured and underinsured Americans, thereby expanding access to health care to nearly all citizens. The bill capped out-of-pocket expenses and required that preventive care be fully covered, and it set rules to rein in certain insurance company practices.

The bill's provisions include the following:

- Insurance companies may not set lifetime limits on health care coverage.
- Insurance companies may not deny coverage based on pre-existing conditions.
- Young adults may remain on their parents' insurance plans to age 26.
- Everyone who can afford it must purchase health insurance (the "individual mandate"); subsidies are available for people with low incomes.
- Employers with more than 50 employees must provide health insurance (the "employer mandate"); tax credits are available to make insurance affordable for small businesses.
- Medicaid will be expanded to cover all low-income individuals and families as determined by each state.

The Affordable Care Act was controversial before its enactment and has continued to be the subject of debate and court appeals; it was a driving factor in the government shutdown in 2013. Supporters point out that under the previous system, access to health care was limited to those who could afford it. Millions of low-income people received poorer or less timely care, using emergency rooms for primary care and putting off treatment until their conditions were dire. The cost of services for the underinsured or uninsured fell to society, in the form of higher taxes or higher insurance premiums. Supporters of the bill believe that health care is a basic right and that everyone should have equal access, regardless of ability to pay. (For a list of essential health benefits that ACA plans must offer, see www.healthcare.gov/what-does-marketplace-health-insurance-cover/.)

Supporters of the act also point out that the U.S. health care system is the most expensive in the world but the health of Americans does not reflect that expenditure. Compared with countries that spend significantly less on health care, the United States has poorer health outcomes; for example, the country ranks 34th in life expectancy. Proponents of the Affordable Care Act assert that high health care costs and worse-than-expected outcomes are caused by the large numbers of uninsured and the fragmented U.S. health insurance system. They point out that skyrocketing health care costs make the system unsustainable, and they believe the act will remedy these problems to a large extent, containing costs and expanding access.

A primary objection to the law by its opponents is that it forces people to buy health insurance, infringing on their personal liberties. They believe that individuals have the right to make their

Continued. . .

Concluded. . .

own decisions about how they spend their money. If they don't want to carry health insurance, they shouldn't have to, and others shouldn't have to pay for them to do so. Opponents also object to the expansion of government involvement in private life and increases in taxes and regulations. Although they acknowledge the unsustainable costs of the existing system, they don't believe "big government" is the answer. Referring to the act as "Obamacare," opponents support repeal of the legislation.

Despite a Supreme Court ruling in June 2012 upholding the individual mandate, the act remains controversial. Is the Affordable Care Act the right way to solve the nation's health care problems? What do you think?

Pros

- Access to health care is a basic right, regardless of ability to pay. The law ensures access for vulnerable segments of the population, including low-income families and children.
- With everyone required to have insurance coverage, costs will be more fairly distributed across the system.
- Preventive care brings down health care costs; by making preventive care free, the bill increases the likelihood that people will be healthier, need less medical care, and have lower expenses.

- The law regulates the most abusive practices of the health insurance industry, expanding access and helping to control costs.
- The law reflects the moral values of our society regarding care and compassion for all.

Cons

- People have the right to choose how to spend their money; if they don't want to pay for health insurance, they shouldn't have to.
- Taxpayers and those who have been successful should not have to pay for people who may be living off the system.
- The health insurance industry operates in the private realm, driven by market forces; government involvement increases bureaucracy, costs, and regulation that stifles competition and job creation.
- If the government is willing to impose these policies on the population, it could also impose policies that are morally objectionable to some, such as using taxpayer money to pay for abortions.
- The law is fundamentally at odds with a founding principle of our country: the right to self-determination.

Sources: "Read the Law: The Affordable Care Act," retrieved October 3, 2013, from www.healthcare.gov/law/full; "International Profiles of Health Care Systems," by S. Thompson, et al., 2011; *The Commonwealth Fund November,* retrieved from www.commonwealthfund.org/Publications/Fund-Reports/2011/Nov/International-Profiles-of-Health-Care-Systems-2011.aspx#citation; *Health, United States, 2009,* by the National Center for Health Statistics, 2010, retrieved from www.cdc.gov/nchs/data/hus/hus09.pdf; *National Federation of Individual Businesses et al. v. Sebelius, Secretary of Health and Human Services,* retrieved from www.supremecourt.gov/docket/ppaaca.aspx.

In Review

How are *health* and *wellness* defined?

Health is defined by the World Health Organization as a state of complete physical, mental, social, and spiritual well-being, not just the absence of disease. *Wellness* is defined as the process of adopting patterns of behavior that lead to better health and greater life satisfaction, encompassing several dimensions: physical, emotional, intellectual, spiritual, interpersonal or social, environmental, and, in some models, occupational. Very often, people want to have good health as a means to achieving wellness, an optimum quality of life.

What factors influence a person's health?

Individual health-related behavior choices play a key role in health, but economic, social, cultural, and physical conditions—referred to as the social determinants of health—are also important, along with the person's individual genetic makeup. Community health and public health actions are needed to ensure the personal health of individuals.

How do genes affect your health?

Although some diseases and disorders are caused by a single gene, most genetic disorders are multifactorial; that is, they are associated with interactions among several genes and interactions of genes with environmental factors, such as tobacco smoke, diet, and air pollution. Even if you have a genetic predisposition for a disease, you may never get that disease if the environmental factors are not present.

What is health-related behavior change?

The process of changing a health behavior (e.g., quitting smoking, changing your diet) has been conceptualized in the Health Belief Model, a framework that shows how people's perceptions affect their health choices, and the Stages of Change Model, which suggests that change has six stages, from precontemplation to maintenance of new behavior.

What challenges do we face in changing our health behavior?

Health challenges for individuals include learning to be more informed consumers of health information and making lifestyle decisions that enhance rather than endanger their health. Health challenges for society include finding a balance between the freedom of individuals to make their own choices and the responsibility of society to protect individuals from poor choices and to offer increasing access to affordable health care.

What health-related trends are occurring in our society?

As the United States becomes more multiethnic and multicultural, advances in medicine and health care have not reached many minority communities in the United States. Eliminating health disparities among different segments of the population is one of the broad goals of the national health initiative *Healthy People 2020.*

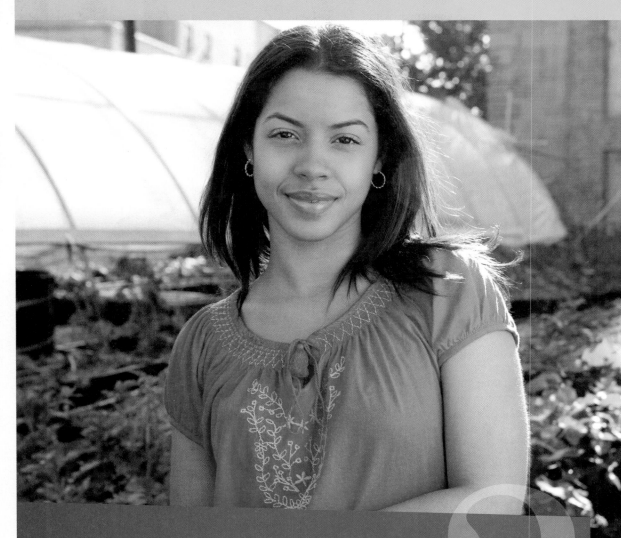

Ever Wonder...

- what it means to be "mentally healthy," as opposed to "mentally ill"?

- how to tell if you are seriously depressed or just feeling down?

- what you can do to reduce the effects of stress in your life?

Mental health encompasses several aspects of overall health and wellness—emotional, psychological, cognitive, interpersonal, and spiritual aspects of a person's life. It includes the capacity to respond to challenges in ways that allow continued growth and forward movement in life. The key to mental health and happiness is not freedom from adversity but rather the ability to respond to adversity in adaptive, effective ways. A mentally healthy person is able to deal with life's inevitable challenges without becoming impaired or overwhelmed by them.

The majority of people are mentally healthy, but many experience emotional or psychological difficulties at some point in their lives, and mental disorders are fairly common. More than 26 percent of the adult American population are affected by a diagnosable mental disorder in a given year, with almost 6 percent identified as having a serious mental illness.[1] An estimated 50 percent of Americans experience some symptoms of depression during their lifetime. Many mental health problems—as well as many general health problems—are triggered or worsened by stress.

WHAT IS MENTAL HEALTH?

Like physical health, mental health is not just the absence of illness; it is also the presence of many positive characteristics.

Positive Psychology and Character Strengths

Psychologists have long been interested in such positive human characteristics as optimism, attachment, love, and emotional intelligence, but in recent years this interest has coalesced in the **positive psychology** movement. Rather than focusing on mental illness and problems, positive psychologists focus on positive emotions, character strengths, and conditions that create happiness—in short, "what makes life worth living."[2] By investigating such topics as gratitude, forgiveness, awe, inspiration, hope, curiosity, humor, resilience, and happiness, positive psychologists strive to understand the full spectrum of human experience. Others have focused on "grit," or an individual's perseverance and passion for achieving long-term goals, as a predictor of life success.[87]

One outcome of this research has been the identification of character strengths and virtues that "enable human thriving" and that are endorsed by nearly all cultures across the world.[3] The six broad virtues are wisdom, courage, humanity, justice, temperance, and transcendence. Related to each virtue are particular strengths that meet various criteria. For example, they contribute to individual fulfillment and satisfaction, they are

positive psychology
Area of interest within the field of psychology that focuses on positive emotions, character strengths, and conditions that create happiness.

self-esteem
Sense of positive regard and valuation for oneself.

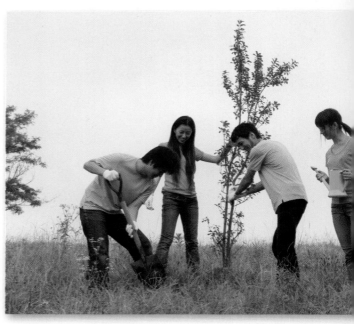

■ Which virtues and character strengths listed in Table 2.1 seem to be expressed in the actions of these young people?

valued in their own right and not as a means to an end, they do not diminish others, and they are deliberately cultivated by individuals and societies. The most commonly endorsed strengths are kindness, fairness, authenticity, gratitude, and open-mindedness. The character strengths and virtues are described in Table 2.1. Which ones are your top strengths? How can you use them more often?

Characteristics of Mentally Healthy People

People who are described as mentally healthy have certain characteristics in common (often expressions of the character strengths and virtues in Table 2.1):

■ They have high **self-esteem** and feel good about themselves.

■ They are realistic and accept imperfections in themselves and others.

■ They are altruistic; they help others.

■ They have a sense of control over their lives and feel capable of meeting challenges and solving problems.

■ They demonstrate social competence in their relationships with others, and they are comfortable with other people and believe they can rely on them.

■ They are not overwhelmed by fear, love, or anger; they try to control irrational thoughts and levels of stress.

■ They are optimistic; they maintain a positive outlook.

Table 2.1   Classification of 6 Virtues and 24 Character Strengths

Virtue and Strengths	Definition
1. Wisdom and knowledge	**Cognitive strengths that entail the acquisition and use of knowledge**
Creativity	Thinking of novel and productive ways to do things
Curiosity	Taking an interest in ongoing experience, openness to experience
Open-mindedness	Thinking things through and examining them from all sides
Love of learning	Mastering new skills, topics, and bodies of knowledge
Perspective	Being able to provide wise counsel to others
2. Courage	**Emotional strengths that involve the exercise of will to accomplish goals in the face of opposition, external or internal**
Authenticity	Speaking the truth and presenting oneself in a genuine way
Bravery	Not shrinking from threat, challenge, difficulty, or pain
Persistence	Finishing what one starts
Zest	Approaching life with excitement and energy
3. Humanity	**Interpersonal strengths that involve "tending and befriending" others**
Kindness	Doing favors and good deeds for others
Love	Valuing close relations with others
Social intelligence	Being aware of the motives and feelings of self and others
4. Justice	**Civic strengths that underlie healthy community life**
Fairness	Treating all people the same according to notions of fairness and justice
Leadership	Organizing group activities and seeing that they happen
Teamwork	Working well as a member of a group or team
5. Temperance	**Strengths that protect against excess**
Forgiveness	Forgiving those who have done wrong
Modesty	Letting one's accomplishments speak for themselves
Prudence	Being careful about one's choices; not saying or doing things that might later be regretted
Self-regulation	Regulating what one feels and does
6. Transcendence	**Strengths that forge connections to the larger universe and provide meaning**
Appreciation of beauty and excellence	Noticing and appreciating beauty, excellence, and/or skilled performance in all domains of life
Gratitude	Being aware of and thankful for the good things that happen
Hope	Expecting the best and working to achieve it
Humor	Liking to laugh and tease; bringing smiles to other people
Religiousness	Having coherent beliefs about the higher purpose and meaning of life

Source: Character Strengths and Virtues: A Handbook and Classification, by C. Peterson and M. Seligman, 2004, Washington, DC: American Psychological Association.

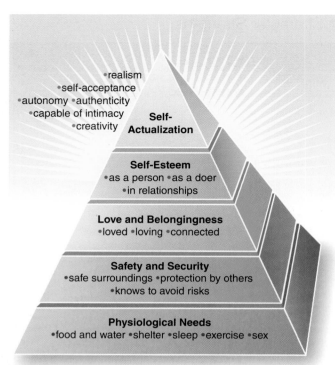

figure 2.1   **Maslow's hierarchy of needs.**
Source: Based on *Motivation and Personality,* by Abraham H. Maslow, ed.
Robert D. Frager and James Fadiman, 3rd ed., New York: Harper & Row.

■ They have a capacity for intimacy; they do not fear commitment.

■ They are creative and appreciate creativity in others.

■ They persevere and take on challenges.

■ They take reasonable risks in order to grow.

■ They bounce back from adversity.

The Self-Actualized Person

Many of these healthy characteristics are found in the self-actualized person. The concept of **self-actualization** was developed by Abraham Maslow in the 1960s as a model of human personality development in his "hierarchy of needs" theory (Figure 2.1). Maslow proposed that once people meet their needs for survival, safety and security, love and belonging, and achievement and self-esteem, they have opportunities for self-exploration and expression that can lead them to reach their fullest human potential. According to Maslow, a self-actualized person is

self-actualization
In Maslow's work, the state attained when a person has reached his or her full potential.

resilience
Ability to bounce back from adversity.

realistic, self-accepting, self-motivated, creative, and capable of intimacy, among other traits. Those who reach this level achieve a state of transcendence, a sense of well-being that comes from finding purpose and meaning in life.

Optimism, Self-Efficacy, and Resilience

A key characteristic of mentally healthy people is *optimism*—the general expectation that things will turn out well. People with an "optimistic explanatory style"—the tendency to see problems as temporary and specific rather than permanent and general—seem to have better physical and mental health than more pessimistic people do.[4,5] Optimistic people react to failures as things they can do something about, as challenges and opportunities for learning and growth. A recent analysis of 83 studies has linked optimism to positive physical health outcomes.[6] Compared with pessimists, optimists have better physical functioning, report less pain, have better outcomes after surgery, experience lower levels of depression, and live longer. Pessimistic people tend to attribute failure to personal defects and react with discouragement and a sense of defeat. Of course, you also need to be realistic and recognize your own limitations; people who disregard the information provided by their successes and failures will end up only with disappointment.[7] For more about balance, see the box, "Is Optimism Overrated?"

Related to optimism is *self-efficacy,* a general sense that you have some control over what happens in your life. Mentally healthy people have a basic belief that they can guide their own lives, and they take unexpected events in stride, adapt, and move on.

This ability to bounce back from adverse events is known as **resilience,** and it is another characteristic of mentally healthy individuals. People who can respond flexibly to life's challenges and redirect their energies toward positive actions tend to be more successful in life. Our lives will always have moments of adversity and vulnerability and be filled with challenging situations. Individuals who are resilient learn ways to respond to these events and situations. Resilience involves patterns of thinking, feeling, and behaving that contribute to a balanced life based on self-esteem, satisfying relationships, and a belief that life is meaningful. To discover more about your own resilience, complete the Chapter 2 Personal Health Portfolio activity at the back of the book.

Happiness and Positive Psychology

The study of happiness is part of the positive psychology movement, which focuses on what makes life worth living. In general, people who are in good romantic relationships, are physically healthier, and attend some form of religious institution seem to be the happiest. Overall, few experiences

Starting the Conversation

Is Optimism Overrated?

Q: Do you wonder if you are optimistic enough to reap the supposed benefits of optimism, like better health outcomes?

Research has consistently found associations between optimism and good health, both physical and mental. The reasons for these associations aren't entirely clear, but one possibility is that optimists have better coping skills in stressful situations, so they avoid some of the damaging effects of stress on their bodies. Another possibility is that optimistic people have healthier lifestyles and take better care of themselves, behaviors linked to the belief that one has some control over future outcomes. It may be that optimism is adaptive in the evolutionary scheme of things, or even hard-wired into our brains, helping people feel confident enough to plan, explore, and pursue goals.

But is it possible to be *too* optimistic? Critics warn against the "optimism bias," the tendency to be overly optimistic about expected outcomes, often as a result of self-delusion, an "illusion of control," or "magical thinking." They point to events like the 2008 financial crisis that swept Wall Street and the 2010 Deepwater Horizon oil spill as cases where optimistic thinking was so overblown that there were no contingency plans, resulting in disasters.

On a personal level, the optimism bias leads individuals to harbor such beliefs as "I can write this paper in one night" (despite previous experience), "My marriage will be happy and long lasting" (despite divorce rates), and "I will not get cancer from smoking" (despite health statistics). One study of undergraduates found that a positive outlook on life was correlated with self-rated abilities and predictions of success but not with GPA, suggesting that many were overestimating their talents.

Being *over*optimistic and *over*confident can bring problems. Overoptimistic people are likely to take more risks (e.g., with alcohol, drugs, cars, or thrill-seeking behaviors) and to practice less preventive care than others. They may neglect threats and dangers that give others pause, and they may be more gullible. They may avoid confronting problems and fail to plan ahead because of their belief that things will somehow work out, and they may be more disappointed by failures than someone with lower expectations. Some research indicates that people experiencing positive emotions are more likely to rely on their pre-existing beliefs, expectations, and stereotypes to evaluate a person or situation, rather than systematically processing the relevant aspects of the environment.

The solution is not to trade in your rose-colored glasses for a more pessimistic outlook. Pessimism—the expectation that things will work out badly—is associated with poorer health outcomes, including depression. Although pessimists have been found to have a more accurate view of reality, they may experience unnecessary suffering and miss out on opportunities for positive feelings like excitement and joy. A better choice is to temper your optimism with a healthy dash of realism—to use your critical thinking skills to weigh the likelihood of different outcomes. Although you may never achieve a truly objective assessment of a situation, your awareness of the optimism bias may help you come to more balanced decisions.

Q: How do you see yourself, as an optimist or a pessimist? Do you think you were born that way? Could you change?

Q: Given that even the founding document of the United States asserts the right to the pursuit of happiness, do you think Americans overvalue optimism and positive thinking?

Sources: "The Optimism Bias," by T. Sharot, 2011, New York: Pantheon; "Positive Affect and College Success," by C. Nickerson, E. Diener, and N. Schwartz, 2011, *Journal of Happiness Studies, 12* (4), pp. 717–746; "A Dark Side of Happiness? How, When, and Why Happiness Is Not Always Good," by J. Gruber, I. Mauss, and M. Tamir, 2012, *Perspectives on Psychological Science, 6* (3), pp. 222–233; "Positive Thinking: Reduce Stress by Eliminating Negative Self-Talk," by the Mayo Clinic, 2011, www.mayoclinic.com/health/positive-thinking/SR00009.

seem to affect us for more than three months; we seem to celebrate or feel bad for awhile and then recover and move on. Most individuals seem to be resilient.[8] According to one poll, wealth, education, IQ, and youth have little impact on happiness: instead, the top sources of happiness are connection with family and friends (Figure 2.2).[9]

In their research, positive psychologists have found that happiness has three components: positive emotion and pleasure (savoring sensory experiences), engagement (being deeply involved with family, work, romance, and hobbies), and meaning (using personal strengths to serve some larger end).[10] The happiest people are those who orient their lives toward all three, but the latter two—engagement and meaning—are the most important in giving people satisfaction and happiness. Accordingly, positive psychologists suggest "happiness exercises," described in the box, "Increase Your Happiness," to help people feel more connected to others.

However, people may have a happiness "set point," determined largely by genetics. That is, no matter what happens in life, people may have a tendency to return to their norm. The notion that people can increase their happiness reinforces Western cultural biases about how individual initiative and a positive attitude can solve complex problems.[7] In addition, because happiness research focuses on internal processes, it pays little or no attention to the very real sources of unhappiness that are connected to social and economic circumstances.

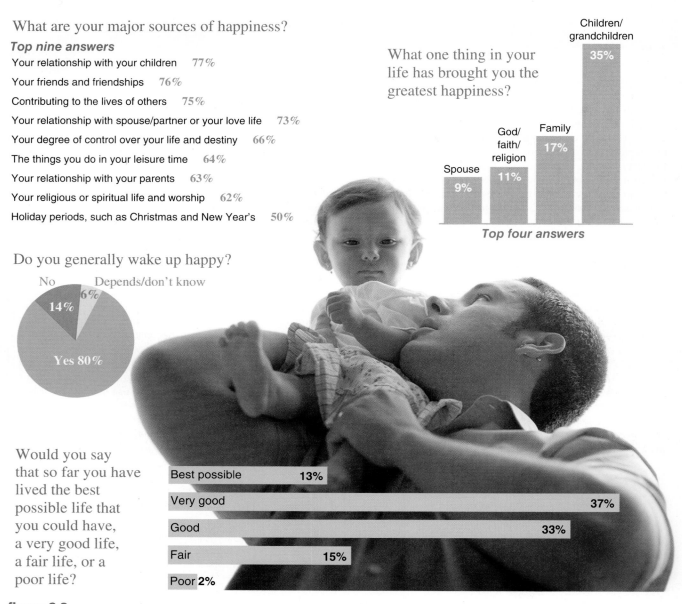

What are your major sources of happiness?

Top nine answers

Your relationship with your children   77%

Your friends and friendships   76%

Contributing to the lives of others   75%

Your relationship with spouse/partner or your love life   73%

Your degree of control over your life and destiny   66%

The things you do in your leisure time   64%

Your relationship with your parents   63%

Your religious or spiritual life and worship   62%

Holiday periods, such as Christmas and New Year's   50%

What one thing in your life has brought you the greatest happiness?

Children/grandchildren 35%

God/faith/religion 11%

Family 17%

Spouse 9%

Top four answers

Do you generally wake up happy?

No 14%

Depends/don't know 6%

Yes 80%

Would you say that so far you have lived the best possible life that you could have, a very good life, a fair life, or a poor life?

Best possible   13%

Very good   37%

Good   33%

Fair   15%

Poor 2%

figure 2.2   **Sources of happiness and other happiness factors reported by Americans.**
Source: Adapted from "The New Science of Happiness," by C. Wallis, January 17, 2007, *Time.*

Emotional Intelligence

Another aspect of mental health, is the concept of **emotional intelligence**. Daniel Goleman argued that such qualities as self-awareness, self-discipline, persistence, and empathy are much more important to success in life than IQ. People who are emotionally intelligent are able to

1. Recognize, name, and understand their emotions.

2. Manage their emotions and control their moods.

3. Motivate themselves.

4. Recognize and respond to emotions in others.

5. Be socially competent.[11]

The last ability involves skills in understanding relationships, cooperating, solving problems, resolving conflicts, communicating assertively, and being considerate and compassionate.[12] Those with more emotional intelligence have more positive relationships, perform better academically, have more adaptive decision-making skills, and tend to be mentally healthy.[13] In addition, it seems that emotional intelligence can reduce the likelihood of participating in risky behaviors.

emotional intelligence
In Goleman's work, the kind of intelligence that includes an understanding of emotional experience, self-awareness, and sensitivity to others.

Action Skill-Builder

Increase Your Happiness

Happiness research has found that people can increase their level of happiness by practicing "happiness exercises." Here are three that you can try:

☐ *Three good things in life.* Every night for a week, write down three things that went well that day and their causes. Research suggests that this can increase happiness and decrease depressive symptoms for up to six months.

☐ *Using signature strengths in a new way.* Using the classification of character strengths and virtues (see Table 2.1), take inventory of your character strengths and identify the top five, your "signature strengths." Use one of these top strengths in a new and different way every day for a week.

☐ *Gratitude visit.* Write a letter of gratitude and then deliver it in person to someone who has been especially kind to you but whom you have never thanked properly. Research suggests that this exercise can significantly increase happiness for one month.

Related research has identified other ways to increase happiness and life satisfaction, including performing acts of kindness, savoring life's joys, and learning to forgive. Positive psychologists say that happiness exercises give meaning to life by helping people feel more connected to others. Almost everyone feels happier when they are with other people, even those who think they want to be alone.

Source: "Positive Psychology Progress: Empirical Validation of Interventions," by M. Seligman, T. Steen, N. Park, and C. Peterson, 2005, *American Psychologist, 60* (5), pp. 410–421.

Like many of the other characteristics of mentally healthy people, emotional intelligence can be learned and improved. Many groups, workshops, and self-help books assist people in learning how to control impulses, manage anger, recognize emotions in themselves and others, and respond more appropriately in social situations.

THE GRIEVING PROCESS: PART OF LIFE

Mental health is determined not by the challenges a person faces but by how the person responds to those challenges. The challenges themselves come in a range of intensities—from being turned down for a date to the death of a loved one—and people's responses also vary in how well they work in allowing the person to maintain an overall sense of balance and well-being.

Coping with the loss of a loved one or acknowledging your own mortality may represent the biggest challenge to mental health you will experience in life. Grieving is an extremely personal experience, yet it is one that you also share with everyone in your community and culture. Life and death are part of the cycle of existence and the natural order of things, and therefore grieving is also a universal process. Understanding more about this process can help you prepare for a situation where you or someone you know experiences a loss.

Bereavement and Healthy Grieving

Grief is a natural reaction to loss; in fact, many of the familiar rituals that surround death and dying are actually for the living, to help people cope with their reactions to loss. Rituals help mourners move through the emotional work of grieving. When a person has been important to us, we never forget that person or lose the relationship. Instead, we find ways of "emotionally relocating" the deceased person in our lives, keeping our bonds with them while moving on. Cultural rituals can facilitate this process.

Cultural rituals aside, grieving is also a very personal process, often expressed by feelings of sadness, loneliness, anger, and guilt. These feelings are part of the process of healing because we do not begin to feel better until we have acknowledged and felt sorrow over our loss.[14]

Physical symptoms of grief may include crying and sighing, aches and pains, sleep disturbances, headaches, lethargy, reduced appetite, and stomach upset. The intense emotions you feel at the time of a loss can have a negative impact on immune system functioning, reducing your ability to fight off illness. Studies have shown that surviving spouses may have increased risk for heart disease, cancer, depression, alcoholism, and suicide.[15,16]

Everyone has higher risk for disease after the loss of a loved one, but those who are more resilient may cope with the loss better. Resilient people seem to be more likely to find comfort in talking and thinking about the deceased and are flexible enough to either suppress or express emotions about a death.[17] It is critical to remember that flexibility is the key: being able to choose when to talk and when it might be more helpful to not share. For example, suppressing an emotion might be useful when it allows you to concentrate on the current task.

Bereavement after the loss of a loved one typically involves four phases:

■ *Numbness and shock.* This phase occurs immediately after the loss and lasts for a brief period. The numbness protects you from acute pain.

■ *Separation.* As the shock wears off, you start to feel the pain of loss, and you experience acute yearning and longing to be reunited with your loved one.

■ *Disorganization.* You are preoccupied and distracted; you have trouble concentrating and thinking clearly. You may feel lethargic and indifferent. This phase can last much longer than you anticipate.

■ *Reorganization.* You begin to adjust to the loss. Your life will never be the same without your loved one, but your feelings have less intensity and you can reinvest in life.

When you experience the death of a loved one, it is important to take care of yourself while you are grieving. During the grieving process, it is vital that you eat a balanced diet, exercise regularly, drink plenty of fluids, and get enough rest. Keeping a journal and talking about the person who has died can also be part of the healing process. Finally, you should not hesitate to ask friends for support because having a nurturing social network is particularly helpful in coping with loss.

There is no right or wrong way to grieve and no specific timetable. Friends who suggest that it's time to move on need to understand that you are on your own journey and cannot be rushed. You need to give yourself permission to

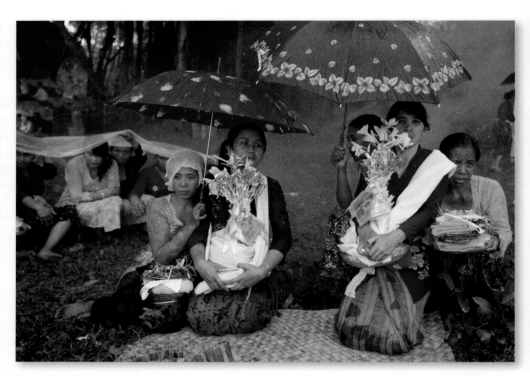

■ Spiritual beliefs and rituals can help people deal with grief and pain when a loved one dies.

feel the loss and take time to heal. Some people cope better if they talk about the death rather than internalizing their feelings.

Approximately 10 to 15 percent of those in grief will experience persistent and intense symptoms related to the loss. If you are in that group, it is important to seek out professional help. One of the changes in the DSM-5 is to allow a diagnosis of depression during the first two months following the death of a loved one; some worry that this change may result in overdiagnosis and overmedication.[18] However, if intense grief persists, or if you find yourself losing or gaining weight or not sleeping, consult a health professional to get a treatment referral. Treatment options include support groups, family therapy, individual counseling, or a psychiatric evaluation.

Facing Death

In 1969, Elisabeth Kübler-Ross published *On Death and Dying,* one of the first books to propose stages that people go through when they believe they are in the process of dying.[19] The five stages are (1) denial and isolation, (2) anger, (3) bargaining, (4) depression, and (5) acceptance. Over time, further study has shown that these stages are not linear—individuals may experience them in a different order or may return to stages they have already gone through—nor are they necessarily universal—individuals may not experience some stages at all.

While the Kübler-Ross model serves as a good baseline for understanding the stages that a dying person might go through, attitudes about mental health have changed drastically since 1969. Health care professionals and patients can now talk more openly about the emotional toll of illness and

death, and this can help shift the focus on ways to *live* with an illness rather than simply looking at the diagnosis as the point at which one begins to prepare for death. The dying person may find comfort and strength in talking through the process with family and friends or with a doctor or counselor. Also, there is often time to repair relationships, to build memories, and to review one's life.

Spiritual and religious beliefs can also help terminally ill people through the final stages of their lives. Many report that because of their personal faith, they do not fear death because they know that their lives have had meaning within the context of a larger plan. In fact, studies suggest that, unrelated to belief in an afterlife, religiously involved people at the end of life are more accepting of death and less anxious about it than those who are less religiously involved.[20]

THE BRAIN'S ROLE IN MENTAL HEALTH AND ILLNESS

The human brain has been called the most complex structure in the universe.[21] This unimpressive-looking organ is the central control station for human intelligence, feeling, and creativity. All behavior, both normal and abnormal, is mediated in some way by the brain and the nervous system.

Since the 1980s, knowledge of the structure and function of the brain has increased dramatically. In fact, the 1990s were called the "decade of the brain" because of the advances made in understanding how the brain works. Most of these discoveries were made possible by advances in imaging technologies, such as computerized axial tomography (CAT scans), positron emission tomography (PET scans), magnetic resonance imaging (MRIs), and functional MRIs (fMRIs).

The Developing Brain

One surprise that recent brain research produced is that the brain continues to change and grow through adolescence into the early 20s. Previously, scientists thought that brain development was completed in childhood, and in fact, 95 percent of the structure of the brain is formed by the age of 6. Scientists discovered, however, that a growth spurt occurs in the **frontal cortex**—the part of the brain where "executive functions" such as planning, organizing, and rational thinking are controlled—just before puberty. During adolescence, these new brain cells are pruned and consolidated, resulting in a more mature, adult brain by the early to mid-20s.

Because structural changes are taking place in the brain into early adulthood, the activities that teenagers engage in can have lifelong effects (Figure 2.3). The brain cells and connections that are used for academics, music, sports, language learning, and other productive activities—or, alternatively, for watching television and playing video games—are the ones that are more likely to be hardwired into the brain and survive.[22]

Some experts have disputed these conclusions about the brain. They argue that the differences seen in brain images are not necessarily the *cause* of erratic or impulsive behaviors, and they point out that young adults in other cultures are often fully ready to regulate and be responsible for their behavior. In addition, some research has indicated a relationship between impulsive, risk-taking behavior and exposure to movies, television, and video games. More research is needed to sort out the effects of biological versus cultural influences on behavior.[23]

Mental Illness and the Brain

Human beings have always experienced mental disturbances: descriptions of conditions called "mania," "melancholia," "hysteria," and "insanity" can be found in the literature of many ancient societies. It wasn't until the 18th and 19th centuries, however, that advances in anatomy, physiology, and medicine allowed scientists to identify the brain as the organ afflicted in cases of mental disturbance and to propose biological causes, especially damage to the brain, for mental disorders.

frontal cortex
The part of the brain where the executive functions of planning, organizing, and rational thinking are controlled.

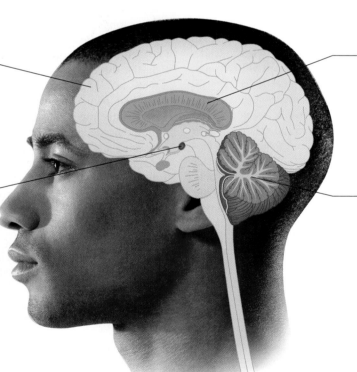

Frontal cortex
Controls planning, organizing, rational thinking, working memory, judgment, mood modulation. Undergoes rapid growth just before puberty, followed by pruning and consolidation during adolescence.

Amygdala
Controls emotional responses and instinctual, "gut" reactions. Adolescents appear to rely more heavily on this part of the brain to interpret situations than adults do. As they mature, the center of brain activity shifts to the frontal cortex.

Corpus callosum
Relays information between the two hemispheres of the brain and is believed to play a role in creativity and problem solving. Grows and changes significantly during adolescence.

Cerebellum
Long known to be involved in motor activity and physical coordination; now understood to coordinate thinking processes, including decision making and social skills. Undergoes dynamic growth and change during adolescence.

figure 2.3   The teenage brain.

Sources: Adapted from "Adolescent Brains Are Works in Progress," by S. Spinks, 2005, *Frontline,* www.pbs.org; "Teenage Brain: A Work in Progress," 2001, National Institute of Mental Health, NIH Publication No. 01-4929, www.nimh.nih.gov.

Since then, other explanations have been proposed, involving, for example, psychological factors, sociocultural and environmental factors, and faulty learning. Debate over the roles of these various categories of causal factors continues to this day although the central role of the brain in mental health and mental illness is beyond doubt. Mental illnesses are diseases that affect the brain.[24]

Nevertheless, mental disorders that are caused specifically by some pathology in the brain are rare. These disorders are referred to as *cognitive disorders;* an example is Alzheimer's disease. More commonly, mental disorders are caused by complex interactions of biological factors, psychological processes, social influences, and cultural factors, especially those affecting a person during early childhood. In addition, some mental disorders, including depression, bipolar disorder, and schizophrenia, have a genetic component.

Research has expanded in recent decades in the physiology of the brain and the function of **neurotransmitters**. These brain chemicals are responsible for the transmission of signals from one brain cell to the next. There are dozens of neurotransmitters, but four seem to be particularly important in mental disorders: norepinephrine (active during the stress response; see later in this chapter); dopamine (implicated in schizophrenia); serotonin (implicated in mood disorders); and gamma-aminobutyric acid, or GABA (implicated in anxiety).[22]

Neurotransmitter imbalances are believed to be involved in a variety of mental disorders. For example, dopamine gives us the positive feelings we experience when eating and participating in sexual activity, among other behaviors. All addictive drugs appear to trigger a dopamine release. Under consistently high levels of dopamine, a person will begin to behave erratically, with increases in sexual desire, aggressiveness, and likelihood of risk taking. Serotonin is associated with emotion and mood. Low levels of serotonin have been shown to be related to depression, problems with anger control and concentration, and a variety of other disorders. High levels of serotonin, which can be an unintended side effect of some migraine medicines and some antidepressants, can result in serotonin syndrome. Symptoms of this syndrome include nausea, vomiting, changes in blood pressure, and agitation. GABA is a chemical messenger that promotes relaxation and inhibits excitation. It is typically found in high concentrations in areas such as the hypothalamus and hippocampus. Symptoms of GABA deficiency include night sweats, reflux, poor verbal memory, restlessness, and a short temper. Many drugs have been developed to correct neurotransmitter imbalances, such as the class of antidepressants that affect levels of serotonin.

neurotransmitters
Brain chemicals that conduct signals from one brain cell to the next.

mental disorder
A pattern of behavior associated with distress (pain) or disability (impairment in an important area of functioning, such as school or work) or with significantly increased risk of suffering, death, pain, disability, or loss of freedom.

MENTAL DISORDERS AND TREATMENT

Although evidence of mental disorders like depression or schizophrenia can be found in the brain, and although many disorders can be treated with drugs that act on the brain, neither of these facts means that all mental disorders originate in the brain. In general, a mental disorder is diagnosed on the basis of the amount of distress and impairment a person is experiencing. According to the *Diagnostic and Statistical Manual of Mental Disorders* (DSM-5), a **mental disorder** is a pattern of behavior in an individual that is associated with distress (pain) or disability (impairment in an important area of functioning, such as school or work) or with significantly increased risk of suffering, death, pain, disability, or loss of freedom.[25] Deciding when a psychological problem becomes a mental disorder is not easy. Nevertheless, a basic premise of the DSM-5 is that a mental disorder is qualitatively different from a psychological problem that can be considered normal, and it can be diagnosed from a set of symptoms.

For example, feelings of sadness and discouragement are common, especially during the college years. These feelings can occur in response to disappointment, loss, failure, or other negative events, or they can occur for no apparent reason. Usually such experiences don't last too long; people recover and go on with their lives. If the feelings *do* go on for a long time and are painful and intense, however, the person may be experiencing depression.

Similarly, worries, fears, and anxieties are common during the college years. Individuals have stresses to deal with, such as grades, relationships, and learning how to live on their own without parental guidance or support. They may be feeling homesick and lonely, or they may be having problems sleeping. Most people gradually make their way, learning who they are and how they want to relate to other people. Some people, however, may develop anxiety disorders or stress-related disorders, experience panic attacks, or be overwhelmed with fears and worries.

People experience many emotional difficulties in the course of daily living that are not a cause for alarm. At the same time, it is important to be able to recognize when a person needs professional help. Far too often, people struggle with mental disorders without knowing that something is wrong or that treatments are available. They don't realize that their problems may be causing them unnecessary distress and that professional treatment can help.

After more than an 11-year effort, the American Psychiatric Association, not without controversy,[26,27] has revised the text that is used to diagnose those with a mental disorder. Among the changes in the recently revised DSM are the inclusion of hoarding as an official mental disorder, the introduction of gambling disorder, and modifications in the diagnosis of those with autism.[28] Here, we discuss the DSM's major categories of mental disorders.

Mood Disorders

Also called depressive disorders or affective disorders, mood disorders include major depressive disorder, dysthymic disorder, and bipolar disorder (formerly called manic depression). They are among the most common mental disorders around the world.

People of all ages can get depressed, including children and adolescents, but the average age of onset for major depressive disorders is the mid-20s. In any one year, more than 20.9 million adults in the United States—about 9.5 percent of the adult population—suffer from a depressive illness. Of these individuals, a significant number will be hospitalized, and many will die from suicide.[1] Women experience depressive episodes twice as frequently as men.

In many of these situations, the illness goes undiagnosed, and people struggle for long periods of time. About two-thirds of depressed individuals seek help, but many are undertreated, meaning that they don't get enough medication or they don't see a therapist on a regular basis. Many

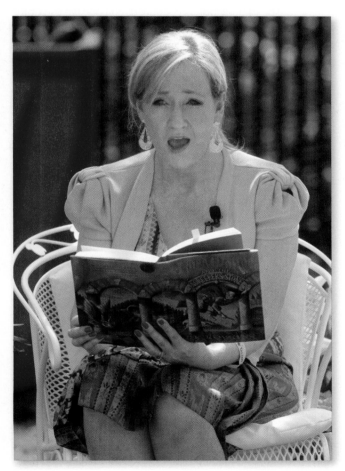

■ J. K. Rowling, author of the Harry Potter books, is one of many talented people who have spoken about their own experiences with depression. Rowling suffered a bout of depression and suicidal thoughts in her mid-20s.

medications for depression take up to four weeks to begin to have an effect, so some people conclude they aren't working and stop taking them before then.

The DSM-5 contains a number of new depressive disorders including disruptive mood dysregulation disorder and premenstrual dysphoric disorder. In addition, dysthymia (neurotic or chronic depression) and chronic major depressive disorder are now included in the DSM-5 as persistent depressive disorder. This change was made because of the difficulty in differentiating between these two conditions.

Major Depressive Disorder Symptoms of **depression** include depressed mood, as indicated by feelings of sadness or emptiness or by behaviors such as crying; a loss of interest or pleasure in activities that previously provided pleasure; fatigue; feelings of worthlessness; and a reduced ability to concentrate. If a person experiences one or more episodes of depression lasting at least two weeks, he or she may be diagnosed with **major depressive disorder**.

Bipolar Disorder A person with **bipolar disorder** experiences one or more manic episodes, often but not always alternating with depressive episodes. A **manic episode** is a distinct period during which the person has an abnormally elevated mood. Individuals experiencing manic episodes may be euphoric, expansive, and full of energy, or, alternatively, highly irritable. They may be grandiose, with an inflated sense of their own importance and power; they may have racing thoughts and accelerated and pressured speech. They may stay awake for days without getting tired or wake from a few hours of sleep feeling refreshed and full of energy. People experiencing a manic episode typically are not aware they are ill.

Bipolar disorder occurs equally in men and women, with an average age at onset of about 20. Family and twin studies offer strong evidence of a genetic component in this disorder.

Anxiety Disorders

Along with depression, anxiety disorders are the most common mental disorders affecting Americans. Almost 40 million Americans 18 and older—more than 18 percent of all people in this age group— have an anxiety disorder.[1]

Many of these disorders are characterized by a **panic attack**,

depression
Mental state characterized by a depressed mood, loss of interest or pleasure in activities, and other related symptoms.

major depressive disorder
Mood disorder characterized by one or more episodes of depression lasting at least two weeks.

bipolar disorder
Mood disorder characterized by one or more manic episodes that may alternate with depressive episodes.

manic episode
An abnormally elevated or irritable mood during a specific period of time.

panic attack
Clear physiological and psychological experience of apprehension or intense fear in the absence of a real danger.

a clear physiological and psychological experience of apprehension or intense fear in the absence of a real danger. Symptoms include heart palpitations, sweating, shortness of breath, chest pain, and a sense that one is "going crazy." There is a feeling of impending doom or danger and a strong urge to escape. Panic attacks usually occur suddenly and last for a discrete period of time, reaching a peak within 10 minutes, but some can last longer. Many people may have only one panic attack in a lifetime.[29]

Panic disorder is characterized by recurrent, unexpected panic attacks along with concern about having another attack. The attacks may be triggered by a situation, or they may "come out of nowhere." Twin studies and family studies indicate that there is a genetic contribution to panic disorder.

A **specific phobia** is an intense fear of an activity, situation, or object, exposure to which evokes immediate anxiety. Examples of common phobias are flying, heights, specific animals or insects (dogs, spiders), and blood. Individuals with phobias realize their fear is unreasonable, but they cannot control it. Usually they try to avoid the phobic situation or object, and if they can't avoid it, they endure it with great distress. Often the phobia interferes with their lives in some way.

A **social phobia** involves an intense fear of certain kinds of social or performance situations, again leading the individual to try to avoid such situations. If the phobic situation is public speaking, individuals may be able to structure their lives so as to avoid all such situations. However, some social phobias involve simply conversing with other people. This is different from shyness; individuals with this disorder experience tremors, sweating, confusion, blushing, and other distressing symptoms when they are in the feared situation.

Excessive and uncontrollable worrying, usually far out of proportion to the likelihood of the feared event, is known as **generalized anxiety disorder**. Adults with this disorder worry about routine matters such as health, work, and money; children with the disorder worry about their competence in school or sports, being evaluated by others, or even natural disasters.

Obsessive-compulsive disorder is now included in the DSM-5 as a separate chapter. It is characterized by persistent, intrusive thoughts, impulses, or images that cause intense anxiety or distress. For example, the person may have repeated thoughts about contamination, persistent doubts about having done something, or a need to have things done in a particular order. To control the obsessive thoughts and images, the person develops compulsions—repetitive behaviors performed to reduce the anxiety associated with the obsession.

Addiction

Addiction—dependence on a substance or a behavior—is classified as a mental disorder. All addictions in the DSM-5 are classified as substance-related and addictive disorders. The key characteristic of addiction is continued, compulsive use of the substance or involvement in the behavior despite serious negative consequences. Individuals with a substance addiction may spend a great deal of time trying to obtain the substance, give up important parts of their lives to use it, and make repeated, unsuccessful attempts to cut down or control their use.

A person with **physiological dependence** on a substance experiences *tolerance,* reduced sensitivity to its effects such that increased doses are needed to give the same high, and *withdrawal,* uncomfortable symptoms that occur when substance use stops. Tolerance and withdrawal are indicators that the brain and body have adapted to the substance. Even without physiological dependence, the person can experience *psychological dependence.*

Typically, a person begins by using a substance to reduce pain or anxiety or to produce feelings of pleasure, excitement, confidence, or connection with others. With repeated use, users can come to depend on being in this altered state, and without the drug, they may feel worse than they did before they ever took it. Although most people don't think they will become addicted when they start, gradually the substance takes over their lives. Research has established that drugs cause addiction by operating on the "pleasure pathway" in the brain and changing brain chemistry (see Chapter 10 for details of this process).

Although addiction is usually associated with drug use, many experts now extend the concept of addiction to other areas in which behavior can become compulsive and out of control, such as gambling. In fact, there appear to be similarities between changes in a gambler's brain when viewing a videotape on gambling and changes in a cocaine user's brain when viewing a video focused on cocaine use.

In the DSM-5, gambling disorder was included as an addictive disorder because recent evidence suggests that the brains of those addicted to substances and to gambling appear to make similar changes. The results in both cases include feelings of euphoria along with a strong desire to repeat the behavior and a craving for the behavior when it stops. Internet use gaming disorder has also been included in the DSM, although it is in a section reserved for conditions that require further study rather than treated as a mental disorder.

Alcohol		AA has more than 2 million members—only a small proportion of those who are dependent on alcohol.
Drugs		More than 8 percent of the population currently use illicit drugs, with marijuana by far the most commonly used.
Tobacco		Smoking rates have declined dramatically since their peak in the 1960s, but one in five Americans still smokes.
Caffeine		The most widely used psychoactive drug in the United States, caffeine is consumed in coffee, soda, and, most recently, energy drinks with names like Red Bull and Full Throttle.
Food		Some people who are addicted to food have binge-eating disorder—a psychological disorder like anorexia or bulimia—and are likely to be overweight or obese.
Gambling		About 3–4 percent of those who gamble are believed to do so compulsively.
Shopping		A cultural emphasis on material goods, fueled by advertising, contributes to compulsive shopping.
Sex		Sex addicts are preoccupied with sexual thoughts and activities much of the time. The vast majority grew up in abusive family environments.
Internet		Internet addicts spend hours online every day instead of spending time on real-life activities and relationships.

figure 2.4 **What we're addicted to: Substances and behaviors.**
The common feature in all addictions is loss of control.

Although pathological gambling and potentially Internet use are the best known of these behavioral disorders, people may also be addicted to sex, shopping, eating, exercising, or other activities (Figure 2.4), but at this time they are not listed in the DSM as addictive disorders. The key characteristic of these conditions is that the person feels out of control and powerless over the behavior. Both psychotherapy and self-help groups are available to assist individuals struggling with these troubling behavior patterns.

Schizophrenia and Other Psychotic Disorders

Psychotic disorders are characterized by delusions, hallucinations, disorganized speech or behavior, and other signs that the individual has lost touch with reality. The most common psychotic disorder is **schizophrenia**. A person with schizophrenia typically has disorganized and disordered thinking and perceptions, bizarre ideas, hallucinations (often voices), and impaired functioning.[30] The symptoms are sometimes so severe that the person becomes socially, interpersonally, and occupationally dysfunctional. Age at onset is usually the early 20s for men and the late 20s for women.

Schizophrenia has a strong genetic component. First-degree relatives of individuals with schizophrenia have a risk for the disorder 10 times higher than that of the general population.[31] All of the brain scanning and visualizing technologies reveal abnormalities in the brains of people with schizophrenia. Studies indicate that these abnormalities are present before the onset of symptoms, suggesting that this illness is the result of problems in brain development, perhaps even occurring prenatally. In most cases, symptoms of the disease can be controlled with medication.

Mental Disorders and Suicide

A major public health concern, particularly among young people, suicide is the second leading cause of death among college students. According to the fall 2012 National College Health Assessment, approximately 30 percent of college students had been so depressed that they could not function, 59 percent felt very sad in the past year, and 50 percent had periods of overwhelming anxiety. About 7 percent of students had seriously considered suicide, and 1 percent had attempted to kill themselves in the past year.[31]

Overall, women in U.S. society are more likely than men to attempt suicide, but men are four times more likely to succeed, probably because they choose more violent methods, usually a firearm. In the United States, firearms are used in 55 to 60 percent

psychotic disorders Mental disorders characterized by signs that the individual has lost touch with reality.

schizophrenia Psychotic disorder characterized by disorganized and disordered thinking and perceptions, bizarre ideas, hallucinations (often voices), and impaired functioning.

of all suicides. Women tend to use less violent methods for suicide, but in recent years they have begun to use firearms more frequently.

What Leads a Person to Suicide? Individuals contemplating suicide are most likely experiencing unbearable emotional pain, anguish, or despair. As many as 90 percent of those who commit suicide are suffering from a mental disorder, often depression.[32] Studies indicate that the symptom linking depression and suicide is a feeling of hopelessness. Depression and alcoholism may be involved in two-thirds of all suicides. Abuse of substances other than alcohol is another factor; the combination of drugs and depression can be lethal. People experiencing psychosis are also at risk.

Besides mental disorders and substance abuse, other major risk factors associated with suicide are a family history of suicide, serious medical problems, and access to the means, such as a gun or pills. The most significant risk factor, however, is a previous suicide attempt or a history of such attempts.

Sometimes, vulnerable individuals turn to suicide in response to a specific event, such as the loss of a relationship or job, an experience of failure, or a worry that a secret will be revealed. Other times there is no apparent precipitating event, and the suicide seems to come out of nowhere. However, suicide is always a process, and certain behavioral signs indicate that a person may be thinking about suicide:

■ Comments about death and threats to commit suicide.

■ Increasing social withdrawal and isolation.

■ Intensified moodiness.

■ Increase in risk-taking behaviors.

■ Sudden improvement in mood accompanied by such behaviors as giving away possessions. (The person may have made the decision to commit suicide.)

---

psychotherapy
Treatment for psychological problems usually based on the development of a positive interpersonal relationship between a client and a therapist.

How to Help If you know someone who seems to be suicidal, it is critical to get the person help. All mentions of suicide should be taken seriously. It is a myth that asking a person if he or she is thinking about suicide will plant the seed in the person's mind. Ignoring someone's sadness and depressed mood only increases the risk. Encourage the person to talk, and ask direct questions:

■ Are you thinking about killing yourself?

■ Do you have a plan?

■ Do you have the means?

■ Have you attempted suicide in the past?

Encourage the person to get help by calling a suicide hotline or seeking counseling. Do not agree to keep the person's mental state or intentions a secret. If he or she refuses to get help or resists your advice, you may need to contact a parent or relative or, if you are a student, share your concern with a professional at the student health center. Do not leave a suicidal person alone. Call for help or take the person to an emergency room.

If you have thought about suicide yourself, we encourage you to seek counseling. Therapy can help you resolve problems, develop better coping skills, and diminish the feelings that are causing you pain. It can also help you see things in a broader perspective and understand that you will not always feel this way. Remember the saying, suicide is a permanent solution to a temporary problem.

Self-Injury

Self-injury, sometimes known as self-harm, self-mutilation, or self-injurious behavior, is defined as any intentional injury to one's own body. Specific behaviors include cutting, burning, scratching, branding, and head banging. Self-injurious behaviors are sometimes mistaken for suicide attempts. Individuals who self-injure often have a history of physical and/or sexual abuse as well as coexisting problems such as substance abuse and eating disorders.

There is evidence that the incidence of self-injury is increasing, particularly among adolescents.[33] It has been estimated that approximately 6 percent of college students have engaged in at least one incident of self-injury within the past 12 months.[34] Many of the college students reporting self-injurious behaviors had never been in therapy and only rarely disclosed their behaviors to anyone.[35] Self-injury seems to be equally prevalent among men and women, and the behavior does not appear to be correlated to race, ethnicity, education, sexual orientation, socioeconomic status, or religion. A variety of treatments can help people who injure themselves, including family therapy and medications. The DSM-5 does not list either nonsuicidal self-injury or personal history of self-harm as a mental illness.

Treatments for Mental Disorders

More than 250 different models of psychotherapy exist for the treatment of mental disorders, and many different drugs can be prescribed. Most of the mild and moderate mental disorders are readily treatable with therapy and, if needed, medications. Currently, hospital emergency rooms are the primary source of treatment for many mentally ill people; see the box, "Emergency Rooms: Overused and Overwhelmed."

Psychotherapy The key feature of most forms of **psychotherapy** (or *counseling*) is the development of a positive interpersonal relationship between a person seeking help (the client or patient) and a therapist—a trained and licensed professional who can provide that help. Most

Public Health Is Personal

Emergency Rooms: Overused and Overwhelmed

In any economic crisis, the most vulnerable tend to be at greatest risk for cutbacks in services. In the last few years, many states have cut back their mental health budgets and closed programs to save money. Emergency rooms are overwhelmed with mentally ill individuals who often have coexisting chronic physical illnesses. Almost 70 percent of emergency rooms indicate that they keep mentally ill individuals for 24 hours and in some cases mentally ill individuals wait in emergency rooms for several days waiting for care or specific placement. Basically, mentally ill individuals are often forced to wait days for care and, at times, are simply warehoused in general medical units where their psychiatric conditions go untreated. At the same time, the overall number of ER patients has risen because many people are using emergency rooms for nonemergency issues, and even those who are newly insured because of health care reform may be high utilizers of emergency rooms.

Continued overuse of the ER will only result in bankrupting medical facilities. What can be done to reduce the use of emergency rooms by mentally ill individuals and ensure that they receive appropriate care? Here are some proposals:

- *Develop patient navigator positions.* When mentally ill individuals are admitted into a hospital setting, they would be assigned a patient navigator who would help them arrange for follow-up services once they leave the hospital.

- *Improve primary care access.* All mentally ill individuals should have primary care providers who can help them with their nonurgent medical situations. This would reduce the use of the emergency room as a primary care clinic.

- *Increase funds for Assertive Community Treatment (ACT) teams.* ACT teams provide multidisciplinary care for the mentally ill, including home visits and follow-up care.

- *Increase funding.* More funding could help provide a variety of outpatient day treatment programs, job training, and housing programs for people with mental illnesses.

connect
ACTIVITY

Sources: "Emergency Rooms Provide Care of Last Resort for Mentally Ill," by J. Gold, April 11, 2013, *Kaiser Health News;* "E.R. Costs for Mentally Ill Soar, and Hospitals Seek Better Way," by J. Creswell, December 25, 2013, *New York Times,* www.nytimes.com/2013/12/26/health/er-costs-for-mentally-ill-soar-and-hospitals-seek-better-way.html; "Medicaid Increases Emergency-Department Use: Evidence from Oregon's Health Insurance Experiment," by S.L. Taubman, H. Allen, B.J. Wright, K. Baicker, and A.N. Finkelstein, January 17, 2014, *Science, 343,* pp. 263–268.

therapy models agree on the central importance of this interpersonal relationship between client and therapist.

Most therapists espouse a particular theoretical orientation, but many take an eclectic approach; that is, they fuse ideas from a variety of different theories and approaches. A number of evidence-based psychotherapies and factors that are part of all effective treatments have been well researched and appear to have a positive impact on those who participate.[36] These include cognitive behavioral therapy (CBT) and the importance of a positive client therapist relationship.

What should you expect if you decide to try therapy? You can expect to be treated with warmth, respect, and an open, accepting attitude. The therapist will try to provide you with a safe place to explore your feelings and thoughts. At the end of the first session, the therapist will probably propose a plan for treatment, such as a series of 10 sessions or a referral to another professional (see the box, "Choosing a Mental Health Care Provider").

Medications Until the 1950s, few effective medications for the symptoms of mental illness existed. Since that time, discoveries and breakthroughs in drug research have revolutionized the treatment of mental disorders. Today, the symptoms of many serious disorders can be treated successfully with drugs.

The symptoms of schizophrenia and other psychotic disorders, especially delusions and hallucinations, can be treated with *antipsychotics.* Symptoms of mood disorders can be relieved with any of several different types of *antidepressants,*

most of which act on the neurotransmitters serotonin and norepinephrine. Prozac, Zoloft, and Paxil are used to treat mood disorders and are among the most frequently prescribed drugs in the United States today. The most frequently prescribed drugs overall are antidepressants. Between 2002 and 2005, prescriptions for antidepressants increased from 154 million to 170 million.[37]

Symptoms of anxiety disorders can be reduced with antianxiety drugs (or *anxiolytics*). Benzodiazepines, the most widely used antianxiety drugs, are believed to act on the neurotransmitter GABA, which has a role in the inhibition of anxiety in the brain during stressful situations. Common antianxiety medications include Valium, Xanax, and Ativan.

The use of medications for mental disorders has increased dramatically in recent years, including the use of drugs for children and adolescents. The controversy over this practice was highlighted in 2004 when a study showed that

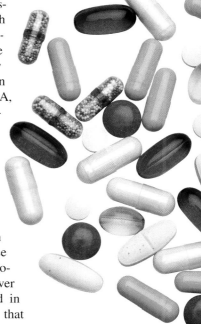

Consumer Clipboard

Choosing a Mental Health Care Provider

Think you might like to talk to a therapist? Wonder if you could benefit from medication? Use these guidelines to get the right care.

Would it be helpful to see a mental health care provider?

Assess your mental and emotional status with these questions:

- Am I feeling sad (homesick, lonely) a lot of the time?
- Am I having trouble studying for exams?
- Am I having difficulty concentrating?
- Do I feel inadequate, guilty, or worthless?
- Am I feeling overwhelmed?
- Have I lost interest in doing the things I usually like to do?
- Is this problem interfering with my everyday life?
- Have my friends and family asked if there's a problem?
- Am I avoiding friends because of the problem?

These are the kinds of problems a counselor can help you with. Many colleges provide free psychological assessments, short-term counseling, and referrals.

What's the difference among kinds of providers?

- Psychiatrists are medical doctors (M.D.s) who have completed medical school and at least a three-year residency in psychiatry. They can independently prescribe medication but often do not have a great deal of training in psychotherapy. If you see a psychiatrist, you will probably be prescribed a medication but will not meet for therapy sessions.
- Psychiatric nurse practitioners (PNPs) have completed training in nursing and have additional qualifications in psychiatry. PNPs can prescribe medications but often have to be supervised by an M.D. Like psychiatrists, they focus on psychiatric diagnosis and medication treatment.

- Licensed psychologists most often have a Ph.D. or Psy.D. (doctor of psychology) and receive four to five years of training following their bachelor's degree. They have to fulfill a specific number of supervised hours before they can be licensed. They cannot prescribe medication but are trained in providing psychotherapy.
- Licensed clinical social workers, counselors, and marriage and family therapists typically have at least a master's degree and have to fulfill a specific number of supervised hours before they can be licensed. Like psychologists, they cannot prescribe medication but are trained in providing psychotherapy.

No matter what type of provider you see, you should feel comfortable and emotionally safe sharing your concerns.

Are there other options?

- Support groups provide the opportunity to share your problems with peers, which may help you put them in perspective. This may be all the help you need.
- Pastoral counseling may be available in your religious community. Pastoral counselors have a professional degree from a seminary, a master's degree or doctorate in the mental health field, and clinical training.

Does insurance cover mental health care?

- Your college tuition fees or health insurance may cover some mental health services. If you choose to go off campus for counseling, those services may not be covered by your college benefits. If your insurance is through your parents, you will need to check with that insurance company about coverage.

Are parents informed about mental health care?

- If you're over 18, most schools leave this decision up to you. Communication between a mental health care provider and a client is considered confidential, with a few exceptions. If you're considered to be at risk for suicide, most counselors will encourage you to inform your parents about the counseling.

---

certain antidepressants increased the risk of suicidal thinking and behavior in adolescents.[38–41] The FDA directed manufacturers of all antidepressants to include "black box" warnings to physicians and parents on their labels.

More recent studies indicate that antidepressants also significantly increase the risk of suicidal thoughts and behaviors in young adults aged 18 to 24, usually during the first one to two months of treatment. The FDA has proposed that warnings on antidepressants be updated to include young adults.[42]

The increase in the use of drug treatments is due not just to improvements in the drugs themselves but also to the growing use of managed health care in the United States. Insurance companies often prefer to pay for medications, which tend to produce faster, more visible, and more verifiable results, than for psychotherapy, which may last for months or years and produce results that are less objectively verifiable.

Drugs treat only the symptoms of mental disorders, however, and although they continue to remain the treatment of choice, research has been mixed about their overall effectiveness.[43] For example, some antidepressants are not recommended for individuals diagnosed with minor depression and should be used only by people who are suicidal or have

a family history of mood disorders.[44] Psychotherapy is usually necessary as a supplement to drug treatment, as it helps the person understand the root causes of problems and change maladaptive patterns of thinking, feeling, and behaving.

WHAT IS STRESS?

Although stress can sometimes trigger a mental disorder, for most people, stress is a fact of life. You experience varying levels of stress throughout the day as your body and mind continually adjust to the demands of living. We often think of stress in negative terms, as an uncomfortable or unpleasant pressure—for example, to complete a project on time or to deal with a traffic ticket. However, stress can also be positive. When you get a promotion at work or when someone throws you a surprise birthday party, you also experience stress.

A survey conducted by the American Psychological Association in 2013 found that 72 percent of American adults regularly experience physical symptoms caused by stress, and 67 percent experience psychological symptoms caused by stress.[45] Such statistics reinforce the need to manage the stress in our lives and to reduce its negative impact

Who's at Risk?

Stress in America

Although stress levels have dropped a bit in recent years, they continue to exceed what many consider to be healthy. All segments of the population apparently experience unhealthy levels of stress on a regular basis, but as the graphs here show, men and women differ somewhat in the stress symptoms they report, and the generations differ somewhat in the types of stress reduction strategies they use.

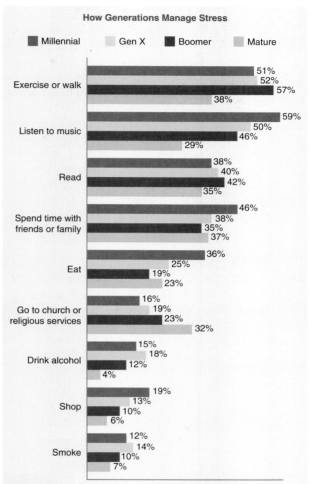

How Generations Manage Stress

Millennial · Gen X · Boomer · Mature

Exercise or walk	51% / 52% / 57% / 38%
Listen to music	59% / 50% / 46% / 29%
Read	38% / 40% / 42% / 35%
Spend time with friends or family	46% / 38% / 35% / 37%
Eat	36% / 25% / 19% / 23%
Go to church or religious services	16% / 19% / 23% / 32%
Drink alcohol	15% / 18% / 12% / 4%
Shop	19% / 13% / 10% / 6%
Smoke	12% / 14% / 10% / 7%

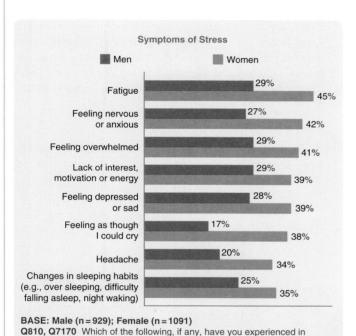

Symptoms of Stress

Men · Women

Fatigue	29% / 45%
Feeling nervous or anxious	27% / 42%
Feeling overwhelmed	29% / 41%
Lack of interest, motivation or energy	29% / 39%
Feeling depressed or sad	28% / 39%
Feeling as though I could cry	17% / 38%
Headache	20% / 34%
Changes in sleeping habits (e.g., over sleeping, difficulty falling asleep, night waking)	25% / 35%

BASE: Male (n = 929); Female (n = 1091)
Q810, Q7170 Which of the following, if any, have you experienced in the last month as a result of stress?

BASE: Millennial (n = 340); Gen X (n = 397); Boomer (n = 1040); Mature (n = 243) Q965 Do you do any of the following to help manage stress? Please select all that apply.

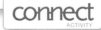

Source: *Stress in America: Missing the Health Care Connection,* by American Psychological Association, released February 7, 2013, pp. 17, 21, www.apa.org/news/press/releases/stress/2012/full-report.pdf

on our well-being. When excessive stress is unavoidable, having a repertoire of stress management techniques to fall back on is invaluable (see the box, "Stress in America").

Events or agents in the environment that cause us stress are called **stressors**. They can range from being late for class to having a close friend die, from finding a parking space to winning the lottery. Your reaction to these events is called the *stress response;* this concept is discussed at length in the next section. Stressors disrupt the body's balance and require adjustments to return systems to normal. **Stress** can be defined as the general state of the body, mind, and emotions when an environmental stressor has triggered the stress response.

Not all stress is bad. Under certain circumstances, stress might even improve recall and performance.[46] Because there is so much variation in individual responses to stressors, stress may be thought of as a *transaction* between an individual and a stressor in the environment, mediated by personal variables that include the person's perceptions and appraisal of the event.[47] When faced with a stressor, you evaluate it without necessarily realizing you are doing

stressors
Events or agents in the environment that cause stress.

stress
The general state of the body, mind, and emotions when an environmental stressor has triggered the stress response.

eustress
Good stress or a positive form of stress.

stress response or fight-or-flight response
Series of physiological changes that activate body systems, providing a burst of energy to deal with a perceived threat or danger.

so: Is it positive or negative? How threatening is it to my well-being, my self-esteem, my identity? Can I cope with it or not? When you appraise an event as positive, you experience **eustress**, or positive stress. When you appraise it as negative, you experience *distress.* Often, it is not the stressor itself that is debilitating, but the feeling that stress is constant and unrelieved by the opportunity to relax.

Regardless of your situation, stressors can make it more difficult for you to achieve your goals. College students report to researchers that stress is the top impediment to academic performance, for example.[34] However, there are tools that anyone can use to reduce stress before it becomes chronic.

The Stress Response

Whether the individual's appraisal of the stressor is negative or positive, all stressors elicit the **stress response** (also known as the **fight-or-flight response**), a series of physiological changes that occur in the body in the face of a threat. All animals, it appears—humans included—need sudden bursts of energy to fight or flee from situations they perceive as dangerous.

The stress response is carried out by the *autonomic nervous system,* which controls involuntary, unconscious functions like breathing, heart rate, and digestion. The autonomic nervous system has two branches: the *sympathetic branch* is responsible for initiating the stress response, and the *parasympathetic branch* is responsible for turning off the stress response and returning the body to normal.

The stress response begins when the cerebral cortex (in the front of the brain) sends a chemical signal to the hypothalamus, which sends a signal to the pituitary gland. The pituitary gland sends adrenocorticotropic hormone (ACTH) to the adrenal glands, which release the hormones cortisol, epinephrine (adrenaline), and norepinephrine (noradrenaline) into the bloodstream. Glucose and fats are released from the liver and other storage sites to provide energy. As stress hormones surge through your body, your heart rate, breathing rate, muscle tension, metabolism, and blood pressure all increase, and other changes occur to prepare you for fight or flight (Figure 2.5). All this happens in an instant.

The Relaxation Response

When a stressful event is over—you decide the situation is no longer dangerous, or you complete your task—the

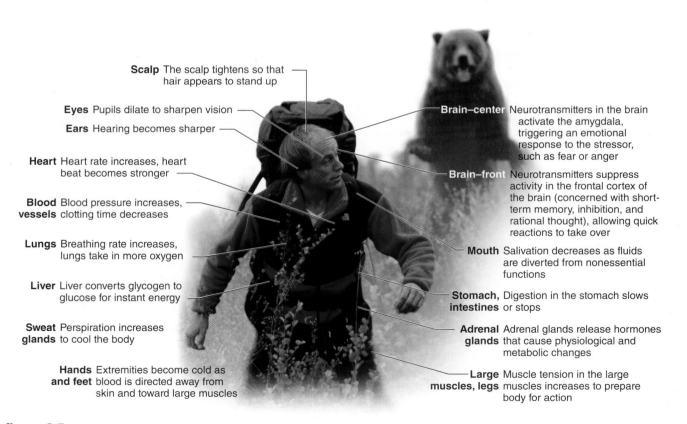

Scalp The scalp tightens so that hair appears to stand up

Eyes Pupils dilate to sharpen vision

Ears Hearing becomes sharper

Heart Heart rate increases, heart beat becomes stronger

Blood vessels Blood pressure increases, clotting time decreases

Lungs Breathing rate increases, lungs take in more oxygen

Liver Liver converts glycogen to glucose for instant energy

Sweat glands Perspiration increases to cool the body

Hands and feet Extremities become cold as blood is directed away from skin and toward large muscles

Brain–center Neurotransmitters in the brain activate the amygdala, triggering an emotional response to the stressor, such as fear or anger

Brain–front Neurotransmitters suppress activity in the frontal cortex of the brain (concerned with short-term memory, inhibition, and rational thought), allowing quick reactions to take over

Mouth Salivation decreases as fluids are diverted from nonessential functions

Stomach, intestines Digestion in the stomach slows or stops

Adrenal glands Adrenal glands release hormones that cause physiological and metabolic changes

Large muscles, legs Muscle tension in the large muscles increases to prepare body for action

figure 2.5 **The stress response: Changes in the body.**

parasympathetic branch of the autonomic nervous system takes over, turning off the stress response.[48] Heart rate, breathing, muscle tension, and blood pressure all decrease. The body returns to **homeostasis**, a state of stability and balance in which functions are maintained within a normal range. This process is called the **relaxation response**, which we will discuss in more detail later in this chapter.

Acute Stress and Chronic Stress

According to evolutionary biology, the fight-or-flight response served an important function for our ancestors. Today, most of us do not live in such dangerous environments, but this innate response to threat is still essential to our survival, warning us when it is time to fight or flee. Although the fight-or-flight response requires a great deal of energy—which is why you often feel so tired after a stressful event—your body is equipped to deal with short-term **acute stress** as long as it does not happen too often and as long as you can relax and recover afterward.

A frequent or persistent stress response, however, can lead to problems. In these instances, the stress response itself becomes damaging. Many people live in a state of **chronic stress**, in which stressful conditions are ongoing and the stress response continues without resolution. Chronic stress increases the likelihood that the person will become ill or, if already ill, that her or his defense system will be overwhelmed by the disease. Prolonged or severe stress has been found to weaken nearly every system in the body.

STRESS AND YOUR HEALTH

Researchers have been looking at the relationship between stress and disease since the 1950s. Chronic stress can weaken body systems, and mediators such as personality traits and attitudes can intensify or diminish the physical effects of stress.

The General Adaptation Syndrome

One of the first scientists to develop a broad theory of stress and disease was Hans Selye.[48] He introduced the **General Adaptation Syndrome (GAS)** as a description and explanation of the physiological changes that he observed and that he believed to be predictable responses to stressors by all organisms. The syndrome has three stages—alarm, resistance, and exhaustion—that are described in Figure 2.6.

Physical Effects of Chronic Stress

Stress plays a role in illness and disease in a variety of ways. For example, stress-triggered changes in the lungs increase the symptoms of asthma and other respiratory conditions. Stress also appears to inhibit tissue repair, which increases the likelihood of bone fractures and is related to the development of osteoporosis (porous, weak bones). Stress can lead to sexual problems, including failure to ovulate and amenorrhea (absence of menstrual periods) in women and sexual dysfunction and loss of sexual desire in both men and women. Some suggest that high levels of stress can even speed up the aging process

homeostasis
State of stability and balance in which body functions are maintained within a normal range.

relaxation response
Series of physiological changes that calm body systems and return them to normal functioning.

acute stress
Short-term stress, produced by the stress response.

chronic stress
Long-term, low-level stress in which the stress response continues without resolution.

General Adaptation Syndrome (GAS)
Selye's classic model used to describe the physiological changes associated with the stress response. The three phases are alarm, resistance, and exhaustion.

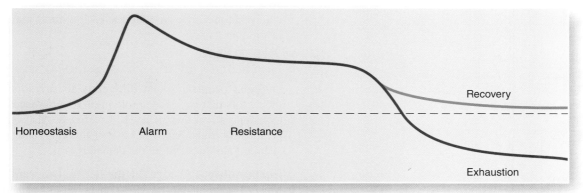

figure 2.6 **General Adaptation Syndrome.**
Selye's model describes the physiological response to stress. In the *alarm stage,* the body's fight-or-flight response is activated, accompanied by reduced immune system functioning. In the *resistance stage,* the body uses energy to cope with the continued stress and stay at peak level. After prolonged exposure to stress, the body may either recover or enter the *exhaustion stage* and become totally depleted, leading to illness and even death.

Stress and the Immune System Since Selye's time, research has definitively shown that stress decreases immune function. One study demonstrated a strong relationship between levels of psychological stress and the possibility of infection by a common cold virus. Other studies have found that both brief and long-term stressors have an impact on the function of the immune system.[49] Stressors as diverse as taking exams, experiencing major life events, and providing long-term care for someone with Alzheimer's disease affect the immune system. Scientists still do not fully understand why the stress response suppresses immune function or whether there is an evolutionary explanation for this suppression.

Stress and the Cardiovascular System The stress response causes heart rate to accelerate and blood pressure to increase. Chronic stress causes heart rate and blood pressure to remain elevated for long periods of time. Chronic hypertension (high blood pressure) makes blood vessels more susceptible to the development of atherosclerosis, a disease in which arteries are damaged and clogged with fatty deposits. Both hypertension and atherosclerosis increase the risk of heart attack and stroke. Overall stress levels are typically higher for individuals who have suffered heart attacks.

Stress and the Gastrointestinal System Although not conclusive, evidence suggests that gastrointestinal problems might be stress related. More specifically, conditions such as acid reflux, indigestion, and stomach pain all seem to be more common in people who have higher levels or more frequent occurrences of stress. Irritable bowel syndrome (IBS) may be an example of individual response differences to the gastrointestinal tract by stress. When IBS patients are under stress, food seems to move more slowly through the small intestine in those individuals who are constipated; the opposite is true for those who suffer from diarrhea.

Type A behavior pattern
Set of personality traits originally thought to be associated with risk for heart disease. Type A individuals are hard driving, competitive, achievement oriented, and quick to anger; further research has identified hostility as the key risk factor in the pattern.

For a long time, stress was commonly believed to cause stomach ulcers. Research suggests, however, that ulcers may be caused or exacerbated by a bacterial infection that irritates the stomach lining. While not causing ulcers, stress may contribute to their development.

Stress and Mental Health Both acute and chronic stress can contribute to psychological problems and the development of psychological illnesses, including anxiety disorders and depression.[50] Overall, chronic stress appears to take a toll on an individual's mental health.[51] In *acute stress disorder,* for example, a person develops

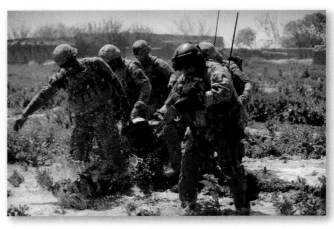

■ The stress and trauma of combat can lead to post-traumatic stress disorder in some individuals.

symptoms after experiencing severe trauma, such as assault, rape, domestic violence, child physical or sexual abuse, terrorist attacks, or natural disasters. Symptoms can include a feeling of numbness, a sense of being in a daze, amnesia, flashbacks, increased arousal and anxiety, and impaired functioning.

If such symptoms appear six months or more after the traumatic event, the person may have *post-traumatic stress disorder (PTSD),* a condition characterized by a sense of numbness or emotional detachment from people, repeated reliving of the event through flashbacks and/or nightmares, and avoidance of things that might be associated with the trauma. In some cases, years may pass after the trauma before PTSD symptoms appear.[24]

Low-level, unresolved chronic stress can also be a factor in psychological problems. An example is *adjustment disorder,* in which a response to a stressor (such as anxiety, worry, and social withdrawal) continues for a longer period than would normally be expected. Stress can diminish wellness and reduce the ability to function at the highest level even without an identifiable disorder. Symptoms such as irritability, impatience, difficulty concentrating, excessive worrying, insomnia, and forgetfulness, like physical symptoms, can be addressed with stress management techniques.

Mediators of the Stress Response

Different people respond differently to stressors. Among the factors that may play a role in these differences are past experiences and overall level of wellness. Also critical are personality traits, habitual ways of thinking, and inborn or acquired attitudes toward the demands of life.

Personality Factors In the 1970s two cardiologists, Meyer Friedman and Ray Rosenman, described and named the **Type A behavior pattern**.[52] Type A individuals tend to be impulsive, need to get things done quickly, and live their lives on a time schedule. They are hard driving, achievement oriented, and highly competitive. Some estimates are that more than 40 percent of the population of the United States—and possibly half of all men—might be Type As.

Individuals who fit this description are prime candidates for stress-related illnesses. The relationship between Type A personality traits and heart disease has been known for some time. More recently, there have been indications that a Type A personality can mean increased risk for a number of other diseases, including peptic ulcers, asthma, headaches, and thyroid problems.

However, not all the characteristics of this personality seem to be harmful. Many Type As are achievement oriented and successful and yet remain healthy. According to recent research, a key culprit is **hostility**, defined as an ongoing accumulation of irritation and anger. Hostile individuals are generally cynical about others, frequently express anger, and display aggressive behaviors.[53] Research has indicated that hostility, by itself, is related to coronary heart disease, and it may also contribute to premature death.[54]

Friedman and Rosenman also described a constellation of personality traits they labeled Type B. In contrast to the Type A personality, the Type B personality is less driven and more relaxed. Type Bs are more easygoing and less readily frustrated. All other things being equal, Type Bs are less susceptible to coronary heart disease.

Other experts have expanded on Friedman and Rosenman's research and have described two additional personality types. Type C personalities are introverted, detail-oriented people who may have trouble communicating and appear to be very cautious and reserved. These individuals might be at greater risk for autoimmune disorders and demonstrate a tendency to please others. Type D individuals appear to hold in negative emotions and are not very expressive. They experience negative emotions like anger, anxiety, and sadness while fearing negative judgments from others. Type Ds are also at risk for negative health outcomes, including arterial disease, heart failure, and poor health ratings.[55–57]

Cognitive Factors Until you decide that an event is actually a threat and beyond your ability to cope, it remains merely a potential stressor. Experts suggest that people create their own distress with their habitual thinking patterns—illogical thinking, unrealistic expectations, and negative beliefs.[25] For example, a person may think she has to get straight As in order to be a worthy human being. If she gets a B, she will experience much more stress than if she had more realistic expectations about herself and was more self-forgiving. Her ideas can transform a relatively neutral event into a stressor.

Other common illogical ideas and unrealistic expectations are "life should be fair," "friends should be there when you need them," "everyone I care about has to love and approve of me," and "everything has to go my way." When everyday experiences don't live up to these ideas, people who hold them end up feeling angry, frustrated, disappointed, or demoralized. Common patterns of distorted thinking include focusing on the negative and filtering out the positive, catastrophizing (expecting the worst), thinking in polarities (black-and-white thinking), and personalizing (thinking everything's about you). With a more realistic attitude, people can take things in stride and reduce the frequency and intensity of the stress response. This doesn't mean they should have unrealistically low expectations. When expectations are too low, people may experience underachievement, depression, resignation, and lowered self-esteem. The goal is a realistic balance.

Resilience and Hardiness Just as resilience is a factor in mental health, it is also a factor in the ability to handle stress. Stress-resistant people also seem to focus on immediate issues and explain their struggle in positive and helpful ways. For example, a poor grade on one exam might motivate the stress-resilient person to study harder, using the grade as motivation. A person who is not so resilient may react to a poor grade by feeling like a failure and giving up.

Another line of research has developed the concept of **hardiness**, an effective style of coping with stress. The researchers suggest that positive ways of coping with stress

hostility
Ongoing accumulation of irritation and anger.

hardiness
Effective style of coping with stress, characterized by a tendency to view life events as challenges rather than threats, a commitment to meaningful activities, and a sense of being in control.

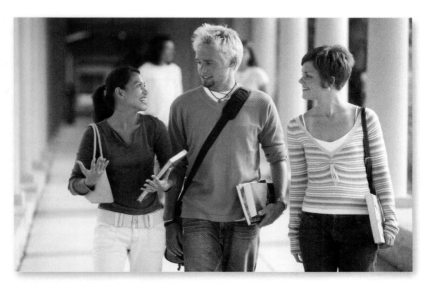

■ Starting college is a major life transition with unique stressors. Individuals with the qualities of resilience and hardiness are able to take the challenges in stride and respond with energy and excitement.

may buffer the body from its effects.[58,59] They call this style *hardiness* and have suggested that people high in hardiness are more resistant to illness.

These researchers found that hardy people (1) perceive the demands of living as a challenge rather than a threat, (2) are committed to meaningful activities, and (3) have a sense of control over their lives. Having a sense of control may be especially critical in avoiding illness and responding to stressful situations.

SOURCES OF STRESS

Contemporary life presents us with nearly limitless sources of stress, ranging from major life events to our interpersonal relationships to some of our own feelings. In this section, we describe some of these stressors; in the next section, we present a variety of tips for handling them.

Life Events

Can stressful life events make people more vulnerable to illness? Thomas Holmes and Richard Rahe, medical researchers at the University of Washington, observed that individuals frequently experienced major life events before the onset of an illness. They proposed that life events—major changes and transitions that force the individual to adjust and adapt—may precipitate illness, especially if several such events occur at the same time.[60] Holmes and Rahe examined medical records to determine if there was a relationship between stressful events and onset of illnesses. From this work, they developed the Holmes-Rahe Social Readjustment Scale, a ranking of life events that require the individual to adjust and adapt to change. The higher a person's score on the scale, the more likely that person is to experience symptoms of illness.

The most stressful event on this scale is the death of a spouse, followed by such events as divorce, separation, a personal injury, and being fired from a job. Less stressful events on the scale include moving, going on vacation, experiencing a change in sleeping habits, and dealing with a minor violation of the law.

Daily Hassles

Surprisingly, everyday hassles can also cause health problems. In fact, daily hassles are related to subsequent illness and disease to a greater degree than are major life events.[61] Examples of daily hassles are arguments, car problems, deadlines, traffic jams, long lines, and money worries. All of these events can lead to a state of chronic, low-level stress, especially if they pile up and you don't have a period of recovery.

College Stress College students experience a great deal of life change, and some studies even suggest that the college years may be the most stressful time in people's lives.[62,63] In one survey of college students, stress was identified as the top health concern, with 28 percent of respondents reporting

that stress affected their academic performance.[34] Considering the health effects of stress, it should not be surprising that colds, mononucleosis, and sexually transmitted diseases are familiar on college campuses.

Besides the effect of this major life transition, common sources of stress for college students include academic work, exams and grades, sleep deprivation, worries about money, relationship concerns, and uncertainty about their futures. The stress of college may be growing even more intense, particularly for young women.[34] Nontraditional college students, including students who have returned to school after a hiatus, face some unique stressors. These can include having to adapt to new technologies on campus, remembering how to study, trying to retrain for a new career, and balancing coursework with the demands of a job or family.

Rising tuition costs also appear to affect stress levels of many students. A record number of students say they have to work to afford college. Concern about the economy and being successful also have an impact on students (see the box, "Jason: A New Financial Reality").

College officials indicate that although more young people are going to college, they might also be less prepared to deal with college stressors and expectations. Almost all college students describe themselves as being depressed during their college experience, although the depression is often moderate and of a short duration. These episodes are often related to specific stressors, such as difficulties in a relationship, poor grades, and general adjustment concerns. When the intensity of the situation increases or the student is unable to find support, symptoms such as changes in appetite or increases in risk-taking behaviors, self-injurious behaviors, and smoking may appear.

Job Pressure Sixty-nine percent of Americans say that work is a significant source of stress, and stress has been found to affect productivity.[45] Half of all employees stated that they lost productivity at work due to stress, and a large portion of young people (60 percent) report being less productive because of work stress.[64] Satisfaction with one's employer remains low, and about one in three workers reports an intention to seek employment elsewhere.[45,64]

Job pressure contributes to many stress-related illnesses, including cardiovascular disease, and may be related to the incidence of back pain, fatigue, muscular pain, and headaches. The costs are high in terms of dollars and worker performance, seen in accidents, absenteeism, turnover, reduced levels of productivity, and insurance costs.

Over the past century, many jobs have become physically easier, but expectations have grown that people will work more. Managers and professionals seem to work the longest days and are subject to associated stresses.[65] They bring work home and thus never really leave the job. Almost 35 percent of American workers cannot afford to take all their allotted vacation time each year, and almost 55 percent

Life Stories

Jason: A New Financial Reality

Jason, a college freshman, was an athlete with a passion for everything having to do with sports, from exercise physiology to sport psychology. He planned to major in exercise science and hoped to eventually become a college professor and football coach.

Jason's parents had been saving money for their children's education for years, and with the help of his scholarship, they had been able to pay nearly all of his first-year expenses. Unfortunately, Jason's dad had been laid off from his management position at a manufacturing company during the recent recession and had not been able to find a comparable job since. His mom worked part-time at a county office and had asked to increase her hours, but she was told there was a freeze on government spending.

With one son in college and two younger children at home, Jason's parents were struggling to make ends meet. They cut back on expenses in every way they could, from gym memberships, magazine subscriptions, and cable to groceries, clothes, and auto maintenance. There was no longer any extra for the kids' guitar lessons, soccer registration, or class trips, and it wasn't clear where more college money was going to come from.

When Jason came home for spring break, he was startled to hear what was going on, especially when he heard that his parents were worried about keeping up with the mortgage payments. The idea that his family could lose their home was shocking to him. He knew his dad hadn't been able to find another job, but he didn't know his parents had been living off their savings and had started dipping into their retirement funds.

Jason and his family sat around the kitchen table talking about options. Jason offered to reduce his course load and get a part-time job at school, though it would take him longer to get his degree. He also had the idea of transferring to a community college to reduce costs and then transferring back to his four-year college after he had his two-year degree. His parents said they didn't want him to do that yet and asked him to talk to someone in the financial aid office about grants, loans, and work-study programs.

When Jason returned to campus, he realized how shaken he was. He felt selfish for "living in a bubble" at school while his family was struggling, and he found himself avoiding friends, especially some whose families were well off. For a few weeks, he found it hard to focus on his schoolwork or his practices, and he had trouble sleeping. He felt that his whole view of the world was shifting, from one in which anything was possible to one in which his dreams might have to be tempered with a dose of reality.

- What would you do if you were in Jason's position? What options would you consider?

- How do you think Jason handled his reaction? What could he have done to help himself handle the stress he was experiencing?

connect ACTIVITY

---

check their e-mail or voicemail while on vacation.[66] Many people who want to be successful become *workaholics,* never taking a break from work and setting themselves up for burnout.

Burnout is an adverse, work-related stress reaction with physical, psychological, and behavioral components.[67] The symptoms of burnout include increasing discouragement and pessimism about work; a decline in motivation and job performance; irritability, anger, and apathy on the job; and physical complaints.[68]

Money and Financial Worries Sixty-nine percent of Americans say that money is a source of stress.[45] Financial worries take a particular toll on young people, with 80 percent of 18- to 30-year-olds, more than any other age group, saying that money is a source of stress.[64]

Many people experience financial stress because their income is not equal to their expenditures. Familiar sources of financial stress are fear of running short of money before the end of the month, carrying too much debt, reduced employment or unemployment, no savings to cover medical emergencies, and unexpected home or car repairs.

burnout
Adverse work-related stress reaction with physical, psychological, and behavioral components.

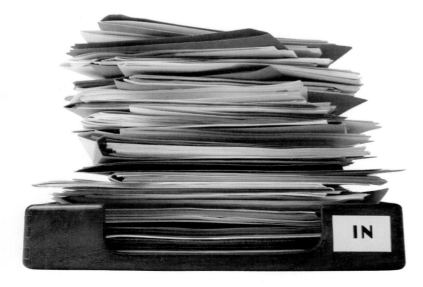

- Work overload and time pressure are major sources of stress and stress-related illnesses, including headaches, stomachaches, and depression.

One of the best ways to relieve financial stress is to plan ahead. Being willing to follow a budget and make the lifestyle changes necessary to live within available funds may be the key to relief from financial stress. Simplifying your life, shedding those items and events that you can live without, can be liberating. Finding ways to ensure financial peace of mind is an excellent stress reduction technique.

Family and Interpersonal Stress Families have to continuously adapt to a series of life changes and transitions. The birth of a baby places new demands on parents and siblings, and families must adapt as a teenager moves through adolescence to adulthood and leaves home. A family may be disrupted by death or divorce, and in fact, a growing number of children spend part of their lives in single-parent households, blended family units, or stepfamily systems.

Families may become weakened by these experiences, or they may become stronger and more resilient. Relationships of all kinds have the potential to be stressful, including intimate partnerships. Many experts agree that the key to a successful relationship is not finding the perfect partner but being able to communicate effectively with the partner you have. Whereas poor communication skills can cause interactions to escalate into arguments and fights (or deteriorate into cold silences), thoughtful communication and conflict resolution techniques can resolve issues before they become problems.

Time Pressure, Overload, and Technology Most of us experience some degree of time pressure in our lives. Many people find that they have more and more to do, despite time-saving devices, and want to compress more activity into less time. Multitasking is common—people talk on the phone while driving and answer e-mail while eating lunch. While many people think they are more productive when they multitask, multitasking actually distracts people and causes them to perform poorly on a variety of tasks.[69] The rush to do things quickly and simultaneously ends up increasing levels of stress.

Many people do not see their overstuffed schedules as a problem. Instead, they go to time management classes to learn how to squeeze more activities into the time they have. Although planning and good use of time are effective stress management techniques, there are limits to how much a person can do. Many times the solution is not to use time more effectively but to do less. Many stressed-out people are not poor stress managers; they are simply overloaded with responsibilities. Sometimes, learning to say no to others' requests is the best way to handle time management issues.

Technology has the effect of making us constantly available and never fully alone. Friends can reach us anytime with a text message or an e-mail, and work knows how to contact us outside of the office. With communication happening so quickly, we feel we must respond right away—even if we are doing something else or trying to relax. We may find that we have more "friends" on social networking sites than we can have meaningful contact with, but we continue to widen our social circles, simply adding stress to our lives. The idea of quality time with one's children has even been compromised. On a typical visit to a playground, you are likely to find parents checking their e-mail and reviewing their fantasy football teams on a smartphone while their children play. See the box, "How 'Connected' Should We Be?" at the end of the chapter for some thoughts about technology's effect on communication.

Anger Sometimes the source of stress is within the individual. Unresolved feelings of anger can be extremely stressful. The idea that blowing off steam, or venting, is a positive way to deal with anger is generally not the case. Releasing anger in an uncontrolled way often reinforces the feeling and may cause it to escalate into rage.[48] Venting can create anger in the person on the receiving end and hurts relationships. Suppressing anger or turning it against oneself is also unhealthy, lowering self-esteem and possibly fostering depression.

If you find yourself in a situation in which you are getting angry, take a time-out, remove yourself from the situation physically, and take some deep breaths. Examine the situation and think about whether your reaction is logical or illogical and whether you could see it another way. Look for absurdity or humor in the situation. Put it in perspective. If you cannot avoid the situation or reduce your reaction, try some of the stress management strategies and relaxation techniques described later in this chapter.

Trauma The effect of traumatic experiences has received a great deal of study. The events of September 11, 2001, and military service in Iraq and Afghanistan are frequently cited as traumatic events of the highest order. Events of this magnitude overwhelm our ability to cope and destroy any sense of control, connection, or meaning. They shake the foundations of beliefs about the safety and trustworthiness of the world.

Some people develop post-traumatic stress disorder (PTSD) in response to trauma, as mentioned earlier in this chapter. Although the triggering event may be overwhelming, often it alone is not sufficient to explain the occurrence of PTSD. For example, fewer than 40 percent of those with war zone experience in Vietnam developed PTSD.[70] Again, this is evidence of the role of mediating factors in the individual experience of stress.

Societal Pressures Intolerance, prejudice, discrimination, injustice, poverty, pressure to conform to mainstream culture—all are common sources of stress for members of modern society. Exposure to racism and homophobia, for example, can cause distrust, frustration, resentment, negative emotions such as anger and fear, and a sense of helplessness and hopelessness. Experiencing racism has been associated with both physical and mental health-related symptoms, including hypertension, cardiovascular reactivity, depression, eating disorders, substance abuse, and violence.[71–73]

Similarly, lesbians, gay males, bisexuals, and transgender individuals experience symptoms of stress when they are the targets of prejudice and homophobia.[74,75] These individuals often have higher rates of school-related problems, substance abuse, criminal activity, prostitution, running away from home, and suicide than do their non-gay peers.

MANAGING STRESS

The effects of unrelieved stress on the body and mind can range from muscle tension to a pervasive sense of hopelessness about the future, yet life without stress is unrealistic if not impossible. The solution is to find effective ways to manage stress.

Healthy and Unhealthy Ways to Manage Stress

There are many ways to manage stress, but some are ineffective, counterproductive, and unhealthy, such as the following:

■ *Use of tobacco.* The chemicals in tobacco can make a smoker feel both more relaxed and more alert. However, nicotine is highly addictive, and smoking causes a host of health problems. Tobacco use is the leading preventable cause of death in the United States.

■ *Use and abuse of alcohol.* Moderate use of alcohol can lower inhibitions and create a sense of social ease and relaxation, but drinking provides only temporary relief without addressing the sources of stress. Heavy drinking and binge drinking carry risks of their own, including the risk of addiction. All too often, what began as a solution becomes a new problem.

■ *Use and abuse of other drugs.* Like alcohol, illicit drugs alter mood and mind without solving problems, and they often cause additional problems. For example, stimulants like methamphetamine and cocaine increase mental alertness and energy, but they can induce the stress response and disrupt sleep. Opiates like oxycodone (OxyContin) and hydrocodone (Vicodin) can relieve pain and anxiety, but tolerance develops quickly, making dependence likely. Marijuana can cause panic attacks, and even caffeine raises blood pressure and levels of stress hormones.

■ *Use of food to manage feelings.* Many people overeat or eat unhealthy foods when they feel stressed. According to one survey, the top "comfort foods" are candy, ice cream, chips, cookies and cakes, fast food, and pizza, in that order.[31] Other people eat less or skip meals in

response to stress. For most of us, eating is a pleasurable, relaxing experience, but using food to manage feelings and stress can lead to disordered eating patterns as well as overweight and obesity.

Other approaches to stress management that are especially popular with college students are listening to music, socializing with friends, going to movies, and reading. Though not unhealthy, these sedentary activities need to be balanced with more active stress management techniques, such as walking or exercising. Colleges usually offer resources to help students deal with stress, and at some major universities 40 percent of all undergraduates visit the counseling center. However, a sign that not enough students are getting the help they need is the fact that suicide is the second leading cause of death on college campuses. More effort must be made to reach and educate students about stress reduction and stress management techniques, including time management, relaxation techniques, exercise, and good nutrition.

No single stress management technique is helpful or comfortable for everyone. For example, some individuals feel comfortable with meditation, while others who need a more active stress reduction method might choose exercise. Some methods are very simple, like scheduling "worry time,"[76] while others, such as yoga, take a great deal more time and practice. As you review the methods described in the following pages, consider how they might fit with your personality and lifestyle. Experiment with a few methods—and try something new—before you settle on something you think will work for you. Whatever methods you choose, we recommend practicing them on a regular basis. They will become second nature to you and part of your everyday life. They will be available during stressful moments and may even be activated naturally.

Sometimes stressful events and situations are overwhelming, and your resources and coping abilities are insufficient to support you. These times call for professional help. Don't hesitate to visit your college counseling center or avail yourself of other resources if you find that you need more support.

Stress Reduction Strategies

Any activity that decreases the number or lessens the effect of stressors is a stress reduction technique. Although you might not think of avoidance as an effective coping strategy, sometimes protecting yourself from unnecessary stressors makes sense. For example, try not listening to the news for a few days. You'll find that world events continue as always without your participation. If certain people in your life consistently trigger negative feelings in you, try not seeing them for a while. When you do see them, you may have a better perspective on your interpersonal dynamics. If you have too many activities going on in your life, assert your right to say no to the next request for your time. Downscaling and simplifying your life are effective ways of alleviating stress.

Time Management Time management is the topic of seminars and books, and some experts have devoted their entire careers to helping people learn how to manage their time. Here, we focus just on two key points: planning and prioritizing.

To improve planning, ask yourself if you are focusing on the things that are most important to you. You may be focusing on the right tasks if

- You're engaged in activities that advance your overall purpose in life.

- You're doing things you have always wanted to do or that make you feel good about yourself.

- You're working on tasks you don't like, but you're doing them knowing they relate to the bigger picture.[77]

To make sure you focus on the things that matter to you, ask whether each task is worthy of your time. Obviously, you need time for sleeping, working, studying, but remember to allow yourself time for maintaining wellness through such activities as relaxing, playing, and spending time with family and friends. A global picture of your goals and priorities provides a perspective that can give you a sense of control and reduce stress.

To manage your time on the everyday level, keep a daily "to do" list and prioritize the items on it. Write the items down, because it's stressful to just keep them in your head! As you look at the list, assign each task a priority:

- Is it something you must get done today, such as turning in a paper?

- Is it something you would like to get done, such as catching up on the week's reading?

- Is it something that can wait until tomorrow, such as buying a new pair of jeans?

Then organize the items into these three categories. Complete the tasks in the first category first, before moving on to tasks in the other two categories. This approach will help you be more purposeful, organized, and efficient about the use of your time, giving you more of a sense of control in your life.

In the course of evaluating your goals and prioritizing your daily tasks, you may find that you have too many commitments. Trying to do more than you have time for and doing the wrong things in the time you have are stressful. Managing your time well is a key to reducing stress.

Social Support Another key to reducing stress, just as it is a key to mental health and to a meaningful spiritual life, is social support. Numerous studies show that social support decreases the stress response hormones in the body. Dr. Dean Ornish points out that people who have close relationships and a strong sense of connection and community enjoy better health and live longer than do those who live in isolation. People who suffer alone suffer a lot.[78]

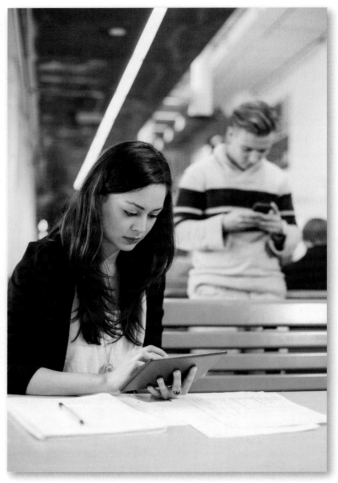

■ Time management skills are effective tools in reducing stress. Keeping a daily planner can help you stay organized and on track throughout your day.

Many people lack the sense of belonging and community that was provided by the extended family and closer-knit society of our grandparents' day. You may have to consciously create a social support system to overcome isolation and loneliness and buffer yourself from stress.[79,80] The benefits make the effort worthwhile. They include a shoulder to lean on and an ear to listen when you need support. Communicating about your feelings reduces stress and helps you to work through problems and feel better about yourself.

The best way to develop a support system is to give support to others, establishing relationships and building trust:

- Cultivate a variety of types of relationships.

- Stay in touch with your friends, especially when you know they're going through a hard time, and keep your family ties strong.

- Find people who share your interests and pursue activities together, whether it's hiking, dancing, or seeing

■ Having a strong social support system is an important ingredient in both the maintenance of psychological health and the reduction of stress.

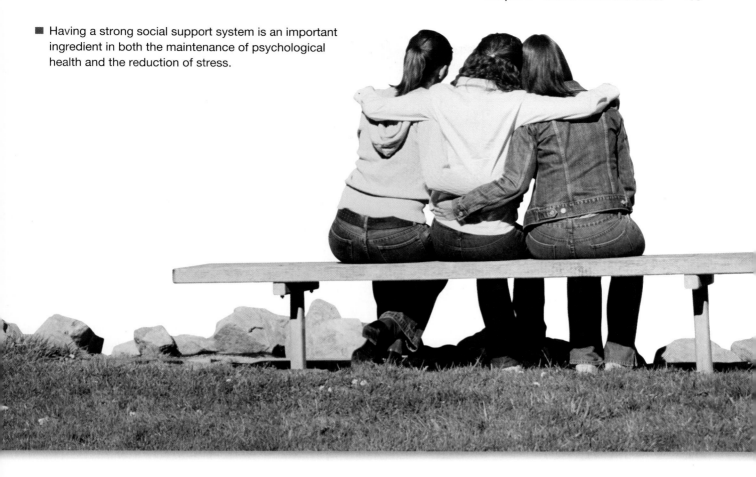

classic movies. You may want to join a group with a goal that interests you, such as a church group, a study group, or a book club.

■ Try to get involved with your community and participate in activities that benefit others.

■ Maintain and improve your communication skills—both listening to other people's feelings and sharing your own.

A Healthy Lifestyle A healthy lifestyle is an essential component of any stress management program. A nutritious diet helps you care for your body and keeps you at your best. Experts recommend emphasizing whole grains, vegetables, and fruits in the diet and avoiding excessive amounts of caffeine (see Chapter 5). Getting enough sleep is also essential for wellness (see Chapter 4), as are opportunities for relaxation and fun.

Exercise is probably the most popular and most effective stress buster available (see Chapter 6). It has a positive effect on both physical and mental functioning and helps people withstand stress. Regular exercisers are also less likely to use smoking, drinking, or overeating as methods for reducing their levels of stress.[81] A growing body of evidence suggests that getting regular exercise is the best thing you can do to protect yourself from the effects of stress. While many people say they "just don't have enough time," all you really need is a jump rope and 15 to 20 minutes each day.

Relaxation Techniques

If you are in a state of chronic stress and the relaxation response does not happen naturally, it is in your best interest to learn how to induce it. Relaxation techniques seem to have an effect on a number of physiological functions, including blood pressure, heart rate, and muscle tension.[82] Here we describe just a few of the many techniques that have been developed.

Deep Breathing One relaxation tool that is simple and always available is breathing. When you feel yourself starting to experience the stress response, you can simply remember to breathe deeply. As you learn to be aware of breathing patterns and practice slowing that process, your mind and body will begin to relax. Breathing exercises have been found to be effective in reducing panic attacks, muscle tension, headaches, and fatigue.

To practice deep breathing, inhale through your nose slowly and deeply through the count of 10. Don't just raise your shoulders and chest; allow your abdomen to expand as well. Exhale very slowly through your nose or through gently pursed lips and concentrate fully on your breath as you let it out. Try to repeat this exercise a number of times during the day even when you're not feeling stressed. Once it becomes routine, use it to help relax before an exam or in any stressful situation.

Progressive Relaxation Progressive muscle relaxation is based on the premise that deliberate muscle relaxation will block the muscle tension that is part of the stress response, thus reducing overall levels of stress. Progressive relaxation has provided relief when used to treat such stress-related symptoms as neck and back pain and high blood pressure.

To practice progressive muscle relaxation, find a quiet place and lie down in a comfortable position without crossing your arms or legs. Maintain a slow breathing pattern while you tense each muscle or muscle group as tightly as possible for 10 seconds before releasing it. Begin by making a fist with one hand, holding it, and then releasing it. Notice the difference between the tensed state and the relaxed state, and allow your muscles to remain relaxed. Continue with your other hand, your arms, shoulders, neck, and so on, moving around your entire body. Don't forget your ears, forehead, mouth, and all the muscles of your face.

If you take the time to relax your body this way, the technique will provide significant relief from stress. You will also find that once your body learns the process, you will be able to relax your muscles quickly on command during moments of stress.

Visualization Also called *guided imagery,* visualization is the mental creation of visual images and scenes. Because our thoughts have such a powerful influence on our reactions, simply imagining a relaxing scene can bring about the relaxation response.[48,50] Visualization can be used alone or in combination with other techniques such as deep breathing and meditation to help reduce stress, tension, and anxiety.

To try visualization, sit or lie in a quiet place. Imagine yourself in a soothing, peaceful scene, one that you find particularly relaxing—a quiet beach, a garden, a spot in the woods. Try to visualize all you would see there as vividly as you can, scanning the scene. Bring in your other senses; what sounds do you hear, what scents do you smell? Is the sun warm, the breeze gentle? If you can imagine the scene fully, your body will respond as if you were really there. Commercial tapes are also available that use guided imagery to promote relaxation, but because imagery is personal and subjective, you may need to be selective in finding a tape that works for you.

Mindfulness-Based Meditation Mindfulness meditation is a form of meditation that involves paying attention to the present moment and letting thoughts and feelings come and go without judging them. Other mindfulness-based practices include yoga and focused breathing. Research on mindfulness meditation indicates that it can lower blood pressure, improve immune system functioning, and alleviate a variety of mental and physical conditions. It may also improve psychological well-being, enhance cognitive functioning, and increase momentary positive emotions.[83–85] The specific components that contribute to positive outcomes include attention regulation, emotional regulation, body awareness, and changes in self-perspective.[85]

Yoga The ancient practice of yoga is rooted in Hindu philosophy, with physical, mental, and spiritual components. It is a consciously performed activity involving posture, breath, and body and mind awareness. In the path and practice of yoga, the aim is to calm the mind, cleanse the body, and raise awareness. The outcomes of this practice include a release of mental and physical tension and the attainment of a relaxed state.

The most widely practiced form of yoga in the Western world is hatha yoga. The practitioner assumes a number of different postures, or poses, holding them while stretching, breathing, and balancing. They are performed slowly and gently, with focused attention. Yoga stretching improves flexibility as well as muscular strength and endurance. For yoga to be effective, the poses have to be performed correctly. If you are interested in trying yoga, we recommend that you begin by taking a class with a certified instructor. There are also commercial videos that can get you started.

T'ai Chi T'ai chi is a form of Chinese martial arts that dates back to the 14th century. Central to this method is the concept of qi, or life energy, and practicing t'ai chi is said to increase and promote the flow of qi throughout the body. T'ai chi combines 13 postures with elements of other stress-relieving techniques, such as exercise, meditation, and deep breathing. Research has shown that t'ai chi is beneficial in combating stress, although exactly how it works is unclear. You can take t'ai chi classes, although these are not as widely available as yoga classes. Using instructional videos to learn t'ai chi is another option.

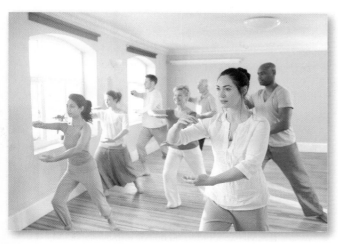

■ T'ai chi is a calming and energizing practice that can be used to elicit relaxation and manage stress.

Biofeedback Biofeedback is a kind of relaxation training that involves the use of special equipment to provide feedback on the body's physiological functions. You receive information about your heart rate, breathing, skin temperature, and other autonomic nervous system activities and thus become more aware of exactly what is happening in your body during both the relaxation response and the stress response. Once you have this heightened awareness, you can use relaxation techniques at the first sign of the stress response in daily life. Biofeedback can be used to reduce tension headaches, chronic muscle pain, hypertension, and anxiety.[86] If you are interested in trying biofeedback, check with your school to see if the special equipment and training are available.

Affirmations Researchers have found that when people have an optimistic attitude and a positive view of themselves, they are less likely to suffer the negative effects of stress. **Affirmations** are positive thoughts that you can write down or say to yourself to balance the negative thoughts you may have internalized over the course of your life. Repeatedly reciting such negative, distorted thoughts can increase stress levels. Although they may seem silly to some people, affirmations can help you shift from a negative view of yourself to a more positive one. The more often you repeat an affirmation, the more likely you are to believe it.

affirmations
Positive thoughts that you can write down or say to yourself to balance negative thoughts.

To create affirmations for yourself, think about areas of your life in which you would like to see improvements, such as health, self-esteem, or happiness, and then imagine what that change would look like. Here are some examples:

■ I make healthy choices for myself.

■ I am the right weight for me.

■ The more grateful I am, the more reasons I find to be grateful.

■ I love and accept myself.

■ I attract only healthy relationships.

■ I have abundant energy, vitality, and well-being.

■ I can open my heart and let wonderful things flow into my life.

We have provided a sampling of stress-reducing techniques; there are many others. Many people choose other relaxation strategies, such as listening to soothing music, going for walks in a beautiful setting, or enjoying the company of a pet. Whatever your preferences, learn to incorporate peaceful moments into your day, every day. You will experience improved quality of life today and a better chance of avoiding stress-related illness in the future.

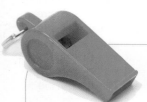

You Make the Call

How "Connected" Should We Be?

Are there times when we would be better off turning off our electronic devices? Can we really multitask and walk and text or sit in a meeting and text, tweet, or e-mail our friends? What do you do when you are socializing with friends and your smartphone tells you that you have a message? Do you answer? Have we forgotten how to have conversations and develop relationships since so much of our lives are handled in 140 characters?

We have created a culture where technology organizes much of what we do and at times can even dominate our lives. But is all this bad? Our level of connectivity allows us to "stay in touch" more easily. We can see pictures of grandchildren instantly and have more face-to-face meetings across states and continents.

Continued. . .

Concluded. . .

However, evidence suggests that when students multitask while doing schoolwork, they are not as focused on the learning activity and they actually learn less. Evidence is also mounting about the dangers of using an electronic device when driving or walking, yet automobiles now come equipped with a GPS, phone system, and other electronic ways to stay connected. In order to have uninterrupted face-to-face time, some people have turned to cell phone stacking. Basically, this means placing all cell phones in the middle of the table, and the first person to check his or her phone is required to buy the next drink or even dinner.

As a culture, we seem to be providing a mixed message. On one hand, we are telling people that technology can distract them and make them less efficient, and on the other we are demanding that people stay connected. Where is the balance? Will we hurt a relationship if we don't stay connected to our friends and lovers? Will our work dominate our lives because we are expected to respond to electronic messages at any time of day or night? Are we less likely to get promoted if we do not respond?

What are the costs and what are the benefits of constant connectivity?

Pros

- Being available by phone allows us to stay more connected to friends and family.
- Geography does not have to be a barrier for either the development or maintenance of social relationships.
- More information is available and easily accessible.

Cons

- We are always expected to be on call and available.
- We are often distracted anticipating the next interruption.
- In-person relationships are having to compete with online friends.

connect ACTIVITY

IN REVIEW

What is mental health?
Mental health is usually conceptualized as the presence of many positive qualities, such as optimism, a sense of self-efficacy, and resilience (the ability to bounce back from adversity). Some specific approaches include positive psychology's focus on "character strengths and virtues," Maslow's self-actualization model, and Goleman's concept of emotional intelligence.

How do we respond to a loss?
Having someone close to you die is part of life, but it is also one of the most difficult life transitions you will face. Grieving is an extremely personal experience, yet it is one that others in your community and culture share. Give yourself the time to recover from the loss of a loved one, and seek out support from friends. If you feel sad or at a loss after many months, consider seeking out professional help.

What is the brain's role in mental health and illness?
Structural changes in the brain until early adulthood affect both learning and behavior. A few mental disorders are caused by some pathology in the brain, but research in recent decades has found that neurotransmitter imbalances lead to a variety of mental disorders, from stress and anxiety to mood disorders and schizophrenia. Typically, mental illness is caused by a complex interaction of biological, genetic, psychological, social, and cultural factors.

What are common mental disorders, and how are they treated?
A mental disorder is a pattern of behavior associated with excessive distress or impaired functioning, and it is not always easy to discern when a common psychological problem becomes a mental disorder. Major categories of mental disorders according to the *Diagnostic and Statistical Manual of Mental Disorders (DSM-5)* include mood disorders, such as depression and bipolar disorder; anxiety disorders, such as panic attacks, phobias, and obsessive-compulsive disorder; addiction; and psychotic disorders, such as schizophrenia. Most people who commit suicide have a mental disorder. The two broad approaches to treatment to mental disorders are medications and psychotherapy. Although some drugs have serious side effects, both treatments can be effective, especially in combination.

What is stress?
Stress is a general state of the body, mind, and emotions when an environmental stressor has triggered the stress response. It is mediated by personal variables that include the person's perceptions and appraisal of the event; stress can be positive (eustress) or negative (distress). The stress response, also known as the fight-or-flight response, is the set of physiological changes that occur in the face of a threat. When the stressful event is over, the body returns to homeostasis in the relaxation response. The human body can handle short-term acute stress, but chronic stress often leads to illness.

How does stress affect health?
Selye's General Adaptation Syndrome (GAS) describes three stages of the physiological response to stress: alarm, resistance, exhaustion. Stress can decrease immune function, increase the heart rate and blood pressure, cause gastrointestinal problems, and contribute to mental disorders, such as post-traumatic stress disorder. Mediators, including personality traits, self-perceptions and expectations, and resilience and hardiness, affect how the body responds to stress.

What are the main sources of stress and the main approaches to managing stress?
Common stressors are life events, both bad and good, daily hassles at school and work, money problems, family and interpersonal problems, time pressures, anger, trauma, and societal pressures.

Healthy alternatives to self-medicating with alcohol, drugs, and tobacco are reducing stress through time management, social support, maintaining a healthy lifestyle, and practicing relaxation techniques, such as deep breathing, progressive relaxation, visualization, mindfulness-based meditation, yoga, t'ai chi, biofeedback, and affirmations.

3 Social Connections

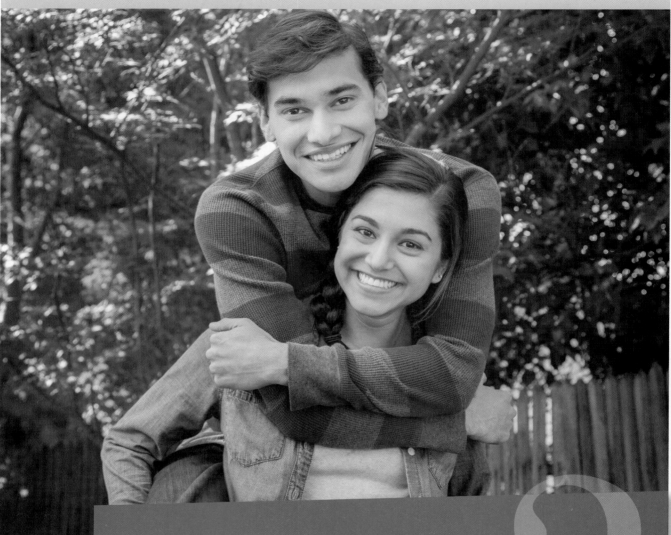

Ever Wonder...

- what you can do to form more satisfying relationships?
- how you can be better at communicating with other people?
- what is important about community?

Relationships are a vital part of wellness. For many of us, close social ties give meaning and significance to our lives. Evidence indicates that an individual's social relationships are important predictors of health and well-being. People with strong social support systems have better mental and physical health, and they are more capable of handling stress and adverse life events. In fact, people with strong social support may even live longer than those without it. Some researchers even believe that some of our personal behaviors, such as food choice and life satisfaction, can spread throughout social networks and greatly influence the behaviors of larger groups of people.[1] Other researchers have found that "extreme giving" is very much related to having a satisfying and successful life.[2] Extreme givers according to Grant are those individuals who say yes to others without an expectation of immediate gain, share credit easily, are willing to mentor others, and are genuinely concerned about others.[2] This chapter addresses the social aspects of health, particularly pertaining to interpersonal relationships and community involvement.

HEALTHY PERSONAL RELATIONSHIPS

Relationships are at the heart of human experience. We are born into a family; grow up in a community; have classmates, teammates, and colleagues; find a partner from among our acquaintances and friends; and establish our own family. Yet for all their importance in our lives, relationships are fraught with difficulties and challenges. About half of all marriages in the United States end in divorce, and many children grow up in a single-parent or blended family of one kind or another. Many people also live alone in the United States, either by choice or by chance. In today's electronically connected world, college students seem to have less of an opportunity to experience real relationships on campuses, where electronic meetings and dating have often become the norm.

Three kinds of important relationships are the one you have with yourself, the ones you have with friends, and the ones you have with intimate partners. In each, certain qualities serve to enhance the relationship's positive effects.

A Healthy Sense of Self

All your relationships begin with who you are as an individual. A healthy sense of self, reasonably high self-esteem, a capacity for empathy, and the ability both to be alone and to be with others are attributes that make successful relationships possible. Many people develop these assets growing up in their families, but people who experience deficits in childhood can still make up for them later in life.

Friendships and Other Kinds of Relationships

Friendship is a reciprocal relationship based on mutual liking and caring, respect and trust, interest and companionship. We often share a big part of our personal history with our friends. Compared with romantic partnerships, friendships are usually more stable and longer lasting. In fact, the bonds created among friends can be so powerful that the mood of one person spreads to the other people in a friendship network. That is, if you are happy and healthy, it is possible that the factors in your happiness might be determined by a friend of a friend of a friend.[3]

A recent survey found that 97 percent of Americans report having people in their lives whom they trust and can turn to when they need support.[4] The average American has four close social contacts, with most having between one and six.[5] Generally, we find and keep friends who are geographically close to us,[6] and we are much more likely to be happy if we have a close friend who lives within a mile.[3] However, social media forums like Facebook and Twitter and communication devices like smartphones may change that.

Like family ties and involvement in social activities, friendships offer a psychological and emotional buffer against stress, anxiety, and depression. People who are surrounded by happy people and those who have high status in any network are most likely to be happy. Overall, friendships and networks can help protect you against illness and help you cope with problems if you do become ill. Friendships and other kinds of social support may also increase your sense of belonging, purpose, and self-worth.[7]

Strengths of Successful Partnerships

An intimate relationship with a partner has many similarities with friendships, but it has other qualities as well. Compared with friendships, partnerships are more exclusive, involve deeper levels of connection and caring, and have a sexual component. The following are some characteristics of successful partnerships:

- The more mature and independent individuals are, the more likely they are to establish intimacy in the relationship. Independence and maturity often increase with age; in fact, the best predictor of a successful marriage is the age of the partners.

- The partners have both self-esteem and mutual respect.

- The partners understand the importance of good communication and are willing to work at their communication skills. They know that listening to the other's feelings and trying to see things from the other's perspective are key in communication, even if they do not ultimately agree.

- The partners have a good sexual relationship, one that includes the open expression of affection and respect for the other's needs and boundaries.

- The partners enjoy spending time together in leisure activities, but they also value the time they spend alone pursuing their own interests.

- The partners are able to acknowledge their strengths and failings and take responsibility for both.

- The partners are assertive about what they want and need in the relationship and flexible about accommodating the other's wants and needs. They can maintain a sense of self in the face of pressure to agree or conform.

- The partners know that disagreement is normal in relationships and that when conflict is handled constructively, it can strengthen the relationship.[8]

- The partners are friends as well as lovers, able to focus unselfish caring on each other.

- The couple has good relationships with family and friends, including in-laws, members of their extended family, and other couples.

- The partners have shared spiritual values.

Developing and maintaining a successful intimate relationship takes time and effort, but it is a challenge worth pursuing (see Table 3.1).

LOOKING FOR A PARTNER

How do we go about finding the right person for a successful intimate partnership, and how do we know when we find him or her? Is it all about magic and chemistry, or is there something more deliberate and purposeful about it?

Attraction

People appear to use a systematic screening process when deciding whether someone could be a potential partner. According to one scholar, love is not blind, and we do not fall in love accidentally.[9] Some of the conscious and unconscious factors that affect this process include proximity, physical attractiveness, and similarity.

Proximity is an often overlooked but significant factor in how we find our romantic partners.[10] Simply being physically close to people makes it more likely that we will establish a relationship with them. Sometimes attraction is a function of familiarity, and proximity determines how often two people are exposed to one another.

Of the people in proximity to us, we are most interested in those we find physically attractive. Only if we find a person attractive are we willing to consider his or her other traits, although "signaling" devices like coy looks and other flirtatious moves are also effective at garnering attention.[11] In general, people who are perceived as attractive in our society have an advantage. They are evaluated more positively by parents, teachers, and potential employers; make more money; and report having better sex with more attractive partners.

We are also drawn to people who are similar to ourselves, usually in characteristics such as age; physical traits such as height, weight, and attractiveness; educational attainment; family, ethnic, and cultural background; religion; political views; and values, beliefs, and interests. We are attracted to people who agree with us, validate our opinions, and share our attitudes. Even though opposites may initially attract, partners who are like each other tend to have more successful relationships. The more differences partners have, the more important communication skills become.

The Process of Finding a Partner: Dating and More

Both in and out of college, many people prefer a flexible approach to finding a life partner rather than traditional dating. For example, some women take the lead in asking men out and play a more assertive role in

Table 3.1 Healthy Versus Unhealthy Relationships

Being in a HEALTHY RELATIONSHIP means . . .	If you are in an UNHEALTHY RELATIONSHIP . . .
Loving and taking care of yourself as well as the other person.	You care for and focus on the other person only and neglect yourself, or you focus only on yourself and neglect the other person.
Respecting individuality, embracing differences, and allowing each person to be themselves.	You feel pressure to change to meet the other person's standards, you are afraid to disagree, and your ideas are criticized. Or you pressure the other person to meet your standards and criticize his or her ideas.
Doing things with friends and family and having activities independent of each other.	One of you has to justify what you do, where you go, and who you see.
Discussing things, allowing for differences of opinion, and compromising equally.	One of you makes all the decisions and controls everything without listening to the other's input.
Expressing and listening to each other's feelings, needs, and desires.	One of you feels unheard and is unable to communicate what you want.
Trusting and being honest with yourself and each other.	You lie to each other and find yourself making excuses for the other person.
Respecting each other's need for privacy.	You don't have any personal space and have to share everything with the other person.
Sharing sexual histories and sexual health status with a partner.	Your partner keeps his or her sexual history a secret or hides a sexually transmitted infection from you, or you do not disclose your history to your partner.
Practicing safer sex methods.	You feel scared about asking your partner to use protection, or he or she has refused your requests for safer sex. Or you refuse to use safer sex methods after your partner has requested, or you make your partner feel scared.
Respecting sexual boundaries and being able to say no to sex.	Your partner has forced you to have sex, or you have had sex when you don't really want to. Or you have forced or coerced your partner to have sex.
Resolving conflicts in a rational, peaceful, and mutually agreed-upon way.	One or both of you yells and hits, shoves, or throws things at the other in an argument.
Having room for positive growth and learning more about each other as you develop and mature.	You feel stifled, trapped, and stagnant. You are unable to escape the pressures of the relationship.

Source: Adapted from "Healthy Vs. Unhealthy Relationships," Copyright © Advocates for Youth. Reprinted with permission.

the development of the relationship. Other people take an indirect approach—they play hard to get or convey interest with a flippant pickup line. However, research generally suggests that indirectness is not an effective strategy and that people who are straightforward and respectful are more likely to get a positive response.[11]

One of the longest-standing ways that people have found potential partners is through their social connections. For example, you may be introduced to someone by your family members, or a friend whom you know from the community center might invite you out for a double-date. However, the Internet is constantly expanding these networks, and therefore, physical proximity may soon be a less significant factor than it has been in the past.[12] Currently, more than one-third of American marriages get their start online, and at least one study has described them as being more satisfying and less likely to end in divorce.[13] It makes sense to cast a wide net in the search for a partner. Even participation in social groups, volunteering, sports, and church may not bring you in contact with a broad range of people. Furthermore, most people

Consumer Clipboard

Know Your Online Dating Site

Since the original online dating site, Match.com, went live in 1995, the number and variety of sites have expanded exponentially, as have the types of technology employed. You can browse photos and profiles, be matched through a personality quiz or a DNA analysis, interact by webcam, or go on virtual dates in online environments. At many sites, you can narrow your search by age, religion, ethnicity and race, sexual orientation, parental status, type of encounter you're seeking, and more. Some controversial dating sites, such as carrotdating.com and WhatsYourPrice.com, involve paying for a date. Most websites charge subscription fees, but some are free. Social networking sites like Facebook and Twitter also account for a large proportion of the time people spend connecting with others.

Regardless of the type of site you use, follow these basic guidelines to stay safe:

- Online dating sites provide access to a much larger pool of potential partners than most people would otherwise encounter. Be prepared to meet a lot of people, and don't take it personally if the chemistry isn't there with most of them.

- Never share personal or financial information online.

- Guard your identity. Remain anonymous until you feel safe enough to share it.

- Protect your online access information if you share a computer.

- Remember that people may lie about themselves and alter their photos.

- When meeting offline, meet in public, tell a friend where you'll be, stay sober, don't leave personal items unattended, and use your own transportation.

- It is wise to transition to face-to-face interactions quickly because that's where two people can get a real sense of their romantic potential.

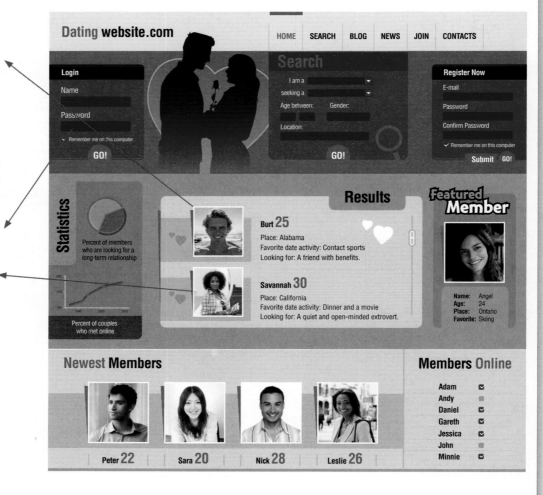

Continued...

lead busy lives, and online approaches to dating enlarge the pool of potential partners.

Still, if you decide to pursue a relationship with someone you meet over the Internet, be cautious (see the box, "Know Your Online Dating Site") because there can be much you do not know about the person. Incidents of "catfishing," where people pretend to be someone else and "hook" a person into an online relationship with exploitive intentions, are all too common.

WHAT IS LOVE?

Passionate love has been defined as "a state of intense longing for union with another."[14] A more biological view of

Know Your Online Dating Site

The following are some of the types of online dating sites available:

- **General:** User browses profiles of a wide range of potential partners. *Examples:* Match.com, PlentyofFish (POF.com)

- **Niche:** User browses profiles of potential partners from specific populations. *Examples:* JDate.com, ChristianMingle.com

- **Self-report algorithm:** User reports data about self, and site uses algorithms to create matches. *Examples:* eHarmony.com, OKCupid.com

- **Non-self-report algorithm:** Site uses non-self-reported data and algorithm to create matches. *Example:* GenePartner.com

- **Video dating sites:** User interacts with potential partners via webcam. *Example:* SpeedDate.com

- **Virtual dating sites:** User creates avatar and goes on virtual date in online setting. *Example:* Weopia.com

- **Smartphone and Facebook apps:** User connects with people via social networks. *Example:* Zoosk.com

In addition to websites, a number of apps create opportunities for people to meet. Lulu is a female-only app with more than 1 million registered users where women share opinions and create reviews of men. Tinder is an app for both men and women that facilitates conversations between people who have an online attraction. It is one of the fastest-growing free dating apps and had more than 13 billion swipe rates one year after it was launched. After signing up and providing information about gender, location, and sexual orientation, users simply swipe through profile pictures based on attraction. Once there is a mutual attraction, a private chat box appears so interested people can get together only minutes after a match. The average Tinder user checks the site 11 times each day, 7 minutes per visit. Grindr is an app for gay, bisexual, and bi-curious men who want to meet potential partners.

Sources: "Online Dating: Critical Analysis from the Perspective of Psychological Science," by E. L. Finkel et al., 2012, *Psychological Science in the Public Interest, 20* (10), pp. 1–64; Top Online Dating Sites of 2012, www.onlinedatingsites.net; Nick Summers, Dating App Tinder Catches Fire, September 5, 2013, *Bloomberg Business Technology*, www.businessweek.com/articles/2013-09-05/dating-app-tinder-catches-fire.

romantic love is that it evolved for the purposes of mating and reproduction.[15] Of all the people we are attracted to and all the potential mates we screen, what makes us fall in love with one or a few in a lifetime?

Some theorists propose that we fall in love with people who are similar to us in important ways *(similarity theory)*. Couples with more similarities seem to have not only greater marital harmony but also higher fertility rates. Other theorists suggest that falling in love and choosing a partner are based on the exchange of "commodities" like love, status, property, and services *(social exchange theory)*. According to this view, we are looking for someone who fills not just our emotional needs but also our needs for security, money, goods, and more.

The Course of Love

The beginning stages of falling in love can feel like a roller-coaster ride, taking the lovers from the heights of euphoria to the depths of despair. They may actually become "lovesick" and find themselves unable to eat, sleep, or think of anything but the object of their desire. These early stages of a love relationship are typically romantic, idealistic, and passionate. The lovers are absorbed in each other and want to spend all their time together, sometimes to the exclusion of other people and everyday responsibilities.

Researchers think this experience of love involves increased levels of the neurotransmitter dopamine in the brain.[10] Dopamine is associated with the experience of pleasure. On the physiological level, this kind of love also causes arousal of the sympathetic nervous system, as evidenced by such physiological signs as increased heart rate, respiration, and perspiration. These responses gradually decrease

as the relationship develops and progresses. Intense passion may subside as lovers become habituated to each other. In some cases, passion continues at a more bearable level and intimacy deepens; the relationship becomes more fulfilling and comes to include affection, empathy, tolerance, caring, and attachment. The partners are able to become involved in the world again, while maintaining their connection with each other. In other cases, the lessening of passion signals the ending of the relationship; the lovers drift apart, seeking newer, more satisfying partnerships.

intimacy
Emotional component of love, including feelings of closeness, warmth, openness, and affection.

passion
Sexual component of love, including attraction, romance, excitement, and physical intensity.

commitment
The decision aspect of a relationship, the pledge to stay with a partner through good times and bad.

Sternberg's Love Triangle

Psychologist Robert Sternberg has proposed a view of love that can give us insight into its various aspects. In this view, love has three dimensions: intimacy, passion, and commitment. **Intimacy** is the emotional component of love and includes feelings of closeness, warmth, openness, and affection. **Passion** is the sexual component of love; it includes attraction, romance, excitement, and physical intensity. **Commitment** is the decision aspect of a relationship, the pledge that you will stay with your partner through good times and bad, despite the possibility of disappointment and disillusionment.[16]

Different combinations of these three components, represented metaphorically as a triangle, produce different kinds of love (Figure 3.1). When there is only intimacy, the

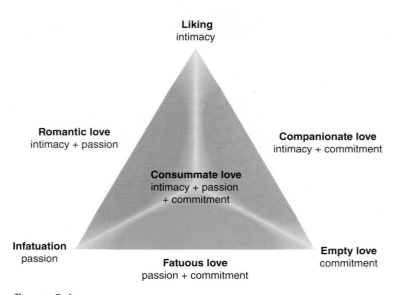

figure 3.1   **Sternberg's triangular theory of love.**
Source: "A Triangular Theory of Love," by Robert J. Sternberg, in *Psychological Review,* 93, pp. 119–135. Copyright © 1986. Reprinted by permission of Robert J. Sternberg.

Nonverbal Behavior and Metamessages

A good deal of communication takes place as **nonverbal communication** through facial expressions, eye contact, gestures, body position and movement, and spatial behavior (how far apart people sit or stand). People tend to monitor their verbal behavior—what they say—much more carefully than their nonverbal behavior, yet nonverbal communication may convey their real message.

Nonverbal behavior is part of the **metamessage**—the unspoken message you send or get when you are communicating. The metamessage encompasses all the conscious and unconscious aspects of a message, including the way something is said, who says it, when and where it is said, or even that it is said at all. It includes the meaning and intent behind a message, rather than just the words someone says. Often, the metamessage is what triggers an emotional response.

relationship is likely to be a friendship. Passion alone is infatuation, the high-intensity early stage of a love relationship. Commitment alone is characteristic of a dutiful, obligatory relationship, one that many people would consider empty. When there is both intimacy and passion, the relationship is a romantic one; commitment may develop in time. When there is passion and commitment, the relationship has probably developed rapidly, without the partners getting to know each other very well; when passion fades, there may not be much substance to this type of relationship. When there is intimacy and commitment but no passion, the relationship may have evolved into more of a long-term friendship; Sternberg calls this relationship *companionate love.* Finally, when all three components are present, the couple has *consummate love.*[16] This type of relationship is what many dream of, but it's difficult to find and even harder to sustain. However love is conceptualized, it is something that enhances happiness and satisfaction in life.

nonverbal communication
Communication that takes place without words, mainly through body language.

metamessage
The unspoken message in a communication; the meaning behind the message, conveyed by nonverbal behavior and by situational factors such as how, when, and where the message is delivered.

COMMUNICATION SKILLS AND STYLES

We establish, maintain, and nourish our relationships—or, alternatively, damage and destroy them—through communication. Clear, positive communication is a key to successful intimate relationships. Complete the activity in this chapter's Personal Health Portfolio to assess how well you communicate to people close to you.

Building Communication Skills

To be an effective communicator when you speak, know what you want to say. Examine your feelings, motives, and intentions before you speak. When you do speak, use "I" statements to state what you feel or want in a clear, direct

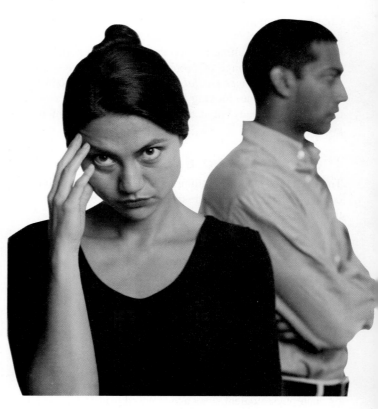

■ When words fail, body language speaks volumes.

way without blaming or accusing the other person. Using "I" statements helps you take responsibility for your own emotions and reactions rather than trying to place responsibility on someone else. For example, it is more productive to say, "I feel . . . when you . . ." than to say, "You make me feel . . ." Saying what you would like to have happen is also more productive than complaining about what isn't happening. Other keys to positive, effective communication are avoiding generalizations, making specific requests, and remaining calm. If you feel yourself starting to get angry, take a time-out and come back to the conversation after you cool off.

When you are the listener, do just that—listen. Don't interrupt, give advice, explain, judge, analyze, defend yourself, or offer solutions. Give the other person the time and space to say fully what is on his or her mind, just as you would like when you are speaking. Attentive listening shows that you respect the other person and care about him or her. It is the cornerstone of good communication.

If you and your partner are experiencing conflict, good communication skills can help you resolve it constructively. Conflict is a normal part of healthy relationships. Often, it is a sign that partners are maintaining their right to be different people and to have different points of view; it can also indicate that the relationship is changing or growing.

When you are trying to resolve a conflict with your partner, keep the topic narrow. Try not to generalize to other topics, incidents, or issues. Avoid being either passive or aggressive; **assertiveness** means speaking up for yourself without violating someone else's rights. Be prepared to negotiate and compromise, but don't give up something that is really important to you (e.g., time to keep up your other friendships). If you feel that demands are being made on you that you cannot or do not want to meet, this may not be the right relationship for you. Communicating clearly about that is important, too.

Gender Differences in Communication Styles

According to linguistics scholar Deborah Tannen, gender differences in communication patterns have a significant impact on relationships (see Table 3.2). Tannen suggests that men are more likely to use communication to compete and women are more likely to use communication to connect.[17]

Although these patterns are broad and general, they are sometimes at the root of misunderstandings between men and women. If you find yourself experiencing confusion or conflict in your communications with the other sex, consider whether gender differences may be involved. Neither style is right or wrong, better or worse—they are just different.

SEX AND GENDER

Most adult partnerships and intimate relationships include not just sexual behavior but also biological, psychological, sociological, and cultural aspects of sexual identity.

Table 3.2 Gender Differences in Communication

Men	Women
Feel oppressed by lengthy discussions	Expect a decision to be discussed first and made by consensus
Do not want to have long discussions, particularly about what they consider to be minor decisions	Appreciate the discussion itself as evidence of involvement
Are inclined to resist what they perceive as someone telling them what to do; do not want to take orders	Are inclined to do what is asked of them
Think every question needs to be answered	Believe a question is not simply a question but the opening for a negotiation
Believe they are showing independence by not asking probing questions	Believe that when men change the subject they are showing a lack of interest and sympathy
Goal is to "fix" the problem	Goal is to share, develop relationships, and listen

Source: Adapted from *You Just Don't Understand: Women and Men in Conversation,* by D. Tannen, 1990, New York: William Morrow.

In this section, we consider two such dimensions—gender roles and sexual orientation.

Although they are often used interchangeably, the terms *sex* and *gender* have different meanings. **Sex** refers to a person's biological status as male or female; it is usually established at birth by the appearance of the external genitals. A person with female genitals usually has XX chromosomes, and a person with male genitals usually has XY chromosomes.

Sex is not always clear-cut, however. For example, chromosomes are sometimes added, lost, or rearranged during the production of sperm and ova, causing such conditions as Klinefelter syndrome (XXY) and Turner syndrome (XO). Sometimes, as a result of genetic factors or prenatal hormonal influences, a baby is born with ambiguous genitals—a condition referred to as **intersex**. Other times, a person experiences a sense of inappropriateness about his or her sex and identifies psychologically or emotionally with the other sex.

assertiveness
The ability to stand up for oneself without violating other people's rights.

sex
A person's biological status as a male or a female, usually established at birth by the appearance of the external genitals.

intersex
Having ambiguous reproductive or sexual anatomy.

Gender refers to the behaviors and characteristics considered appropriate for a male or a female in a particular culture. "Masculine" and "feminine" traits are learned largely via the process of socialization during childhood.

Gender Roles and Gender Identities

A **gender role** is the set of behaviors and activities a person engages in to conform to society's expectations. Gender role stereotypes suggest that a masculine man is competitive, aggressive, ambitious, power-oriented, and logical and that a feminine woman is cooperative, passive, nurturing, supportive, and emotional.

gender
Masculine or feminine behaviors and characteristics considered appropriate for a male or a female in a particular culture.

gender role
Set of behaviors and activities a person engages in to conform to society's expectations of his or her sex.

transgender
Having a sense of identity as a male or female that conflicts with one's biological sex.

gender identity
Internal sense of being male or female.

sexual orientation
A person's emotional, romantic, and sexual attraction to a member of the same sex, the other sex, or both.

Today, we commonly assume that both genders are capable and can be successful in a variety of roles at home and at work. However, gender roles and gender stereotypes are learned in childhood and are hard to change, even when we are aware of them. For example, both men and women have been shown to play the stereotyped role assigned to their gender in order to appear romantically attractive to the other sex, and both men and women may be initially attracted to romantic partners because they fit the gender role stereotype.[18]

In long-term relationships, both sexes tend to prefer a partner who integrates so-called masculine and feminine traits. The term *androgynous* is applied to a person who displays characteristics or performs tasks traditionally associated with both sexes; sometimes it is also applied to a person who does not display overt characteristics associated with either sex.

Individuals who experience discomfort or a sense of inappropriateness about their sex (called *gender dysphoria*) and who identify strongly with the other sex are referred to as cross-gender identified, transsexual, or **transgender**. The term *transgender* can describe anyone whose **gender identity** differs from the sex of his or her birth. Many transgender individuals dress in the clothes of the other gender *(cross-dressing)* and live in society as the other gender. Some undergo surgery and hormone treatments to experience a more complete transformation into the other sex, and others do not. Transgender individuals have typically experienced gender dysphoria since earliest childhood, but there is controversy about using the gender identity disorder diagnosis with children.[19] Most children who do not fit the cultural stereotype of masculinity or femininity do not

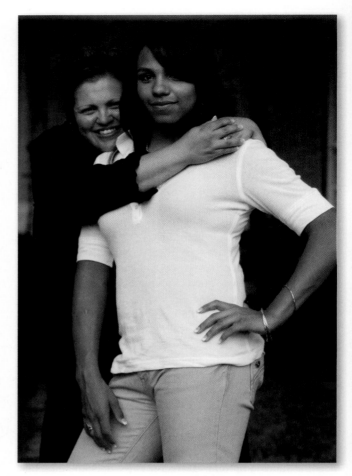

■ Rochelle Evans, shown here with her mom, is a transgender teen living in Texas. She started high school as Rodney Evans and fought a public battle to be allowed to wear women's clothes to school.

grow up to be transgender. According to the National Center for Transgender Equality, fewer than 1 percent of the population in the United States (between 750,000 and 3,000,000 people) is transgender (http://transequality.org/).

Sexual Orientation

Sexual orientation refers to a person's emotional, romantic, and sexual attraction to a member of the same sex, the other sex, or both. It exists along a continuum that ranges from exclusive heterosexuality through bisexuality to exclusive homosexuality. Although the role of genes in sexual orientation is not clearly understood, sexual orientation is known to be influenced by a complex interaction of biological, psychological, and societal factors, and these factors may be different for different people.

Sexual orientation involves a person's sense of identity. Most experts believe that it is not a choice and does not change (perhaps more so for men than for women). A person's sexual orientation may or may not be evidenced in his or her appearance or behavior, and the person may choose not to act on his or her sexual orientation.

Heterosexuality is emotional and sexual attraction to members of the other sex. Heterosexuals are often referred to as *straight.* Throughout the world, laws related to marriage, child rearing, health benefits, financial matters, sexual behavior, and inheritance generally support heterosexual relationships. **Homosexuality** is emotional and sexual attraction to members of one's own sex. In today's usage, homosexual men are typically referred to as *gay,* and homosexual women are referred to either as gay or as *lesbian.*

Homosexuality occurs in all cultures, but researchers have generally had difficulty determining exactly what proportions of the population are straight and gay. Sex researcher Alfred Kinsey estimated that about 4 percent of American males and 2 percent of American females were exclusively homosexual.[20,21] The popular media tend to place the combined figure for gays and lesbians at about 10 percent of the population.

Emotional and sexual attraction to both sexes is referred to as **bisexuality**. Bisexuals may date members of both sexes, or they may have a relationship with a member of one sex for a period of time and then a relationship with a member of the other sex for a period of time. After having relationships with members of both sexes, a bisexual may move toward a more exclusive orientation, either heterosexual or homosexual.

COMMITTED RELATIONSHIPS AND LIFESTYLE CHOICES

In this section, we consider marriage—one of the most important social and legal institutions in societies throughout the world—along with other relationship and lifestyle choices that many people make today.

Marriage

Marriage is not only the legal union of two people but also a contract between the couple and the state. In the United States, each state specifies the rights and responsibilities of the partners in a marriage. Although marriage has traditionally meant the union of a man and a woman, many same-sex couples are interested in marriage, and some states now issue marriage licenses to same-sex couples.

One of the most noticeable changes in marital patterns since the mid-1980s has been the increase in the age at first marriage. Since the 1950s, the median age of first marriage has risen from 23 for men and 20 for women to 28 for men and 26 for women.[22] The delay in getting married along with the increase in cohabiting couples and the decrease in the number of people getting married for a second time contribute to a decline in the number of people

who are married. The percentage of women cohabiting went from 3 percent in 1982 to 11 percent in the period 2006–2010.[22] Overall 48 percent of women cohabited with a partner as a first union. One-third of these relationships resulted in marriage, and one-third dissolved within five years.[22]

Marriage confers benefits in many domains. Partnerships and family relationships provide emotional connection for individuals and stability for society. Married people live longer than single or divorced people, partly because they lead a healthier lifestyle. Marriage may also be a protective factor for patients with cancer; married individuals are 12 to 33 percent more likely to survive than those who are not married.[23] Married people report greater happiness than do single, widowed, or cohabiting people. Married couples have sex more frequently and consider their sexual relationship more satisfying emotionally and physically than do single people. Married people are more successful in their careers, earn more, and have more wealth. Children brought up by married couples tend to be more academically successful and emotionally stable.

What makes a marriage successful? One predictor of a successful marriage is positive reasons for getting married. Positive motivations include companionship, love and intimacy, supportive partnership, sexual compatibility, and interest in sharing parenthood. Poorer reasons for getting married, those associated with less chance of having a successful marriage, include premarital pregnancy, rebellion against parents, quest for independence, desire for economic security, family or social pressure, and rebounding from another relationship.

Love alone is not enough to make a marriage successful. Research has found that the best predictors of a happy marriage are realistic attitudes about the relationship and the challenges of marriage, satisfaction with the personality of the partner, enjoyment of communicating with the partner, ability to resolve conflicts together, agreement on religious and ethical values, egalitarian roles, and a balance of individual and joint leisure activities. The characteristics associated with successful and unsuccessful marriages are typically present in a couple's relationship before they are married.[24]

Infidelity mars some marriages, though it does not necessarily end them. It is the reason most reported for divorce. Men are twice as likely as women to have a sexual affair during marriage, but women are more likely to have an affair to end a bad marriage.[25] Men are more threatened if their partner has a sexual affair than if she falls in love with someone else, whereas women are more distressed if their partner falls in love with someone else.

heterosexuality
Emotional and sexual attraction to members of the other sex.

homosexuality
Emotional and sexual attraction to members of the same sex.

bisexuality
Emotional and sexual attraction to members of both sexes.

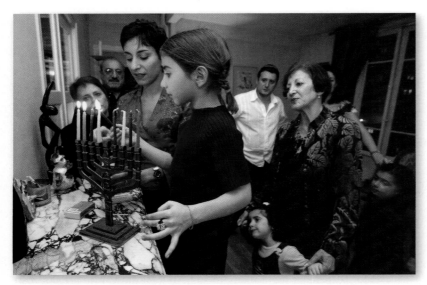

■ Relationships are more likely to be strong and lasting when partners share important values, including spiritual values.

Gay and Lesbian Partnerships

Like heterosexual couples, same-sex couples desire intimacy, companionship, passion, and commitment in their relationships. Because they often have to struggle with "coming out" and disapproval from their families, many gays and lesbians have communication skills and strengths that are valuable in relationships. These qualities include flexible role relationships, the ability to adapt to a partner, the ability to negotiate and share decision-making power, and effective parenting skills among those who choose to become parents.[26,27]

Unfortunately, gays and lesbians often have to deal with discrimination and **homophobia** (irrational fear of homosexuality and homosexuals). Same-sex relationships do not receive the same level of societal support and acceptance as heterosexual relationships. The options of domestic partnership, civil union, and marriage have become available for same-sex partners in some states. The issue of gay marriage has become a hot political topic in the United States in recent years, with one side asserting that marriage must be defined as a union between a man and a woman and the other side arguing that denying marriage to gays and lesbians is a violation of their civil rights.[28]

Recent decisions by the Supreme Court of the United States found that married same-sex couples were entitled to federal benefits and allowed same-sex marriage in California. As of November 2013, 14 states allowed same-sex marriage, and that number is likely to increase. The debate over same-sex marriage will continue on a state-by-state basis. Polling information seems to suggest

homophobia
Irrational fear of homosexuality and homosexuals.

cohabitation
Living arrangement in which two people of the opposite sex live together as unmarried partners.

that younger individuals are more comfortable with same-sex marriage and that, overall, around 50 percent of adults in the United States believe it should be available.

Cohabitation

The U.S. government defines **cohabitation** as two people of the opposite sex living together as unmarried partners. Since the 1960s, cohabitation has become one of the most rapidly growing social phenomena in the history of our society. The rate of cohabitation has increased more than tenfold since the 1960s, with almost 50 percent of women entering a cohabiting relationship in their lifetime and more than 60 percent of marriages being preceded by a cohabiting relationship. Many of these cohabiting relationships resulted in marriage, yet almost one-third dissolved within five years.[22]

For many couples, cohabitation is an accepted part of the process of finding a mate (see the box, "Isabel and Paul: Living Together . . . Happily Ever After?"). Most couples today believe it is a good idea to live together in order to decide if they should get married, though cohabiting couples report higher levels of conflict and less commitment than couples who do not live together. While some studies have shown that cohabitation decreases the likelihood of success in marriage, recent studies suggest that cohabiting couples in engaged, fast-moving relationships are more successful than other types of couples.[29] Some might suggest that the differences in divorce rate between those who cohabit and those who do not might be attributable to the age at which they choose to cohabit. Those who cohabit in their late 20s were less likely to get divorced than those who cohabited in their late teens

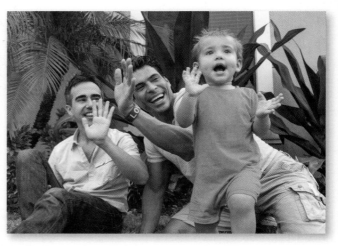

■ Gay and lesbian partnerships are very similar to heterosexual partnerships, but same-sex couples often have to deal with bias and discrimination.

Life Stories

Isabel and Paul: Living Together . . . Happily Ever After?

Isabel and Paul were both 24 years old and had just graduated from a university in the Northeast. They had been in an exclusive relationship with each other for the past two years. They felt committed to each other but hadn't talked about their long-term plans or the future of their relationship. Neither of them had really thought about marriage. Paul was interviewing for jobs in New York City and hoping to move there. He asked Isabel to come live with him—she hadn't found a job yet, and it would be easier to find one in a big city rather than in the mid-sized city where their university was. They could save money by living together, he said, and besides, they cared about each other.

Isabel wasn't so sure. She hadn't planned to move to New York, but she didn't have any definite direction in her life yet. Paul was right that it would be easier to find a job there, and she wasn't sure what would happen to their relationship if she didn't move with him. She did love him, and the prospect of living in New York was exciting, so she said yes. They agreed to split rent and utilities in proportion to their earnings once they both found jobs.

Isabel turned out to really enjoy living in New York—and living with Paul. They bought furniture together and developed a social circle with old friends from school and new friends from work. A year passed quickly and Isabel found herself thinking about their future together. More and more of their friends were getting engaged. Isabel was ready to make a commitment to Paul. But when she brought up the subject of marriage or the future, Paul always seemed to deflect the conversation. He said he didn't know what the rush was and didn't know why they needed to get married. They were still young and enjoying their life together—why change a good thing? He was happy just living with her.

Isabel felt hurt by his responses and began to wonder if he really wanted to spend his life with her. She knew that she wanted to be married—but did he? She wondered if he found living together convenient until something better came along. She thought about it more and more but felt reluctant to initiate further conversations about it for fear she would push him away. Because she didn't bring it up again, Paul thought that everything was fine between them.

Finally, Isabel felt she had to talk to someone about the growing distance she was experiencing in the relationship and decided to make an appointment with a therapist. When she told Paul she was going to see someone about "some issues," he was surprised and concerned and asked why she was going. She hesitantly told him. Paul had had no idea that she had so many doubts about their relationship and their future. He apologized for giving the appearance that he didn't want to talk about their future plans—he could now see that it was an important issue to her. He told her he knew he had some fears about marriage based on his parents' relationship and that he wasn't sure he felt ready to get married yet. Still, he said, he would be happy to go to counseling with her so that they could talk more about the issue in a healthy way.

- Do you think Paul and Isabel made the right decision when they decided to live together? Why or why not?

- What happened in their communication with each other? How could they have prevented this from happening?

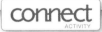

---

or early 20s.[30] Others have found that cohabitation improves psychological well-being and, on a range of outcomes, might be very similar to marriage.[31] Overall, it seems that cohabitation is a form of social attachment that many individuals are now choosing as either a path to marriage or an end in itself.

Divorce

For a large percentage of couples, the demands of marriage prove too difficult, and the couple choose to divorce. The current divorce rate is nearly twice what it was in 1960, although it has declined since reaching its highest point in the 1980s. The lifetime probability that a couple in their first marriage will divorce is between 40 and 50 percent.[32] For a closer look at divorce rates during the first 20 years of marriage, see the box, "Divorce Rates by Ethnic Group."

Why do so many couples divorce in our society? Many couples simply cannot handle the challenges of married life.

They may not have the problem-solving skills, or they may not be sufficiently committed to the relationship. Many people enter marriage with unrealistic expectations, and some people choose an unsuitable mate.

Although divorce may seem to be a single event in a person's life, the termination of a marriage is almost always a traumatic process lasting months or years. Divorce is a leading cause of poverty, leaving many children in impoverished homes headed by a single parent, often the parent with the lower income. Most single-parent families cannot maintain the same lifestyle that they had before the divorce.

Divorce is one of the most stressful life events a person can experience. It is especially hard on children, leading to different kinds of problems for children of different ages. Counseling can help both children and adults deal with the stress of divorce and adjust to a new life. Children are best served by continuing to have contact with both parents as long as the adults can get along.

Who's at Risk?

Divorce Rates by Ethnic Group

What is the likelihood that a marriage in the United States will last? There will always be individual circumstances and exceptions that affect any married couple, but some factors are statistically linked to higher divorce rates. Couples are more likely to divorce if the partners are poor, uneducated, have had premarital births, are victims or perpetrators of domestic violence, or are unfaithful to each other. What does the following graph indicate about cultural background and the likelihood of divorce?

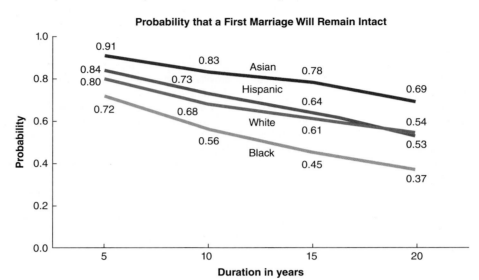

Probability that a First Marriage Will Remain Intact

Source: "First Marriages in the United States: Data from the 2006–2010 National Survey of Family Growth," by C. E. Copen, K. Daniels, J. Vespa, and W. D. Mosher, March 22, 2012, *National Health Statistics Reports, 49.* www.cdc.gov/nchs/data/nhsr/nhsr049.pdf.

Blended Families

Many divorced people eventually remarry, and **blended families**, in which one or both partners bring children from a previous marriage, are becoming a common form of family.

Just as it takes time for a family to reorganize and stabilize itself after a divorce, it also takes time for a blended family to achieve some measure of cohesion after parents remarry. It can take two years or more for stepparents and stepchildren to build relationships. Adults should allow time for trust and attachment to develop before they take on a parenting role with their stepchildren. When children regularly see their noncustodial parent, they are better able to adjust to their new family. Children also adjust better if the parents in the blended family have a low-intensity relationship and if the relationships between ex-spouses are civil.

blended families
Families in which one or both partners bring a child or children from a previous marriage.

Singlehood

Although marriage continues to be a popular institution, a growing number of people in our society are unmarried. Many young adults are delaying marriage to pursue educational and career goals, but an increasing number of people view singlehood as a legitimate, healthy, and satisfying alternative to marriage. Some people, including some highly educated professionals and career-oriented individuals, prefer to remain unmarried. In singlehood they find the freedom to pursue their own interests, spend their money as they wish, invest time in their careers, develop a broad network of friends, have a variety of sexual relationships, and enjoy opportunities for solitude. For them, being single is a positive choice.

Keeping Your Relationships Strong and Vital

A characteristic of relationships—both partnerships and families—is that they change over time. No matter what specific challenges come up, three basic qualities seem to make partnerships and families strong: cohesion, flexibility, and communication.[33]

Cohesion is the dynamic balance between separateness and togetherness in both couple and family relationships. Relationships are strongest when there is a balance between intimacy and autonomy. There are times when partners and

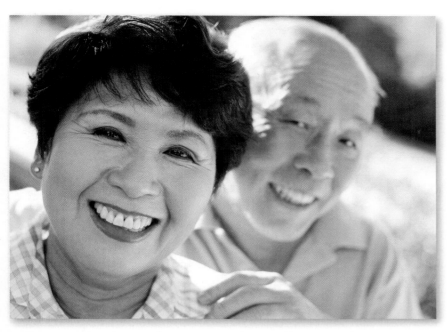

■ Some couples discover the secrets to a long and happy marriage.

family members spend more time together and other times when they spend more time apart, but they come back to a comfortably cohesive point.

Flexibility is the dynamic balance between stability and change. Again, relationships are strongest when there is a balance. Too much stability can cause rigidity; too much change can cause chaos. Communication is the tool that partners and families use to adjust levels of cohesion or flexibility when change is needed. It is important that communication with a partner include expressions of appreciation, healthy complaining, and the recognition of both partners' levels of sensitivity.[8]

When relationship problems persist for two or three months and the partners are not able to resolve them, the couple should probably seek help. Couples who receive help with difficulties before they become too severe have a better chance of overcoming the problems and developing a stronger relationship than do those who delay. Marriage and family therapists are specifically trained to help couples and families with relationship problems. Look for a therapist who is licensed by your state or who is a certified member of the American Association for Marriage and Family Therapists. Your physician or clergyperson may be able to recommend a qualified professional. A couples' therapist can help you develop the strengths and resources you need to nourish and enhance this vital part of your life.

COMMUNITIES

Connection with others within a community as well as with a partner, family, and friends promotes personal health and growth. Healthy relationships in all cases involve a balance between closeness and separateness and are characterized by mutual support, respect, good communication, and caring actions. Having strong personal relationships improves health and self-esteem and gives greater meaning to life.[34]

community
A group of people connected by values, purpose, and goals.

A **community** is a group of people connected in a way that transcends a casual attachment. Although a physical neighborhood can be a community, we are using the term here in a larger sense, as an association of like-minded people or people with a common goal.[35] Participating in a spiritual practice, volunteer service, a political campaign, intramural sports, or in any type of hobby-focused club are examples of community involvement and social connectedness.

Being active in a community is usually has a positive impact on people's health. Several studies have demonstrated links between social connectedness and individual health and well-being.[36,37] In general, the size of a person's social network and his or her sense of connectedness are inversely related to risk-related behaviors such as alcohol and tobacco consumption, physical inactivity, and behaviors leading to obesity.[34,38] Evidence also shows that social participation and engagement are related to the maintenance of cognitive function in older adulthood and to lowered mortality rates.

A sense of trust among individuals who belong to communities can promote social stability and strong collaborative

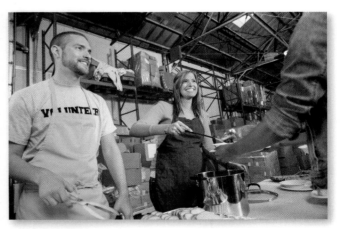

■ Participating in community activities can reinforce feelings of connectedness with others and enhance a person's sense of well-being.

Public Health Is Personal

Individual Freedom Versus the Common Good

By definition, public health involves areas in which individual health is connected to the health of others. In these cases, the government makes decisions that can sometimes be seen as restricting individual freedom. Such decisions are justified as supporting community health and promoting the common good. They represent what might be our strongest social connection—our dependence on one another for good health, longer life, and a better quality of life.

The following examples are just a few of the many public health issues that affect all of us:

- *Child abuse.* Should families be allowed to discipline their children in whatever way they see fit, or should society set standards and limits on these actions? In all states, child abuse and neglect are crimes and must be reported by those identified as mandatory reporters, including therapists and physicians. Every day, more than 2,000 children are abused or neglected, and 5 die at the hands of their abusers.

- *Smoking.* Should people be allowed to smoke wherever and whenever they want? Research clearly indicates that smoking is bad for your health, and it also shows that secondhand smoke damages the health of children and others who live or work with smokers. The U.S. surgeon general has determined that there is no safe level of exposure to secondhand smoke. Across the United States, a growing number of states and localities ban smoking in workplaces, restaurants, or bars, or some combination of these places.

- *Syringe exchange.* Should communities provide drug users with syringes so they can inject drugs with less risk of disease? Syringe exchange programs are now legal in many states, but the federal government and some states still decline to provide funds for these programs. Research suggests that syringe exchange programs reduce HIV and hepatitis C transmission and are cost effective without resulting in any increase in drug abuse. While the positive impact of syringe exchange programs has been supported by the literature, they are not legal in all localities and the federal government refuses to provide support.

- *Vaccinations.* Should parents be required to have their children vaccinated against infectious diseases? Many school districts require specific vaccinations before a child can enter school. Colleges also often require proof of vaccination against specific contagious diseases, such as measles, mumps, and hepatitis B. Some parents refuse to have their children vaccinated because of fears of complications, relying instead on "herd immunity." If they claim religious objections, the state cannot force them to comply.

- *"Presenteeism."* Should people stay home when they are sick with a cold or other contagious illness or when they have a sick child? Many people fear "absenteeism"—staying home from work—out of concern that they will lose a day's pay or even their job. Instead, by going to work sick or sending a sick child to school, they expose others to contagious diseases and even risk contributing to epidemics. The government encourages people with the flu to stay home and avoid contact with others, but many people still go to work, and many employers have not adjusted their sick leave policies to accommodate such absences.

To participate in the conversation about public health issues like these, become educated about the facts, support programs that make sense to you, and vote from an informed perspective.

connect ACTIVITY

---

networks. For example, unpaid work done by a group of people results in an improved environment for all, whether that means organizing a block party, producing a community newsletter, or working with friends to repaint the local library. People with a strong sense of their community also have more social capital than those who do not— that is, they are more likely to share and exchange resources with others whom they trust in their communities.

values
Set of criteria for judging what is good and bad that underlies moral decisions and behavior.

Public health is an arena in which the connections between individuals and community become concrete, and decisions about regulating personal behaviors for the good of the community sometimes lead to debate and controversy. For some examples, see the box, "Individual Freedom Versus the Common Good."

Community Starts Within

In the act of joining a community, you bring your deepest beliefs and intentions into the world. Participation in a community requires that you understand your beliefs and how you fit into a particular community. Figuring out what your values are, what gives meaning to your life, and what you want to accomplish will help you identify the communities whose members share your values and in which you will feel most personally fulfilled.

Values Your personal value system is a set of guidelines for how you want to live your life. **Values**, the criteria for judging what is good and bad, underlie moral principles and behavior. Your value system shapes who you are as a person, how you make decisions, and what goals you set for yourself. When you develop a way of life that makes sense and enables you to navigate the world effectively, the many choices

Action Skill-Builder

Live Your Values

Many people are unaware of their own core values and the guiding principles by which they live their lives. We seldom think through our values until we are faced with a difficult choice, and even then we may make a choice without understanding our values. Instead, we may make a "gut decision" without knowing why. For inspiration, we often look to people who stood up for their values despite enormous pressure or took action even if it put their own lives at risk. They may be whistle blowers, social activists, or people who started foundations in support of particular causes. We see many of these individuals as courageous because they spoke up while others remained silent or did nothing.

Living your values doesn't have to be on a grand scale, however. In fact, you live your values every day, when you listen to a friend, speak up to a bigoted comment, or treat the environment with respect. How would you articulate your own core values? How do you express them in your daily life? What guiding principles do you derive from them?

Consider the following list of values and identify those that are important to you. If some of your values aren't on the list, add them. Take some time to consider how you can embody them in your life and what kinds of communities share them. What steps can you take to bring your behaviors into line with your values? What opportunities arise each day for you to put your values into action?

☐ achievement	☐ home
☐ autonomy	☐ honesty
☐ care for the environment	☐ integrity
☐ compassion	☐ learning
☐ connectedness	☐ love
☐ creativity	☐ personal growth
☐ determination	☐ prestige
☐ education	☐ relationships
☐ fairness	☐ respect
☐ family	☐ service
☐ financial well-being	☐ social justice
☐ freedom	☐ spirituality
☐ hard work	☐ status
☐ health	

Purpose Why am I here? What gives my life meaning? These questions have been asked by people all over the world, in all eras, and at all stages of life. Searching for answers to these questions is part of life's journey. For some, the answers may involve developing relationships and connections. For others, it could be caring for others, or working for a healthier planet. Positive psychology (discussed in Chapter 2) contributes the idea that meaning in life comes from using one's personal strengths to serve some larger end.

Goals When you identify and pursue your personal goals, you are taking responsibility for yourself and taking charge of your life. Personal growth and achievement of goals is an incremental process through which you develop a reservoir of inner strengths, self-esteem, and fulfillment. A community can help you reach your goals. For example, if you want to learn to play chess, you can join a chess club and learn from people who are passionate about the game—and probably happy to share their knowledge. In addition, the mere process of participating in a community can help you achieve broader goals for personal improvement, such as becoming more compassionate or learning, being a better listener, developing a more optimistic attitude, or simply becoming less self-absorbed.

What is most important to you in life? If you were to write a personal statement of purpose, what would it be? It could be as simple as "to live and learn" or "to know my higher being and teach and express love."

Finding a Community That Works for You

Community involvement provides a feeling of participation in something greater than yourself and a sense of unity with your surroundings and neighbors. No matter what your values and purpose in life are, you can be confident that there is a community out there for you.

Religious and Spiritual Communities For thousands of years, one of the most significant realms in which humans have found personal and social connectedness has been religious or spiritual communities. Spirituality involves different paths for different people, so it has been defined in many ways. In health promotion literature, **spirituality** is commonly defined as a person's connection to self, significant others, and the community at large. Many experts also agree that spirituality involves a personal belief system or value system that gives meaning and purpose to life.[39]

spirituality
The experience of connection to self, others, and the community at large, providing a sense of purpose and meaning.

For some individuals, this personal value system may include a belief in and reverence for a higher power, which may be expressed through an organized religion.

you face each day become much less complex and easier to handle. Your value system becomes your map, providing a structure for decision making that allows flexibility and the possibility of change (see the box, "Live Your Values").

Worldwide, there are more than 20 major religions and thousands of other forms of spiritual expression. Many individuals count religion or spirituality as an important part of their lives; according to recent surveys, more than 8 in 10 Americans identify with a religion and believe in God or a universal spirit or higher power.[40]

While there is no definitive scientific proof that religious involvement has positive health benefits, the connection between spirituality and health is gaining serious attention from the medical and scientific communities.[41,42] There are many scientific articles focused on the relationship between spirituality and health,[43,44] and more than half the nation's medical schools now offer courses on spirituality and medicine, whereas only three did 25 years ago. The pursuit is not without its skeptics, however, and the connection between spirituality and health remains an area of controversy and debate (see the box, "Is Research on the Associations Between Spirituality and Health Worthwhile?" at the end of the chapter).

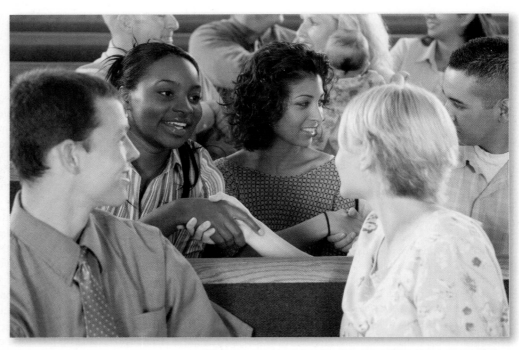

■ People who have strong ties to a religious or community group are more likely to have a network of people who can support and help them in time of need.

One of the most consistent research findings is that spiritually connected people stay healthier and live longer than those who are not connected.[45,46] One study found that people who attend church regularly live an average of seven years longer than their non-churchgoing counterparts.[47] An important reason for this outcome is that people who are religious or spiritually connected generally have healthier lifestyles. They smoke less, drink less alcohol, have better diets, exercise more, and are more likely to wear seat belts and to avoid drugs and unsafe sex. However, these factors don't seem to account for all of the health-related benefits of religious and spiritual commitment. Studies find that the positive differences in death rates persist even after controlling for factors such as age, health, habits, demographics, and other health-related variables.[45]

Another explanation for better health among people who are spiritually involved is that they react more effectively to health crises. People who are religious or spiritual seem to be more willing than those who are not spiritually connected to alter their health habits, to be proactive in seeking medical treatment, and to accept the support of others. People who have strong ties to a religious group or another community segment may receive help and encouragement

from that community in times of crisis.[48] Friends may transport them to the doctor and to church, shop for them, prepare meals, arrange child care, and encourage them to get appropriate medical treatment.

Studies have shown that spiritual connectedness appears to be associated with high levels of *health-related quality of life*—the physical, psychological, social, and spiritual aspects of a person's daily experience. Spiritual connectedness is especially important when a person is coping with serious health issues such as cancer, HIV infection, heart disease, limb amputation, or spinal cord injury.[45] This positive relationship persists even as physical health declines with serious illness.[49]

In addition, spiritual practices such as meditation, prayer, and worship seem to promote positive emotions such as hope, love, contentment, and forgiveness, which can result in lower levels of anxiety. Studies have also shown that prayer and relaxation techniques such as meditation, yoga, and hypnotherapy reduce the secretion of stress hormones and their harmful side effects. This in turn may help to minimize the stress response, which suppresses immune functioning.[50–53] Many people may even turn to religion in times of stress.[54]

Social Activism and the Global Community Some people connect with their communities—local, national, and global—through social activism. A social cause, such as overcoming poverty or fighting illiteracy, can unite people from diverse backgrounds for a common good (see the box, "Who Joins Social Movements, and Why?"). Many people find it meaningful to participate in global citizenship by joining organizations through which they can put their values into practice in the world. Here are a few:

- The Peace Corps was inspired by President John F. Kennedy's call to college students to give two years of their lives to help people in developing nations. Today, it is still sending people to developing nations from Ecuador to Ghana to the Ukraine with the goal of promoting world peace and friendship. The services its volunteers provide include helping teachers develop their teaching methodologies, raising awareness about health issues like HIV/AIDS, teaching environmental conservation strategies, and teaching computer skills.

- Habitat for Humanity is widely known for its work providing housing for needy people in the United States, but it also works to eliminate poverty and homelessness on a global level. So far, the organization has built more than 350,000 houses in more than 90 countries.

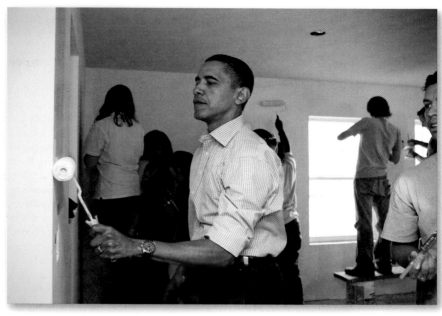

- Volunteers benefit others and themselves when they serve their communities. President Obama has emphasized the importance of volunteering by participating in several community service projects since his inauguration, and his administration created a website, www.serve.gov, to put people in touch with volunteer opportunities in their communities.

- Greenpeace focuses on the most crucial worldwide threats to the planet's biodiversity and environment. Greenpeace has been campaigning against environmental degradation since 1971, bearing witness in a nonviolent manner.

- Clowns Without Borders offers laughter to relieve the suffering of all people, especially children, who live in areas of crisis including refugee camps, conflict zones, and territories in crisis situations.

Recently, Aaker and Smith coined the term "the dragonfly effect" to describe how social media has been used to facilitate social change.[55] The reach of the Internet has dramatically changed how social change can occur. From facilitating governmental reform to providing funding for non-profits to getting a friend a bone marrow transplant donor, the possibilities of social media are limitless. This includes using media such as blogs, Twitter, and crowdsourcing to reach people quickly, tell your story, and get an electronic audience to become "team members" who become devoted to your cause.

If you are interested in social activism, look for ways to participate through your school, your religious community, or groups you locate on the Internet or through social media. When you volunteer for such an organization, you commit yourself to building a foundation for a better world, making a contribution through service to others, and creating opportunities for mutual understanding.

Volunteering Volunteering is another way to find social connectedness and personal fulfillment. It seems that most students who volunteer do it because they have compassion for those in need. Those, however, who volunteer to "pad their résumé" invest fewer hours in the activity and may not get the maximum benefit of participation.[56] Volunteers may experience a "helper's high," similar to a "runner's high."[57] Research shows that people who give time, money, and support to others are likely to be more satisfied with their lives and less depressed.[58]

Not all kinds of volunteering have the same effect, however. One-on-one contact and direct involvement significantly increase the effects of volunteering on the volunteer. Working closely with strangers appears to confer potential health benefits. Liking the volunteer work, performing it consistently, and having unselfish motives increase the helper's high and the health benefits associated with it.[59,60] Simply donating money or doing volunteer work in isolation does not seem to have the same positive effect.

Just as the high of helping may create enjoyable immediate benefits, volunteering may result in significant long-term health benefits. For example, volunteering may reduce the negative health effects of living with high levels of stress for long periods of time. It may also reduce arthritis pain, lupus symptoms, asthma attacks, migraine headaches, colds, and episodes of the flu. Volunteering may even result in longer life for the volunteer.[61,62]

Starting the Conversation

Who Joins Social Movements, and Why?

Q: Have you ever been drawn into a social movement, such as the Occupy movement?

In September 2011, people gathered in Zuccotti Park in lower Manhattan to protest the greed, corruption, and corporate influence represented by the nearby Wall Street financial institutions. They were particularly protesting the growing economic inequality between the wealthiest 1 percent of the population and the 99 percent that represented everyone else. The Occupy Wall Street movement resonated with people everywhere, and within weeks, the Occupy movement had spread to major cities and colleges campuses across the country.

This grassroots movement drew participants from many sectors of the population, but the typical protester had a particular profile. He or she was young but not necessarily college-aged (average age: 33), White (but other races and ethnicities were represented), employed (only 13 percent unemployed), and on the left-leaning side of the political spectrum (but 70 percent identified themselves as Independents, compared with 27 percent who identified as Democrats). Although diverse, members shared a basic set of values and beliefs about the current social, economic, and political direction of the United States.

Another grassroots movement appeared on the American scene a couple years earlier, in 2009. The Tea Party movement coalesced around conservative and libertarian themes of reduced government spending, reduced national debt, lower taxes, and smaller government overall. The Tea Party had a significant impact on the 2010 midterm elections, upsetting more moderate Republican candidates in primaries and establishing a voting bloc in Congress. A typical Tea Party member is 45 or older, White, male, married, a member of the Republican Party (though self-described as more conservative than Republicans generally), and better educated and wealthier than the general population. Like members of the Occupy movement, Tea Party members share a basic set of values and beliefs—albeit one very different from that embraced by Occupy members.

Occupy and the Tea Party are examples of social movements—groups organized around a particular issue or common cause and working for social change. Other examples in recent U.S. history include the civil rights movement, the women's movement, the gay rights movement, and the environmental movement. Social movements usually crystallize around a grievance that leads to public outrage and a major shift in public attitudes. To succeed, social movements need a means of communication to spread ideas, and in all recent cases, this communication has been via the Internet, social networking sites, and mobile phones.

Social movements have both positive and negative effects. They bring together like-minded people who find support, affirmation, and a sense of belonging and collective identity. They amplify the voice of the individual and provide a forum for a segment of the population that otherwise goes unheard. They promote social change and reform at times when those in charge of existing social institutions want only to preserve the status quo.

On the other hand, social movements can narrow perspectives and promote extremism because people are exposing themselves only to the ideas they already embrace. Shared beliefs can be reinforced without question, and debate between proponents of different points of view can disappear. Social movements can polarize segments of the population and make compromise more difficult. They may also promote radical change that is beyond the scope of what the general population wants. Nevertheless, social movements appear to be an important way that social change is gradually incorporated into mainstream society.

Q: Do you identify more with the profile of the Occupy member or the profile of the Tea Party member? Which group would you be more likely to join?

Q: What impact do you think being part of a social movement has on a person's values and beliefs?

Sources: "Who is Occupy Wall Street?" by G. Goodale, 2011, *The Christian Science Monitor,* www.csmonitor.com/USA/Politics/2011/1101/Who-is-Occupy -Wall-Street-After-six-weeks-a-profile-finally-emerges; "The Demographics of Occupy Wall Street," by S. Captain, 2011, *Fast Company,* from www.fastcompany .com/1789018/occupy-wall-street-demographics-statistics#disqus_thread; "Poll Finds Tea Party Backers Wealthier and More Educated," by K. Zernike and M. Thee-Brenan, April 14, 2010, *The New York Times,* www.nytimes.com/2010/04/15/us/politics/15poll.html?_r=1&src=me&ref=general.

service learning
Form of education that combines academic study with community service.

Service Learning One way that people can connect classroom activities to community service and community building is through **service learning**. The purpose of integrating community service with academic study is to enrich learning, teach civic responsibility, and strengthen communities. Students are encouraged to take a positive role in their community, such as by tutoring, caring for the environment, or conducting oral histories with senior citizens. All of these activities are meant to teach students how to extend themselves beyond their enclosed world, taking the risk of getting involved in the lives of others. In this way they learn about caring and taking care of—two particularly important concepts for personal growth.

The Arts Experiencing the arts—whether sculpture, painting, music, poetry, literature, theater, storytelling, dance, or some other form—is another way to build connections with your community. Experiencing great art can inspire you, through felt experience, to think about the purpose of life and the nature of reality.[63] By engaging your heart, mind, and spirit, art can give you fresh insights, challenge preconceptions, and trigger inner growth. Scholar Joseph Campbell

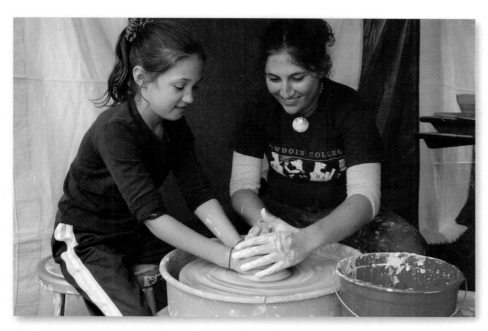

■ Engagement in meaningful activities—such as sharing one's expertise and passion with a younger person—is a major source of happiness and satisfaction for most people.

once asserted, "The goal of life is rapture. Art is the way we experience it. Art is the transforming experience."

When you enjoy and appreciate the arts, you embrace diverse cultures past and present and frequently discover in them the universal themes of human existence—love, loss, birth, death, isolation, community, continuity, change. When you express yourself creatively, you may be able to experience a spiritual connection between your inner core and the natural world beyond yourself. Both experiences—art appreciation and artistic expression—can be transforming. If the visual

or performing arts are not part of your life right now, try to schedule time to visit a museum or attend a concert. Make notes or sketches in a journal reflecting on your experiences. Doing so may stimulate a new sense of fulfillment in your life.

Internet Communities The Internet provides an opportunity unprecedented in human history for people all over the world to connect with others and be part of communities. The number of online communities is virtually limitless, as is the range of interests and conversation topics. You can follow blogs by theme, participate in discussion groups and threaded conversations, join Twitter to follow experts and celebrities, and create your own circle of friends on Facebook. Websites like Meetup help you find and form groups around your interests—from Android developers to Zen meditation centers—based on your zip code. Sites like idealist.org help you find volunteer opportunities, start an organization or business, and connect with like-minded people interested in social and environmental problems. Globally, people are using the Internet to join social and political movements and to garner support for their struggles from the international community. The social connections that begin at your doorstep now extend around the world.

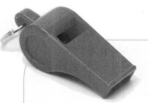

You Make the Call

Is Research on the Associations Between Spirituality and Health Worthwhile?

A recent research review found that more than 3,000 studies have been conducted over the years on whether there is a relationship between religion or spirituality and health. Some findings have been positive, others negative, still others inconclusive.

Many people believe research into the relationship between religion/spirituality and health is worthwhile. They believe that when positive associations are found, people are encouraged to build or improve their spiritual practices, if only because they want to stay healthy or become healthier. Research has shown that people with spiritual beliefs and practices have healthier lifestyles and exercise greater self-control. They may be better

able to manage stress and anxiety through prayer or meditation; they may be more optimistic, which contributes to mental health; they may participate more in their community, both giving and receiving aid; and they may be more successful at finding peace of mind and acceptance when facing illness, loss, or death. Because of their healthier lifestyles, their health care costs are lower, which benefits society. Thus, investigations into possible associations between health and religion/spirituality are important because findings can have a very positive effect on people.

Skeptics, on the other hand, think this type of research is a waste of time and money. In their opinion, these studies are really inquiring into the supernatural arena, which is beyond the scope of science. Furthermore, results can have damaging effects. When

Continued...

Concluded...

positive associations are found, they say, people with a health problem who don't have religious or spiritual beliefs may experience stress and anxiety about their lack of belief. They may even blame themselves—or others may blame them—for their illness. As suggested by one study, people with religious questions and doubts experience more stress and anxiety when ill and thus may have worse health outcomes. Even people with strong religious beliefs may suffer unnecessarily if they believe their prayers were not answered (rather than looking for a biologically based explanation). Skeptics ask whether the outcomes of these studies, positive or negative, will make a difference in what health care providers do or how people live their lives. They suggest that the money and resources devoted to these studies could be better used on research with more direct, scientifically supported applications to health and well-being.

Is research on health and religion/spirituality a good use of money, time, and energy? What do you think?

Pros

- It's important to conduct these studies because positive research findings encourage people to attend to their spiritual health.

- Positive research findings also support the health practices of religiously or spiritually oriented people, which include healthier lifestyles, more self-control, better stress management, more optimism, more community participation, and more acceptance and peace of mind.
- Positive research findings indirectly lead to lower health care costs.

Cons

- The findings of these studies are open to misinterpretation and misapplication and can have damaging effects. People may experience stress about their lack of belief, they may blame themselves for their illness, or they may feel their prayers were not answered.
- These research findings do not make a difference in what health care providers do or how people live their lives.
- These studies are inquiring into the realm of the supernatural, which is by definition unknowable through the methods of science.
- These studies are a waste of time and money, which could be better directed toward well-known health problems.

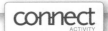

Sources: "Why Do Research on Spirituality and Health, and What Do the Results Mean?" by H. Koenig, 2012, *Journal of Religion and Health*, January, e-pub; "Religion, Self-Regulation, and Self-Control: Associations, Explanations, and Implications," by M. E. McCullough and B. L. B. Willoughby, 2009, *APA Psychological Bulletin, 135* (1), pp. 69–93.

In Review

What kinds of relationships are important for health?
People are social beings and need connections with friends and intimate partners to live fully functioning lives. People with strong social support networks tend to enjoy better health than do those with fewer connections. Healthy relationships allow people to be themselves and to grow.

Two important kinds of relationships are friendships and intimate partnerships. Friendships are reciprocal relationships based on mutual liking. Intimate partnerships have additional qualities, usually including exclusivity, commitment, and sexuality.

How do people attract and find intimate partners?
Proximity, physical attractiveness, and similarity are key factors in attraction, although today proximity may be electronic rather than physical. Finding a potential life partner is more likely to be successful with a direct, respectful approach and a social connection.

What makes people fall in love and fall out of love?
According to the similarity theory, we fall in love with people who are similar to us in important ways. According to the social exchange theory, we fall in love with people who can fulfill emotional and other needs, such as security, money, and status. The early stage of a love relationship is romantic, idealistic, and passionate. Physiological changes, such as increased dopamine, gradually decrease. Sometimes intimacy increases as passion lessens; for other couples, the end of passion is the end of the relationship. According to Sternberg's love triangle, different kinds of love have different combinations of intimacy, passion, and commitment.

What are different communication skills and styles?
Clear, positive communication is key to successful intimate relationships. Communication is both conscious and unconscious, verbal and nonverbal—together they constitute the metamessage. Effective communicators use "I" statements, make specific requests, remain calm, and listen thoughtfully to the other person. Gender difference in communication style can cause misunderstandings; men tend to use communication to compete, and women to connect.

What are the differences between *sex* and *gender?*
Sex is a person's biological status as female or male. *Gender* refers to the qualities a particular culture considers appropriate for males and females. A *gender role* is the set of attributes and activities defined by a society as masculine or feminine. Individuals who integrate masculine and feminine traits are androgynous; individuals who feel their gender identity does not match their biological sex are transsexual. *Sexual orientation* depends on the sex of those to whom a person is emotionally, romantically, and sexually attracted; people can be heterosexual, homosexual, or bisexual.

What are different types of relationship choices?
The most common type of committed relationship is marriage. Research has found that successful marriages are based on positive reasons for getting married and realistic, shared expectations of marriage. Gay and lesbian couples have the options of domestic partnership, civil union, and, in some states, marriage. Cohabitation is an option for couples; for two thirds, it leads to marriage. Research findings have been varied about the effect of cohabitation on the relationship. About 40 to 50 percent of first marriages now end in divorce, and many single-parent families struggle with poverty. Many people who remarry bring their children to the new relationship, creating a blended family. A growing number of young adults are postponing marriage, and older adults are choosing to remain single. Cohesion, flexibility, and communication are key to maintaining any kind of partnership or family.

What are the benefits of connecting with a community?
Community involvement provides a feeling of participation in something greater than yourself and a sense of unity with your surroundings and neighbors. Recognizing your values and goals in life is key to finding a community that works for you. Communities can be based on religion, social activism, volunteering, service learning, or the arts. Increasingly, the Internet is a way for people to locate others of a like mind.

4 Sleep

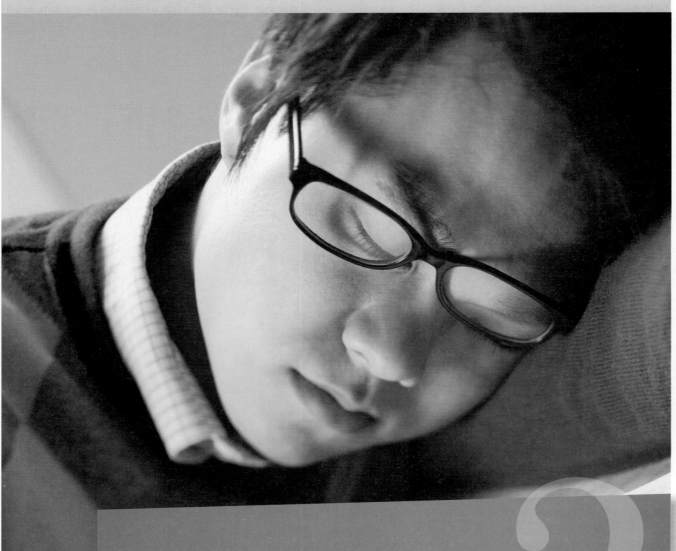

Ever Wonder...

- if pulling an all-nighter is worth it?
- how often you should replace your mattress?
- if it's okay to exercise right before sleep?

College students often have a reputation for missing early-morning classes or falling asleep in class. It doesn't necessarily mean that they've been out partying. Most young adults have a **circadian rhythm**—an internal daily cycle of waking and sleeping—that tells them to fall asleep later in the evening and to wake up later in the morning than older adults. These circadian rhythms, accompanied by a demanding college environment, make college students vulnerable to chronic sleep deprivation. Most adults need about 8 to 9 hours of sleep each night, but the typical college student sleeps only 6 to 7 hours a night on weekdays.[1] Lack of sufficient sleep impairs academic performance. According to a survey by the American College Health Association, 23 percent of college men and 25 percent of college women rated sleep difficulties as the third major impediment (after stress and illness) to academic performance.[2] To help their sleep-deprived students, some colleges and universities include programs on sleep and health as part of summer orientation for freshmen.

According to the Sleep in America Poll conducted by the National Sleep Foundation (NSF), many Americans are not sleeping enough to sustain optimum health.[3,4] Of the poll's respondents—adults aged 18 to 54—72 percent reported sleeping less than 8 hours on weekdays, and 20 percent said they slept less than 6 hours. On average, the respondents reported sleeping about 6.7 hours on weekdays and 7.1 hours on weekends.[4] Many people are unaware of the vital role that adequate sleep plays in good health. See the box, "Insufficient Sleep Is a Public Health Epidemic."

SLEEP AND YOUR HEALTH

Sleep is commonly understood as a period of rest and recovery from the demands of wakefulness. It can also be described as a state of unconsciousness or partial consciousness from which a person can be roused by stimulation (e.g., as distinguished from a coma). We spend about one-third of our lives sleeping, a fact that in itself indicates how important sleep is.

Health Effects of Sleep

Sleep is strongly associated with overall health and quality of life. During the deepest stages of sleep, restoration and growth take place. Growth hormone stimulates the growth and repair of the body's tissues and helps to prevent certain types of cancer. Natural immune system moderators increase during deep sleep to promote resistance to viral infections. When sleep time is deficient, a breakdown in the body's health-promoting processes can occur. Sleeping less than 7 hours—sometimes called *short sleep*—increases the risk for negative health outcomes in both men and women. Sleeping 10 hours or more—*long sleep*—has not been found to have negative health outcomes.[5] Sleep deprivation and other sleep behaviors disruption are often associated with serious physical and mental health conditions, which are summarized in Figure 4.1.[5–10]

Sleep and Metabolism Adults who sleep less than 7 hours a night are at a higher risk for obesity than adults who sleep 7 to 8 hours. One study found that women who sleep less than 6 hours were 32 percent more likely to gain 30 pounds or more over the next 16 years than women who slept at least 7 hours. Scientists believe the association between weight and sleep is caused by four factors: (1) altering of glucose metabolism so that the body does not metabolize food effectively; (2) hormone imbalance involving ghrelin (increases appetite) and leptin (suppresses appetite); (3) less time in rapid-eye movement (REM) sleep (burn more calories in REM); and (4) increased production of cortisol, which encourages food binges for high-calorie, high-fat foods.[5] Obesity is a primary risk factor associated with diabetes.

Sleep and Safety Motor vehicle safety will be discussed in detail in Chapter 16. Here, however, it is important to note that even small increases in sleep deprivation can cause driving drowsiness. For example, the loss of 1 hour of sleep caused by the shift to daylight saving time in the spring coincides with about a 20 percent increase in motor vehicle accidents the day or two after implementation.[5]

Sleep and Heart Disease People who chronically sleep less than 6 hours a night are at higher risk for heart disease, stroke, and high blood pressure than people who sleep more than 6 hours a night. For example, a person's risk for a heart attack increases by 5 percent for three weeks after the start of spring daylight saving time. The metabolic causes associated with heart disease include increased fat in the blood and pro-inflammatory processes, which will be discussed in Chapter 14.

Sleep and Immune Function Inadequate sleep reduces the effectiveness of the immune system in a number of ways. It suppressed the production of cells that help fight infections, so if you are sleep deprived, you are more likely to catch an infection such as a cold or the flu, and it will take your body longer to recover. In addition, inadequate sleep causes an increase in cells associated with inflammation, including C-reactive protein, which is described in more detail in Chapter 14. Inflammation is a healthy response to an acute infection or injury, but over the long term, chronic, low-level inflammation can damage tissues and organs and increase risk for a variety of chronic diseases. Adequate sleep is needed for effective functioning of the immune system.[5,8]

circadian rhythm Daily 24-hour cycle of physiological and behavioral functioning.

sleep Period of rest and recovery from the demands of wakefulness; a state of unconsciousness or partial consciousness from which a person can be roused by stimulation.

Sleep and Cancer Research on sleep and cancer has primarily focused on shift-workers. Shift-workers experiencing extreme sleep disruption disorders have a 50 percent increase risk for breast cancer in women and prostate cancer in men.

Public Health Is Personal

Insufficient Sleep Is a Public Health Epidemic

Ten years ago if you gave college students a list of 20 personal health topics, sleep would have ranked near the bottom in terms of importance and interest. Today, the topic of sleep has significantly increased in popularity of topics to cover in personal health courses. Sleep deprivation is also receiving more attention as an important public health issue due to its association with motor vehicle accidents, industrial disasters, medical and occupational errors, and medical costs due to chronic diseases. Increased mortality, reduced quality of life, and reduced productivity are also tied to insufficient sleep. Health experts estimate that 50 to 70 million U.S. adults have sleep or wakefulness disorders.

The basal sleep need for adults is about 7 to 8 hours. However, the optimal sleep need for adults is 8 to 9 hours. Overall, more than 35 percent of adults report getting less than 7 hours of sleep in a 24-hour period. The National Health and Nutrition Examination Survey (NHANES) found insufficient sleep to be more prevalent among adults ages 20 to 39 (37 percent) than among adults ages 60 or older (32 percent). More non-Hispanic blacks (53 percent) reported getting less than 7 hours of sleep than did non-Hispanic whites (34.5 percent), Mexican Americans (35.2 percent), or those of other races/ethnicities (41.7 percent). Insufficient sleep for adults is mainly due to lifestyles, work schedules, or sleep disorders.

The public health burden for sleep deprivation is enormous. There is substantial information on the neurobiology of sleep and sleep disorders, but much less work has been done on effective strategies that promote sleep. A report by the International Office of Medicine (IOM), *Sleep Disorders and Sleep Deprivation: An Unmet Public Health Problem,* calls for action that increases public awareness of the role that sleep plays in quality of life. This action includes more effective public education on the need for healthy sleep, more training for public health providers and primary health care providers on counseling and screening for healthy sleep behaviors, and use of surveillance and monitoring tools addressing the health and economic burdens of a sleepless American society. The bottom line of these campaigns is that sleep is essential for quality of life. To attain these objectives, federal agencies, public health organizations, and private organizations are partnering to employ strategies identified by the IOM report. The National Sleep Awareness Roundtable (www.nsart.org) is a good example of such collaboration efforts. Multisectoral public health campaigns, similar to those used to reduce alcohol consumption and tobacco consumption, are educating the public about the importance of sleep and the health consequences of sleep deprivation.

The IOM report identified the major obstacles to getting the help people need for insufficient sleep problems as the general lack of awareness by the public on the importance of avoiding sleep deprivation and the detection of sleep disorders of patients by primary health care professionals. The bottom line of this report is that the cumulative effects of sleep loss and sleep disorders is a widely unrecognized public health problem that cost billions of dollars spent directly on health care costs and lost productivity.

Sources: "Insufficient Sleep Is a Public Health Epidemic," Centers for Disease Control and Prevention, www.cdc.gov/Features/dsSleep; Centers for Disease Control and Prevention. "Raising Awareness of Sleep as a Healthy Behavior," Centers for Disease Control and Prevention, www.cdc.gov/pcd/issues/2013/13_0081.htm; *Sleep Disorders and Sleep Deprivation: An Unmet Public Health Problem,* National Academies Press, full text available at www.nap.edu.

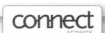

The causes for this increased risk are thought to include changes in hormonal and metabolic systems, immune system suppression, and decreased melatonin levels.[5,12]

Mental Health and Neurodegenerative Diseases

Sleep complaints are also symptoms of various mental disorders. They are regularly reported by people with bipolar disorder, schizophrenia, depression, and substance abuse.[10] Abnormal sleep is also associated with such neurodegenerative diseases as dementia, Alzheimer's, Huntington's, Parkinson's, and multiple sclerosis. The specific mechanisms causing abnormal sleep for people with mental health disorders and neurodegenerative diseases are not known.[5]

sleep deprivation
Lack of sufficient time asleep, a condition that impairs physical, emotional, and cognitive functioning.

Sleep Deprivation

Sleep deprivation refers to sleep shorter than what a person actually needs to feel vibrant. Most of us know what it feels like when we don't get enough sleep—we feel drowsy,

our eyes burn, we find it hard to pay attention. The effects of sleep deprivation can be much more serious than this, however. Studies have shown that individuals with severe sleep deprivation (e.g., staying awake for 19 to 24 hours) score worse on performance tests and alertness scales than do people with a blood alcohol concentration (BAC) of 0.1 percent—legally too drunk to drive.

Sleep deprivation has effects in all domains of functioning. Heightened irritability, lowered anger threshold, frustration, nervousness, and difficulty handling stress are some of the emotional effects. Reduced motivation may affect school and job performance, and lack of interest in socializing with others may cause relationships to suffer. Performance of daily activities is affected as is the brain's ability to learn new material. Reaction time, coordination, and judgment are all impaired. Individuals who are sleep deprived may experience microsleep—brief episodes of sleep lasting a few seconds at a time—which increases their risk of being involved in accidents.[4,5]

The impact of sleep deprivation on memory is well documented. Sleep scientists believe sleep is the time when the hippocampus and neocortex (two brain memory systems) communicate with each other. Initial memories are formed

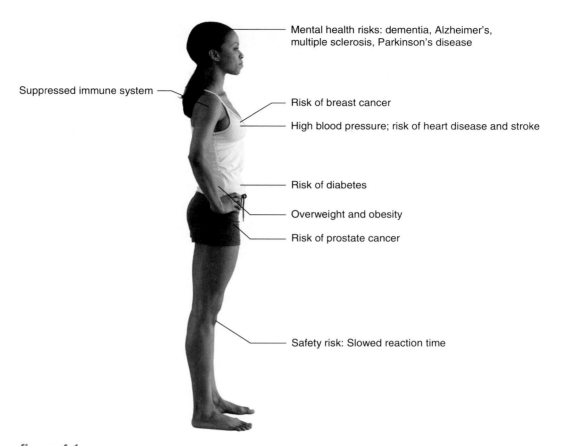

Mental health risks: dementia, Alzheimer's, multiple sclerosis, Parkinson's disease

Suppressed immune system

Risk of breast cancer

High blood pressure; risk of heart disease and stroke

Risk of diabetes

Overweight and obesity

Risk of prostate cancer

Safety risk: Slowed reaction time

figure 4.1   **Sleep and health.**
Physical and mental health conditions associated with sleep deprivation and sleep disorders.

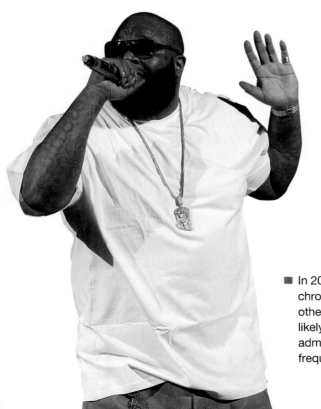

in the hippocampus. To be retained, the formed memory must be transmitted from the hippocampus to the neocortex, where it is stored as a long-term memory.[13–15] The strengthening of neuron links between the two areas is called "sleep-dependent memory processing." Sleep provides the optimal time for this transmission. Some sleep experts believe that for every 2 hours a person stays awake, his or her brain will need an hour of sleep to support communication between the hippocampus and neocortex.[16]

According to scientific research, if you sleep after learning a finger-tapping sequence, the memory of this motor task will be imprinted in your brain so that you become better at the task. Deep sleep is needed for this imprint to occur. If you do not attain deep sleep, your brain does not have the opportunity to solidify what you have learned. This is why pulling an all-nighter for an exam results in short-term memory but not long-term memory.[5]

■ In 2011, rapper Rick Ross suffered two seizures. After tests for chronic illnesses like cancer, diabetes, and HIV confirmed that he was otherwise healthy, Ross's doctors identified sleep deprivation as the likely cause of the seizures. Ross reflected on his hectic schedule, admitting that he hadn't gotten a full night's sleep in five years—and frequently got as little as 2 hours of sleep a night.

Life Stories

Dylan: Underground Adderall

Dylan, a devoted political science major, hoped to get accepted to a prestigious law school after he earned his bachelor's degree. He carried a full semester course load, worked 20 hours a week in a bookstore, was president of his fraternity, and was active in student government. Dylan spent his weekends preparing for the LSAT, and he usually managed to squeeze in some socializing. He averaged about 6 hours of sleep on weekdays and 7 hours on weekends.

Early in the fall semester of his senior year, sleep deprivation caught up with Dylan, and he started feeling stressed and tired. Dylan's roommate, Henry, who had a prescription of Adderall for attention deficit/hyperactivity disorder (ADHD), offered to share one of his pills with Dylan. With a looming due date for a paper and midterms to study for, Dylan decided to try it. The Adderall pill relieved Dylan's fatigue almost immediately. Suddenly, he was able to concentrate for hours at a time, remember more of what he read, and maintain energy for his work at the bookstore.

Dylan scored very high on the LSAT. His GPA that fall was fantastic. Dylan attributed these successes to his use of Adderall, but he had become aware of the fact that taking it was risky. He knew it was illegal for him to take it without a prescription and, in fact, a felony for Henry to give or sell it to him. He also learned in psychology class that although Adderall can help patients with real medical problems, such as ADHD, depression, and narcolepsy, it increases blood pressure and thus increases the risk for sudden death, heart attack, and stroke. Dylan's psychology professor also warned that chronic use of Adderall, especially without the supervision of a doctor, could cause amphetamine psychosis. Despite the serious potential side effects of Adderall, Dylan felt that the boost he got from the drug was vital to his ability to compete with other students and win admission to a top law school. Dylan decided to keep using the drug. After all, he suspected that many other students were also off-label users of Adderall.

- Do you think Dylan's use of Adderall is cheating?

- What percentage of students at your school do you think use stimulant drugs like Adderall for studying? Partying? Do you think most students are aware of the health risks associated with these stimulants? Are these stimulants more likely to be used at schools with high competitive academic environments?

- Should your school implement discipline policies for students who use or sell off-label stimulant drugs?

- Many students succeed in achieving their goals without resorting to illegal use of stimulants. What healthy strategies can a motivated, high-achieving student take to reduce fatigue and successfully manage his or her many commitments?

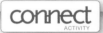

connect ACTIVITY

Sleeping less than you need causes a **sleep debt**.[14] Your sleep debt accumulates over time. For example, sleeping one hour less than you need every night for a week makes your body feel as if you have been staying up all night, and sleeping less than 6 hours each day for two weeks is equivalent to 24 hours of no sleep. If you sleep less than 4 hours a night for one week, this is equivalent to 48 to 72 hours without sleep. College students are especially vulnerable to building up a sleep debt, especially when they pull all-nighters to prepare for an exam. It is not known how many nights of extended sleep are needed to offset these sleep debts. However, the occasional sleep-in weekend is not enough.[5]

Many college students and others who build up a sleep debt during the week—night-shift workers, for example—try to cancel the debt by sleeping more on the weekends. This "solution," however, can actually worsen sleep deprivation during the week by disrupting sleep structure.[8,16] Consistently getting a sufficient amount of sleep strengthens sleep structure (which will be described shortly, in the section "The Structure of Sleep").

Prescription stimulants—which are used to treat a variety of ailments including asthma and attention deficit/ hyperactivity disorder (ADHD)—are not a healthy solution to sleep deprivation. They work by increasing the amount of norepinephrine and dopamine in the brain. These chemicals increase blood pressure and heart rate, constrict blood vessels, increase respiration rate, and increase blood glucose. Their effects are increased alertness, attention, and energy and a sense of euphoria. However, side effects include cardiovascular failure and deadly seizures. High doses can cause feelings of hostility or paranoia, dangerously high body temperature, irregular heart beat, and addiction. Today, college students are using prescription stimulants like Adderall, Ritalin, and Provigil as study aids, party aids, and weight loss aids. See the boxes, "Dylan: Underground Adderall," and at the end of the chapter, "Should College Campuses Conduct Random Drug Tests for Adderall?"

How can you tell if you are getting enough sleep? A prime symptom of sleep deprivation is daytime drowsiness. If you feel alert during the day, you are probably getting enough sleep. If you are sleepy in sedentary situations such as reading, sitting in class, or watching television, you may be sleep deprived. Another measure of sleep deprivation is how long it takes you to fall asleep at night. A well-rested person will need 15 to 20 minutes to fall asleep.[8] If you fall asleep the instant your head hits the pillow, there is a good chance that you are sleep deprived.

sleep debt
The difference between the amount of sleep attained and the amount needed to maintain alert wakefulness during the daytime, when the amount attained is less than the amount needed.

WHAT MAKES YOU SLEEP?

Over the course of the day, your body undergoes rhythmic changes that help you move from waking to sleep and back to waking. These *circadian rhythms* are maintained primarily by two tiny structures in the brain, the *suprachiasmic nuclei* (SCN), which are located in the hypothalamus directly behind the optic nerve (Figure 4.2). This internal "biological clock" controls body temperature and levels of alertness and activity. These controls are active in the daytime, increasing wakefulness, and inactive at night, allowing the body to relax and sleep. They are also less active in the early afternoon. In addition, the SCN control the release of certain hormones. They signal the pineal gland to release **melatonin**, a hormone that increases relaxation and sleepiness, and they signal the pituitary gland to release growth hormone during sleep, to help repair damaged body tissues.[16]

Also important in maintaining circadian rhythms are external, environmental cues, especially light. Neurons in the SCN monitor the amount of light entering the eyes so that as daylight increases, the SCN slow down the secretion of melatonin and begin to be more active.[14] This process keeps your sleep/wake cycles generally synchronized with the changing lengths of day and night. The process is sensitive to artificial light as well as natural light, so even relatively dim lights in the evening (e.g., from a lamp or a computer screen) may delay when your biological clock induces sleepiness.

The biological clock operates even without the cues of daylight or darkness, though not in perfect synchrony with a 24-hour day. Without the stimulation of light and dark, human beings would have a daily cycle several minutes longer than 24 hours. Every morning your body resets your biological clock to adjust to the next 24-hour period.[1] Your body may tolerate a 1-hour adjustment. However, when bedtimes and awakening times differ greatly from their established norms, the adjustment is more difficult. Working the night shift or flying across several time zones, for example, can wreak havoc with your biological clock.[16] Because the powerful sleep-regulating cues from sunlight are missing for shift workers, they are at increased risk for heart disease, digestive disorders, and mood problems. Similarly, many totally blind people experience a misalignment of the circadian clock called "non-24-hour sleep-wake disorder" because their retinas are not able to sense light. Their circadian clock is dysfunctional, so it is as if they have a permanent jet lag and periodic insomnia.[5]

melatonin
A hormone that increases relaxation and sleepiness, released by the pineal gland during sleep.

THE STRUCTURE OF SLEEP

Studies have revealed that sleep consists of distinct stages in which muscle relaxation and nervous system arousal vary, as do types of brain waves and levels of neural activity. The brain cycles into two main states of sleep: non–rapid eye movement sleep, which has four stages, and rapid eye movement sleep.

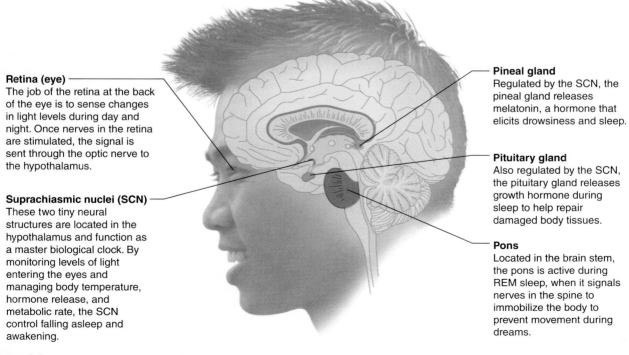

Retina (eye)
The job of the retina at the back of the eye is to sense changes in light levels during day and night. Once nerves in the retina are stimulated, the signal is sent through the optic nerve to the hypothalamus.

Suprachiasmic nuclei (SCN)
These two tiny neural structures are located in the hypothalamus and function as a master biological clock. By monitoring levels of light entering the eyes and managing body temperature, hormone release, and metabolic rate, the SCN control falling asleep and awakening.

Pineal gland
Regulated by the SCN, the pineal gland releases melatonin, a hormone that elicits drowsiness and sleep.

Pituitary gland
Also regulated by the SCN, the pituitary gland releases growth hormone during sleep to help repair damaged body tissues.

Pons
Located in the brain stem, the pons is active during REM sleep, when it signals nerves in the spine to immobilize the body to prevent movement during dreams.

figure 4.2 **Brain structures involved in sleep and waking.**

NREM Sleep

You spend about 75 percent of your sleep time in **non–rapid eye movement (NREM) sleep**, a time of reduced brain activity with four stages.

Stage 1 of NREM sleep is a transitional, light sleep—a relaxed or half-awake state. Your heart rate slows and your breathing becomes shallow and rhythmic. This stage may last from 10 seconds to 10 minutes and is sometimes accompanied by visual imagery. People awakened in stage 1 often deny that they were asleep.[7,8]

In stage 2, your brain's activity slows further, and you stop moving. This lack of movement decreases muscle tension and brain stem stimulation so that sleep is induced. Stage 2 lasts about 10 to 20 minutes and represents the beginning of actual sleep. You are no longer consciously aware of your external environment. People awakened in stage 2 readily admit that they were asleep.[7,8]

During stages 3 and 4 your blood pressure drops, your heart rate and respiration slow, and the blood supply to your brain is minimized. If you were suddenly awakened during stage 4, referred to as *deep sleep,* you would feel momentarily groggy. You usually spend about 20 to 40 minutes at a time in deep sleep, and most of your deep sleep takes place in the first third of the night.[7,8]

REM Sleep

Rapid eye movement (REM) sleep begins about 70 to 90 minutes after you have fallen asleep. As you enter this stage, your breathing and heart rate increase, and brain wave activity becomes more like that of a waking state. REM sleep is characterized by noticeable eye movements, usually lasting between 1 and 10 minutes. During this period, you are most likely to experience your first dream of the night. Although dreams may occur in all stages of sleep, they generally happen in REM sleep.[8,17]

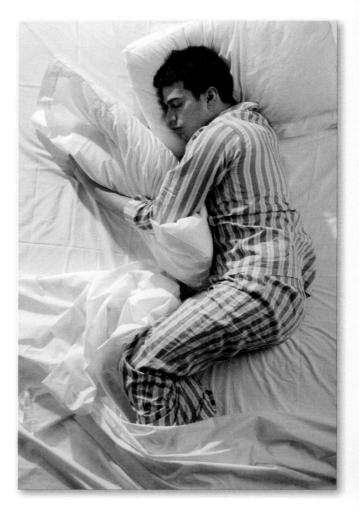

When you dream, there are periods when you have no muscle tone and your body cannot move, except for your eyes, diaphragm, nasal membranes, and erectile tissue (such as penis or clitoris).[16] This state is referred to as *REM sleep paralysis.* If you were not immobilized, there is a danger that you would act on—or act out—your dreams. REM sleep is sometimes called *paradoxical sleep* because the sleeper appears peaceful and still but is in a state of physiological arousal.

Many people believe that dreams have some meaning and relevance to daily life, often reflecting changes or shifts in emotions. By examining your dreams, according to this view, you may gain insight into the mental and emotional processes you are applying to problems or events in your life. Most dreams involve people who are familiar to the dreamer. Dreams are visual and rarely involve taste or smell. However, the dreams of people who have been blind since birth are dominated by sound and emotional feelings. If people lose sight at age 7 or later, their dreams tend to be visually dominated.[5]

Besides giving us time to dream, REM sleep also appears to give the brain the opportunity to "file" important ideas and thoughts in long-term storage, that is, in memory. This reorganization and consolidation may account for the fact that we are able to solve problems in our dreams. Scientists further believe that creative and novel ideas are more likely to flourish during REM sleep because we have easier access to memories and emotions.

Because ideas are filed in long-term storage during REM sleep, memory may be impaired if sleep time is insufficient. As a result of such memory impairment, the ability to learn new skills is also impaired. Performance in learning a new skill does not improve until an individual has had 6 hours of sleep; performance improves even more after 8 hours of sleep.[7,8]

non–rapid eye movement (NREM) sleep
Type of sleep characterized by slower brain waves than are seen during wakefulness as well as other physiological markers; divided into four stages of increasingly deep sleep.

rapid eye movement (REM) sleep
Type of sleep characterized by brain waves and other physiological signs characteristic of a waking state but also characterized by reduced muscle tone, or sleep paralysis; most dreaming occurs during REM sleep.

The importance of REM sleep to the brain is demonstrated by what is called the **REM rebound effect**. If you get inadequate sleep for several nights, you will have longer and more frequent periods of REM sleep when you have a night in which you can sleep longer.[7,16]

Sleep Cycles

After your first REM period, you cycle back and forth between REM and NREM sleep stages. These cycles repeat themselves about every 90 to 110 minutes until you wake up. Typically, you experience four or five sleep cycles each night. After the second cycle, however, you spend little or no time in NREM stages 3 and 4 and most of your time in NREM stage 2 and REM sleep (Figure 4.3). After each successive cycle, the time spent in REM sleep doubles, lasting from 10 to 60 minutes at a time.[7,16]

The sleep cycle pattern changes across the lifespan, with children and young adolescents experiencing large quantities of NREM stages 3 and 4 sleep (deep sleep). Sleep needs are constant across adulthood, but as people get older, high-quality sleep may become more elusive, and older adults may experience less deep sleep and REM sleep and more NREM stage 1 sleep and wakefulness.[18] The production of melatonin and growth hormone declines with age, and the body temperature cycle may become irregular. All of these changes decrease total nighttime sleep.[8,18]

Although the structure of sleep is essentially the same for men and women, women tend to have more slow-wave sleep (NREM stages 3 and 4) than men do and to experience more insomnia. Men have more REM periods. Men and women also tend to have some differences in habits and behaviors related to sleep. For example, women tend to get less sleep than they need in order to feel alert during the week, and men tend to get more sleep than they need. A majority of women (60 percent) say they do not get enough sleep most nights of the week. However, men and women get about the same amount of sleep on the weekends.[7]

SLEEP DISORDERS

The National Sleep Foundation estimates that at least 40 million Americans suffer from long-term sleep disorders each year; another 20 million experience occasional sleep problems. Because many sleep disorders are undiagnosed or not reported to physicians, many people who are chronically exhausted may not know why. Common sleeping disorders affecting college students include insomnia, sleep apnea, sleep walking, and nocturnal eating disorders.

Insomnia

In a poll conducted by the National Sleep Foundation (NSF), 30 percent of adult women and 40 percent of adult men reported experiencing one or more symptoms of **insomnia**—defined as difficulty falling or staying asleep—at least a few nights a week.[3] Clinical symptoms of insomnia include

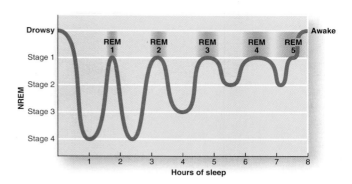

figure 4.3   One night's sleep cycles.

(1) taking longer than 30 minutes to fall asleep, (2) experiencing five or more awakenings per night, (3) sleeping less than a total of 6½ hours as a result of these awakenings, and/or (4) experiencing less than 15 minutes of deep/slow-wave sleep.[8]

Insomnia can be caused by stress, anxiety, medical problems, poor sleep environment, noisy or restless partners, and schedule changes (e.g., due to travel across time zones or shift work).[19,20] For adult women, more than half of whom report symptoms of insomnia during any given month, additional causes may include depression, headaches, effects of pregnancy, premenstrual syndrome, menopausal hot flashes, and overactive bladder. Insomnia causes for men include depression, headaches, and overactive bladder. Often, people with insomnia become distressed by their inability to fall asleep, which increases arousal and

REM rebound effect
Increase in the length and frequency of REM sleep episodes that are experienced when a person sleeps for a longer time after a period of sleep deprivation.

insomnia
Sleep disorder characterized by difficulty falling or staying asleep.

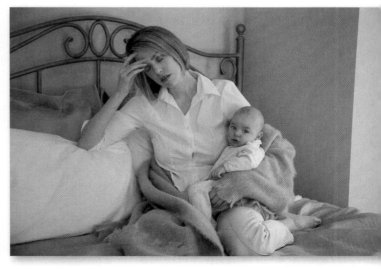

■ Women are more likely than men to get insufficient sleep. New mothers are particularly at risk for sleep deprivation.

Action Skill-Builder

Get a Better Night's Sleep

College students are at high risk for insomnia due to varying class times, demanding work schedules, and busy social lives. Because insomnia can impair memory and reduce concentration, it can affect your GPA. Take the following actions, discussed in detail later in the chapter, to ensure you get a good night's sleep:

☐ **Maintain a regular sleep schedule.**

☐ **Establish realistic, achievable daily goals.**

☐ **Relax with deep, slow breathing once you are in bed.** Focus on opening up your lungs and breathing so deeply that your chest moves.

☐ **Make your bedroom conducive to sleeping.**

☐ **Avoid naps in late afternoon or early evening.** They can disrupt the body's sleep cycle.

☐ **Get regular exercise, but not close to bedtime.**

☐ **If you drink alcohol, reduce or limit it.** Excess alcohol causes restless sleep.

☐ **Avoid stimulants in the evening, or cut them out entirely.**

☐ **Use a sleep journal to track your habits.** Each time you wake up, record the time and how many hours you slept. Also record events of the day that may have hindered your sleep, such as extra stress, a nap, or a late coffee.

If insomnia persists over several weeks, or if you experience distress and discomfort as a result of insomnia, make an appointment at your school's student health clinic. A health professional will ask about your sleep experience, sleep schedule, and daily routine to determine if behavioral therapies or medication can help.

Sources: "College Students & Sleep," by Geneseo Education, 2011, www.geneseo.edu/health/sleep; "Insomnia Significantly Affects the School Performance of College Students," by AASM News Archive, 2011, www.aasmnet.org/articles.aspx?id=884.

sleep apnea
Sleep disorder characterized by periods of nonbreathing during sleep; also known as breathing-related sleep disorder.

body temperature post-exercise is the likely reason why exercise is beneficial. See the box, "Get a Better Night's Sleep" for strategies and tips on dealing with insomnia.

Sleep Apnea

Also known as breathing-related sleep disorder, **sleep apnea** is a condition characterized by periods of nonbreathing during sleep. Some health experts estimate that almost 40 percent of the U.S. population has some form of sleep apnea and that half of those afflicted may have a severe condition. Some 80 to 90 percent of these cases are undiagnosed. The condition occurs in all ethnic, age, and socioeconomic groups, although men are more at risk for developing sleep apnea than women are.[21]

Scientists have distinguished two main types of sleep apnea: central sleep apnea and obstructive sleep apnea. In *central sleep apnea,* a rare condition, the brain fails to regulate the diaphragm and other breathing mechanisms correctly. In *obstructive sleep apnea,* by far the more common type, the upper airway is obstructed during sleep.[21] Individuals with obstructive sleep apnea are frequently overweight and have an excess of bulky soft tissue in the neck and throat. When the muscles relax during sleep, the tissue can block the airway (Figure 4.4).

In obstructive sleep apnea, the individual stops breathing many times during sleep, often for as long as 60 to 90 seconds. The person's breathing pattern is usually characterized by periods of loud snoring (when the airway is

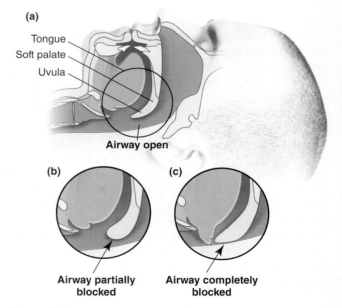

figure 4.4 Obstructive sleep apnea.
(a) Normally, the airway is open during sleep. (b) When the muscles of the soft palate, tongue, and uvula relax, they narrow the airway and cause snoring. (c) If these structures collapse on the back wall of the airway, they close the airway, preventing breathing. The efforts of the diaphragm and chest cause the blocked airway to become even more tightly sealed. For breathing to resume, the sleeper must rouse enough to cause tension in the tongue, which opens the airway.

makes it even harder to fall asleep. In time, the bedroom, bedtime, or sleep itself become associated with frustration instead of relaxation, and a vicious cycle sets in.

Chronic insomnia is difficult to treat, but individuals may be able to break the cycle and experience relief through such approaches as improving their sleep habits and sleeping environment and using relaxation techniques such as deep breathing and massage. Exercise has also been shown to significantly improve sleep quality for chronic insomnia. The exact mechanism for this benefit is not known. Scientists conjecture that an increase in core

partially blocked), alternating with periods of silence (when the airway is completely blocked), punctuated by sudden loud snores or jerking body movements as the person awakens for a few seconds and gasps for air. The individual is usually not aware of this pattern of snoring and gasping, although bed partners and other members of the household often are. The chief complaint of those with obstructive sleep apnea is daytime sleepiness, not nighttime awakening. Other symptoms include difficulty concentrating, depression, irritability, sexual dysfunction, and learning and memory difficulties.

Obstructive sleep apnea is a potentially dangerous condition; occasionally, it is even fatal. It is frequently seen in association with high blood pressure, and it can increase the risk of heart disease and stroke. Oxygen saturation of the blood decreases and levels of carbon dioxide rise when a person stops breathing, increasing the likelihood that heart and blood vessel abnormalities may occur. If sufficient oxygen is not delivered to the brain, death may occur during sleep.[21–23]

In children, sleep apnea is usually associated with enlarged tonsils. In adults, obstructive sleep apnea occurs most often in overweight, middle-aged men, although it becomes almost equally common in women after menopause. It is associated with larger neck circumferences (greater than 17 inches in men and 16 inches in women). People with the disorder often smoke, use alcohol, and/or sleep on their backs. There is sometimes a family history of sleep apnea, suggesting a genetic link.

If sleep apnea is not severe, it can be addressed with a variety of behavioral strategies. They include losing weight, forgoing alcoholic nightcaps and sedatives, avoiding allergens, not smoking, using a nasal decongestant spray, using a firm pillow and mattress, and not sleeping on the back. In addition, adjustable mouthpieces are available that extend the lower jaw, adding room to the airway. They are expensive, however, and may not be covered by health insurance.[8]

In cases of severe sleep apnea, one treatment option is a continuous positive airway pressure (CPAP) machine. Through a comfortable mask, a CPAP machine gently blows slightly pressurized air into the patient's nose. Other treatment options include surgery to cut away excess tissue at the back of the throat and a newer technique called *somnoplasty* that involves shrinking tissue in the back of the throat with radio-frequency energy.[8,15]

Sleepwalking Disorder

People with **sleepwalking disorder** rise out of an apparently deep sleep and act as if they are awake. They do not respond to other people while in this state, or, if they do, it is with reduced alertness. Sleepwalking affects between 1 and 15 percent of the general population.[8] Sleepwalking takes place during the first third of the night's sleep. Episodes typically last less than 10 minutes.[15] If sleepwalkers are awakened, they are often confused for several minutes; if they are not awakened, they may return to bed and have little or no memory of the episode the next day.[24]

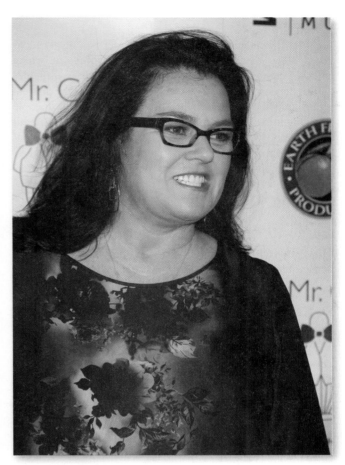

■ When she was a host on *The View*, Rosie O'Donnell announced that she has obstructive sleep apnea and uses a CPAP (continuous positive airway pressure) mask at night.

Although there may be a genetic link to sleepwalking, most sufferers do not have a family history of this disorder. Episodes may be brought on by excessive sleep deprivation, fatigue, stress, illness, excessive alcohol consumption, and the use of sedatives.[25]

Sleep-Related Eating Disorder

A person with **sleep-related eating disorder (SRED)** rises from bed during the night and eats and drinks while asleep. About three-quarters of people with this disorder are female. The person may consume bizarre concoctions but has no memory of these experiences in the morning. Fifty percent of people suffering from this disorder binge eat without awakening. Although they may binge up to six times a night, they do not experience indigestion or feelings of fullness after the binge.[12,25]

sleepwalking disorder
Sleep disorder in which a person rises out of an apparently deep sleep and acts as if awake.

sleep-related eating disorder
Sleep disorder in which a person rises from bed during the night and eats and drinks while asleep.

Night Eating Syndrome

Distinct from sleep-related eating disorder is a newly identified sleep disorder, **night eating syndrome**, in which affected persons binge eat late at night, have difficulty falling asleep, repeatedly awaken during the night and eat again, and then eat very little the next day. Some people with night eating syndrome consume more than 50 percent of their daily calories at night. Sleep experts estimate that the syndrome's frequency is about 1.5 percent in the general population and up to 10 percent among obese people seeking treatment for their weight. Treatments include medications and behavior management techniques.[12,25]

Evaluating Your Sleep

How can you tell if you have a sleep problem? First, get a sense of your general level of daytime sleepiness by taking the **sleep latency** test (a measure of how long it takes you to fall asleep) in Part 1 of the Personal Health Portfolio activity for Chapter 4 at the end of the book. Next, check to see if you have any symptoms of a sleep disorder by completing Part 2 of the activity. Then take a look at the various behavior change strategies in the next section of the chapter and make any appropriate improvements. Of course, the most basic recommendation is to make sure you are getting enough hours of sleep every night. If you still experience a sleep problem after following these recommendations, you may want to consult your physician. If the problem is serious enough, your physician may refer you to a sleep clinic or lab or a sleep disorder specialist.

night eating syndrome
Condition in which a person eats excessively during the night while awake.

sleep latency
Amount of time it takes a person to fall asleep.

Multiple Sleep Latency Test
Test of sleep latency, administered as an index of daytime sleepiness and usually given five times during the day in a sleep clinic.

If you are referred to a sleep clinic or lab, you may be asked to monitor your sleeping habits at home by keeping a sleep diary for a week or more. You will record the times you go to bed, awaken during the night, and wake up in the morning, as well as what and when you eat in the evening, any alcohol, tobacco, or drugs you consume, and so on. Alternatively, you may be evaluated at the lab. You may take a **Multiple Sleep Latency Test**, in which you lie down in a dark room and are told not to resist sleep. This test, repeated five times during the day, measures sleep latency as an index of daytime sleepiness.

GETTING A GOOD NIGHT'S SLEEP

At times, most people experience what is called disordered sleep. Disordered sleep includes the symptoms of sleep disorders, but these symptoms are less frequent and much less severe. What is the best way to ensure healthy sleep patterns over the course of your lifespan? In this section, we provide several strategies and tips that will help you get a good night's sleep.

Establishing Good Sleep Habits

Several habits and behaviors concerning when and where you sleep and what you do before you sleep can help you sleep better and solve sleep problems.

Maintain a Regular Sleep Schedule Try to get about 8 hours of sleep every night, seven days a week. With a regular sleep schedule, you fall asleep faster and awaken more easily because you are psychologically and physiologically conditioned for sleep and waking. Most students have an irregular sleep schedule.[8] As noted earlier, such a schedule throws off your internal biological clock and disrupts the structure of sleep.

Create a Sleep-Friendly Environment Your bedroom should be a comfortable, secure, quiet, cool, and dark place for inducing sleep.

- *Mattress.* Your mattress should be hard enough to allow you to get into a comfortable sleep position. If it is too hard, however, it may not provide an adequate cushion to prevent painful pressure on your body.[9] Your body and mattress condition change over time. Bed mattresses should be replaced every seven to eight years. You should use mattress pads that can protect against liquid spills, urine, blood, and allergens such as dust mites.

- *Pillow.* Picking the ideal pillow is important so that the pillow is properly aligned with your cervical spine. Proper cervical alignment will help prevent tightness in your neck muscles. Pillow thickness should be based on your preferred sleep position. Side sleepers need a pillow that fills the space between the ears and shoulders (5 to 6 inches). Back sleepers need a pillow thin enough so that the chin points straight ahead (1 to 2 inches). And, stomach sleepers should use pillows that do not put pressure on the head, neck, or lower back (1 to 2 inches).[9]

- *Quiet.* Noise can reduce restful sleep. Research on people who live near airports has found that excessive noise may jog individuals out of deep sleep and into a lighter sleep. Street noises, such as the sound of a motorcycle revving its engine, have a similar effect.[14,26] Measurable effects of noise begin at about 35 decibels (dB); significant health problems from sleep disruption occur at 55 dB and higher with long-term exposure. (A normal conversation is about 60 dB; a vacuum cleaner, about 80.) College residence halls and apartment complexes often have noise levels that exceed 35 decibels.

Nighttime noise isn't just annoying—it's bad for your health. Noise affects sleep quality, which in turn affects your overall health and quality of life. Your body responds physiologically to loud noise while you're asleep even if it doesn't wake you up. For example, the noise from an airplane can increase your blood pressure and affect your heart rate and breathing rate although you remain asleep. When your sleep is disturbed, you may feel lethargic, irritable, or anxious the next day and not be able to function at your usual level. Disturbed sleep and sleep deprivation are stressful, and stress is known to be a factor in such conditions as heart disease and depression.[26]

Earplugs and earphones can reduce noise levels by as much as 90 percent. Earplugs with a noise reduction rating of 32 decibels or below are recommended so that you can still hear a fire alarm or a crying child.[8] If it isn't possible to reduce or eliminate noise, try creating *white noise,* a monotonous and unchanging sound such as that of an air conditioner or a fan. White noise generators that create soothing sounds such as falling rain, wind, and surf have also been proven effective in protecting sleep.[15] If you can't find an inexpensive noise generator, start with a fan.[27] Intelligent sound machines use sensors that determine sounds that are audible in a room and then produce the appropriate masking sound. These machines typically have a timer that can be selected to turn off the machine after a designated time period.

■ *Temperature.* The ideal temperature for a bedroom is usually 62° F to 65° F, but you will sleep best when the temperature is within your specific comfort zone.

■ One key to getting a good night's sleep is creating a pleasant environment and establishing a relaxing bedtime routine.

A temperature below or above that zone often causes fragmented sleep or wakefulness. Generally, temperatures above 75° F and below 54° F cause people to awaken.

Before bed, a normal sleeper has a lower body temperature than a person with insomnia. The temperature will increase in the sleeper's hands and feet after the onset of sleep.[9] This temperature disrupts sleep as it struggles to reset the body thermostat to a comfortable temperature. For a normal sleeper, blood vessels will dilate to radiate heat as the core body temperature drops.[14] If you have trouble sleeping, keep your room temperature at the cool end of your comfort zone. Placing a hot water bottle or using a heating pad by your feet may also help by lowering your core body temperature and increasing blood flow to the extremities.[27]

■ *Body position.* Don't expect to get a good night's sleep if you cannot lie down. Research has shown that people sleeping in an upright position have poorer quality sleep than those sleeping in a horizontal position. The amount of slow-wave sleep a person experiences in a sitting position is almost zero. If you fall asleep while standing up, your body begins to sway so that you quickly awaken. Perhaps the brain operates in a similar fashion when you are sleeping in a seated position. With your body mainly upright, your brain may interpret this position as not sufficiently safe to allow deep sleep.[8]

■ *Pain and sleep.* About 15 percent of the American population suffers from chronic pain. This percentage increases to 50 percent for older adults. Two-thirds of people with chronic pain report poor sleep quality.[5] Common pain medications, such as morphine and codeine, complicate the problem by causing fragmented sleep. The primary sources of pain include headaches, back pain, joint pain, muscle pain, and pain around the ears and jaw. Women are more likely to experience abdominal pain caused by premenstrual cramping. If chronic pain disrupts your sleep quality, you should visit your health professional.

Avoid Caffeine, Nicotine, and Alcohol

Caffeine, a stimulant, disrupts sleep, whether it comes in coffee, tea, chocolate, or soda. Caffeine enters the bloodstream quickly and reaches a peak in about 30 to 60 minutes. It may take 4 to 6 hours for half of caffeine intake to clear the blood system of a young adult. A single cup of coffee may double the amount of time it takes an average adult to fall asleep. It may also reduce the amount of slow-wave or deep sleep by half and quadruple the number of nighttime awakenings.[14] Avoiding caffeine intake 6 to 8 hours before going to bed may improve sleep quality. For late-night studying, you could choose instead to take a quick walk or to eat some fruit. Exercise stimulates acetylcholine, which improves memory, and fruit contains sugar, which can provide an energy boost.

Starting the Conversation

Caffeinated Energy Drinks and Sleep

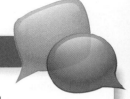

Q: Do you consume energy drinks for late-night studying? Partying? Do these drinks impede your ability to attain deep, reenergizing sleep every night?

Beverages marketed as energy drinks are a popular form of stimulants used by college students for late-night studying and partying. Caffeine is the primary stimulant ingredient in energy drinks. They contain between 50 to 500 milligrams of caffeine. Five hundred milligrams of caffeine is equivalent to 4.5 or more cups of coffee. Doctors generally recommend a maximum intake of 200 to 250 milligrams per day.

How does caffeine work? Caffeine looks like adenosine to nerve cells, so they let caffeine bind to their adenosine receptors. Adenosine causes drowsiness by slowing down nerve cell activity and dilating blood vessels to deliver oxygen to the brain during sleep. In contrast, caffeine speeds up nerve cell activity and constricts blood vessels to the brain. Caffeine causes the release of the "fight or flight" stress hormones cortisol and adrenaline discussed in Chapter 2. The result is a boost in energy and mental alertness.

Caffeine affects people differently, depending on dosage level. For many people, consuming as little as 200 milligrams per day of caffeine (two cups of coffee) increases stress levels. Too much caffeine in a short period of time causes a "caffeine crash": loss of focus, irritability, anxiety, racing heart rate, elevated blood pressure, headache, nausea, and jittery feelings. Some people even experience panic attacks and ringing in the ears.

Caffeine's effects can make relaxation difficult and impede the ability to enter stage 2 in NREM (light sleep). Caffeine is also a diuretic, causing more frequent trips to the bathroom during the night. A study of soldiers in war zones found those who consumed three or more energy drinks daily reported significantly more disrupted sleep than soldiers who consumed fewer or no energy drinks.

Q: Should the FDA mandate that energy drinks not contain more than 50 milligrams of caffeine?

Q: Energy drinks can be addictive due to high caffeine levels. What steps can you take to reduce your dependence on energy drinks?

Sources: "Energy Drink Consumption and Its Association With Sleep Problems Among U.S. Service Members on a Combat Deployment–Afghanistan 2010," *Morbidity and Mortality Weekly Report,* Centers for Disease Control and Prevention, November 9, 2012, www.cdc.gov/mmwr/preview/mmwrhtml/mm6144a3. htm; "Caffeinated Energy Drinks—A Growing Problem," by C. J. Reissig, E. C. Strain, and R. R. Griffiths, 2009, *Drug and Alcohol Dependence, 99,* pp. 1–10; "How Caffeine Works," by M. Brain, C. W. Bryant, and M. Cunningham, http://science.howstuffworks.com/caffeine.htm; *Sleep: A Very Short Introduction,* by S. W. Lockley and R. G. Foster, 2012, New York: Oxford University Press.

Energy drinks are especially high in caffeine. The Food and Drug Administration limits caffeine content in soft drinks to 71 milligrams per 12 fluid ounces, but caffeine levels in energy drinks can be much higher, and they often contain additional stimulants such as taurine. For more about the effects of high levels of caffeine, see the box, "Caffeinated Energy Drinks and Sleep."

Like caffeine, nicotine is a stimulant that can disrupt sleep. People who smoke a pack of cigarettes a day have been shown to have sleep problems. Brain-wave-pattern analysis indicates that they do not sleep as deeply as nonsmokers.[28]

Smoking also affects the respiratory system by causing congestion in the nose and swelling of the mucous membranes lining the throat and upper airway passages. These physiological factors increase the likelihood of snoring and aggravate the symptoms of sleep apnea. They also decrease oxygen uptake, which leads to more frequent awakenings.[9,16]

Alcohol induces sleepiness and reduces the amount of time it takes to fall asleep, but it causes poorer sleep and restlessness later in the night. Even if consumed 6 hours before bedtime, alcohol can increase wakefulness in the second half of the night, probably through its effect on serotonin and norepinephrine, neurotransmitters that regulate sleep. Because alcohol is a depressant, it prevents REM sleep from occurring until most of the alcohol has been absorbed. After

absorption, vivid dreams are more likely. Sleep experts call this an *alcohol rebound effect,* in which the body seems to be trying to recover REM sleep that was lost earlier.[29]

Additionally, alcohol can aggravate sleep disorders such as obstructive sleep apnea and trigger episodes of sleepwalking, sleep-related eating disorders, and other disorders. The impact of alcohol on sleep apnea is of particular concern; it can even be deadly. Alcohol consumption makes throat muscles even more relaxed than during normal sleep; it also interferes with the ability to awaken.[29]

Get Regular Exercise but Not Close to Bedtime
Regular exercise during the day or early evening hours may be beneficial for sleep. Exercising within 3 hours of going to bed, however, is not recommended, because exercise stimulates the release of adrenaline and elevates core body temperature. It takes 5 to 6 hours for body temperature to drop enough after vigorous exercise for drowsiness to occur and deeper sleep to take place.[27] See the box "Exercise and Sleep" for information about the effect of different amounts of exercise.

Manage Stress and Establish Relaxing Bedtime Rituals Stress increases physiological arousal and can adversely affect sleep patterns. Stress management and stress reduction techniques, such as those described in

Who's at Risk?

Exercise, Sleep, and Health

People who exercise moderately or vigorously report better quality of sleep than those who get light or no exercise. Similarly, moderate or vigorous exercisers report better health than people who are sedentary.

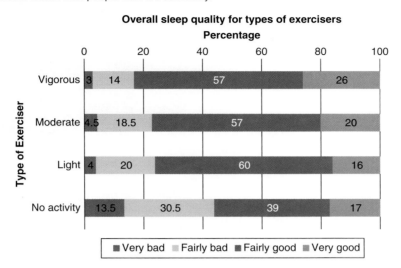

Overall sleep quality for types of exercisers

Percentage

Type of Exerciser	Very bad	Fairly bad	Fairly good	Very good
Vigorous	3	14	57	26
Moderate	4.5	18.5	57	20
Light	4	20	60	16
No activity	13.5	30.5	39	17

■ Very bad ■ Fairly bad ■ Fairly good ■ Very good

Overall health quality for types of exercisers

Percentage

Type of Exerciser	Poor	Fair	Good	Excellent
Vigorous	1	8	44	47
Moderate	1	10	59	30
Light	2	19	64	15
No activity	12	30	51	7

■ Poor ■ Fair ■ Good ■ Excellent

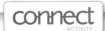

Source: "2013 Sleep in America Poll: Exercise and Sleep," National Sleep Foundation, 2013, www.sleepfoundation.org/2013poll.

Chapter 2, can be used to help induce sleepiness. For example, keep a worry book by your bedside and record bothersome thoughts and problems in it that keep you awake at night. Once you've written them down, tell yourself you'll work on them during daylight hours, and then let go of them. Use your notes to focus energy and attention on these problems over the course of the next few days.

It can also be helpful to develop a bedtime ritual, such as reading, listening to soothing music, or taking a warm (but not too hot) bath; your mind and body will come to associate bedtime with relaxation and peacefulness. Avoid stressful or stimulating activities before bedtime, such as working or paying bills, and dim the lights to let your internal clock know that drowsiness is appropriate. Experiment until you find a method of calming down and relaxing at bedtime that works for you.

If you do have a hard time falling asleep, don't stay in bed longer than 30 minutes. Get up, leave the room, and listen to soothing music or read until you feel sleepy. Listening to classical music 45 minutes before bedtime has been found to help people get to sleep faster and to experience fewer sleep disturbances during the night.[25]

Avoid Eating Too Close to Bedtime Try not to eat heavy meals within 3 hours of bedtime, particularly meals with high fat content. When you are lying down, the force of gravity cannot assist the movement of food from the stomach into the small intestine to complete digestion, and you may experience acid indigestion, often known as heartburn.

Also avoid caffeinated beverages, citrus fruits and juices, and tomato-based products such as pasta sauce because these foods can temporarily weaken the esophageal sphincter. When weakened, this sphincter allows stomach contents to move back into the esophagus, a condition known as *acid reflux*. If you have acid reflux, try raising the head of your bed 6 to 8 inches, which will allow gravity to help empty stomach contents into the small intestine. Tilting the bed is more effective than elevating the upper body with pillows. For those who are overweight, moderate weight loss may reduce discomfort because excessive stomach fat can cause abdominal pressure that contributes to heartburn.[8]

Take a Break from Technology The artificial blue light from computers, televisions, and phones blocks the production of melatonin, the hormone that induces sleep.[30] As a result, those who watch TV or surf the Web too close to bedtime may have a hard time drifting off unless they purchase a computer or TV screen that filters out blue light. Melanopsin is a photopigment expressed by optical cells. Scientists believe melanopsin is a primary regulator of the circadian clock and melatonin (sleep hormone). Melanopsin reacts most strongly to blue light.

The best way to prevent blue light from disturbing sleep is to turn off your electronic devices at least 2 hours before going to sleep. Because this is impractical for most college students, dimming your computer screen's brightness level as it becomes dark outside can help maintain normal melatonin levels. Wearing glasses with orange lenses at night can effectively filter out blue light. A similar strategy is to turn off the blue in your screen's color palette, which will give the screen a red hue. Red hue does not interfere with melatonin.[31]

The 2011 Sleep in America Poll examined which age groups were more likely to use electronics like cell phones, computers, and televisions within an hour of bedtime.[20] The poll identified four groups: generation Z (age 13 to 18 at the time of the poll), generation Y (age 18 to 29), generation X (age 30 to 45), and baby boomers (age 46 to 64). Overall, 39 percent of Americans brought their smartphones with them to bed and used them while trying to go to sleep. Those in generation Z (72 percent) and generation Y (67 percent) were more likely to do so. Twenty-two percent of the respondents in all age groups left their cell phone ringer on while they slept, which probably explains why 1 in 10 of the respondents were awakened at least a few nights every week by phone calls, text messages, or e-mails. About 61 percent of those polled said they used their computers or laptops a few nights a week within an hour of trying to go to sleep. This habit was more prevalent in generations Z (77 percent) and Y (73 percent) than generation X (59 percent) and baby boomers (51 percent). Television use before sleeping was also higher among generations Z and Y.[30,31]

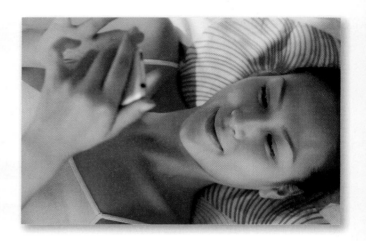

Some college students are so addicted to their smartphone that they text and update their social media while they're half-asleep. This behavior not only interrupts sleep architecture, it can lead to awkward and embarrassing texts. It takes about 30 seconds for people who are awakened from sleep to realize that they are awake. This means sleeping students who text in response to the beep of their smartphone are likely to send a garbled message and have no memory of sleep texting the next morning.[32]

Communicating during sleep is not a new activity. Texting has just replaced the phone. People have long answered phone calls in the middle of the night with no memory of the conversation in the morning. This has been referred to as the "on-call" effect because doctors are especially prone to this behavior.[32] In other words, sleep texting is an arousal disorder; the person is awakened by an outside stimulus and responds while being half-consious.[32] For a good night's sleep, turn off the phone.

Remember Air Quality Irritating agents such as allergens in the air disrupt sleep and increase the risk of upper respiratory infections. Typical air irritants include cigarette smoke, pollen, dust mites, and pet dander. Poor ventilation will aggravate the effects of the irritants, so open your bedroom windows at least once a week to allow fresh air to flow through your dwelling. Replace filters in air conditioners and air purifiers every three months.

Get Rid of Dust Mites Dust mites are microscopic insects that feed on dead skin cells. They live primarily in pillows and mattresses. Dust mite droppings become airborne and are inhaled while people are sleeping, causing allergic reactions and asthma in sensitive individuals. If you experience itchy or watery eyes, sneezing, wheezing, congestion, or difficulty breathing in your bedroom, the culprit may be dust mites. Wash your bed linen regularly. You may also using dust mite prevention sheets and bed linens.

Be Smart About Napping The typical North American adult takes one or two naps a week, and about a third of adults nap more than four times a week. About a fourth never take a nap. If you are a napper, sleep experts recommend naps of only 15 to 45 minutes, which can be refreshing and restorative. If you nap longer than 45 minutes, your body can enter stage 4 deep sleep. It is more difficult to awaken from this stage, and you are likely to feel groggy.[33]

If you know you will be going to bed later than usual, you may want to take a "preventive nap" of 2 to 3 hours. Research suggests that people who take preventive naps increase their alertness by about 30 percent over that of people who do not nap. Napping 15 minutes every 4 hours until you attain 2 hours of preventive napping is also recommended. This short-nap strategy has been effectively used by physicians and law enforcement officers, who must perform in emergency situations for long hours.[33]

Consider Your Bed Partner Thirty-seven percent of Americans snore regularly. More men snore than women. However, after menopause women snore as much as men.[9] Snoring is a major disrupter of partners' sleep, and body movement during sleep can also be a problem for partners. Avoiding alcohol before bedtime, using nasal sprays, sleeping on your side, and using a humidifier may help reduce snoring.

Men tend to thrash around in bed more than women do, and older couples tend to move in less compatible ways than do younger couples. A firm mattress with low motion transfer may help prevent sleep disruption caused by a partner's movement. Sleep can also be disrupted if a partner has a different sleep schedule or has a sleep disorder. If your partner's sleep habits create a problem for you, encourage your partner to improve his or her sleep habits or to see a sleep disorder specialist. As a last resort, you or your partner may have to sleep in different beds or rooms.

Using Sleep Aids

Because sleep is so influential in daily functioning, and because sleep problems are so common, it should not be surprising that many people resort to sleep aids of one kind or another to help them get a good night's sleep. About 15 percent of adults use a prescription sleep medication and/or an over-the-counter sleep aid a few nights a week.[34]

Prescription Medications About 4 percent of adults aged 20 and older use prescription sleep medications like Lunesta and Ambien. The safest and most effective sleep medications are ones that you can take at various doses, are not addictive, do not produce serious side effects, and wear off quickly so that you are not drowsy the next day. Sleep experts disagree about whether today's sleep medications meet these criteria.[27] No sleep medication should be used for longer than two weeks without consulting a physician.

The most frequently prescribed longer-acting sleep medications are the benzodiazepines Restoril, Dalmon, and Doral. These drugs induce sleep but suppress both deep sleep and REM sleep. Their effects can last from 3 to 24 hours, and daytime side effects include decreased memory and intellectual functioning. People quickly build tolerance to long-lasting benzodiazepines, which are addictive and lose

their effectiveness after 30 nights of consecutive use. There are some shorter-acting benzodiazepines on the market that do not suppress deep sleep and REM sleep.[34] A new category of sleep medications is the imidazopyridines. The National Sleep Foundation (NSF) considers these drugs the best prescription sleeping aids.[34] One drug in this category, zolpidem, sold under the trade name Ambien, has become the best-selling prescription sleep aid in the United States, but it has been associated with some disturbing side effects. Although the NSF endorses imidazopyridines as the best category of sleep medications, it has major concerns about Ambien. Ambien has been required to more specifically identify cognitive distortion side effects on its label, such as sleep driving and sleep-related binge eating disorder.

rebound insomnia
Insomnia that occurs after a person stops taking sleep medication and that is worse than it was before the medication was started.

Over-the-Counter Medications
Nonprescription, or over-the-counter, medications can be useful for treating transient or short-term insomnia, such as may occur under conditions of great stress or trauma. They should be discontinued once the cause of the problem has been eliminated, ideally within two weeks. The recommended maximum use is four weeks.

Many over-the-counter sleep products contain antihistamine, a type of drug developed to treat allergies. The effects of antihistamines are general throughout the body; besides drowsiness, they cause dehydration, agitation, and constipation. Additionally, you can quickly develop tolerance to antihistamines, and when you stop taking them, you may experience **rebound insomnia**— insomnia that is worse than what

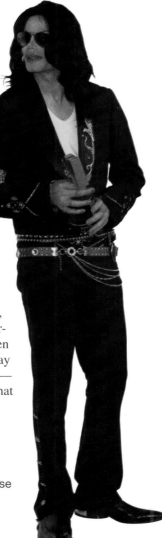

■ Pop star Michael Jackson became dependent on powerful anesthetics, which he used to help himself fall asleep. He died of an overdose of propofol, an anesthetic normally used to sedate patients for major surgery.

Consumer Clipboard

Insomnia and Sleep Aids

About 20 percent of college students report that they have insomnia, and in most cases the easiest and safest cure is simply to correct poor sleep habits. However, many people resort to over-the-counter (OTC) sleep aids, especially when all other measures have failed to help them get to sleep. OTC sleep aids can be a safe way to combat insomnia in the short term, but it is important to be a smart consumer when choosing and using a sleep aid. Compare the labels before you buy.

Keep in mind that no matter what the label tells you, a sleep aid is only a short-term solution. It is vitally important to make an appointment with your student health clinic or family physician if your insomnia persists for two or three weeks.

Know that "natural" does not always mean safer.
Herbal products are typically labeled upfront as supplements, not drugs. Active ingredients typically include valerian and melatonin, which also induce sleep. It is important to remember that these supplements do not undergo the same rigorous testing required by prescriptive medications for FDA approval.

Check the inactive ingredients.
If there is any ingredient that you know you are allergic to or should not ingest, do not take this medication.

Read the warnings.
Do not drink alcohol with sleep medications. Take sleep medication only within half an hour of going to sleep. Do not take sleep medications if you have sleep apnea or any other conditions that are listed in this section on the label. Use the label to confirm that any medications you currently take will not conflict with the sleep aid.

Know what the active ingredients do.
Most FDA-approved sleep aids contain either doxylamine or diphenhydramine, both of which are antihistamines. Aside from combating allergies by blocking histamines in the brain, these drugs are known to promote sleep.

Begin with the lowest possible effective dose recommended on the label.

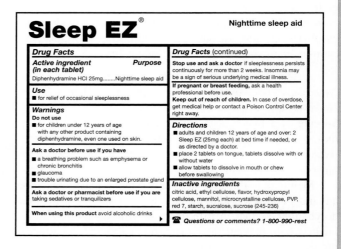

Source: "Sleep Aids and Insomnia," by the National Sleep Foundation, www.sleepfoundation.org/article/sleep-related-problems/sleep-aids-and-insomnia.

you experienced before you started taking the medication.[27] Rebound insomnia can be avoided by gradually reducing the dose. Over-the-counter products like Tylenol PM that contain acetaminophen should also be used with caution. Large doses of acetaminophen are toxic to the liver and can cause severe liver damage. Learn what to look for when shopping for sleep aids in the box, "Insomnia and Sleep Aids."

Complementary and Alternative Products and Approaches Complementary and alternative products and approaches to sleep problems include herbal products, dietary supplements, aromatherapy, and relaxation drinks. The herbal product most commonly used for insomnia is valerian, which has a tranquilizing or sedative effect. Hops is another product currently receiving attention as a possible sleep aid. Both are widely available in health food stores. Herbal products can interact with other medications and drugs, including caffeine and alcohol; it is strongly recommended that you consult with your physician before trying any herbal remedies.[34]

The dietary supplement melatonin has been marketed as a sleep aid, but health experts are divided on its effectiveness. As noted earlier in this chapter, melatonin is a hormone naturally secreted by the pineal gland in response to darkness. It lowers body temperature and causes drowsiness. Most experts agree that the 3-milligram dose of synthetically produced melatonin available in health food stores is too high and that a dose of 0.1 milligram is as effective as a higher dose.[27,34] Potential side effects, interactions with drugs, and long-term health effects of melatonin supplements have not been studied extensively. Take caution because some studies have reported increased risk of heart attack, infertility, fatigue, and depression with melatonin use.

In aromatherapy, certain essential oils, such as jasmine and lavender, are used to induce relaxation and sleepiness. Aromatherapists believe these oils relieve insomnia by reducing stress, enhancing moods, and easing respiratory or muscular problems, but no strong scientific evidence supports these claims.[27] Aromatherapy oils may be applied to the skin by full body massage, or a drop may be placed on the wrist or at the base of the throat so the scent is inhaled during sleep. Scented sprays can be used on bed linens, but aromatherapy candles should not be burning when you are sleeping. Aromatherapy products are generally available in health food stores. If you are interested in trying this approach, however, it is recommended that you consult a trained aromatherapist before making any purchases.

Relaxation drinks, also known as anti-energy drinks, are being marketed to high school and college students as a product to facilitate relaxation and sleep. Examples include Drank, Mary Jane's Relaxing Soda, Koma Unwind, Chill, and Slow Cow. They commonly contain herbal ingredients or dietary supplements such as kava, valerian root, rose hips, passionflower, theanine, and melatonin. Some relaxation drinks contain warnings that they can cause drowsiness and discourage driving after use. It is important to remember that this is an emerging market and relaxation drinks have not received sufficient scientific research as to safety and benefits. The Food and Drug Administration (FDA) does not strictly regulate dietary supplements like these. The FDA, however, is critical of melatonin in drinks because it is a hormone. Canna Cola is also grabbing attention—it is a marijuana-infused soft drink that contains THC, which is the hallucinogenic ingredient in marijuana. Canna Cola sales are restricted to medical marijuana dispensaries.[35,36]

It is not surprising that people go to great lengths to get enough high-quality sleep. Nothing is as refreshing and restorative as a good night's sleep, giving us a fresh perspective and renewed energy for facing the demands of the day. Shakespeare called sleep the "balm of hurt minds, chief nourisher in life's feast." Sleep, he wrote, "knits up the ravell'd sleeve of care." Conversely, almost nothing is as distressing as being unable to avail ourselves of the respite provided by sleep. Chronic sleep deprivation can interfere with physical, emotional, and cognitive functioning and leave us fatigued, depressed, and more susceptible to illness and disease. As with so many other facets of lifestyle, good sleep habits and practices, established early in life, can help you maintain wellness in both younger and older adulthood.

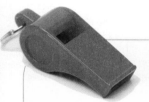

You Make the Call

Should Colleges Conduct Random Drug Tests for Adderall?

Between 4 and 35 percent of students say that they use stimulant medications like Ritalin, Adderall, and Provigil to help them study, which qualifies as an off-label (illegal) use. Adderall has become the stimulant of choice for most college students because it has fewer side effects than Ritalin and produces a steadier, longer-lasting effect than Ritalin.

Students suffering from ADHD have trouble focusing on a single task for any length of time; Adderall enhances concentration. Because many students with ADHD do not want a perpetual state of mental arousal, they use Adderall only for studying. This means that they are likely to have a surplus of Adderall pills. According to the law, they are supposed to legally discard surplus pills. However, some students choose to give them away to friends or sell them to other students.

Some college administrators believe that students on their campuses fake symptoms of ADHD to obtain a prescription for Adderall for their own use, to share with friends, or to sell to other students, even though selling a prescribed stimulant drug is a felony. On some campuses, physicians will not prescribe stimulants or will prescribe only a 15- or 30-day supply at a time.

Many students resist the message that stimulant drugs like Adderall can be dangerous. They view the illegal use of such drugs as morally acceptable because they are primarily used for academic performance rather than social recreation. They say the drugs help them focus better, give them an extra edge, and help meet the demands of active social lives and academic schedules. Health experts warn that the risks aren't worth it.

When Bill Haas ran for Congress in Missouri in 2010, he promised voters that he would push for legislation to require random drug testing on college campuses at state-funded colleges and universities. He believed that such tests would detect the off-label use of prescription drugs. He lost the election. But a growing chorus of voices is calling for such legislation. So, should random drug testing for off-label use of drugs like Adderall be conducted on college campuses and universities?

Pros

- The health side effects for Adderall for a student who does not have ADHD are risky.
- Off-label use of a prescribed drug is a felony under the Federal Controlled Substances Act.
- One study found that as many as 34 to 60 percent of undergraduate students are taking stimulants like Adderall as a "study buddy." At least 97 percent are using these stimulants illegally or without medical supervision.
- Students illegally using stimulants like Adderall have a mental advantage over students who do not use them. It is a form of cheating and amoral.

Cons

- A lot of things should be banned from college campuses, including alcohol, illegal drugs, smoking, and guns. It is not fair to specifically target off-label use of prescription stimulants.
- Drug manufacturers have developed a slow-release version of Adderall (Adderall XR), which they claim has less potential for abuse.

Continued…

Concluded...

- This is just another example of "nanny" controls that are not needed. The focus should be on students selling Adderall to other students.
- If Adderall was banned on college campuses, it would result in an underground market for this drug. Not all students can afford Adderall. An underground market would place even more students at an unfair advantage in the academic marketplace.

Sources: Data from "Illicit use of Prescription ADHD Medications on a College Campus: A Methodological Approach," by A. D. DeSantis, E. M. Webb, and S. M. Noar, 2008, *Journal of American College Health, 57* (30), pp. 315–323; Pro's and Con's of Adderall, http://storka1.wordpress.com/anti-adderall/; Are Drug Tests for Adderall Coming to a College Near You? http://voices.yahoo.com/are=drug-tests-adderall-coming-college-near-5951862.html?cat=5; "Prescription Stimulants in Individuals with and without Attention Deficit Hyperactivty Disorder: Misuse, Cognitive Impact, and Adverse Effects," by S. E. Lakhan and A. Kirchgessner, 2012, *Brain and Behavior, 2* (5), pp. 661–677, doi:10.1002/brb3.78.

In Review

How does sleep affect your health?

Quantity and quality of sleep are strongly associated with overall health and quality of life. Adequate sleep gives the body time for repair, recovery, and renewal. Sleep deprivation is associated with a wide range of health problems, ranging from cardiovascular disease to depression to overweight and obesity.

What makes you sleep?

Sleep is induced by the activity of a specific set of structures in the brain, in combination with environmental cues such as darkness. Humans have a circadian rhythm slightly longer than 24 hours; every morning the body resets this biological clock to adjust to the next 24-hour cycle.

What is the structure of sleep?

Every night, people cycle through several stages of sleep, characterized by different brain waves, different states of muscle relaxation, and different nervous system activity. NREM sleep includes stages of deep sleep, whereas REM sleep includes dreaming and brain activity related to the consolidation of learning and memory.

What are common sleep disorders?

Insomnia, or difficulty falling or staying asleep, is experienced by 30 to 40 percent of adults. Sleep apnea, or periods during sleep when breathing stops, is almost as common, but men are more at risk for it than women. About 1 to 15 percent of the population sleepwalk. Nighttime eating disorders are somewhat less common; if the person is unaware that he or she is eating, it is a sleep disorder, but if the person wakes up frequently during the night to eat, it is an eating disorder. Sleep problems can be diagnosed with sleep latency tests, sleep diaries, or evaluation in a sleep lab.

How can you enhance the quality of your sleep?

The key to a good night's sleep is good sleep habits, such as a regular sleep schedule, a sleep-friendly environment, avoiding stimulants late in the day, exercising regularly, managing stress, not eating heavy meals close to bedtime, turning off electronics 2 hours before you plan to go to sleep, and being considerate of your sleep partner. Sleep aids, whether prescription, over the counter, or alternative, can help with situational sleep problems but shouldn't be used long term. Alternative approaches to sleep include herbal products, dietary supplements, and aromatherapy. Valerian and hops are examples of herbal products. Melatonin is a common but controversial dietary supplement to promote sleep. Jasmine and lavender are oils that induce sleep by reducing stress, relaxing muscles, and enhancing mood. Relaxation drinks are a relatively new product containing herbal products or dietary supplements.

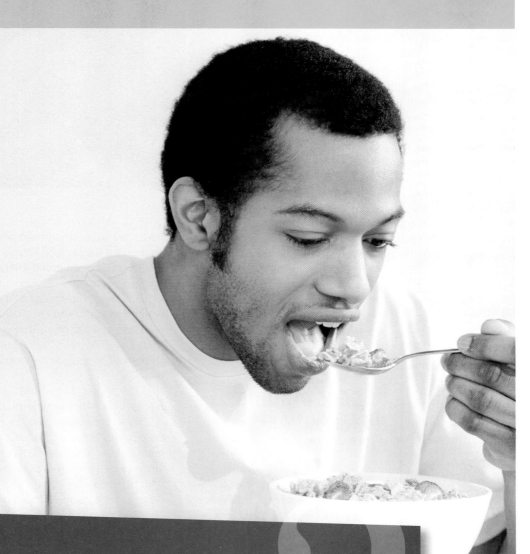

Ever Wonder...

- why some fats are good for you and others aren't?
- if organic food is better for you than conventional food?
- if multivitamins make people healthier?

Your day begins with a bagel spread with cream cheese and a jolt of caffeine from freshly brewed coffee. Mid-morning hunger pangs are relieved by an energy bar and an energy drink. Lunch at the local fast-food place includes a cheeseburger, fries, and a soda. Another energy bar in mid-afternoon, accompanied by a bottle of water, tides you over to dinner. Still, you're so hungry when you get to the campus food court that you overindulge, downing several soft tacos with salsa, shredded lettuce, and sour cream. Late-night studying is supported by the consumption of popcorn, cookies, and another energy bar. Welcome to college dining!

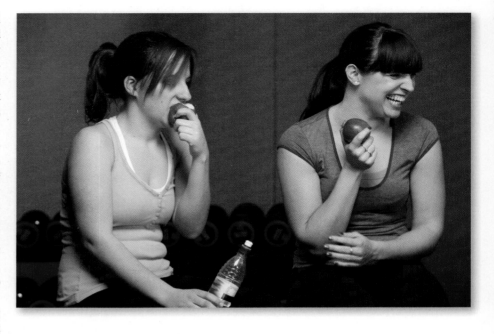

Unfortunately, healthy dining can be a challenge in a culture that promotes the consumption of fast foods and convenience foods in shopping malls, sports arenas, airports, and college dining halls. Many people have acquired a taste for the high-calorie, full-fat, heavily salted foods so plentiful in our environment. It *is* possible to choose a healthy diet, however, and this chapter will help you see how, starting with research-based guidelines for healthy eating.

UNDERSTANDING NUTRITIONAL GUIDELINES

In 1997, the National Academies' Food and Nutrition Board introduced the **Dietary Reference Intakes (DRIs)**, a set of recommendations designed to promote optimal health and prevent both nutritional deficiencies and chronic diseases like cancer and cardiovascular disease. The DRIs, developed by American and Canadian scientists, encompass four kinds of recommendations. The *Estimated Average Requirement (EAR)* is the amount of nutrients needed by half of the people in any one age group, for example, teenage boys. Nutritionists use the EARs to assess whether an entire population's normal diet provides sufficient nutrients. The

EARs are used in nutrition research and as a basis for recommended dietary allowances.[1,2]

The **Recommended Dietary Allowance (RDA)** represents the average daily amount of any one nutrient an individual needs to protect against nutritional deficiency. If there is not enough information about a nutrient to set an RDA, the Food and Nutrition Board provides an *Adequate Intake (AI)*. The *Tolerable Upper Intake Level (UL)* is the highest amount of a nutrient a person can take in without risking toxicity.

The Food and Nutrition Board also provides the **Acceptable Macronutrient Distribution Range (AMDR)**. AMDRs represent intake levels of essential nutrients associated with reduced risk of chronic disease while providing adequate nutrition. If your intake exceeds the AMDR, you increase your risk of chronic disease. For example, the AMDR for dietary fat for adult men is 20 to 35 percent of the calories consumed in a day. A man who consumes more than 35 percent of his daily calories as fat increases his risk for chronic diseases [1,2]

Whereas the DRIs are recommended intake levels for individual nutrients, the *Dietary Guidelines for Americans* provide scientifically based diet and exercise recommendations designed to promote health and reduce the risk of chronic disease. The *Dietary Guidelines*, first published in 1980 and revised every five years by the U.S. Department of Agriculture (USDA) and the U.S. Department of Health and Human Services, is the cornerstone of U.S. nutrition policy. The most recent version was published in 2010. These guidelines will be discussed in detail later in the chapter.

To translate DRIs and the *Dietary Guidelines* into healthy food choices, the USDA publishes **MyPlate**, a graphic nutritional tool that can be customized for different calorie needs. The Food and Drug Administration (FDA)

Dietary Reference Intakes (DRIs)
An umbrella term for four sets of dietary recommendations: Estimated Average Requirement, Recommended Dietary Allowances, Adequate Intake, and Tolerable Upper Intake Level; designed to promote optimal health and prevent both nutritional deficiencies and chronic diseases.

Recommended Dietary Allowance (RDA)
The average daily amount of any one nutrient an individual needs to protect against nutritional deficiency.

Acceptable Macronutrient Distribution Range (AMDR)
Intake ranges that provide adequate nutrition and that are associated with reduced risk of chronic disease.

developed the **Daily Values** used on food labels to indicate how a particular food contributes to the recommended daily intake of major nutrients in a 2,000-calorie diet.[1,2]

Before we explore how you can use these tools to choose a healthy diet, we take a look at the major nutrients that make up our diet. For each nutrient, we include general recommendations for intake based on either the DRIs or the AMDRs.

TYPES OF NUTRIENTS

As you engage in daily activities, your body is powered by energy produced from the food you eat. Your body needs the **essential nutrients**—water, carbohydrates, proteins, fats, vitamins, and minerals—contained in these foods, but not only to provide fuel. They are also needed to build, maintain, and repair tissues; regulate body functions; and support the communication among cells that allows you to be a living, sensing human being.

We need large quantities of *macronutrients*—water, carbohydrates, protein, and fat—for energy and important functions like building new cells and facilitating chemical reactions. We need only small amounts of *micronutrients*—vitamins and minerals—for regulating body functions. People who fail to consume adequate amounts of an essential nutrient are likely to develop a nutritional deficiency disease, such as kwashiorkor from inadequate protein or scurvy from lack of vitamin C. Nutritional deficiency diseases are seldom seen in developed countries because most people consume an adequate diet.

Water—The Unappreciated Nutrient

You can live without the other nutrients for weeks, but you can survive without water for only a few days. We need water to digest, absorb, and transport nutrients. Water helps regulate body temperature, carries waste products out of the body, and lubricates our moving parts.[1]

The right *fluid balance*—the right amount of fluid inside and outside each cell—is maintained through the action of substances called **electrolytes**, minerals that carry electrical charges and conduct nerve impulses. Electrolytes include sodium, potassium, and chloride. Water and a balanced diet, replaces electrolytes lost daily through sweat.[2]

Many people assume bottled water is purer and safer than tap water, but for the most part the water supply in the United States is well regulated and very safe. The Environmental Protection Agency (EPA) sets standards for water quality and inspects water supplies for bacteria and toxic chemicals. (Some bottled water is drawn from municipal water supplies, including Coca-Cola's Dasani and Pepsi's Aquafina, despite ads and labels showing pristine springs and snowy mountain peaks.) You can check the quality of your community's water supply at the National Drinking Water Database (www.ewg.org/tap-water/whats -in-yourwater.php).

In contrast, the FDA regulates bottled water only if it is shipped across state lines. About 70 percent is bottled and sold within the same state, so it is exempt from FDA inspection. Federal regulations do not require bottled water companies to list how their water was purified, the results of any contaminant tests, or any other safety information. Bottled water has been found to contain contaminants, and health experts warn that it lacks fluoride, which is added to most water supplies and prevents tooth decay. Additionally, Americans typically discard and do not recycle water bottles.

What about water that's been enhanced with vitamins, minerals, and other nutrients? Although they offer a colorful and flavorful alternative to plain water, they add little nutritional value to the typical American diet because the average American adult consumes 100 percent of the DRI for most vitamins. They do pack a wallop when it comes to

Dietary Guidelines for Americans
Set of scientifically based recommendations designed to promote health and reduce the risk for many chronic diseases through diet and physical activity.

MyPlate
Graphic nutritional tool developed by the USDA that can be customized depending on your calorie needs.

Daily Values
Set of dietary standards used on food labels to indicate how a particular food contributes to the recommended daily intake of major nutrients in a 2,000-calorie diet.

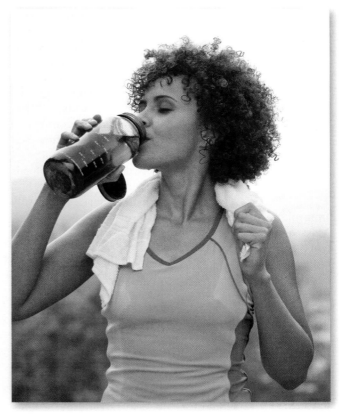

■ Water is an essential nutrient. In most communities in the United States, the quality and safety of tap water are equal or superior to the quality and safety of bottled water.

essential nutrients
Chemical substances used by the body to build, maintain, and repair tissues and regulate body functions. They cannot be manufactured by the body and must be obtained from foods or supplements.

electrolytes
Mineral components that carry electrical charges and conduct nerve impulses.

simple carbohydrates
Easily digestible carbohydrates composed of one or two units of sugar.

glycogen
The complex carbohydrate form in which glucose is stored in the liver and muscles.

added sugars
Sugars that are added to foods when they are processed.

complex carbohydrates
Carbohydrates that are composed of multiple sugar units and that must be broken down further before they can be used by the body.

starches
Complex carbohydrates found in many plant foods.

added sugars, however. A 20-ounce bottle of Vitaminwater, for example, has 31 to 32 grams of sugar (two heaping tablespoons) and 120 calories, about the same as a soft drink.

Adults generally need 1 to 1.5 milliliters of water for each calorie spent in the day. If you expend 2,000 calories a day, you require 2 to 3 liters—8 to 12 cups—of fluids.[3] Heavy sweating increases your need for fluids. You obtain fluids not only from the water you drink, but also from the water in foods, particularly fruits such as oranges and apples. Caffeinated beverages and alcohol are not good sources of your daily fluid intake because of their dehydrating effects, although some recent research suggests that the water in such beverages may offset these effects to some extent.[3]

Carbohydrates— Your Body's Fuel

Carbohydrates are the body's main source of energy.[3] They fuel most of the body's cells during daily activities; they are used by muscle cells during high-intensity exercise; and they are the only source of energy for brain cells, red blood cells, and some other types of cells. Athletes in particular need to consume a high-carbohydrate diet to fuel their high-energy activities.

Carbohydrates are the foods we think of as sugars and starches. They come almost exclusively from plants (the exception is lactose, the sugar in milk). Most of the carbohydrates and other nutrients we need come from grains, seeds, fruits, and vegetables.[2] Carbohydrates are divided into simple carbohydrates and complex carbohydrates.

Simple Carbohydrates **Simple carbohydrates** are easily digestible carbohydrates composed of one or two units of sugar. Six simple carbohydrates (sugars) are important in nutrition: glucose, fructose, galactose, lactose, maltose, and sucrose. Sugars are absorbed into the bloodstream and travel to body cells, where they can be used for energy. Glucose is the main source of energy for the brain and nervous system. Glucose also travels to the liver and muscles, where it can be stored as **glycogen** (a complex carbohydrate) for future energy needs.

When you eat food containing large amounts of simple carbohydrates, sugar enters your bloodstream quickly, giving you a burst of energy, or a "sugar high." It is also absorbed into your cells quickly, leaving you feeling depleted and craving more sugar; see the box, "Is Sugar Addictive?" Foods containing **added sugars**, such as candy bars and sodas, have an even more dramatic effect. Consumption of sugar has been linked to the epidemic of overweight and obesity in the United States and to the parallel increase in the incidence of diabetes, a disorder in which body cells cannot use the sugar circulating in the blood. Similar health concerns have been raised about high fructose corn syrup (HFCS), a highly processed alternative sweetener made from corn. HFCS has replaced sugar in hundreds of foods, ranging from sodas to breads to lunch meats. It has the same effects on the body as sugar.

The Food and Nutrition Board recommends that no more than 10 percent of calories come from added sugars, and many health professionals recommend only 10 percent.[4] According to the American Heart Association, most American women should consume no more than 100 calories per day of sugar (about 6 teaspoons) and men no more than 150 calories per day (9 teaspoons). See the box, "Sugar Consumption Among Adults by Age, Gender, and Income."

To cut back on sugar, check for food label ingredients like sugar, corn syrup, fructose, dextrose, molasses, and evaporated cane juice. You may be surprised at the relatively high sugar content of many foods. For example, two servings of spaghetti sauce can contain almost five-and-a-half teaspoons of sugars.[4,5]

Because of the negative health effects of sugar, particularly weight gain and tooth decay, sugar substitutes have been developed as alternative low-calorie sweeteners. Some are naturally occurring (e.g., stevia, sorbitol, xylitol), but most are synthetic and are usually referred to as artificial sweeteners (e.g., saccharin, aspartame, sucralose). Many artificial sweeteners are intensely sweet— hundreds of times sweeter than sugar—so very small amounts can be added to foods or beverages without adding calories. Concerns have been raised about the safety of artificial sweeteners, but the FDA has determined that they are safe if used in recommended amounts. Still under investigation is the possibility that alternative sweeteners actually result in weight gain due to their effect on appetite and insulin response, a factor in feelings of hunger and fullness.

Complex Carbohydrates The type of carbohydrates called **complex carbohydrates** is composed of multiple sugar units and includes starches and dietary fiber. **Starches** occur in grains, vegetables, and some fruits. Most starchy foods also contain ample portions of vitamins, minerals, proteins, and water. Starches must be broken down into single sugars in the digestive system before they can be absorbed into the bloodstream to be used for energy or stored for future use.

Starting the Conversation

Is Sugar Addictive?

Q: Is sugar toxic?

This question was posed in a recent *60 Minutes* episode. The experts who were interviewed claimed that sugar is not only toxic, but addictive. A neuroscientist on the program used MRI scans to show that sugar activates the same regions in the brain as cocaine does. Your brain releases dopamine after you eat sugar. Dopamine controls pleasure in the brain. Eating something with sugar triggers a cycle that increases craving for sugar. The more sugar you consume, the higher your tolerance level to prevent a sugar rush. Tolerance is one of the symptoms of a substance dependence. Consuming lots of sugar causes a spike in insulin, which is followed by a glucose crash. People generally compensate for the glucose crash by consuming more sugar. The up-and-down cycle of a sugar crash can disrupt your body's ability to metabolize sugar, which can lead to diseases like diabetes.

According to the medical community, a substance is addictive if it meets four criteria: (1) induces a pleasant state or relieves stress; (2) causes long-term changes in brain chemistry; (3) leads to adaptation changes in the brain that trigger tolerance, physical dependence, and uncontrollable cravings; and (4) causes substance dependence so that abstaining causes severe physical and mental reactions. Many neuroscientists argue that sugar does not meet the four criteria, particularly physical dependence.

Research does suggest that calorie-dense food that is high in sugar can elicit brain-chemistry changes that mirror addiction. Cravings are powerful desires to pursue natural rewards such as food pleasure. Your brain has a "stop" circuitry that serves as a brake on cravings. People with a weak brake circuitry are likely to have more difficulty in managing cravings. Food high in sugar can serve as a cue (signal) that activates the brain circuitry "go" system even if a person is not conscious of the cue. Still, some food scientists view sugar as habit-forming and potentially toxic but not addictive.

Research on food addiction is in its infancy. Most of this research has focused on sugar. Studies on rats do suggest that overeating sugar may dampen the dopamine response and cause changes in the dopamine system that also leads to changes in the brain cortex. The functions of the cortex include exerting control, making decisions, and exercising judgment. These changes in brain chemistry for humans who overconsume sugar have not been empirically established.

There are endless websites and anecdotal reports claiming sugar is addictive. But empirical evidence has not yet validated this claim. The key word is "yet." Do you think growing research on sugar will conclude that it is addictive?

Q: What do we do with this information about sugar addiction? Would giving up sugar be as difficult as giving up smoking? Alcohol? Cocaine? Should we advocate for an abstinence model of sugar?

Q: Do you think you are addicted to sugar? What steps can you take to limit sugar intake?

Sources: "Is Sugar Toxic?" by S. Gupta (interviewing Robert Lustig, Kimber Stanhope, Lewis Cantley, Eric Stice, and Jim Simon), April 1, 2012, *60 Minutes,* retrieved from www.cbsnews.com/8301-18560_162-57407294/sugar/; "Food Addiction: Can Some Foods Hijack the Brain?" by B. Liebman, May 2012, *Nutrition Action Healthletter,* pp. 3–7; "Probing Question: Is Sugar Addictive?" by L. Duchene, January 16, 2006, *Penn State News,* retrieved from http://news.psu.edu/story/141336/2006/01/16/research/probing-question-sugar-addictive.

Whole grains are often refined to make them easier to digest and more appealing to the consumer, but the refining process removes many of the vitamins, minerals, and other nutritious components. Refined carbohydrates include white rice; white bread, pasta, and other products made from white flour; and sweet desserts. About 90 percent of the grains Americans consume are refined.[1] Like sugar, refined carbohydrates can enter the bloodstream quickly and just as quickly leave you feeling hungry again. Whole grains (such as whole wheat, brown rice, oatmeal, and corn) are preferred because they provide more nutrients, slow the digestive process, and make you feel full longer. The consumption of whole grains lowers the risk of diabetes, obesity, heart disease, and some forms of cancer.[6–8]

The RDA for carbohydrates is 130 grams for males and females aged 1 to 70 years. The AMDR for carbohydrates is 45 to 65 percent of daily energy intake, which amounts to 225 to 325 grams in a 2,000-calorie diet (even though only about 130 grams per day are enough to meet the body's needs). In the typical American diet, carbohydrates contribute about half of all calories, and most of them are in the form of simple sugars or highly refined grains. Instead, carbohydrates should come from a diverse spectrum of whole grains and other starches, vegetables, and fruits.[9]

Fiber **Dietary fiber**, a complex carbohydrate found in plants, cannot be broken down in the digestive tract. A diet rich in dietary fiber makes stools soft and bulky. They pass through the intestines rapidly and are expelled easily, helping to prevent hemorrhoids and constipation.[8,10] Some foods contain **functional fiber**, natural or synthetic fiber that has been added to increase the healthful effects of the food. **Total fiber** refers to the combined amount of dietary fiber and functional fiber in a food.

dietary fiber
A complex carbohydrate found in plants that cannot be broken down in the digestive tract.

functional fiber
Natural or synthetic fiber that has been added to food.

total fiber
Combined amount of dietary fiber and functional fiber in a food.

Who's at Risk?

Sugar Consumption Among Adults by Age, Gender, and Income

Compare these graphs to the recommendations of the Food and Nutrition Board and the American Heart Association about consumption of sugar.

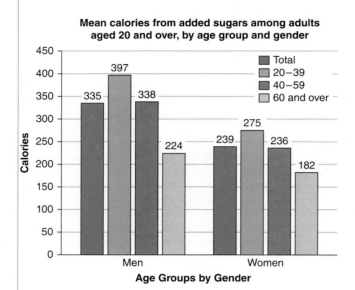

Mean calories from added sugars among adults aged 20 and over, by age group and gender

Legend: Total, 20–39, 40–59, 60 and over

Men: 335, 397, 338, 224
Women: 239, 275, 236, 182

Y-axis: Calories (0–450)
X-axis: Age Groups by Gender

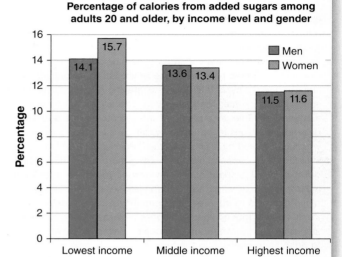

Percentage of calories from added sugars among adults 20 and older, by income level and gender

Legend: Men, Women

Lowest income: 14.1, 15.7
Middle income: 13.6, 13.4
Highest income: 11.5, 11.6

Y-axis: Percentage (0–16)
X-axis: Income Level

connect ACTIVITY

Source: "NCHS Data Brief. Consumption of Added Sugars Among Adults, 2005–2010," by B. Ervin and C. L. Ogden, May 2013, *NCHS Data Brief* no. 122, Centers for Disease Control and Prevention, www.cdc.gov/nchs/data/databriefs/db122.htm.

---

protein
Essential nutrient made up of amino acids, needed to build and maintain muscles, bones, and other body tissues.

Dietary fiber that dissolves in water, referred to as *soluble fiber,* is known to lower blood cholesterol levels and can slow the process of digestion so that blood sugar levels remain more even. Dietary fiber that does not dissolve in water, called *insoluble fiber,* passes through the digestive tract essentially unchanged. Because it absorbs water, insoluble fiber helps you feel full after eating and stimulates your intestinal wall to contract and relax, serving as a natural laxative.

The RDAs for fiber are 25 grams for women aged 19 to 50 and 38 grams for men aged 14 to 50 (or 14 grams of fiber for every 1,000 calories consumed). For people over 50, the RDA is 21 grams for women and 30 grams for men.[1] The typical American diet provides only about 14 or 15 grams of fiber a day. If you want to increase the fiber in your diet, it is important to do so gradually. A sudden increase in daily fiber may cause bloating, gas, abdominal cramping, or even a bowel obstruction, particularly if you fail to drink enough liquids to easily carry the fiber through the body.[2]

Fiber is best obtained through diet. Pills and other fiber supplements do not contain the nutrients found in high-fiber foods.[2] Excessive amounts of fiber (generally 60 grams or more per day) can decrease the absorption of important vitamins and minerals such as calcium, zinc, magnesium, and iron.[10] Fruits, vegetables, dried beans, peas and other legumes, cereals, grains, nuts, and seeds are the best sources of dietary fiber.

Protein—Nutritional Muscle

Your body uses **protein** to build and maintain muscles, bones, and other body tissues. Proteins also form enzymes that in turn facilitate chemical reactions. Proteins are constructed from 20 different amino acids. There are nine amino acids that your body cannot produce on its own. These are called **essential amino acids**, and they must be supplied by foods. Those that can be produced by your body are called nonessential amino acids.

Food sources of protein include both animals and plants. Animal proteins (meat, fish, poultry, milk, cheese, and eggs) are usually a good source of **complete proteins**, meaning they contain ample amounts of all the essential amino acids. Vegetable proteins (grains, legumes, nuts, seeds, and vegetables) provide **incomplete proteins**, meaning they contain small amounts of essential amino acids or some, but not all, of the essential amino acids. If you do not consume sufficient amounts of the essential amino acids, body organ functions may be compromised.

People who eat little or no animal protein may not be getting all the essential amino acids they need. One remedy is to eat plant foods with different amounts of incomplete proteins. For example, beans are low in the essential amino acid methionine but high in lysine, and rice is high in methionine and low in lysine. In combination, beans and rice form *complementary proteins*. Eating the two over the course of a day provides all the essential amino acids.[2] The matching of such foods is called *mutual supplementation*.

The AMDR for protein is 10 to 35 percent of daily calories consumed.[3] The need for protein is based on body weight: the larger your body, the more protein you need to take in. A healthy adult typically needs 0.8 gram of protein for every kilogram (2.2 pounds) of body weight, or about 0.36 gram for every pound.[3] At the upper end of the AMDR range, the percentages provide a more than ample amount of protein in the diet.

Fats—A Necessary Nutrient

Fats are a concentrated energy source and the principal form of stored energy in the body. The fats in food provide essential fatty acids, play a role in the production of other fatty acids and vitamin D, and provide the major material for cell membranes and for the myelin sheaths that surround nerve fibers. They assist in the absorption of the fat-soluble vitamins (A, D, E, and K) and affect the texture, taste, and smell of foods. Fats provide an emergency reserve when we are sick or our food intake is diminished.

Types of Fat Fats, or lipids, are composed of fatty acids. Nutritionists divide these acids into three groups—saturated, monounsaturated, and polyunsaturated—on the basis of their chemical composition. **Saturated fats** remain stable (solid) at room temperature; **monounsaturated fats** are liquid at room temperature but solidify somewhat when refrigerated; **polyunsaturated fats** are liquid both at room temperature and in the refrigerator. Liquid fats are commonly referred to as oils.

Saturated fatty acids are found in animal sources, such as beef, pork, poultry, and whole-milk dairy products. They are also found in certain tropical oils and nuts, including coconut and palm oil and macadamia nuts. Monounsaturated and polyunsaturated fatty acids are found primarily in plant sources. Olive, safflower, peanut, and canola oils, as well as avocados and many nuts, contain mostly monounsaturated fat. Corn and soybean oils contain mostly polyunsaturated fat, as do many kinds of fish, including salmon, trout, and anchovies.

Cholesterol Saturated fats pose a risk to health because they tend to raise blood levels of **cholesterol**, a waxy substance that can clog arteries, leading to cardiovascular disease. More specifically, saturated fats raise blood levels of low-density lipoproteins (LDLs), known as "bad cholesterol," and triglycerides, another kind of blood fat. Unsaturated fats, in contrast, tend to lower blood levels of LDLs, and some unsaturated fats (monounsaturated fats) may also raise levels of high-density lipoproteins (HDLs), known as "good cholesterol."[11]

Cholesterol is needed for several important body functions, but too much of it circulating in the bloodstream can be a problem. The body produces it in the liver and also obtains it from animal food sources, such as meat, cheese, eggs, and milk. It is recommended that no more than 300 milligrams of dietary cholesterol be consumed per day. The effects of cholesterol on cardiovascular health are discussed in detail in Chapter 15.

Trans Fats Another kind of fatty acid, **trans fatty acid**, is produced through **hydrogenation**, a process whereby liquid vegetable oils are turned into more solid fats. Food manufacturers use hydrogenation to prolong a food's shelf life and change its texture. Peanut butter is frequently hydrogenated, as is margarine. With some hydrogenation, margarine becomes semisoft (tub margarine); with further hydrogenation, it becomes hard (stick margarine).[12]

Trans fatty acids (or trans fats) are believed to pose a risk to cardiovascular health similar to or even greater than that of saturated fats because they tend to raise LDLs and

essential amino acids
Amino acids that the body cannot produce on its own.

complete proteins
Proteins composed of ample amounts of all the essential amino acids.

incomplete proteins
Proteins that contain small amounts of essential amino acids or some, but not all, of the essential amino acids.

fats
Also known as lipids, fats are an essential nutrient composed of fatty acids and used for energy and other body functions.

saturated fats
Lipids that are the predominant fat in animal products and other fats that remain solid at room temperature.

monounsaturated fats
Lipids that are liquid at room temperature and semisolid or solid when refrigerated.

polyunsaturated fats
Lipids that are liquid at room temperature and in the refrigerator.

cholesterol
A waxy substance produced by the liver and obtained from animal food sources; essential to the functioning of the body but a possible factor in cardiovascular disease if too much is circulating in the bloodstream.

trans fatty acids
Lipids that have been chemically modified through the process of hydrogenation so that they remain solid at room temperature.

hydrogenation
Process whereby liquid vegetable oils are turned into more solid fats.

omega-3 fatty acids
Polyunsaturated fatty acids that contain the essential nutrient alpha-linolenic acid and that has beneficial effects on cardiovascular health.

omega-6 fatty acids
Polyunsaturated fatty acids that contain lin-oleic acid and that have beneficial health effects.

minerals
Naturally occurring inor-ganic micronutrients, such as magnesium, calcium, and iron, that contribute to proper functioning of the body.

vitamins
Naturally occurring organic micronutrients that aid chemical reac-tions in the body and help maintain healthy body systems.

lower HDLs. Foods high in trans fatty acids include baked and snack foods like crackers, cookies, chips, cakes, pies, and doughnuts, as well as deep-fried fast foods like french fries.[13] In packaged foods, the phrase "partially hydrogenated veg-etable oil" in the list of ingredients indicates the presence of trans fats. In 2006, the FDA began requiring that trans fat be listed on nutrition labels if a food contains more than 0.5 gram, and many food manufac-turers and restaurants have stopped using trans fats in their products. Some cities, including Philadelphia and New York City, have enacted laws to ban or phase out the use of trans fats in restaurants. In 2010, California became the first state to ban the use of trans fats in restau-rants. To date, no other states have followed California's lead in ban-ning trans fatty acids in restaurants.

Omega-3 and Omega-6 Fatty Acids Unlike trans fats, two kinds of polyunsaturated fatty acids—omega-3 and omega-6 fatty acids—provide health benefits. **Omega-3 fatty acids**, which contain the essential nutrient alpha-linolenic acid, help slow the clotting of blood, decrease triglyceride levels, improve arterial health, and lower blood pressure. They may also help protect against autoimmune diseases such as rheumatoid arthritis.[13,14] **Omega-6 fatty acids**, which contain the essential nutrient linoleic acid, are also impor-tant to health, but nutritionists believe that Americans con-sume too much omega-6 in proportion to omega-3.[1] They recommend increasing consumption of omega-3 sources— fatty fish like salmon, trout, and anchovies; vegetable oils like soybean, walnut, and flaxseed; and dark green leafy vegetables—and decreasing consumption of omega-6 sources, mainly corn and cottonseed oils.

Although the USDA recommends two servings of fish per week, there are concerns about contamination with mer-cury and other industrial pollutants, which can accumulate in the tissue of certain types of fish. Mercury may cause fetal brain damage, and high levels of mercury may damage the hearts of adults. Polychlorinated biphenyls (PCBs) and dioxin may be associated with cancer. In 2004, the FDA and the EPA issued a joint warning stating that pregnant women, women planning to become pregnant, nursing mothers, and young children should consume no more than 12 ounces of fish and shellfish per week, should avoid certain types of fish (king mackerel, golden bass, shark, and swordfish), and should vary the kinds of fish they eat. (For more informa-tion, see the EPA fish advisory site at http://water.epa.gov/ scitech/swguidance/fishshellfish/fishadvisories/.)

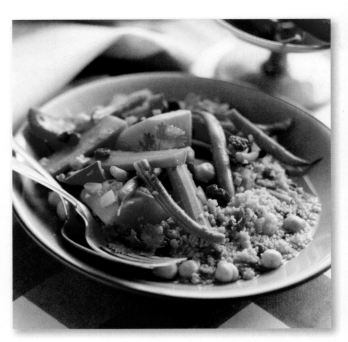

■ You can reduce your risk of chronic diseases by building your diet around colorful meals that include whole grains, legumes, two or more vegetables, and small quantities of chicken or fish.

Dietary Recommendations for Fat How much of your daily caloric intake should come from fat? The AMDR is 20 to 35 percent.[2] The American Heart Association recom-mends that less than one-third of that (7 to 10 percent) come from saturated fats and trans fats; in a 2,000-calorie diet, that's about 22 grams. Most adults need only 15 percent of their daily calorie intake in the form of fat, whereas young children should get 30 to 40 percent of their calories from fat to ensure proper growth and brain development, accord-ing to the American Academy of Pediatrics. A tablespoon of vegetable oil per day is recommended for both adults and children.[1]

These recommendations are designed to help improve cardiovascular health and prevent heart disease. On average, fat intake in the United States is about 34 percent of daily calorie intake.[1] You can limit your intake of saturated fat by selecting vegetable oils instead of animal fats, reducing the amount of fat you use in cooking, removing all visible fat from meat, and choosing lean cuts of meat over fatty ones and poultry or fish over beef. Limit your consumption of fast-food burgers and fries because these foods are loaded with saturated fats.

Minerals—A Need for Balance

Minerals are naturally occurring inorganic substances that are needed by the body in relatively small amounts. Miner-als are important in building strong bones and teeth, helping vitamins and enzymes carry out many metabolic processes, and maintaining proper functioning of most body systems.

Our bodies need 20 essential minerals. We need more than 100 milligrams daily of each of the six *macrominerals*—calcium, chloride, magnesium, phosphorus, potassium, and sodium. We need less than 100 milligrams daily of each of the *microminerals,* or *trace minerals*—chromium, cobalt, copper, fluorine, iodine, iron, manganese, molybdenum, nickel, selenium, silicon, tin, vanadium, and zinc. Other minerals are present in foods and the body, but no requirement has been found for them.[1] Table 5.1 provides an overview of food sources and DRIs for the most important vitamins and minerals.

A varied and balanced diet provides all the essential minerals your body needs, so mineral supplements are not recommended for most people.[2] (Exceptions are listed in the next section.) These insoluble elements can build up in the body and become toxic if consumed in excessive amounts.

Vitamins—Small but Potent Nutrients

Vitamins are organic substances needed by the body in small amounts. They serve as catalysts for releasing energy from carbohydrates, proteins, and fats; they aid chemical reactions in the body; and they help maintain components of the immune, nervous, and skeletal systems.

Our bodies need at least 11 specific vitamins: A, C, D, E, K, and the B-complex vitamins—thiamine (B_1), riboflavin (B_2), niacin, B_6, folic acid, and B_{12}. Biotin and pantothenic acid are part of the vitamin B complex and are also considered important for health. Choline, another B vitamin, is not regarded as essential.

Four of the vitamins—A, D, E, and K—are fat soluble (they dissolve in fat), and the rest are water soluble (they dissolve in water). The fat-soluble vitamins can be stored in the liver or body fat, and if you consume larger amounts than you need, you can reach toxic levels over time. Excess water-soluble vitamins are excreted in the urine and must be consumed more often than fat-soluble vitamins. Most water-soluble vitamins do not cause toxicity, but vitamins B_6 and C can build to toxic levels if taken in excess. Toxicity usually occurs only when these substances are taken as supplements.

Nearly half the people in the United States take vitamin and mineral supplements. The 2010 *Dietary Guidelines for Americans* recommends that people get all their nutrients from food, although there are some population groups for whom vitamin and mineral supplements may be needed, including

- People with nutrient deficiencies.

- People with low energy intake (less than 1,200 calories per day).

- Individuals who eat only foods from plant sources.

- Women who bleed excessively during menstruation.

- Individuals whose calcium intake is too small to preserve strength.

- People in certain life stages (infants, older adults, women of childbearing age, and pregnant women).

Taking supplements to enhance your energy level or athletic performance or to make up for perceived inadequacies in your diet is not generally recommended.[1] Many foods provide, in one serving, the same amounts of nutrients found in a vitamin supplement pill. However, there is some debate about multivitamins. Because many Americans have diets deficient in certain nutrients, some public health experts do advocate taking a daily multivitamin as a kind of nutritional insurance policy.[3] The dietary supplement industry promotes this practice as well, to sell more vitamin pills. There is little evidence that taking a daily multivitamin makes people healthier,[15] but they probably do no harm and may have some benefit. If you decide to take a multivitamin, follow the guidelines shown in the box, "What Your Multivitamin Should Contain," and refer to Table 5.1. For a concise summary of recommended daily intakes of all the categories of macronutrients and micronutrients, see Table 5.2.

Other Substances in Food: Phytochemicals

One promising area of nutrition research is **phytochemicals**, substances that are naturally produced by plants. In the human body, phytochemicals may keep body cells healthy, slow down tissue degeneration, prevent the formation of carcinogens, reduce cholesterol levels, protect the heart, maintain hormone balance, and keep bones strong.[16] A large European study recently found that people who ate eight or more servings of fruits and vegetables per day were 22 percent less likely to die from heart disease than those who ate three servings or less. Eight servings is about 23 ounces, which can sound like a lot until you realize that a large orange or apple weighs about 8 ounces.[17]

Antioxidants Every time you take a breath, you inhale a potentially toxic chemical that could damage your cell DNA: oxygen. If you breathed 100 percent oxygen over a period of days, you would go blind and suffer irreparable damage to your lungs. The process of oxygen metabolism in the body produces unstable molecules, called **free radicals**, which can damage cell structures and DNA. The production of free radicals can also be increased by exposure to certain environmental elements, such as cigarette smoke and sunlight, and even by stress. Free radicals are believed to be a contributing factor in aging, cancer, heart disease, macular degeneration, and other degenerative diseases, although some of the research supporting these claims may be questionable.[1]

Antioxidants are phytochemicals in foods that neutralize

phytochemicals Substances that are naturally produced by plants to protect themselves and that provide health benefits in the human body.

free radicals Unstable molecules that are produced when oxygen is metabolized and that damage cell structures and DNA.

antioxidants Substances in foods that neutralize the effects of free radicals.

Table 5.1 Key Vitamins and Minerals

Vitamins/ Minerals	Food Sources	Adult Daily DRI*	
		Men	Women
Vitamin A	Liver, dairy products, fish, dark green vegetables, yellow and orange fruits and vegetables	900 μg	700 μg
Vitamin C	Citrus fruits, strawberries, broccoli, tomatoes, green leafy vegetables, bell peppers	90 mg	75 mg
Vitamin D	Vitamin D–fortified milk and cereals, fish, eggs	5 μg	5 μg
Vitamin E	Plant oils, seeds, avocados, green leafy vegetables	15 mg	15 mg
Vitamin K	Dark green leafy vegetables, broccoli, cheese	120 μg	90 μg
Vitamin B_1 (thiamine)	Enriched and whole-grain cereals	1.2 mg	1.1 mg
Vitamin B_2 (riboflavin)	Milk, mushrooms, spinach, liver, fortified cereals	1.3 mg	1.1 mg
Vitamin B_6	Fortified cereals, meat, poultry, fish, bananas, potatoes, nuts	1.3 mg	1.3 mg
Vitamin B_{12}	Fortified cereals, meat, poultry, fish, dairy products	2.4 μg	2.4 μg
Niacin	Meat, fish, poultry, peanuts, beans, enriched and whole-grain cereals	16 mg	14 mg
Folate	Dark green leafy vegetables, legumes, oranges, bananas, fortified cereals	400 μg	400 μg
Calcium	Dairy products, canned fish, dark green leafy vegetables	1,000 mg	1,000 mg
Iron	Meat, poultry, legumes, dark green leafy vegetables	8 mg	18 mg
Magnesium	Wheat bran, green leafy vegetables, nuts, legumes, fish	420 mg	320 mg
Potassium	Spinach, squash, bananas, milk, potatoes, oranges, legumes, tomatoes, green leafy vegetables	4,700 mg	4,700 mg
Sodium	Table salt, soy sauce, processed foods	1,500 mg	1,500 mg
Zinc	Fortified cereals, meat, poultry, dairy products, legumes, nuts, seeds	11 mg	8 mg

*For a complete listing, see the website of the Food and Nutrition Information Center (http://fnic.nal.usda.gov/dietary-guidance/dietary-reference-intakes/dri-tables).

Source: "Dietary Reference Intakes," by the Food and Nutrition Board, Institute of Medicine of the National Academies, retrieved from www.iom.edu/About-IOM/Leadership-Staff/Boards/Food-and-Nutrition-Board.aspx.

Table 5.2 Overview of Recommended Daily Intakes of Macronutrients and Micronutrients

Water	1–1.5 ml per calorie spent; 8–12 cups of fluid
Carbohydrates Added sugars Fiber	AMDR: 45–65% of calories consumed No more than 10–25% of calories consumed 14 g for every 1,000 calories consumed; 21–25 g for women, 30–38 g for men
Protein	AMDR: 10–35% of calories consumed; 0.36 g per pound of body weight
Fat Saturated fat Trans fat	AMDR: 20–35% of calories consumed Less than 10% of calories consumed As little as possible
Minerals 6 macrominerals 14 trace minerals	More than 100 mg Less than 100 mg
Vitamins 11 essential vitamins	Varies

the effects of free radicals. Antioxidants are found primarily in fruits and vegetables, especially brightly colored ones (yellow, orange, and dark green), and in green tea. Vitamins E and C are antioxidants, as are some of the precursors to vitamins, such as beta carotene.

Fifty-two percent of Americans take large doses of antioxidant supplements daily. The American Heart Association and the American Diabetes Association advise that antioxidants should not be taken except to treat a vitamin deficiency.[3] Most nutritionists do not recommend supplements as a source of antioxidants because vitamin megadoses have the potential to cause fertility problems, reduce the benefits of exercise, and aggravate illnesses.[1] The best source is whole foods. The top antioxidant-containing foods and beverages include blackberries, walnuts, strawberries, artichokes, cranberries, brewed coffee, raspberries, pecans, blueberries, cloves, grape juice, unsweetened baking chocolate, sour cherries, and red wine. Açai berries have been heavily marketed as a superior source of antioxidants. These berries, however, are no better than blueberries or any other berries. Also high in antioxidants are brussels sprouts, kale, cauliflower, and pomegranates.

Phytoestrogens *Phytoestrogens* are plant hormones similar to human estrogens but less potent. Research

Consumer Clipboard

What Your Multivitamin Should Contain

Multivitamin labels tell you the amount per serving and the percentage of Daily Value (% DV) provided by that amount. Daily Values are the FDA standards that also appear on food labels. When you choose a multivitamin, look for one that contains amounts similar to those shown in the Supplement Facts label here.

Refer to the Tolerable Upper Intake Level (UL) column to the right of the Supplement Facts label to make sure the product does not exceed the maximum daily amounts that you can take without risking toxicity. ULs do not appear on labels.

Supplement manufacturers load their multivitamins with excessive levels of metals that may be linked to brain damage. Copper and iron are of particular concern. Excessive amounts can damage the brain, particularly for people at higher risk for dementia and Alzheimer's. Because meats and vegetables contain copper and iron, you can easily get as much as you need from your diet.

Choose brands from nationally recognized pharmacies or supermarkets.
Don't be fooled by a brand name that suggests the ingredients are "natural"—vitamins from whole foods are no better than synthetic vitamins.

Check the price.
Multivitamins should cost no more than 10 cents per pill.

Look for a U.S. Pharmacopeia (USP) seal, which means the manufacturer has paid an independent lab to test the product and affirm that it contains what the label says it does and that it will disintegrate or dissolve for GI absorption.

Ignore health claims—the FDA doesn't recognize them.
They usually have an asterisk referring to a disclaimer somewhere else on the label.

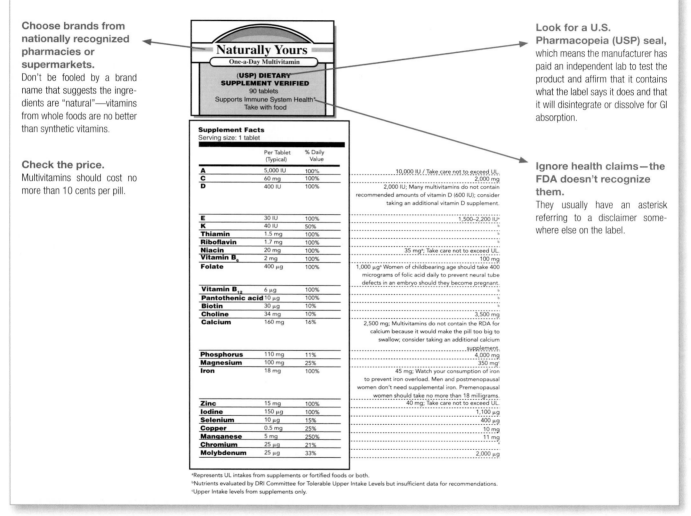

Naturally Yours
One-a-Day Multivitamin
(USP) DIETARY SUPPLEMENT VERIFIED
90 tablets
Supports Immune System Health*
Take with food

Supplement Facts
Serving size: 1 tablet

	Per Tablet (Typical)	% Daily Value	
A	5,000 IU	100%	10,000 IU / Take care not to exceed UL.
C	60 mg	100%	2,000 mg
D	400 IU	100%	2,000 IU; Many multivitamins do not contain recommended amounts of vitamin D (600 IU); consider taking an additional vitamin D supplement.
E	30 IU	100%	1,500–2,200 IU*
K	40 IU	50%	b
Thiamin	1.5 mg	100%	b
Riboflavin	1.7 mg	100%	b
Niacin	20 mg	100%	35 mg*; Take care not to exceed UL.
Vitamin B₆	2 mg	100%	100 mg
Folate	400 μg	100%	1,000 μg* Women of childbearing age should take 400 micrograms of folic acid daily to prevent neural tube defects in an embryo should they become pregnant.
Vitamin B₁₂	6 μg	100%	b
Pantothenic acid	10 μg	100%	b
Biotin	30 μg	10%	b
Choline	34 mg	10%	3,500 mg
Calcium	160 mg	16%	2,500 mg; Multivitamins do not contain the RDA for calcium because it would make the pill too big to swallow; consider taking an additional calcium supplement.
Phosphorus	110 mg	11%	4,000 mg
Magnesium	100 mg	25%	350 mg°
Iron	18 mg	100%	45 mg; Watch your consumption of iron to prevent iron overload. Men and postmenopausal women don't need supplemental iron. Premenopausal women should take no more than 18 milligrams.
Zinc	15 mg	100%	40 mg; Take care not to exceed UL.
Iodine	150 μg	100%	1,100 μg
Selenium	10 μg	15%	400 μg
Copper	0.5 mg	25%	10 mg
Manganese	5 mg	250%	11 mg
Chromium	25 μg	21%	b
Molybdenum	25 μg	33%	2,000 μg

°Represents UL intakes from supplements or fortified foods or both.
bNutrients evaluated by DRI Committee for Tolerable Upper Intake Levels but insufficient data for recommendations.
cUpper Intake levels from supplements only.

Source: Adapted from *Nutrition: Science & Applications,* by L. A. Smolin and M. B. Grosvenor, 2010, Hoboken, NJ: Wiley; Center for Science in the Public Interest; Multi dilemma: Should you take one. *Nutrition Action Healthletter.* November 2013, pp. 2–7.

suggests that some phytoestrogens may lower cholesterol and reduce the risk of heart disease. Other claims—that they lower the risk of osteoporosis and some types of cancer and reduce menopausal symptoms like hot flashes—have not been supported by research.

Phytoestrogens have been identified in more than 300 plants, including vegetables of the cabbage family such as brussels sprouts, broccoli, and cauliflower. Phytoestrogens are also found in plants containing lignin (a woody substance like cellulose), such as rye, wheat, sesame seed, linseed, and flaxseed, and in soybeans and soy products. Foods containing phytoestrogens are safe, but, as with all phytochemicals, research has not established the safety of phytoestrogen supplements.[1]

kilocalorie
Amount of energy needed to raise the temperature of 1 kilogram of water by 1 degree centigrade; commonly shortened to calorie.

Phytonutraceuticals *Phytonutraceuticals* are substances extracted from vegetables and other plant foods and used in supplements. For example, lycopene is an antioxidant found in tomatoes that may inhibit the reproduction of cancer cells in the esophagus, prostate, and stomach.[18] A group of phytochemicals known as *bioflavonoids* are believed to have a beneficial effect on the cardiovascular system.[19]

To date, the FDA has not allowed foods containing phytochemicals to be labeled or marketed as agents that prevent disease. Nutritionists do not recommend taking phytochemical supplements.[1] In 2007, the FDA announced that manufacturers of all dietary supplements, including vitamins and herbs, must evaluate the identity, purity, strength, and composition of their products and accurately label them so that consumers know what they are buying.[20]

National campaigns such as "Reach for It" in Canada and "Fruits and Veggies—More Matters" in the United States encourage consumers to select fruits and vegetables high in phytochemicals.[2] Because different fruits and vegetables contain different phytochemicals, a color-coded dietary plan has been developed that helps you take full advantage of all the beneficial phytochemicals available (Figure 5.1).

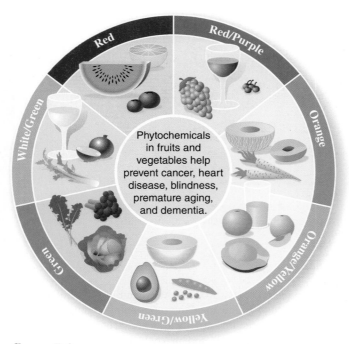

figure 5.1 **The color wheel of foods.**
An optimal diet contains fruits and vegetables from all seven groups.
Source: Adapted from *What Color Is Your Diet?* by D. Heber, 2001, New York: HarperCollins, p. 17.

PLANNING A HEALTHY DIET

When food is *metabolized*—chemically transformed into energy and wastes—it fuels our bodies. The energy provided by food is measured in kilocalories, commonly shortened to *calories*. One **kilocalorie** is the amount of energy needed to raise the temperature of 1 kilogram of water by 1 degree centigrade. The more energy we expend, the more kilocalories we need to consume. We get the most energy from fats—9 calories per gram of fat. Carbohydrates and protein provide 4 calories per gram. In other words, fats provide more calories than do carbohydrates or proteins, a factor to consider when planning a balanced diet that does not lead to weight gain.

Knowing your daily nutritional requirements in grams and percentages is not enough to ensure a healthy diet; you also need to know how to translate DRIs, RDAs, and AMDRs into healthy food choices and appealing meals. In this section we look at several tools that have been created to help you do that.

Dietary Guidelines for Americans

The 2010 *Dietary Guidelines for Americans* notes that two-thirds of Americans are now overweight or obese. As a result, these guidelines focus on stopping and reversing the spread of overweight and obesity through individual, environmental, and food supply changes. Key areas addressed by the Dietary Guidelines Advisory Committee are described in Table 5.3.

The committee also outlined four main goals for Americans:

- Reduce calorie intake and increase physical activity.

- Move toward a more plant-based diet composed of nutrient-dense foods.

- Reduce intake of foods containing added sugars and solid fats and reduce overall sodium and refined grain consumption.

- Meet the 2008 Physical Activity Guidelines provided by the U.S. Department of Health and Human Services.

MyPlate In 2010, the USDA introduced MyPlate, a visual icon that illustrates the five food groups and is intended as a reminder to Americans about maintaining balanced diets (Figure 5.2). MyPlate replaced the food pyramid, which had been introduced in 1992 and was designed to raise awareness and health literacy among consumers about the different food groups.[21] Most nutrition experts were pleased to see the retirement of the pyramid model because it was complicated and sometimes implied misleading information about foods (e.g., that all fats are bad).

Visit the MyPlate website and use the interactive tools to assess your current diet, calculate your calorie needs, develop a customized food plan, and learn strategies for achieving a healthy weight. The Personal Health Portfolio

Table 5.3 2010 *Dietary Guidelines for Americans:* Key Messages

Energy balance and weight management	Increase physical activity to balance calorie intake. Limit time spent in front of the television and computer. Consume smaller portions.
Nutrient adequacy	For most people, nutrients should come from foods, not supplements. Favor nutrient-dense foods over calorie-dense foods.
Fatty acids and cholesterol	Limit saturated fat to less than 7 percent of total calories and avoid consuming any amount of trans fats. Consume two servings of fish per week to obtain heart-healthy omega-3 fatty acids.
Protein	Animal sources of protein are the highest quality sources, but combinations of legumes and grains can also supply complete proteins.
Carbohydrates	Choose fiber-rich carbohydrates (including whole grains, vegetables, fruits, and cooked dry beans) over high-energy, non-nutrient dense carbohydrates (such as sugar-sweetened beverages and pastries).
Sodium and potassium	Reduce daily sodium consumption to 2,300 mg, and further reduce consumption to 1,500 mg if you are African American or 51 or older or have hypertension, diabetes, or chronic kidney disease. Increase potassium consumption (good sources are potatoes, plain yogurt, and bananas).
Alcohol	Adults should limit alcohol consumption to an average of up to two drinks per day for men and up to one drink per day for women. Men should consume no more than four drinks on any single day; women, no more than three drinks.
Food safety and technology	Pay greater attention to food safety when preparing meals in the home. The health benefits of consuming cooked seafood outweigh the food safety concerns surrounding it. There are special recommendations for pregnant women and children.

Source: Dietary Guidelines for Americans: 2010 by the U.S. Department of Agriculture, www.dietarygudielines.gov.

Activity for this chapter will also help you assess your food intake. Estimate your calorie requirements based on your gender and age at three activity levels, as shown in Table 5.4. The activity levels are defined as

- *Sedentary.* Only light physical activity associated with typical day-to-day life.

- *Moderately active.* Physical activity equivalent to walking about 1.5 miles per day at 3 to 4 miles per hour.

- *Active.* Physical activity equivalent to walking more than 3 miles per day at 3 to 4 miles per hour.

The *Dietary Guidelines* and MyPlate differ significantly from current eating patterns in the United States. Specifically, they encourage more consumption of whole grains, vegetables, legumes, fruits, and low-fat milk products and less consumption of refined grain products, total fats, added sugars, and calories. They emphasize foods high in **nutrient density**—proportion of vitamins and minerals to total calories. Especially in a lower calorie diet, the goal is that all calories consumed provide nutrients (as opposed to "empty calories" in sodas, sweets, and alcoholic beverages). Otherwise, you reach your maximum calorie intake without having consumed the nutrients you need.

If you choose nutrient-dense foods from each food group, you may have some calories left over—your discretionary calorie allowance—that can be consumed as added fats or sugars, alcohol, or other foods. At the 2,000-calorie level, your discretionary calorie allowance is 267 calories.

The DASH Eating Plan The *Dietary Guidelines* also recommends the DASH Eating Plan, originally developed to reduce high blood pressure. (DASH stands for Dietary Approaches to Stop Hypertension.) The DASH plan is similar to MyPlate, but it also has a nuts, seeds, and legumes group. For more information, visit www.nhlbi.nih.gov/health/public/heart/hbp/dash/new_dash.pdf.

nutrient density
The proportion of nutrients to total calories in a food.

Recommendations for Specific Groups The *Dietary Guidelines* also includes recommendations, where relevant, for specific population groups, including children and adolescents, older adults, pregnant and breastfeeding women, overweight adults and children, and people with chronic diseases or special medical problems. For example, women of childbearing age and women in the first trimester of pregnancy are advised to consume adequate synthetic folic acid daily in addition to eating foods rich in folate. Individuals with hypertension and those from groups who are prone to hypertension such as African Americans, and middle-aged and older adults are advised to consume no more than 1,500 milligrams of sodium per day. The box, "10 Tips for Eating Healthy in the College Dining Hall," offers advice for students who eat on campus.

Limiting Red Meat Consumption Research strongly supports a link between red meat consumption and heart disease, cancer, and diabetes.[22] The Nurses Health Study found

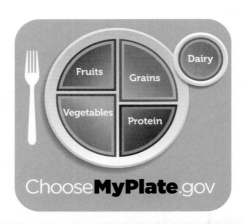

Vegetables	Fruits	Grains	Dairy	Protein Foods
Eat more red, orange, and dark-green veggies like tomatoes, sweet potatoes, and broccoli in main dishes. Add beans or peas to salads (kidney or chickpeas), soups (split peas or lentils), and side dishes (pinto or baked beans), or serve as a main dish. Fresh, frozen, and canned vegetables all count. Choose "reduced sodium" or "no-salt-added" canned veggies.	Use fruits as snacks, salads, and desserts. At breakfast, top your cereal with bananas or strawberries; add blueberries to pancakes. Buy fruits that are dried, frozen, and canned (in water or 100% juice), as well as fresh fruits. Select 100% fruit juice when choosing juices.	Substitute whole-grain choices for refined-grain breads, bagels, rolls, breakfast cereals, crackers, rice, and pasta. Check the ingredients list on product labels for the words "whole" or "whole grain" before the grain ingredient name. Choose products that name a whole grain first on the ingredients list.	Choose skim (fat-free) or 1% (low-fat) milk. They have the same amount of calcium and other essential nutrients as whole milk, but less fat and calories. Top fruit salads and baked potatoes with low-fat yogurt. If you are lactose intolerant, try lactose-free milk or fortified soymilk (soy beverage).	Eat a variety of foods from the protein food group each week, such as seafood, beans and peas, and nuts as well as lean meats, poultry, and eggs. Twice a week, make seafood the protein on your plate. Choose lean meats and ground beef that are at least 90% lean. Trim or drain fat from meat and remove skin from poultry to cut fat and calories.
For a 2,000-calorie daily food plan, you need the amounts below from each food group. To find amounts personalized for you, go to Choose**MyPlate**.gov.				
Eat 2½ cups every day **What counts as a cup?** 1 cup of raw or cooked vegetables or vegetable juice; 2 cups of leafy salad greens	**Eat 2 cups every day** **What counts as a cup?** 1 cup of raw or cooked fruit or 100% fruit juice; ½ cup dried fruit	**Eat 6 ounces every day** **What counts as an ounce?** 1 slice of bread; ½ cup of cooked rice, cereal, or pasta; 1 ounce of ready-to-eat cereal	**Get 3 cups every day** **What counts as a cup?** 1 cup of milk, yogurt, or fortified soymilk; 1½ ounces natural or 2 ounces processed cheese	**Eat 5½ ounces every day** **What counts as an ounce?** 1 ounce of lean meat, poultry, or fish; 1 egg; 1 Tbsp peanut butter; ½ ounce nuts or seeds; ¼ cup beans or peas

figure 5.2   The USDA MyPlate.

Introduced in 2010, MyPlate promotes a dietary balance of five basic food groups: fruits, grains, vegetables, protein, and dairy. The MyPlate website, ChooseMyPlate.gov, contains resources and interactive tools that give specific information on which foods to eat and which to avoid. MyPlate, 2010, U.S. Department of Agriculture, Center for Nutrition Policy and Promotion.

Table 5.4 Estimated Calorie Requirements at Three Levels, by Age and Gender

| Gender | Age (years) | Activity Level | | |
		Sedentary	Moderately Active	Active
Female	14–18	1,800	2,000	2,400
	19–30	2,000	2,000–2,200	2,400
	31–50	1,800	2,000	2,200
	51+	1,600	1,800	2,000–2,200
Male	14–18	2,200	2,400–2,800	2,800–3,200
	19–30	2,400	2,600–2,800	3,000
	31–50	2,200	2,400–2,600	2,800–3,000
	51+	2,000	2,200–2,400	2,400–2,800

Source: Dietary Guidelines for Americans: 2010, by the U.S. Department of Agriculture, www.dietaryguidelines.gov/.

that people who ate two servings a day (3-ounce servings of cooked steak, hamburger, or other unprocessed meats; or 1-ounce servings of processed meat such as bacon and sausage) had a higher risk of heart disease than people who ate a half serving a day. About 8 percent of deaths in women and 10 percent of death in men could be prevented if people ate no more than a half serving of red meat a day.[22] The primary compounds of concern in red meat are heme iron, nitrites, salt, and compounds that cluster when red meat is cooked at high temperatures.

The American Cancer Society (ACS) recommends no more than 18 ounces (cooked weight) of red meats per week and to avoid or strictly limit process meat consumption. The ACS estimates that the risk for colon and rectal cancers increases when people eat more than 18 ounces of red meat per week. Studies also suggest an increased risk for pancreatic, prostate, and esophagus cancers. Processed meats have long been linked to diabetes. Recent research is now linking unprocessed red meats to diabetes. Scientists believe the cause may be heme iron.

The bottom line is to minimize red meat consumption. Beans, nuts, soy-based veggie meats, poultry, and fish are recommended substitutes.[22]

Vegetarian Diets

Vegetarian diets may offer protection against obesity, heart disease, high blood pressure, diabetes, digestive disorders, and some forms of cancer, particularly colon cancer,[1]

depending on the type of vegetarian diet followed. Some research suggests that vegetarians live longer than non-vegetarians. Despite the potential benefits of vegetarian diets, however, vegetarians need to make sure that their diets provide the energy intake and food diversity needed to meet dietary guidelines.[1] Vegetarians should visit the food plan for vegetarians available on MyPlate.

Daily Values on Food Labels

Daily Values are based on a variety of dietary guidelines and used on the food labels on packaged foods. Food labels are regulated by the FDA (labeling of meat and poultry products is regulated by the USDA).[23] The information in the Nutrition Facts panel on a food label tells you how that food fits into a 2,000-calorie-a-day diet that includes no more than 65 grams of fat (30 percent of total calories) (Figure 5.3).

The top of the label lists serving size and number of servings in the container. The second part of the label gives the total calories and the calories from fat. A quick calculation will tell you whether this food is relatively high or low in fat. Look for foods with no more than 30 percent of their calories from fat.

The next part of the label shows how much the food contributes to the Daily Values established for important nutrients, expressed as a percentage. The bottom part of the label, which is the same on all food labels, contains a footnote explaining the term "% Daily Value" and shows recommended daily intake of specified nutrients in a 2,000- and a 2,500-calorie diet.[23]

Packaged foods frequently display food descriptors and health claims, some of which are also regulated by the FDA to help consumers know what they are getting. For example, the term *light* can be used if the product has one-third fewer calories or half the fat of the regular product. Other claims are not yet well regulated, as discussed in the next section. To find out more about common nutritional claims, visit the FDA website.

Front-of-Package Food Labels

Because dietary supplements are subject to less regulation than foods, their manufacturers have been able to include a wide variety of health claims on product labels, asserting everything from support of heart health to promotion of muscle growth. Food and beverage manufacturers have pressured Congress to allow similar health claims on their labels,[24,4] but the FDA's authority to regulate such claims is limited. As a result, health claims on food and beverage products have proliferated without much oversight. Today, there are more than 12 different symbols, logos, and icons that appear on the front of food product packaging to

Action Skill-Builder

10 Tips for Eating Healthy in the College Dining Hall

Although the "Freshman 15" is a myth, eating healthy at the college dining hall may seem as difficult as getting an A+ in an advanced chemistry course. College dining halls typically include plenty of options that are very high in calories, fat, sodium, and sugar. Still, there are many healthy choices. MyPlate provides 10 recommendations for choosing the rights foods to put on your tray.

1. *Know What You Are Eating.* Many college dining rooms post menus with nutrition information. Looking at the menus ahead of time can help choose healthy balanced meals. The Super Tracker in ChooseMyPlate.gov can help you select healthy foods.

2. *Enjoy Your Food, But Eat Less.* The all-you-can-eat dining room can make it challenging to resist large portions of food. Take smaller plates and servings.

3. *Make Half Your Grains Whole Grains.* Choose whole-grain foods when making your selections. Whole-grain bread and whole-grain cereals, for example, are good options.

4. *Re-think Your Drink.* The typical American consumes 400 calories in beverages a day. Avoid or limit sugary drinks such as sodas, energy drinks, cappuccinos, fruit beverages, sweetened teas, and sports drinks. Water is a good alternative.

5. *Make Half Your Plate Fruits and Veggies.* Fruits and veggies make for a healthy meal. Add them to pastas, pizza, sandwiches, and soups. Try spinach in a wrap or add pineapple to your pizza. Select diverse colors of fruits and veggies.

6. *Make It Your Own.* You do not need to choose premade plates. Design your own meal, for example, by combining fresh veggies from the salad bar with your omelet.

7. *Slow Down on the Sauces.* Sauces, gravies, and dressings are usually high in calories and sodium. Be cautious of foods prepared with a lot of oil, butter, or topped with heavy condiments, such as mayonnaise. You can limit condiments by asking that they be placed on the side.

8. *Be on Guard at the Salad Bar.* Limit foods high in fat and sodium such as olives, bacon bits, fried noodles, croutons, and pasta or potato salads that are made with mayonnaise and oil. Choose fat-free or low-fat dressings on the side.

9. *Make Dessert Special.* Choose desserts only on special occasions. If you cannot resist dessert, choose something healthy like fruit-and-yogurt parfait.

10. *Don't Linger.* Limit socializing at dining halls. Staying for long periods of time increases your temptation to keep eating.

Source: "10 Tips for Healthy Eating in the Dining Hall," *DG Tip Sheet* No. 26, USDA Center for Nutrition Policy and Promotion, www.ChooseMyPlate.gov.

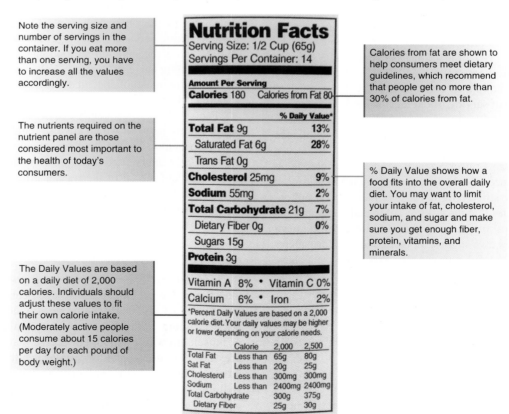

figure 5.3 **Nutrition Facts panel on a food label.**

communicate nutrition information to consumers—none of which has yet been officially designed or endorsed by the FDA. Some of these front-of-package (FOP) labels provide straightforward informational facts on nutrient content, but others can be misleading and confusing.[25]

To clear up this dilemma, the CDC and the FDA asked the Institute of Medicine (IOM) to review FOPs. The IOM found that FOPs tend to provide only basic information and little guidance for consumers about actual healthfulness of products. Unregulated FOPs also cause confusion among consumers and promote unnecessary nutrient fortifications in food and beverage products. The IOM recommended that the FDA develop, test, and implement a single standard FOP system on all food and beverage products to replace the labels currently used.[25,26]

Figure 5.4 shows one of the IOM's recommended standards for FOP labels. Instead of focusing on calories alone, the model provides information about saturated and trans fats, sodium, and added sugars. Products with three checkmarks have amounts of fat, sodium, and added sugar that are considered to be within a healthy range. Products that exceed an upper limit of any of these three nutrients are disqualified from receiving any points at all; soup crackers, for example, contain healthy levels of fats and sugars but are disqualified by their very high sodium content. Until the new standard is in place, some nutrition experts would like FOPs banned.

Proposed Changes to the Nutrition Facts Label

In 2014, the FDA proposed to update the Nutrition Facts label for packaged foods. The proposed changes draw from new scientific evidence that establishes a link between diet and chronic diseases, particularly obesity and heart disease. Key changes include: mandating inclusion of information on added sugars, updating reference amounts, specifying calorie and nutrition information based on whole package and not just serving size, declaring potassium and vitamin D on the label if contained in the packaged food, revision of the daily Percent Daily Values for such nutrients as calcium, dietary fiber, and vitamin D, and altering the label format to emphasize important diet elements such as calories, serving size, and Percent Daily value. The underlying purpose of these changes is to make it easier for the consumer to identify health packaged food products. These changes would apply to all packaged foods, except for meat, poultry, and processed egg products.[26]

Restaurant Menu Labels

Can menu labeling make us healthier? The 2010 Patient Protection and Affordable Care Act (the 2010 health care reform legislation) includes a requirement that all chain restaurants (restaurants with more than 20 locations) provide calorie labeling on their menus. The law does not require a list of fat grams, sodium, or other general information. The National Restaurant Association supports the law but opposes adding information beyond calorie content.

Proponents of menu labeling believe it will help people make healthier decisions and manage their weight more successfully. Opponents argue that people choose unhealthy foods because they lack self-control, not because they lack information. Preliminary research suggests that the latter is true: consumers are not more likely to choose healthier menu items when presented with calorie information. Other methods of guiding consumers may prove to be more effective than providing nutrition

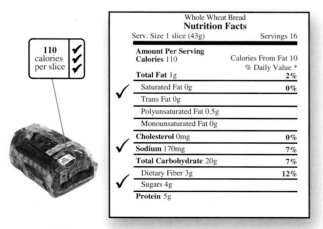

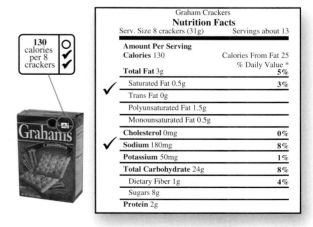

figure 5.4 How front-of-package labeling works.

New informational icons on the front of packaged foods will give you more information about what kinds of nutrients are in the foods that you choose. As shown here, the symbol on the front of a package clearly displays the number of calories in a single serving of this product. A points system—represented here with checkmarks—indicates whether the product has healthful levels of saturated fats, sodium, and sugar. The loaf of bread does not contain excessive amounts of saturated or trans fats, sodium, or added sugars; therefore, it gets three points. The graham crackers have healthy amounts of fats and sodium, but have added sugars (more added sugars than recommended by the FDA), so they get only two points.

information alone. One such method is including information on the health and weight effects of specific ingredients in menu items. Another method is designing menus to encourage healthier eating, for example, by listing healthy choices on the front page of a menu and less healthy items further back.[26,27]

The American Heart Association and the American Public Health Association believe that menu labeling will encourage restaurants to serve smaller portion size and healthier ingredients. These associations do acknowledge the difficulty of precise listings for nutrition information because most people customize their meals by adding condiments such as mustard, mayonnaise, and ketchup, as well as salt and butter. Although they agree that restaurants should not be responsible for labeling nutrition information beyond the basic food product, one recommendation is that restaurants provide a range of potential calories.[27]

CURRENT CONSUMER CONCERNS

The most common food-related topics that you are likely to hear about in the media are related to obesity and poor health because of overconsumption of soft drinks, high-sodium diets, and fast foods. These topics are important because obese young adults and middle-aged adults are likely to live almost a decade less on average than those who maintain a healthy weight.

Overconsumption of Soft Drinks

Americans consume an average of 22.2 teaspoons (335 calories) of sugar each day; as we saw earlier in the chapter, the American Heart Association recommends no more than 6 teaspoons for women and 9 teaspoons for men. Sugar is believed to promote and maintain obesity; cause and aggravate diabetes; increase the risk of heart disease; and cause dental decay, gum disease, osteoporosis, and kidney stones. It should be noted, however, that scientific evidence suggests that moderate levels of sugar (no more than 10 percent of total calories) pose no health risk.[1]

Much of this sugar consumption comes from soft drinks. These beverages represent the largest contributor of daily calories, about 7 percent of calories consumed. Soft drinks account for one in every four beverages consumed in the United States. Some experts attribute the surge in overweight and obesity among American children and adults largely to the increase in the consumption of soft drinks.[28,29]

Equally important is the decreased consumption of milk, which is a major source of calcium, protein, vitamin A, and vitamin D, as well as decreased consumption of orange juice and other fruit juices.[30] Soft drinks contain about the same number of calories as milk and juice but none of the nutrients.

Fat-free and low-fat milk are more nutrient-dense choices than heavily sweetened beverages, and many varieties of milk are available to fit people's different needs:[15]

- Omega-3 fortified milk, which contains small amounts of healthy omega-3 fatty acids.

- Ultra-pasteurized milk, which is treated to have an especially long shelf life when unopened, beneficial for those who shop ahead or in bulk.

- Lactose-free milk, which contains no milk sugar (lactose), which is hard for about 6 percent of adults to digest.

- "Plus" or "deluxe" milk, which is fortified with milk powder, stabilizers, and/or fiber to increase the nutrient content and produce a creamier consistency that some people find closer to whole milk.

- Nondairy milk, which are "milks" made from soy, rice, almonds, and so on; appropriate for anyone but particularly for vegans and those who are lactose-intolerant.

In addition to sugar, soft drinks also contain relatively high levels of caffeine, which is mildly addictive and can lead to nervousness, irritability, insomnia, and bone demineralization. Although soft-drink manufacturers claim that caffeine is added for its flavoring effects, its primary effect is to stimulate the central nervous system.[30] Nutritionists recommend limiting soft drinks in the diet and drinking water and low-fat milk instead.

What about diet sodas? Diet soft drinks don't contain sugar, but like regular soft drinks, they fill you up without providing any nutrients. In addition, diet soda does not help people lose weight. Artificial sweeteners disrupt the ability of the body to regulate calorie intake based on food sweetness. The body is tricked into thinking that sugar is being consumed and thus leads to sugar craving. An 11-year study of 3,000 women found that drinking two or more diet sodas a day may also be associated with a two-fold risk for kidney decline. Because this decline is not associated with sugar-sweetened sodas, scientists believe that the cause is likely diet sweeteners. In addition, another study found that even one diet soda a day may increase the risk for metabolic syndrome (high blood pressure, high LDL, low HDL, belly fat), which places a person at risk for heart disease. Many diet sodas also contain preservatives called mold inhibitors (sodium benzoate, potassium benzoate) that are not found in regular sodas. Mold inhibitors can damage DNA and have been linked to allergic reactions such as hives and asthma as well as mild irritations to the skin, eyes, and mucous membranes. Finally, diet soda has a pH of 3.2, which is very acidic. Acid dissolves tooth enamel. Not surprisingly, a third study found that people who drink three or more diet sodas a day are at higher risk for tooth decay.[31]

High-Sodium Diets

Another current concern is the amount of sodium in our diet. American adults consume an average of 3,400 milligrams per day,[32] men more and women less. Sodium is an essential nutrient, but we need only about 500 milligrams per day—about ¹⁄₁₀ of a teaspoon. Although many foods contain sodium, we get most of our sodium—about 90 percent—from salt (which is made up of sodium and chloride). The 2010 *Dietary Guidelines* recommend no more than 2,300 milligrams of sodium per day for the general population and no more than 1,500 milligrams per day for African Americans; people who are 51 or older; and people who have hypertension, diabetes, or chronic kidney disease. The American Heart Association recommends no more than 1,500 milligrams per day for *all* Americans.

Salt may be a factor in causing hypertension (high blood pressure) in some "salt-sensitive" people. According to CDC findings, two of three adults are at risk for sodium sensitivity, including those who are 40 or older, are African American, or have high blood pressure.[32] New research suggests that salt can damage the brain and hinder cognitive function even in people without hypertension, so people who are not salt-sensitive can also benefit from reducing the sodium in their diets.[33]

Many packaged foods, convenience foods, fast foods, and restaurant foods are heavily salted, primarily to enhance flavor. Some contain more than 5,000 milligrams of sodium in a serving. Canned soups, lunch meats, pickles, soy sauce, teriyaki sauce, catsup, mustard, salad dressing, and barbecue sauce are especially high in sodium.[34]

You can reduce the amount of salt in your diet by emphasizing whole foods, like grains, vegetables, and fruits, which are naturally low in sodium. Remove the salt shaker from your table, and don't use salt in cooking. When buying packaged foods, read the labels to check for salt content and look for descriptors such as "reduced sodium" or "low sodium." Highly salted food is an acquired taste; if you use less salt, you will gradually rediscover the natural taste of the food. Although scientists have found substitutes for sugar, substitutes for salt are much more elusive because it has a distinct taste. Potassium has been used as a salt substitute, but some people find it too bitter.

Food Allergies and Food Intolerances

Food allergies occur when the immune system overreacts to specific proteins in food; they affect about 7 percent of children and 2 percent of adults. More than 200 food ingredients can cause an allergic reaction, but eight foods are responsible for 90 percent of food allergies—milk, eggs, peanuts, tree nuts, fish, shellfish, soy, and wheat. Allergic reactions to these foods cause 30,000 emergency room visits each year and 150 to 200 deaths.[35] The Food Allergen Labeling and Consumer Protection Act of 2004 requires that these allergens be clearly identified below the list of ingredients on all packaged foods. Currently, restaurants are not required to provide information about allergens in their menu items, but many health experts are calling for menu labeling by restaurants, not only for health reasons but also for personal, cultural, and religious reasons.

Typical symptoms of allergic reactions include skin rash, nasal congestion, hives, nausea, and wheezing. Most children eventually outgrow food allergies, except for allergies to peanuts, nuts, and seafood.[1] Food allergies that develop during adulthood are typically lifelong. Many food allergies are associated with other diseases, such as asthma, eczema, and esophagitis.

Generally, people suffer temporary discomfort, but approximately 30,000 people each year in the United States have an *anaphylactic shock* reaction to a food they have eaten—the throat swells enough to cut off breathing.[2] A person experiencing this type of allergic reaction needs immediate medical attention because symptoms can worsen rapidly and sometimes result in death, Therefore, the National Institute of Allergy and Infectious Diseases stresses the importance of having an emergency plan in case of an anaphylactic allergic reaction.[35] You can attain an example of an emergency plan from the American Academy of Allergy, Asthma, and Immunology.

Most food reactions are not caused by allergies, however; most are caused by food intolerances.[3] Such intolerances are less severe than allergies and can be triggered by almost any food. Lactose intolerance, a condition that results from an inability to digest the milk sugar lactose, is especially prevalent.

There is no treatment or cure for food allergies or intolerances. If you experience these reactions, the best you can do is try to avoid the offending food.[1] It can be especially hard to avoid allergenic foods when eating out because restaurants are not required to reveal this information. Many health experts are now calling for menu labeling by restaurants, not only for health reasons but also for personal, cultural, and religious reasons. For example, vegetarian groups and Muslim associations have brought class action suits against McDonald's for flavoring french fries with small amounts of meat, milk, and wheat products without informing customers.

Gluten-Free Diets

Celiac disease, an immune reaction to people who eat gluten, has been getting increasing attention in recent years. About 1 percent of the American population has celiac disease.[36] Gluten is a form of protein found in wheat, barley, rye, and triticale (a cross between wheat and rye). Over time, the immune system reaction to gluten causes inflammatory damage to the small intestine lining. As the box, "Ricardo: Celiac Disease," indicates, this damage can result in many symptoms, including weight loss, bloating, and occasionally diarrhea. If damage persists, there is an increased risk for osteoporosis, intestinal cancers, infertility, and other diseases and disorders. People with celiac disease are at higher risk for other autoimmune diseases.

In 2013, the FDA released a new labeling law that makes it much easier for people with celiac disease to avoid gluten.

Life Stories

Ricardo: Celiac Disease

Ricardo started noticing frequent rumbling in his stomach at age 17. By his sophomore year in college, the rumblings had graduated into severe stomach pain. He felt tired, cranky, and his body hurt all over. Ricardo also noticed that he was often experiencing tingling and numbness in his hands and legs, especially after he had eaten. An itchy skin rash had also appeared. Ricardo felt bloated and frequently felt an urge to go to the bathroom. He lost appetite for food and lost 10 pounds in six weeks. He found it increasingly difficult to sleep. His roommate advised Ricardo that he most likely had a stomach bug and should see a doctor.

Ricardo decided to visit a walk-in health clinic. He was given a blood test. The blood test revealed that he was severely deficient in iron and was anemic. Iron supplementation was prescribed. After several months of high iron supplement dosage, Ricardo's level of iron in his blood had not increased. Ricardo decided to consult a GI specialist. The GI specialist suspected celiac disease. There is no cure for celiac disease. A strict gluten-free diet is the treatment of choice.

This was a very difficult diagnosis for Ricardo. After all, he had grown up his entire life being able to eat any type of food. Adopting a gluten-free diet was a huge lifestyle change. Even a minor slip, such as eating a biscuit, would trigger a severe immune system reaction. If left untreated, Ricardo's brain, nervous system, bones, liver, and other organs could be deprived of needed nourishment.

Because celiac disease can be inherited, Ricardo advised his other family members to be tested. A family history of thyroid problems, arthritis, and diabetes may be an indicator of possible celiac disease. Surgery, pregnancy, childbirth, a viral infection, or traumatic stress may trigger the onset of celiac disease in people who are prone to it.

- Are you or a friend on a gluten-free diet?
- What types of food must be avoided in a gluten-free diet?
- Do your local grocery stores sell gluten-free foods?
- Should restaurants be required to label gluten-free items on their menus?

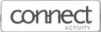

Foods labeled "gluten-free" must contain less than 20 parts per million of the gluten protein. This is about an eighth of a teaspoon of flour. This is low enough for people with mild to severe gluten allergies to avoid an immune reaction. If you are just starting a gluten-free diet, it is recommended that you consult a registered dietician.[36]

Energy Bars and Energy Drinks

Energy bars are a convenient source of calories and nutrients for people with busy schedules or intense exercise regimens. Luna Bars, Power Bars, and Balance Bars are examples of these. Most are low in saturated and trans fats and contain up to 5 grams of fiber. They are better for you than candy bars and other snack foods high in saturated fat, but they can also be high in calories and sugar. Healthier alternatives are whole foods like fruits and vegetables, with their abundant vitamins, minerals, and phytochemicals. If you do buy energy bars, check the labels for calories, total fat, saturated fat, protein, fiber, and sugar and choose the healthiest ones.[37,38]

In addition, Americans consume about four quarts of energy drinks each year per person. Energy drinks are marketed as a source of instant energy, improved concentration and memory, and enhanced physical performance. They have names like Red Bull, 5-Hour, Full Throttle, and Monster. Energy drinks are not considered a health risk if consumed in recommended amounts, but there are no long-term studies on their side effects, if any.

In addition to water, sodium, and glucose, many energy drinks contain caffeine and a variety of dietary supplements, such as ginseng, guarana, and B vitamins. Caffeine can stimulate mental activity and may increase cardiovascular performance, but caffeine consumption should not exceed 300 milligrams per day. Caffeine levels above 400 milligrams are likely to produce negative effects, including loss of focus, racing heart rate, nausea, and anxiety. For most other additives in energy drinks, little or no empirical research either supports their effectiveness or details their potential dangers.[38] The FDA does not monitor energy drinks, but it is beginning to take an interest in doing so.[39]

Mixing hard alcohol and energy drinks has become popular with young adults. Combining a stimulant (caffeine and other herbal ingredients) with a depressant (alcohol) disguises the intoxication effects of alcohol by helping the drinker feel alert and sober. In a recent study, people who had been drinking energy drinks with liquor were three times more likely to be drunk than those who drank only alcohol and were four times more likely to say they planned to drive within the hour.[37] Multiple cocktails of energy drinks and liquor can also pose a danger to heart muscle fibers and cause extreme dehydration.

If you consume energy drinks, your maximum intake should be two 20-ounce cans a day. Consuming more than 20 ounces in an hour can cause an increase in arterial pressure and in blood sugar levels. Energy drinks should not be consumed immediately after a vigorous workout or in combination with alcohol. They should not be consumed by pregnant women, children, young teens, older adults, or people with cardiovascular disease, glaucoma, or sleep disorders. The bottom line, according to many health experts, is that the risks associated with energy drinks outweigh any perceived benefits.

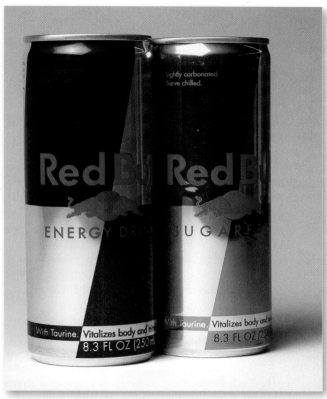

■ Energy drinks are popular because they provide a brief burst of alertness, typically fueled by caffeine, but they are usually followed by a crash.

people who live in *food deserts* do not have adequate access to healthy, affordable food, and fast food is often their only alternative (food deserts are discussed in detail in the next section). Fast-food meals tend to be high in calories, fat, sodium, and sugar and low in vitamins, minerals, and fiber. A single fast-food meal can approach or exceed the recommended limits on calories, fat, saturated fat, and sodium for a whole day's meals (Figure 5.5).

The United States food revolution has called for Americans to eat more fruits and vegetable, less red meat, less processed foods, less food additives, and less fast food that is high in calories, salt, and sugar.[41] Consequently, many fast-food restaurants (and restaurants in general) are offering healthier choices these days. So if you know what to order, it's possible to make healthier choices:

■ Don't supersize or order extra-large servings. Standard-size orders are already very large.

■ Go easy on sauces, toppings, and condiments like sour cream, guacamole, tartar sauce, mayonnaise, and gravy.

■ Order grilled chicken or fish on a whole wheat roll, but have them hold the "special sauce."

■ Order a salad with dressing on the side or a fat-free dressing. A dinner salad without dressing may have about 150 calories, but a Caesar salad with dressing may have almost 1,000 calories.

■ Order a baked potato with vegetables instead of butter or sour cream.

Probiotics, Prebiotics, and Synbiotics

Probiotics are living bacteria that may help with digestion and ease gastrointestinal conditions. Prebiotics are non-digestible carbohydrates that serve as fuel for probiotics. A product that combines probiotics and prebiotics is called a synbiotic. Probiotics are available in pills, powders, and a variety of different foods, including baby formula, yogurt, juices, and granola bars.

Manufacturers claim that probiotics can treat a range of problems, including diarrhea, yeast and urinary infections, irritable bowel syndrome, and eczema. Some products are said to prevent or reduce cold and flu symptoms. Scientific studies have not thoroughly confirmed the health benefits of probiotics, and it may be several more years before they do so. The American Academy of Pediatrics has concluded that probiotics and prebiotics should not be thought of as "wonder cures." However, if you want to try these products, they are inexpensive, natural, and generally considered safe.[1,2]

Fast Foods

Americans eat out more than four times a week, and every day, one in four Americans eats fast food.[40] Although plenty of people choose to eat fast food over healthier options,

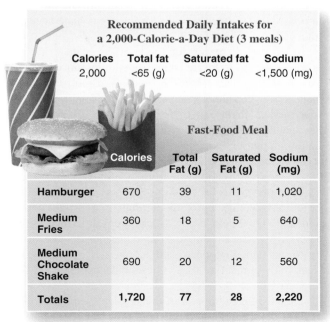

Recommended Daily Intakes for a 2,000-Calorie-a-Day Diet (3 meals)			
Calories	**Total fat**	**Saturated fat**	**Sodium**
2,000	<65 (g)	<20 (g)	<1,500 (mg)

Fast-Food Meal

	Calories	Total Fat (g)	Saturated Fat (g)	Sodium (mg)
Hamburger	670	39	11	1,020
Medium Fries	360	18	5	640
Medium Chocolate Shake	690	20	12	560
Totals	1,720	77	28	2,220

figure 5.5 **A fast-food meal compared with recommended daily intakes.**

- Instead of a soda, order orange juice, low-fat milk, or iced water.

- Instead of pie or cake, order yogurt and fruit.

The least healthy options are fried fish or fried chicken sandwiches, chicken nuggets, croissants and pastries, onion rings, and large fries. Most fast-food restaurants will give you a nutritional brochure if you ask for it, or it may be posted; choose the healthiest options.

Food Deserts

For many years, health experts have been looking at lack of access to affordable and nutritious food as a contributing factor in increasing levels of overweight and obesity among low-income Americans and the related increase in diet-related diseases like diabetes. There are typically many more supermarkets in affluent neighborhoods than in low-income neighborhoods and more convenience stores and fast-food restaurants in low-income neighborhoods than in affluent ones. When fresh produce and other healthy foods aren't available, people cannot choose a healthy diet even if they want to.[41]

food desert
Low-income area where more than 500 people or 33 percent of the population has low access to a supermarket or large grocery store.

Areas where there are no stores with healthy foods are known as food deserts. The USDA defines **food deserts** as low-income areas where more than 500 people or 33 percent of the population have low access to a supermarket or large grocery store, with "low access" defined as more than 1 mile from a store in urban areas and more than 10 miles in rural areas. Other definitions also take into account whether people in such areas have access to transportation to get to a store.[42]

The primary reason for food deserts is the reluctance of food retailers to locate chain stores in low-income areas, usually for business reasons such as lower return on investment, lower consumer demand, or high crime rates. Large supermarket chains have been criticized for abandoning low-income communities, primarily African American and Latino, in densely populated urban areas. Government land use policies have also facilitated the migration of supermarkets to the suburbs and away from inner-city areas.

The prevalence of food deserts increases as economic conditions decline. For example, half of Detroit's population of 900,000 people now live in areas described as food deserts. A related problem is *food insecurity*—the inability to get enough food to support an active, healthy life. Nearly 15 percent of U.S. households experienced food insecurity in 2012.

The Obama administration has addressed the problem of food deserts with several programs. The 2010 Healthy Food Financing Initiative (HFFI) provides financial support to grocery stores and small food retailers in low-income communities to help them offer healthy food to consumers. The HFFI was passed in concert with Michelle Obama's Partnership for a Healthier America (PHA). The mission of PHA is to confront childhood obesity among the 23.5 million Americans living in areas where access to affordable, healthy foods is limited. In conjunction with PHA, executives from several large supermarket chains pledged to open or expand stores in communities designated as food deserts.

In addition, states and cities are entering into partnerships with public and private entities to help defray the costs of developing supermarkets in low-income areas. For example, the Pennsylvania Fresh Food Financing Initiative facilitates grants and loans between public and private financers and supermarkets. As another example, New York City's Food Retail Expansion Program offers property tax abatements and sales tax exemption for full-service grocery stores that locate in underserved areas.

Unfortunately, the supermarket industry is risk-averse, so it is an uphill battle to persuade them to locate stores in low-income neighborhoods. In addition, there is evidence that availability alone is not enough to change people's eating habits. Telling Americans to eat healthier is not going to work by itself. Perhaps, reengineering junk food to be healthier is needed. The food industry is being challenged to find ways to deliver healthier food options to non-health-conscious food consumers. This means using food processing technology that trims unhealthy ingredients while preserving the taste sensations that consumers desire. For example, we generally care most about the first bite and last bite of food. Bites in between do not matter as much. Slipping healthier ingredients into the middle of a food product, such as a candy bar, may work to fool taste buds. Food manufacturers are tinkering with food ingredients to accomplish this objective.[40]

FOOD SAFETY AND TECHNOLOGY

Although the FDA is charged with monitoring the safety of the U.S. food supply, consumers, too, need to learn to distinguish between safe and unsafe foods and understand key elements of food safety.

Organic Foods

Plant foods labeled "organic" are grown without synthetic pesticides or fertilizers,[2] and animal foods labeled organic are from animals raised on organic feed without antibiotics or growth hormones. Organic foods appeal to health- and environment-conscious consumers.[1] They tend to be more expensive than foods grown using conventional methods, however, and consumers cannot always determine exactly how some foods were grown.

The USDA regulates the use of terms related to organic foods on the labels of meat and poultry products. The label "100% organic" means that all contents are organic;

"organic" means that contents are at least 95 percent organic; "made with organic ingredients" means the contents are at least 70 percent organic. Meat and poultry manufacturers who comply with the USDA standards can place the seal "USDA Organic" on their labels.

Although it seems that organic foods ought to be healthier and safer than foods produced conventionally, no research has demonstrated that this is the case. Conventional food products do contain pesticide residues that can be toxic at high doses, but research has not documented ill effects from them at the levels found in foods, nor is there any evidence that people who consume organic food are healthier than those who don't.[1]

A disadvantage of organic foods is that they may place consumers at higher risk of contracting foodborne illnesses. If you purchase organic food, buy only the amount you need immediately, store and cook the food properly, and wash organic produce thoroughly before eating it.[1]

What has been documented is that organic farming is beneficial to the environment. It helps maintain biodiversity of crops; it replenishes the earth's resources; and it is less likely to degrade soil, contaminate water, or expose farm workers to toxic chemicals. As multinational food companies get into the organic food business, however, environment-conscious consumers should look for foods that are not only organic but also locally grown. The average food item currently travels at least 1,500 miles to its destination, requiring massive amounts of oil for transportation. In addition, locally grown food tastes fresher, keeps money in the local economy, and cuts down on the consumption of processed food. The burgeoning popularity of farmers' markets is a sign of growing interest in locally grown food.

Some experts recommend that budget-conscious consumers spend their money on organic fruits and vegetables when those that are grown conventionally carry higher pesticide residues (the "dirty dozen"): apples, bell peppers, celery, cherries, imported grapes, nectarines, peaches, pears, potatoes, red raspberries, spinach, and strawberries. Fruits and vegetables that carry little pesticide residue whether grown conventionally or organically include asparagus, avocados, bananas, broccoli, cauliflower, corn, kiwi, mangoes, onions, papaya, pineapples, and peas.

Foodborne Illnesses

The Centers for Disease Control and Prevention (CDC) estimates that 48 million Americans, or about 1 in 6, get sick every year from foodborne illness, 128,000 are hospitalized, and 3,000 die.[43] The CDC and state health departments play a critical role in tracking foodborne outbreaks. Foodborne illnesses may be caused by food intoxication or by food infection; both types are commonly referred to as *food poisoning.*

Food poisoning causes flu-like symptoms such as diarrhea, abdominal pain, vomiting, fever, and chills. More serious complications can include rheumatoid arthritis, kidney or heart disease, meningitis, *hemolytic uremic syndrome (HUS),* and death. Some symptoms are cause for immediate medical attention:

■ Bloody diarrhea or pus in the stool.

■ Fever that lasts more than 48 hours.

■ Faintness, rapid heart rate, or nausea when standing up suddenly.

■ Significant drop in the frequency of urination.[3]

Food intoxication occurs when a food is contaminated by natural toxins or by microbes that produce toxins. Botulism is an example of food intoxication. When food has been contaminated with the botulism bacterium and then improperly prepared or stored, the bacterium releases a dangerous and potentially fatal toxin. Warning signs of botulism poisoning are double vision, weak muscles, difficulty swallowing, and difficulty breathing.[1] Immediate medical treatment is needed.

food intoxication
A kind of food poisoning in which a food is contaminated by natural toxins or by microbes that produce toxins.

food infection
A kind of food poisoning in which a food is contaminated by disease-causing microorganisms, or pathogens.

Food infection is caused by disease-causing microorganisms, or pathogens, that have contaminated the food. Some commonly contaminated foods are ground beef, chicken, turkey, salami, hot dogs, ice cream, lettuce and other greens, sprouts, cantaloupe, and apple cider. Leafy

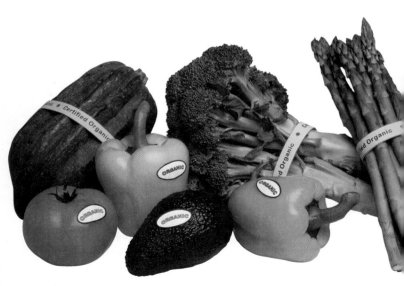

■ Organic foods aren't necessarily healthier, but organic farming is better for the environment. Many consumers are now choosing organic, locally grown produce and other foods.

green vegetables are the top source for food infection, about one in five of food infections. Half of food infections are attributed to fruits and all vegetables. Most of vegetable-related food infections come from norovirus, which is most often spread by cooks and food handlers. This means food infection is usually caused by unsanitary food production or preparation and not by the food itself. Although vegetable-related food infections are the most common, most deaths are caused by poultry (one in five).[44]

In addition to norovirus, three other common pathogens that cause food infection are *Escherichia coli (E. coli),* salmonella, and campylobacter. *E. coli* occurs naturally in the intestines of humans and animals. Raw beef, raw fruits and vegetables, leafy greens, sprouts, and unpasteurized juices and cider are the foods most commonly contaminated by it. In 2011, the USDA investigated a multistate outbreak of *E. coli* infections linked to romaine lettuce. Among the 45 people infected, 30 were hospitalized, and 2 developed HUS.[45,46] One strain, *E. coli* 0157:H7, is especially dangerous because it can cause HUS, which can lead to kidney failure, a potentially fatal condition. The CDC estimates that *E. coli* 0157:H7 causes nearly 73,000 illnesses each year in the United States and kills 250 to 500 people.[47] Young children and older adults are particularly at risk. *E. coli* is a hearty microbe, thriving in moist environments for weeks and on kitchen countertops for days. One study found that 72 percent of grocery carts tested had fecal matter on them, and 50 percent had *E. coli.* After multiple trips to the grocery store, reusable shopping bags may become a "bacterial swamp" and should be cleaned after each use.[46]

Most people who suffer an *E. coli* 0157:H7 infection recover within a few days. One or two in 20 people develop HUS. However, a new strain, 0104:H4, swept across Europe in 2011. More than one-fourth of people infected with this strain developed HUS. *E. coli* 0104:H4 contains many segments of DNA not found in other *E. coli* strains and is especially potent because its new genes are resistant to antibiotics. There is no evidence that this deadly *E. coli* is likely to reach the United States. However, the potential still exists.[45]

Salmonella enteritis can contaminate raw eggs, poultry and meat, fruits and vegetables, and other foods. Eggs containing salmonella enteritis are the number-one cause of food poisoning outbreaks in the nation. The best way to prevent salmonella infection is to thoroughly cook eggs, chicken, and other foods to kill the bacterium. Avoid eating raw or undercooked eggs, such as in raw cake batter or cookie dough, salad dressings, and eggnog.[46] New federal safeguards implemented in 2012 are expected to reduce salmonella infections by 80,000 per year and deaths by 30 per year. The safeguards focus on mandating rodent control programs on egg-producing farms and requiring eggs to be refrigerated during storage.

Many people do not realize that pet food can contain salmonella. Anyone with an impaired immune system is very vulnerable to salmonella infections and should take extra caution when handling pet foods. This includes young children, whose immune systems are still developing, and older adults, whose immune systems become compromised with age. To protect against potential salmonella infection, make sure that canned or bagged dry pet food product has no visible signs of damage to packaging, such as dents, tears, or discoloration. After handling pet food, wash your hands thoroughly before preparing, serving, or eating food. Children under the age of 5 years should not be allowed to touch dry pet foods and should be kept away from pet feeding areas.[47]

Campylobacter occurs in raw or undercooked poultry, meat, and shellfish, in unpasteurized milk, and in contaminated water. Campylobacter from contaminated poultry can spread when juices from packages spill onto kitchen surfaces and other foods; it can also be spread by hand.[46] Campylobacter and salmonella together cause 80 percent of the illnesses and 75 percent of the deaths associated with meat and poultry practices.[46]

A growing concern is the use of antibiotics in food-producing animals to prevent, control, and treat disease and to promote growth. The increasing use of antibiotics for both people and animals is causing the spread of antibiotic-resistant bacteria. According to a 2013 report by the Centers for Disease Control and Prevention, every year more than 2 million people in the United States are getting infections that are resistant to antibiotics, and at least 23,000 of them die from these infections. The CDC recommends that antibiotics be used in farm-producing animals only under veterinary oversight and only to address animal health needs, and not to promote growth.[48] For information about antibiotic-resistant bacteria and public health legislation proposed in 2013, see the box, "Preservation of Antibiotics for Medical Treatment Act."

Although only about 20 percent of food poisoning cases originate at home, the best defense against foodborne illness is the use of safe food preparation and storage practices in your own kitchen (Figure 5.6).

Recent foodborne-illness outbreaks, such as salmonella-tainted chicken from California, cucumbers from Mexico, and peanut butter from New Mexico, have prompted continued food safety concerns. Until passage of the Country-of-Origin Law (COOL) in 2009, consumers had little idea where everyday foods originated. COOL requires retailers to notify consumers of the country of origin of common unprocessed foods such as raw beef, veal, lamb, vegetables, frozen fruits, and many other foods. However, processed foods are not included under COOL; for example, raw pork chops have to be labeled, but ham and bacon do not. Butcher shops selling meat and/or seafood are also exempt.[49]

Are food trucks and food vendors safe? Food trucks and food vendors are required to be licensed so that local health departments can track them for inspections. Most operators are required to post their licenses on the

Public Health Is Personal

Preservation of Antibiotics for Medical Treatment Act (PAMTA)

Antibiotics attack bacteria by killing them or stopping their growth. But, as will be discussed in Chapter 13, bacteria can become resistant to antibiotics. What does this mean for human health? The World Health Organization warns that infectious diseases like strep throat could return to kill people. Resisting the overuse of antibiotics in humans is a principal strategy to confront bacteria resistance. This strategy, however, will not be enough. The inappropriate use of antibiotics in animal agriculture must also be confronted.

Seventy-five to 80 percent of the antibiotics used in the United States are given to animals and not people. The use of antibiotics on food animals can result in bacteria resistance spread to the food supply and end up in people. The National Antimicrobial Resistance Monitoring Systems in 2011 found resistant bacteria in tested samples of 12 percent of chickens (salmonella), 12 percent of ground turkey (salmonella), 40 percent of pork (*E. coli*), and 62 percent of beef (*E. coli*). In other words, the use of antibiotics in farming and raising livestock has resulted in the emergence of new "superbugs" in the food supply that are resistant to some antibiotics.

In 2013, the Food and Drug Administration warned that low-dose levels of antibiotics in animals to promote growth or improve food efficiency needlessly contributes to the emergence of antibiotic-resistant bacteria in the food supply and is an urgent threat to public health. The FDA proposed legislation entitled Preservation of Antibiotics for Medical Treatment Act (PAMTA); it was introduced in March 2013 to confront this problem. PAMTA calls for phasing out the non-therapeutic use in livestock of medically important antibiotics and rigid standards on new applications for approval of animal antibiotics. It does not restrict use of antibiotics to treat sick animals or to treat pets or other animals not used for food.

More than 300 organizations support PAMTA, including the American Public Health Association, and the American Medical Association. In contrast, the American Veterinary Association (AVMA) is vehemently opposed to PAMTA. The AVMA argues that the health risks associated with low-dose use of antibiotics are low and that promoting efficient food production and food safety outweighs the risk of developing more antibiotic resistance.

Companies that sell antibiotics to be used on livestock claim that there is not sufficient empirical evidence to make a connection between resistant bacteria found in animals and humans. Most microbiologists disagree and contend that there are decades of studies linking antibiotic use in food production with the emergence of drug resistance that has spread from animals to humans. The debate centers on whether society views antibiotics as too important for treating sick people to squander on using as a food production tool for raising animals.

Sources: "Antibiotic Resistance: Wasting a Precious Life Saver," by D. Schardt, May 2013, *Nutrition Action Health Letter*, pp. 9–11; "On Antibiotic Resistance in Food Animals," by R. Loglisci, *Food Safety News*, www.foodsafetynews.com/2010/07/on-antibiotic -resistance-in-food-animals; "Antibiotics in Your Food: What's Causing the Rise in Antibiotic-Resistant Bacteria in Our Food Supply and Why You Should Buy Antibiotic-Free Food," by B. Eastbrook, 2013, *Food and Environment Reporting Network*, http://thefern.org/2013/05/whats-causing-the-rise-in-antibiotic -resistant-bacteria/.

---

window so they can be easily seen by customers. Some states require operators to post their inspection grade on the window as well. Illegal operators are less likely to follow food safety laws. Here are some other red flags you need to check. Food handlers should be wearing gloves and changing gloves frequently to prevent bacteria cross-contamination. In cities that do not require food handlers to wear gloves, they are required to wash their hands frequently. You can get a good idea of hand cleanliness by looking at their nails. Dangling hair is another red flag. Hot food should be served hot and not lukewarm. Cold foods such as salads should feel like they were just taken out of the refrigerator.

Genetically Modified Foods

Farmers, scientists, and breeders have long been tinkering with the genetic makeup of plants and animals to breed organisms with desirable traits, a process known as *selective breeding*. Compared with modern techniques, however, selective breeding is slow and imprecise. Using biotechnology to produce **genetically modified (GM) organisms** is a faster and more refined process. Genetic modification involves the addition, deletion, or reorganization of an organism's genes in order to change that organism's protein production. Research on genetic modification in agriculture has focused on three areas:

genetically modified (GM) organisms Organisms whose genetic makeup has been changed to produce desirable traits.

- New strains of crops and animals with improved resistance to disease and pests (e.g., corn plants that resist blights).

- Strains of microorganisms that produce specific substances that occur in small amounts or not at all in nature (e.g., bovine somatotropin, a growth hormone used in cattle to produce more meat).

- Crops that resist destruction by herbicides (e.g., soybean plants that can survive herbicides used to kill weeds).

Many crops have already been genetically modified, and 60 percent of processed foods currently sold in supermarkets contain one or more GM ingredients.[3]

Proponents of GM crops and animals say we must develop new agricultural technologies that increase crop and

119

Clean

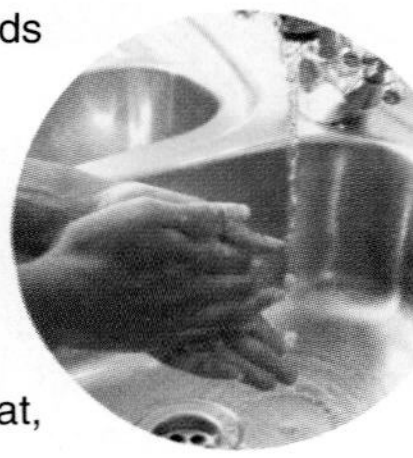

- Before you handle food, wash your hands for 20 seconds with soap and running water
- Wash cutting boards, countertops, and cooking utensils after each use. Clean sponges and dish towels regularly with a bleach solution
- Wash fruits and vegetables, but not meat, poultry, or eggs

Separate

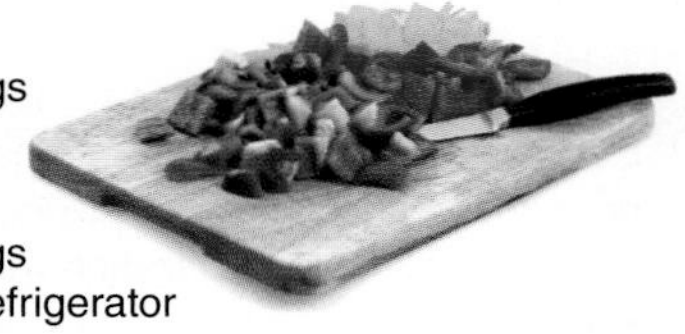

- Use separate cutting boards and plates for produce and for meat, poultry, seafood, and eggs
- Keep meat, poultry, seafood, and eggs separate from all other foods at the grocery
- Keep meat, poultry, seafood, and eggs separate from all other foods in the refrigerator

Cook

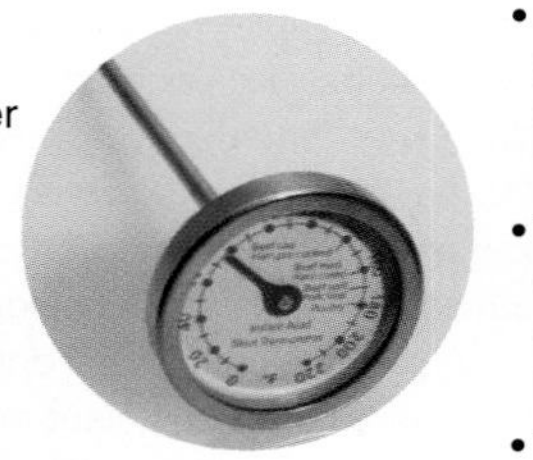

- Because the bacteria that cause food poisoning multiply quickest between 40° and 140° F, use a food thermometer to be sure food cooked in the oven or on top of the stove is done
- Microwave food to 165° F or above. Let the food sit for a few minutes if the directions call for it. The extra time lets heat reach the colder areas of the food
- Never thaw or marinate foods on the counter. Thaw meat in the refrigerator, in cold water, or in the microwave. Marinate food in the refrigerator

Chill

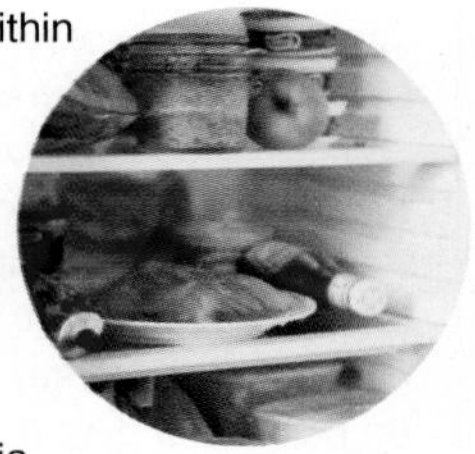

- Refrigerate perishable food, including leftovers, within 2 hours, or within 1 hour if temperature is above 90° F. Store leftovers in shallow containers to facilitate cooling
- The refrigerator temperature should be 40° F or below, and the freezer at 0° F. Don't pack your refrigerator too full because cool air must flow freely to keep food safe
- Throw food out before it goes bad; harmful bacteria start multiplying before food starts getting moldy or sour smelling. Consult the Storage Times chart at www.foodsafety.gov/keep/charts/storagetimes.html.
- In a power outage, food in the refrigerator is usually safe (under 40°) for 4 hours; food in a full freezer will stay frozen for 48 hours, and in a half full freezer for 24 hours. To maintain the cold temperatures, keep refrigerator and freezer doors closed as much as possible. For the length of time specific foods are safe above 40° F, see USDA Food Safety and Inspection Service's chart at www.fsis.usda.gov/wps/portal/fsis/topics/food-safety-education/get-answers/food-safety-fact-sheets/emergency-preparedness/keeping-food-safe-during-an-emergency/CT_Index.

figure 5.6   **Food safety in the kitchen.**
Sources: "Check Your Steps," n.d., by FoodSafety.gov (U.S. Department of Health and Human Services), retrieved from www.foodsafety.gov/keep/basics/index.html; "Keeping Food Safe during an Emergency," July 30, 2013, by USDA FSIS, retrieved from www.fsis.usda.gov/wps/portal/fsis/topics/food-safety-education/get-answers/food-safety-fact-sheets/emergency-preparedness/keeping-food-safe-during-an-emergency/CT_Index.

animal productivity and support food growers and producers economically while not harming the environment. They see genetic modification as a promising agricultural technology that may meet these needs, and many in the food and biotechnology industries have hailed the benefits of GM organisms.[3]

On the other hand, a growing number of consumers, animal rights supporters, national consumer watchdog organizations, and environmentalists have expressed concerns about GM foods. They fear that agriculture driven by biotechnology without restraint will destroy natural ecosystems, create new viruses, increase cruelty to animals, and reduce biodiversity.[3] They have called for all foods containing GM ingredients to be labeled. Connecticut and Maine have passed mandatory GM labeling. About 30 other states are also considering GM mandatory labeling.

The safety of food products produced by biotechnology is assessed by the FDA's Center for Food Safety and Applied Nutrition (CFSAN). To date, the center has held that GM foods do not require any special safety testing—nor do they have to be labeled as GM foods—unless they differ significantly from foods already in use.[1]

The American Dietetic Association and many other scientific organizations support the FDA position on GM foods, citing the potential benefits. For biotechnology in agriculture to achieve the objectives of ensuring safe, abundant, and affordable food, however, it must be accepted by the public. Surveys suggest that consumers are not well informed about this technology but are cautiously optimistic about its potential benefits in food production and processing.[3]

North Americans enjoy the safest and most nutritious food supply in the world. We also enjoy immense choice in what we eat. With choice comes responsibility—the responsibility to be informed, to make wise decisions, to consume foods that promote health and prevent disease. After reading this chapter, you have sufficient information to make nutrition choices that support your own lifelong health and, by extension, the well-being of society at large. We encourage you to make those healthy choices!

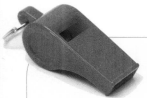

You Make the Call

Should Unhealthy Foods Be Taxed?

Poor diet and inactivity contribute to an estimated 310,000 to 500,000 premature deaths from cardiovascular disease, cancer, and diabetes each year in the United States. High-calorie, high-fat, and high-sodium foods are key components of many people's poor diets, particularly low-income consumers, because unhealthy foods tend to cost less than fresh and unprocessed foods. Public health campaigns aimed at educating the public about healthy diets are unable to keep up with the marketing campaigns of the food and beverage industries. For example, the National Cancer Institute spends about $1 million annually on its "Fruits and Veggies, More Matters" campaign, while the soft-drink industry spends more than 600 times that amount marketing its products. Another example is the efforts by the American Beverage Association that have successfully defeated proposals by various cities to pass a soft-drink tax.

Some health experts want the federal government to impose an excise tax on certain high-calorie, high-fat, and high-sodium foods. An excise tax is a tax on the manufacturer or seller of a product, as opposed to a sales tax, which the consumer pays when purchasing the product. Manufacturers typically pass the extra cost on to consumers in the form of higher prices. Thus, the excise tax would have the effect of making unhealthy food items cost more and would, theoretically, discourage consumers from buying them and possibly steer them to healthier foods.

Advocates of an excise tax believe that consumption of healthier foods would lead to reduced calorie intake by consumers, resulting eventually in better weight management and better overall health among Americans. One study found that a 10 percent increase on soft drinks and pizza resulted in a 7 percent reduction in calories from soft drinks and a 12 percent reduction in calories from pizza. The study authors conjectured that an 18 percent tax increase on soft drinks and pizza could result in an average weight loss of 5 pounds per person per year. Advocates of this tax also propose that the revenue generated could be used to promote healthy foods and physical activity.

Research by the Rudd Center for Food Policy and Obesity at Yale University suggests that a tax equal to about a penny per ounce is significant in changing consumer purchasing behavior. If a 20-ounce bottle of soda costs $1.50, a one-cent-per-ounce tax would increase the cost to $1.70 per bottle. This would result in additional tax revenue of $13.2 billion, which would cover about 8 percent of the health costs associated with obesity. Another study found that a two-cent-per-ounce tax on sugar-sweetened beverages would reduce obesity by 18 percent, save nearly $350 million each year, and bring in $800 million annually to promote healthy nutrition and physical activity.

Opponents of a tax on high-calorie, high-fat, and high-sodium foods argue that it would be a regressive tax, meaning that it would unfairly burden poor people because they buy more unhealthy food than more affluent people and because they spend a larger proportion of their income on food. Proponents counter that the tax would reduce medical expenses among low-income people, who have a higher incidence of diet-related diseases than the general population. Opponents also believe such a tax would represent an unwarranted government intrusion into the rights of individuals to make their own choices. Proponents respond that public health is a government responsibility.

Should the federal government tax unhealthy foods to influence consumer behavior, or should the government take a hands-off approach to individuals' dietary choices? What do you think?

Pros

- Consumer behavior may be more responsive to price increases than to nutrition education. Research suggests that a one-cent-per-ounce tax on sugar-sweetened beverages might reduce consumption of these beverages by 25 percent.
- An excise tax on high-calorie, high-fat, and high-sodium foods would reduce diet-related diseases and medical expenses among low-income Americans.
- Several other countries are now using tax measures to discourage consumption of unhealthy foods and to promote access to healthy foods. The World Health Organization supports this approach.
- In a nationally representative opinion poll, 45 percent of respondents supported a one-cent-per-ounce excise tax on soft drinks, chips, and butter to generate funds for healthy diet programs.
- Public health is a government responsibility, so the government has the right to take actions to protect the health of citizens.

Cons

- There is evidence that obese individuals are less responsive to changes in the price of food than people who are not obese. Thus, a tax on high-calorie, high-fat, and high-sodium food would not have the desired effect of discouraging the purchase of these items by the people who could benefit the most.
- Carelessly imposed food taxes could have unintended negative consequences, such as causing people to eat more highly salted foods to make up for the loss of certain tastes in their diets when they reduce their intake of high-fat foods.
- A tax on packaged and processed foods unfairly targets the low-income population. No one has proposed a tax on high-fat foods consumed by affluent people, like Brie cheese.
- It's impossible to pinpoint a few food items and blame them for the obesity epidemic. Diets include hundreds or thousands of different foods, and no single food is responsible for the problem. A multifaceted, ecological approach is needed to address the problem.
- Most Americans want the freedom to buy and eat whatever they want. They don't want "big brother" interfering with their choices.

connect ACTIVITY

Sources: "Impact of Targeted Beverage Taxes on Higher- and Lower-Income Households," by E. A. Finkelstein, C. Zhen, J. Nonnemaker, et al. 2010, *Archives of Internal Medicine 170* (22), pp. 2028–2034; "Bad Food? Tax It, and Subsidize Vegetables," by M. Bittman, 2011, *The New York Times,* July 23, pp. 1, 6–7; "Should the Government Impose a 'Fat Tax' on Junk Food?" by B. McCuen, 2011, retrieved from http://speakout.com/activism/issue_briefs/1332b-1.html.

In Review

What kinds of nutritional guidelines are established by the federal government?

Used by nutritionists, researchers, and the food industry, the Dietary Reference Intakes (DRIs) encompass four kinds of recommendations: the Estimated Average Requirement (EAR) of nutrients needed by different age groups; the Recommended Dietary Allowance (RDA), which is the average daily amount needed of a particular nutrient; the Tolerable Upper Intake Level (UL), which is the largest amount that can be ingested without risking toxicity; and the Acceptable Macronutrient Distribution Range (AMDR), or the range between the amount of an essential nutrient needed for adequate nutrition and the amount associated with the risk of some kind of chronic disease.

What are the categories of nutrients?

The macronutrients are water, carbohydrates, proteins, and fats. The micronutrients are vitamins and minerals. A balanced diet includes adequate intake of all the nutrients, primarily from nutrient-rich foods (as opposed to dietary supplements). Whole foods and especially plant foods contain additional important substances, such as antioxidants.

How do you plan a healthy diet?

The *Dietary Guidelines for Americans* translates the findings of nutritional research into daily dietary recommendations, and MyPlate customizes these recommendations to the individual, based on activity levels and calorie needs. There are numerous other sets of guidelines and types of labeling as well, including food labels, front-of-package labels, and restaurant menu information.

What are the main nutrition-related concerns currently affecting our society?

Americans overall do not eat a very healthy diet compared to what is recommended, and overweight and obesity are significant problems. The American diet tends to include too many calories; too much sugar, salt, and fat; and too few vegetables, fruits, and whole foods. Current concerns include the overconsumption of soft drinks, high-sodium diets, food allergies and intolerances, overuse of energy bars and energy drinks, unsubstantiated claims about probiotics, the prevalence of fast food, and the existence of food deserts.

What are the main food-safety issues?

Although organic foods are sometimes preferable because pesticides can cause health problems, the main safety issue is food poisoning typically caused by pathogens such as *E. coli,* salmonella, and campylobacter. The American food supply is safe overall, but increasing centralization of food production and distribution creates the conditions for widespread outbreaks of foodborne illness from a single source of contamination. A growing concern is the common use of antibiotics in food-producing animals and the spread of antibiotic-resistant bacteria. Another issue of interest to consumers is genetically modified foods.

Fitness

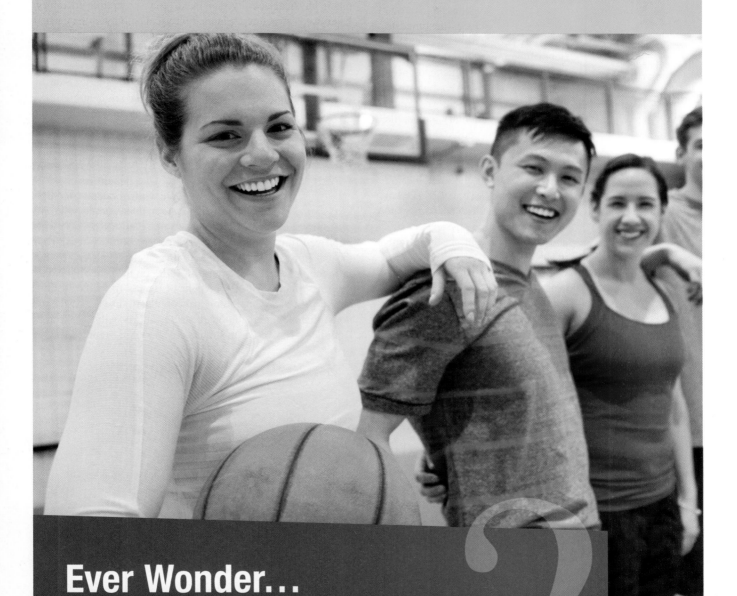

Ever Wonder...

- how much exercise you should be getting?
- what counts as moderate or vigorous physical activity?
- how long it takes to burn off the calories from a burger and fries?

You are jogging through the airport to make a flight on another concourse on your way home for winter break. Your Nike iPod Sport Kit shoe is blaring your favorite song into your earbuds when a voice suddenly interrupts the music: "5 minutes completed. 0.30 mile. Pace, 5 miles per hour. Calories burned, 45." The Nike iPod shoe is just one of many new devices designed to motivate people to exercise, particularly young adults.

Unfortunately, Americans need a lot of motivation. Although many public health campaigns are aimed at Americans' sedentary habits, the fact is that most people don't exercise, as the box, "Adults Meeting 2008 Physical Activity Guidelines for Aerobic and Muscle-Strengthening Activity" shows. Thirty-six percent of American adults do not participate in any leisure-time physical activity, and only 48 percent get the recommended amount of exercise each week.[1] Of college students, 55 percent do not get the recommended amount of cardio activity.[2]

The good news is that there are simple and enjoyable ways to build physical activity into your lifestyle and to increase the amount of exercise you get. This chapter will show you how.

physical fitness
Ability of the body to respond to the physical demands placed upon it.

skill-related fitness
Ability to perform specific skills associated with various sports and leisure activities.

health-related fitness
Ability to perform daily living activities with vigor.

physical activity
Activity that requires any type of movement.

Exercise
Structured, planned physical activity, often carried out to improve fitness.

WHAT IS FITNESS?

Physical fitness, in general, is the ability of the body to respond to the physical demands placed upon it. It is closely related to good health, which means having sufficient energy and vitality to accomplish daily living tasks and leisure-time physical activities without undue fatigue. When we talk about *fitness,* we are really talking about two different concepts: skill-related fitness and health-related fitness.[3] **Skill-related fitness** refers to the ability to perform specific skills associated with various sports and leisure activities. Components of skill-related fitness include agility, speed, power, balance, coordination, and reaction time. **Health-related fitness** refers to the ability to perform daily living activities (like shopping for groceries) and other activities with vigor.[3] Components of health-related fitness are cardiorespiratory fitness, musculoskeletal fitness, and body composition. Musculoskeletal fitness, in turn, includes muscular strength, muscular endurance, and flexibility. Shortly, the chapter will look at each of these fitness components in detail.

Benefits of Physical Activity and Exercise

Physical activity—activity that requires any type of movement—is necessary for good health. Any kind of physical activity is better than no activity at all, and benefits increase as the level of physical activity increases, up to a point. Too much physical activity can make you susceptible to injury. **Exercise** is structured, planned physical activity, often carried out to improve fitness.

Why should you be physically active? Your answers to this question may include having fun, looking good, and feeling good. Beyond these, however, is another reason to be physically active: people who are active are healthier than those who are not.[3] There are benefits in the domains of physical, cognitive, psychological, and emotional health and at the molecular level. The box, "Physical Activity: The Human Capital Model," describes the value of these benefits to society.

Physical Benefits of Exercise One benefit of physical activity is a longer lifespan: people with moderate to high levels of physical activity live longer than people who are sedentary. Physical activity and exercise are associated with improved functioning in just about every body system, from the cardiorespiratory system to the skeletal system to the immune system. A sedentary lifestyle, on the other hand, has been associated with 28 percent of deaths from the leading chronic diseases, including cancer, heart disease, osteoporosis, diabetes, high blood pressure, and obesity.[4–11] Results from just a few research studies are shown in Figure 6.1.

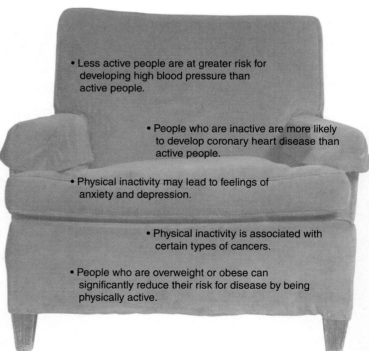

- Less active people are at greater risk for developing high blood pressure than active people.

- People who are inactive are more likely to develop coronary heart disease than active people.

- Physical inactivity may lead to feelings of anxiety and depression.

- Physical inactivity is associated with certain types of cancers.

- People who are overweight or obese can significantly reduce their risk for disease by being physically active.

figure 6.1   **Health risks and physical inactivity.**
Source: www.hopkinsmedicine.org/healthlibrary/conditions/adult/cardiovascular_diseases/risks_of_physical_inactivity_85,P00218/

Who's at Risk?

Adults Meeting 2008 Physical Activity Guidelines for Aerobic and Muscle-Strengthening Activity

Why do you think non-Hispanic black adults are more likely to meet the physical activity guidelines than non-Hispanic white adults and Hispanic adults? Why are adult men more likely to meet the guidelines than adult women?

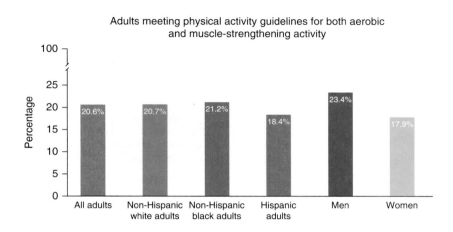

Adults meeting physical activity guidelines for both aerobic and muscle-strengthening activity

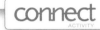

Source: Centers for Disease Control and Prevention. (2013). Adult participation in aerobic and muscle-strengthening physical activities—United States, 2011. *MMWR, 62* (17), 326–330.

Cognitive Benefits of Exercise Although there is no conclusive evidence to suggest that short-term exercise training significantly improves cognitive functioning, some studies on animals and humans suggest that physical activity can be beneficial to the brain.[12,13] Exercise stimulates the growth of new brain cells in the hippocampus (the part of the brain where learning is centered) and in the frontal cortex (the center for decision making, planning, and other executive functions). Exercise encourages brain cells to branch out, join together, and communicate with each other in new ways, and it prompts nerve cells to form denser, more interconnected webs that enable the brain to operate more quickly and efficiently.

Other research has shown that aerobic fitness may prevent or slow down the loss of cognitive functions associated with advancing age,[12] and it may help prevent cognitive disorders like Alzheimer's disease in older adults. Some studies found that inactive individuals were twice as likely to develop Alzheimer's disease as those who participated in aerobic exercise at least 30 minutes a day three times a week. Running, and even nonstrenuous walking, may also improve learning, concentration, and abstract reasoning.[14]

Psychological and Emotional Benefits of Exercise
Moderate to intense levels of physical activity have been shown to influence mood, decrease the risk of depression

and anxiety, relieve stress, and improve overall quality of life.[15] (On the other hand, excessive exercise has the potential to become addictive; see the box, "Colleen: Obsessed With Running.") Although biological explanations have been proposed for the improved sense of well-being associated with physical activity; other explanations are improved self-esteem, improved quality of sleep, and more opportunities for social interaction.

Scientists are currently looking at the benefits of "green exercise"—exercising outdoors in natural settings. Research findings suggest that if you walk, run, or hike in a greenspace area, in the city or countryside, you are more likely to feel better all around than if you exercise indoors. Green exercise provides the brain with a respite from the multitasking of everyday life and increases awareness of the sounds, smells, and colors of the natural landscape. Benefits of green exercise may include improved mood and overall well-being, as well as reduced feelings of anger, tension, confusion, and depression. In one study, improvements in mood occurred regardless of activity chosen or duration of exercise. Green exercisers performed better on tests requiring memory and attention, had lower blood pressure, and felt more spiritually connected than people who did not exercise outdoors.[16,17]

Benefits of Exercise at the Molecular Level Research is challenging what scientists once believed were the reasons

Public Health Is Personal

Physical Activity: The Human Capital Model

Nike brought together a group of sports scientists, medical researchers, and psychologists to develop a conceptual model that validated the importance of physical activity to society as well as individuals, the Human Capital Model (HCM). Most scientific attention has focused on the impact of physical activity on chronic diseases and mortality; for example, research has shown that participation in regular physical activity may reduce all-cause mortality by 20 to 40 percent. Although this disease-mortality defense of physical activity has been an effective tool for engaging and empowering individuals and communities to become more physically active, the cognitive, emotional, social, and economic benefits of physical activity need to receive comparable attention.

The HCM conceptualizes six domains of capital associated with physical activity: (1) *physical capital*—prevention and mitigation of chronic diseases; (2) *emotional capital*—psychological and mental health benefits; (3) *individual capital*—character skills;

(4) *social capital*—networks between and among people, groups, communities, organizations; (5) *intellectual capital*—cognitive function, educational achievements; and (6) *financial capital*—reduced health care costs and increased job productivity and personal earning power.

At a time when governments and institutions are searching for high-return solutions for today's health and social issues, HCM provides a framework for informing public policy. It presents investments in physical activity as having much greater benefit to personal and public health than is commonly assumed. There are many mediating factors that nudge people in the direction toward or away from participation in physical activity. The positive potential capital returns of the HCM captures a more holistic view of physical activity. The bottom line is that the HCM presents investment in physical activity as a powerful catalyst for both personal and social change.

connect ACTIVITY

Sources: "Physical Activity as an Investment in Personal and Social Change: The Human Capital Model," by R. Bailey, C. Hillman, S. Arent et al., 2012, *Journal of Physical Activity and Health, 9,* pp. 1053–1055; "Physical activity: An underestimated investment in human capital," by R. Bailey, C. Hillman, S. Arent et al., 2013, *Journal of Physical Activity and Health, 10,* 289–308.

exercise is beneficial for preventing heart disease. Conventional wisdom suggested prevention benefits were due to decreasing blood pressure, lowering LDL, increasing HDL, and creating collateral blood vessel branches to the heart. But, the impact of exercise on blood pressure is marginal. Exercise has been shown to increase the size of LDL and decrease the number of small LDL. As you will learn in Chapter 14, large LDL is less toxic to the heart than small LDL.[4]

Exercise also affects blood glucose. Your liver, pancreas, and skeletal muscles work in concert so that each part of your body receives glucose as needed while you are at rest or active. Exercise demands on skeletal muscles increases their demand for glucose. Prolonged exercise enables muscle fibers to become more efficient in using glucose. This helps your body keep blood glucose levels between 70 to 140 milligrams/deciliter (mg/dL). Blood glucose needs to be above 70 mg/dL in order to provide your brain with sufficient energy. Prolonged blood glucose levels above 140mg/dL clog your arteries and causes cells to die prematurely. Exercise makes muscle cells more sensitive to insulin, which helps reduce the workload on your pancreas in maintaining stable blood glucose levels. Stable blood glucose levels are especially important for people with Type-2 diabetes. Recent research also suggests that exercise provides a second pathway to remove glucose from the blood that does not depend on insulin by stimulating muscle cells to make a protein called PGC-1a. PGC-1a signals muscles cells to develop new mitochondria. The addition of new mitochondria enables muscle cells to convert more glucose into energy. This new pathway may provide a valuable medical pathway for treating people with diabetes.[4]

An overview of the health benefits associated with physical activity is presented in Figure 6.2.

General Guidelines for Physical Activity

In 2008 the Department of Health and Human Services (HHS) issued a widely accepted set of guidelines aimed at promoting and maintaining health and preventing chronic diseases and premature mortality. These physical activity guidelines recommend that for substantial health benefits, adults should accumulate 150 minutes (2 hours and 30 minutes) of moderate-intensity exercise, or 75 minutes (1 hour and 15 minutes) of vigorous-intensity exercise a week.[18]

The American College of Sports Medicine (ACSM) released its own guidelines in 2013, which are similar to those given by the HHS. The ACSM recommends that adults do moderate-intensity exercise for at least 30 minutes on 5 or more days a week (for a minimum of 150 minutes of moderate-intensity exercise a week), or vigorous-intensity for 20 to 25 minutes on 3 or more days a week (for a minimum of 75 minutes of moderate-intensity exercise a week).[19]

Moderate-intensity activity is defined as activity that noticeably accelerates the heart rate; an example is a brisk walk (see Table 6.1 for more examples). Vigorous-intensity

Colleen: Obsessed With Running

Colleen was an intense, high-achieving perfectionist and a running devotee. She had begun running in high school, and now, as a college sophomore, she tried to run at least 5 miles every day, usually alone. Colleen tried to get to bed no later than 9 p.m. so she could get her run in before her early morning classes. She ran no matter what the weather, even when the temperature was below freezing and the roads were covered in black ice. She ran when she had a cold and when her back and legs ached from fatigue. On days she didn't run, she felt irritable and anxious.

Colleen's family and friends were supportive of her running at first and impressed with her determination, though they weren't surprised, because Colleen did everything all-out. But by the middle of her sophomore year, people were becoming more and more concerned about her preoccupation with daily runs. She would miss family and social events if they interfered with her running schedule or her early-to-bed routine. She didn't have time to date or to socialize with her friends. When she wasn't running she was planning her next run, reading running blogs, or checking out running gear online.

When confronted about her preoccupation with running, Colleen responded, "Running is my life. It gives me my sense of identity. I'm proud of having goals and being committed to a healthy activity. A lot of people don't get any exercise at all. What's wrong with trying to be healthy?"

In April, Colleen was diagnosed with stress fractures in both feet. She had no choice but to stop running for a few months. In the first week after the diagnosis, she was anxious and on edge, beset by worries and feelings of dread and hopelessness. She started having crying spells and felt reluctant to leave her room. She realized that the only time she really felt in control of her life was when she was running.

Concerned about what was going on with her, Colleen made an appointment with a counselor at the campus health clinic. The counselor told her that if running interfered significantly with her personal and school life, it had become a mental health issue. He told her about recent research suggesting that running can become an addiction. Like cocaine or opium, running can cause a spike in levels of the neurotransmitter dopamine, stimulating reward centers in the brain and giving the runner a sensation of pleasure. What Colleen was going through was like withdrawal from a drug.

The first step in overcoming any addiction is acknowledging the problem. This was hard for Colleen to do, and it was only in her third session that she was able to admit to herself that running had become a problem for her. With more counseling, Colleen was able to develop a more balanced approach to her physical, emotional, and psychological health.

■ What do you think about the idea that healthy activities can become unhealthy addictions? What do you think could cause such a shift?

■ What do you think are the signs that an activity has become an addiction?

■ If you had to speculate, what needs do you think Colleen was trying to meet by running so much? What do you think she was trying to avoid?

connect ACTIVITY

---

activity causes rapid breathing and a substantial increase in heart rate, as exemplified by jogging. The recommended activity is in addition to the light activities associated with daily living.[19]

Whether vigorous or moderate, activity should be done in bouts of 10 minutes or more and spread throughout the week. For example, a person can meet the HHS guidelines by doing 30 minutes of moderate-intensity exercise 5 days a week, or by doing 50 minutes of moderate-intensity exercise 3 days a week. Combinations of moderate-intensity activity and vigorous-intensity activity may be used to meet the recommendation. For example, you could walk briskly on a flat surface for 30 minutes 2 days a week and jog for 20 minutes 2 days a week.

These are minimum recommendations; exercise levels beyond the minimum can confer additional health benefits, such as the prevention of unwanted weight gain.[19] In general, people with disabilities should follow the same recommendations as people without disabilities. The HHS and ACSM guidelines also include recommendations for improving muscular strength and endurance; we describe these recommendations later in the chapter. The Personal Health Portfolio Activity for this chapter will help you assess your current level of physical activity.

COMPONENTS OF HEALTH-RELATED FITNESS

Fitness training programs can improve each of the components of health-related fitness—cardiorespiratory fitness, musculoskeletal fitness (muscular strength, muscular endurance, and flexibility), and body composition. In this section, we discuss each component separately.

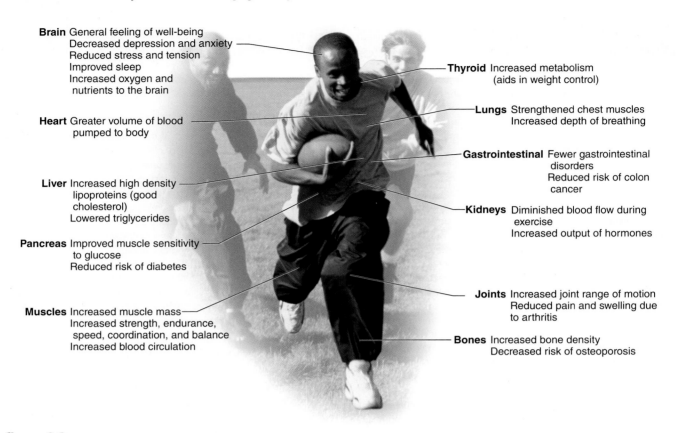

Brain General feeling of well-being
Decreased depression and anxiety
Reduced stress and tension
Improved sleep
Increased oxygen and
nutrients to the brain

Heart Greater volume of blood
pumped to body

Liver Increased high density
lipoproteins (good
cholesterol)
Lowered triglycerides

Pancreas Improved muscle sensitivity
to glucose
Reduced risk of diabetes

Muscles Increased muscle mass
Increased strength, endurance,
speed, coordination, and balance
Increased blood circulation

Thyroid Increased metabolism
(aids in weight control)

Lungs Strengthened chest muscles
Increased depth of breathing

Gastrointestinal Fewer gastrointestinal
disorders
Reduced risk of colon
cancer

Kidneys Diminished blood flow during
exercise
Increased output of hormones

Joints Increased joint range of motion
Reduced pain and swelling due
to arthritis

Bones Increased bone density
Decreased risk of osteoporosis

figure 6.2   **Health benefits of physical activity.**

Table 6.1   Examples of Light-, Moderate-, and Vigorous-Intensity Activities

Light	Moderate	Vigorous
Slow walking	Walking 3.0 mph	Walking 4.5 mph
Canoeing	Cycling leisurely	Cycling moderately
Golf with cart	Golf, no cart	Jogging 7 mph
Croquet	Table tennis	Tennis singles
Fishing—sitting	Slow swimming	Moderate swimming
Billiards	Boat sailing	Volleyball
Darts	Housework/gardening	Basketball
Playing cards	Calisthenics	Competitive soccer
Walking the dog	Tennis doubles	Rope skipping
Grocery shopping	Yoga	Martial arts
Laundry	Playing with children	Snowboarding

The key to fitness training is the body's ability to adapt to increasing demands by becoming more fit—that is, as a general rule, the more you exercise, the fitter you become. The amount of exercise, called *overload,* is significant, however. If you exercise too little, your fitness level won't improve. If you exercise too much, you may be susceptible to injury. When you are designing an exercise program, you need to think about four dimensions of your exercise sessions that affect overload:

- Frequency (number of sessions per week).
- Intensity (level of difficulty of each exercise session).
- Time (duration of each exercise session).
- Type (type of exercise in each exercise session).

You can remember these dimensions with the acronym FITT.

Cardiorespiratory Fitness

Cardiorespiratory fitness is the ability of the heart and lungs to efficiently deliver oxygen and nutrients to the body's muscles and cells via the bloodstream. Cardio fitness should be at the center of any fitness program. It is developed by activities that use the large muscles of the body in continuous movement, such as jogging, running, cycling, swimming, cross-country skiing, and aerobic dance.

Cardiorespiratory Training Benefits of cardiorespiratory training are an increase in the oxygen-carrying capacity of the blood, improved extraction of oxygen from the bloodstream by muscle cells, an increase in the amount of blood the heart pumps with each heartbeat, and increased speed of recovery back to a resting level after exercise. Cardiorespiratory training improves muscle and liver functioning and decreases resting heart rate, resting blood pressure, and heart rate at any work level.

How do you go about developing a cardiorespiratory training program to improve your level of fitness? Start by using the FITT acronym (frequency, intensity, time, and type of activity).

Frequency In general, you must exercise at least twice a week to experience improvements in cardiorespiratory functioning. The ideal frequency for training is three times a week. Exercising five or six times a week is appropriate if weight control is a primary concern.[19]

Intensity The point at which you are stressing your cardiorespiratory system for optimal benefit but not overdoing it is called the **target heart rate (THR) zone**. The ACSM recommends that people set their THR at 55 to 80 percent of their maximum heart rate (MHR)—that is, that they exercise at 55 percent to 80 percent of their maximum heart rate. The most accurate way to find your THR zone is to calculate your heart rate reserve, or the difference between your MHR and your resting heart rate:

1. To determine your resting heart rate (RHR), take your pulse at the carotid (neck) or radial (wrist) artery while you are at rest. Use your middle finger or forefinger or both when taking your pulse; do not use your thumb because it has a pulse of its own. Take your pulse for 15 seconds and multiply by 4.

2. To determine your maximum heart rate (MHR), subtract your age from 220.

3. To determine your THR objective, use the maximal **heart rate reserve (HRR)** formula. The THR is usually 60 to 80 percent for young adults and 55 to 70 percent for older adults. Here is the HRR formula:

$$THR = X\% (MHR - RHR) + RHR$$

Example: Serena is 20 years old and just starting a cardiorespiratory training program. Her THR goal is 60 to 80 percent, and she has a resting heart rate of 70. For a 60 percent threshold, the THR would be calculated as follows:

$$0.6(200 - 70) + 70 = 0.6(130) + 70 = 78 + 70 = 148$$

For an 80 percent threshold, the THR would be calculated as follows:

$$0.8(200 - 70) + 70$$
$$= 0.8(130) + 70 = 104 + 70 = 174$$

Thus, Serena's THR zone is between 148 and 174.

A quicker way to determine your target heart rate is the maximum heart rate formula: 220 (MHR) minus your age times your desired intensity. For example, if you are 20 years old and want to work out at 60 to 80 percent intensity, you would subtract 20 from 220 and multiply by 0.60 and 0.80. Your target heart rate zone would be 120 to 160.

The Harvard Health Studies recommend a more precise maximum heart rate formula: 208 minus (0.7 times age) times intensity. Cardiologist Martha Gulati suggests that because women have a different exercise capacity than men, they should calculate their THRs differently than men.[20] See Table 6.2 for a comparison of the two methods.

cardiorespiratory fitness
Ability of the heart and lungs to efficiently deliver oxygen and nutrients to the body's muscles and cells via the bloodstream.

target heart rate (THR) zone
Range of exercise intensity that allows you to stress your cardiorespiratory system for optimal benefit without overloading the system.

heart rate reserve (HRR)
Difference between maximum heart rate and resting heart rate.

Heart rate alone should not determine your workout intensity: to ensure that intensity is not too low or high, use the breathing test and perceived exertion test. The breathing test is a simple measure of whether you can speak in complete sentences without breathing hard as you exercise.

Table 6.2 Standard Target Heart Rate Formula Compared to the Gulati Heart Rate Formula

	Standard Fitness Guideline	Gulati Formula
Aimed at:	Men/Women	Women Only
To find maximum heart rate:	Subtract age from 220	Subtract 88% of your age from 206
Example, for a 20-year-old	220 − 20 = **200**	206 − 18 = 188 (88% of 20 = 17.6)
Target low for a 20-year-old	200 × 0.70 = **140**	188 × 0.70 = 132 (rounded)
Target high for a 20-year-old	200 × 0.85 = **170**	188 × 0.85 = 160 (rounded)

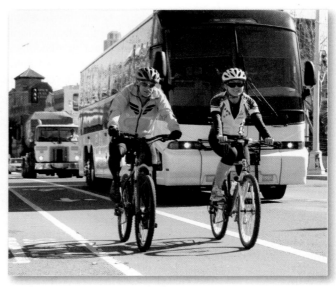

■ Cycling is an excellent way to develop cardiorespiratory fitness. The most effective cardio training is exercise that involves continuous movement by the large muscles of the body.

The perceived exertion test is a subjective measure of how you feel when you are exercising. Moderate intensity would be perceived as "somewhat hard."

Time Generally, exercise sessions should last from 15 to 60 minutes; 30 minutes is a good average to aim for. Duration and intensity of exercise have an inverse relation with each other so that a shorter, higher intensity session can give your cardiorespiratory system the same workout as a longer, lower intensity session.

Type of Activity Aerobic exercise is brisk physical activity that increases the circulation of oxygen through the blood vessels and is associated with increased respiration. There are two types of aerobic exercise: (1) exercises that require sustained intensity with little variability in heart rate response, such as running and rowing, and (2) exercises that involve stop-and-go activities and do not maintain continuous exercise intensity, such as basketball, soccer, and tennis. Stop-and-go activities usually have to be done for a longer period of time than do sustained-intensity activities before they confer cardiorespiratory benefits. Both types of activity can be part of a cardiorespiratory training program.

Training Progression To receive the maximum benefit from exercise, you need to adjust your level of activity by altering duration and intensity every so often. After you have obtained a satisfactory level of cardiorespiratory fitness and are no longer interested in increasing your conditioning workload, you can maintain your fitness level by continuing the same level of workout.[18]

As a general rule, people between the ages of 20 and 29 need two weeks to adapt to a cardiorespiratory activity workload. At that point, they need to increase their activity workload. Older people need to add 10 percent to adaptation time for each decade after age 30. A 20-year-old, for example, can expect to adjust workload every two weeks. A 70-year-old would adjust workload about every three weeks (40 percent longer is about six days).

High-Intensity Interval Training (HIT). The primary reason people give for not exercising is not enough time. HIT is a cardio program that provides a way to receive fitness benefits in less time. Research has shown that 20 minutes of HIT has similar benefits as 40 minutes of continuous aerobic training. High- and low-intensity intervals of exercise are alternated. Your body is never given the chance to plateau; getting used to one setting is common in most forms of cardio activity. The common HIT workout uses combinations of 30 seconds of "hard" interval, followed by either 30, 60, or 90 seconds "easy" intervals that are repeated 10 times. *Hard* (high intensity) is defined as getting your heart rate up to 80 to 90 percent maximum heart rate (MHR), or 8 to 9 on the perceived exertion scale. *Easy* (low intensity) is defined as 40 to 50 percent MHR, or 5 on the perceived exertion scale. Another example is simply getting out of your comfort zone. For example, when walking across campus, you may walk at a very fast rate (4.2 to 4.4 mph) for a block, and then slow down to 3.5 mph for a block. If it hard for you to talk when walking, then you are out of your comfort zone.[21]

Developing Your Own Program To develop your own regular cardiorespiratory training program, start out slowly to avoid injury and gradually build up your endurance. If you have any medical conditions, or if you have been sedentary and are over the age of 40, see your physician for a checkup before starting. To ensure that you will stick with your program, select activities that you enjoy and that are compatible with the constraints of your schedule, budget, and lifestyle. Whether you choose running, swimming, cycling, a team sport, or another aerobic activity, try to build sessions of at least 30 minutes' duration into your schedule three times a week. If you make these sessions part of your life, they can be the foundation of a lasting fitness program.

Muscular Fitness

Health-related fitness also includes muscular fitness. Benefits of improved muscular fitness are increased lean body mass, which helps prevent obesity; increased bone mineral density, which prevents osteoporosis; improved glucose metabolism and insulin sensitivity, which prevent diabetes; and decreased anxiety and depression, which improves quality of life.[19] Muscular fitness improves posture, prevents or reduces low back pain, enables you to perform the tasks of daily living with greater ease, and helps you to look and feel better.[21,22]

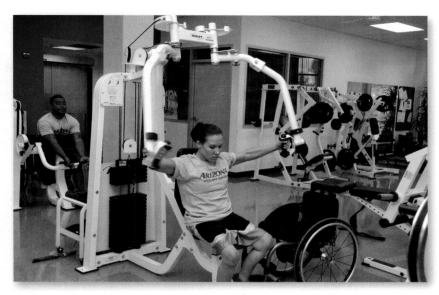

■ Muscular strength and endurance, important components of a fitness program, are developed by weight training, using either weight machines, free weights, or the weight of the body (as in calisthenics).

Muscular fitness has two main components: muscular strength and muscular endurance. **Muscular strength** is the capacity of a muscle to exert force against resistance. It is primarily dependent on how much muscle mass you have. Your muscular strength is measured by how much you can lift, push, or pull in a single, all-out effort. **Muscular endurance** is the capacity of a muscle to exert force repeatedly over a period of time, or to apply and sustain strength for a period lasting from a few seconds to a few minutes.

Strength Training Muscular strength and endurance are developed by strength training, also known as weight training or resistance training. This is a type of exercise in which the muscles exert force against resistance, such as free weights (dumbbells, barbells) or exercise resistance machines.

Frequency and Type of Activity Two to three resistance training sessions a week are sufficient for building muscle strength and endurance. The primary muscle groups targeted in resistance training are the deltoids (shoulders), pectorals (chest), triceps (back of upper arms), biceps (front of upper arms), quadriceps (front of thighs), hamstrings (back of thighs), gluteus maximus (buttocks), and abdomen. Other areas to exercise are the upper back, the lower back, and the calves. Whether you choose free weights or weight machines, try to exercise every muscle group during your strength training sessions.

Intensity and Duration: The Strength-Endurance Continuum The same exercises develop both strength and endurance, but their intensity and duration vary. To develop strength, you need to exercise at a higher intensity (greater resistance or more weight) for a shorter duration; to develop endurance, you need to exercise at a lower intensity for a longer duration. Duration is measured in terms of repetitions—the number of times you perform the exercise (e.g., lift a barbell). If you lift a heavy weight a few times (e.g., 1 to 5 repetitions), you are developing strength. If you lift a lighter weight more times (e.g., 20 repetitions), you are developing endurance.

muscular strength Capacity of a muscle to exert force against resistance.

muscular endurance Capacity of a muscle to exert force repeatedly over a period of time.

Gender Differences in Muscle Development The amount of muscle that can be developed in the body differs by gender. Muscle mass growth is influenced by the male sex hormone testosterone, and although women do produce this hormone, they do so at levels that are only about 10 percent of the levels seen in men. Women can increase muscle mass through strength training programs, but the increase will be less than that achieved by men.[22]

There is also a wide range of individual variability in both men and women. Regardless of gender, some people can develop significantly more muscle than others can. Body type (*somatotype*) plays a role in some of these differences. People with a *mesomorphic* body type (stocky, muscular) gain muscle more easily than those with an *ectomorphic* body type (tall, thin) or *endomorphic* body type (short, fat). Both men and women with mesomorphic bodies have higher levels of testosterone, and thus a greater ability to build muscle, than do those with the other two body types.

Other Types of Muscular Fitness Training and Equipment In addition to strength training, there are many other ways of developing the physical capabilities of the body. The amount of work that can be performed in a given period of time is known as **muscular power**. Power is determined by the amount and quality of muscle; it requires great strength and the ability to produce that strength quickly. You can train for muscular power by performing any exercise faster.

One type of exercise program developed specifically for muscular power is *plyometrics,* a program that trains muscles to reach maximum force in the shortest possible time. A muscle that is stretched before contracting will contract more forcefully and rapidly. For example, you can jump higher if you initiate the jump from a crouched position.[22]

Another type of training is **core-strength training**, also called *functional strength training,* which conditions the body torso from the neck to the lower back. The objectives of core-strength training are to lengthen the spine, develop balance, reduce the waistline, prevent back injury, and sculpt the body without bulking it up. Scientific evidence in support of these claims is sparse. Exercise experts, however, argue that training programs increase muscle mass, and metabolic expenditure provides health benefits.[22]

Probably the most popular core-strength training program being taught in health clubs today is *Pilates* (pi-*lah*-teez), an exercise system developed in the 1920s by physical trainer Joseph Pilates. The exercises, performed on special apparatus and a floor mat, are based on the premise that the body's "powerhouse" is in the torso, particularly the abdomen. Exercises are taught by trained instructors and are tailored to the individual.

Other exercise programs incorporate *unstable surfaces* like balance boards, tilt disks, and trampolines. The theory is that balancing on an unstable surface forces you to make sudden, inconsistent motions that exercise your nervous system's ability to send sensory information to muscles and joints. Uneven surfaces also produce co-contraction of muscles, meaning that muscles on opposite sides of a joint contract simultaneously and build strength more efficiently. However, because the use of unstable surfaces for lower and upper body strength training and core body training is relatively new, there is little evidence that it is more beneficial than exercise on stable surfaces. Moreover, movements like hopping, jumping, and leaping on unstable surfaces increase risk of injury from a fall or excess impact on joints.[23]

Resistance cords are convenient and useful devices for strength training and flexibility. These cords are designed for different age groups and with different strength levels. Cords can be used with other equipment, such as exercise bars and medicine balls. The most important benefit of resistance cords is that then allow you to proceed gradually through your exercise.

muscular power
Amount of work performed by muscles in a given period of time.

core-strength training
Strength training that conditions the body torso from the neck to the lower back.

Stability balls help the user develop balance, strength, and postural awareness. In particular, stability balls help to develop core muscles (abdomen, lower back, gluteals, and thighs). They are versatile, inexpensive, and portable. Stability balls come in four basic sizes: 45 cm, 55 cm, 65 cm, and 75 cm. To determine the optimal ball size for you, sit on it with your feet on the floor. Your legs need to be at 90 degrees with hips even with your knees and thighs parallel to the floor. The ball is too small for your body frame if your hips sink below your knees when you sit down.[24]

Gaining Weight and Muscle Mass Safely When people want to gain weight, it is usually to improve appearance, health, or performance. Gaining weight simply by eating more is not a productive strategy because the weight gain will be nearly all fat. The goal is to increase muscle tissue with little or no increase in body fat stores. The healthy way to attain such a gain is through physical activity, particularly strength training, combined with a high-calorie diet. Gaining a pound of muscle and fat requires consuming about 3,000 extra calories.[25] To build muscle, you need to consume 700 to 1,000 calories a day above energy needs or take in sufficient calories to support both the added activity energy requirements and the formation of new muscle.[26] A gain of a half pound to a pound a week is a reasonable goal. Your primary exercise activity to gain muscle should be weight training.

Drugs and Dietary Supplements Some people, especially athletes, attempt to gain muscle tissue by using drugs, dietary supplements, or protein supplements. Most of these substances are expensive and ineffective; some are dangerous, and some are illegal. People who use performance-enhancing drugs and dietary supplements may enhance their athletic performance by building bigger muscles, but they also may be heading for health problems that can shorten their lives. Unfortunately, any discussion of the risks and benefits of these substances is clouded by a lack of scientific data. Scientists often don't know who is using them, what the effects of different doses are, how long they can be taken before causing side effects, or what happens when they are taken with other drugs.[26] An overview of some of the major performance-enhancing drugs and dietary supplements, along with their possible benefits and side effects, is shown in Table 6.3.

The sports and fitness industry is experiencing a boom in protein supplements,[26] such as Clif Bars. The protein in these products is from natural protein sources, such as soy, eggs, milk, or chicken. Other substances, such as purified amino acids, are often added. Commercial protein supplements are expensive and do not carry all the nutrients of natural fuels. They can serve as a convenient adjunct to a balanced diet for people who are too busy to obtain enough protein in their diet, but most Americans, including athletes, get more than enough protein from their diets.

Table 6.3   Selected Performance-Enhancing Drugs and Dietary Supplements and Their Effects

Substance or Dietary Supplement	Effects	Side Effects
Anabolic steroid, testosterone	Promotes muscle growth by improving ability of muscle to respond to training and to recover.	Masculinization of females; feminization of males; acne; mood swings; sexual dysfunction.
Human growth hormone	Promotes muscle growth.	Widened jawline and nose, protruding eyebrows, buck teeth; increased risk of high blood pressure, congestive heart failure.
Ephedrine	Boosts energy, promotes weight loss (stimulates metabolism).	High blood pressure; irregular heartbeat; increased risk of stroke and heart attack.
Androstenedione (Andro)	Promotes muscle growth.	Decreased good cholesterol (HDL); increased levels of estrogen, breast enlargement in men; increased risk of pancreatic cancer; may significantly increase testosterone levels in women (little known about Andro effects in women).
Dehydroepiandrosterone (DHEA)	May promote muscle growth.	Body hair growth; liver enlargement; aggressive behavior; long-term health effects not known.
Creatine monohydrate	May increase performance in brief high-intensity exercises; promotes increased body mass when used with resistance training.	Diarrhea; dehydration and muscle cramping; muscle tearing; long-term health effects not known.
Chromium picolinate	May build muscle tissue, facilitate burning of fat, and boost energy.	Chromium buildup with large doses and possible liver damage and other health problems; long-term health effects not known.

Sources: www.mayoclinic.com/health/creatine/NS_patient; *Nutrition for Health, Fitness, and Sport,* 10th ed., by M.H. Williams, New York: McGraw-Hill. 2013.

Developing a Strength Training Program The ACSM recommendations for strength training vary by level of experience. Novices (people who have never done resistance training or who have not done resistance training for several years) and intermediates (people who have done six months or more of resistance training) should perform 8 to 12 repetitions per set using sufficient resistance to fatigue the muscles.

Novices are advised to do two to three full-body workouts a week consisting of 8 to 10 exercises that work all major muscle groups.

Intermediates and more advanced people often do a split routine, where they exercise different muscle groups on different days. Intermediates can do four workouts per week on a split routine.

People who have been doing strength training for several years can also do as many as 12 repetitions per set using sufficient resistance to fatigue the muscles, or as few as 1 repetition using the maximum amount of weight they can lift. They can train four to six times a week doing a split routine.

Sets and rest periods for all levels of experience will vary based on goals (strength, power, endurance), but in general, two to four sets should be done with 1 to 2 minutes of rest between sets.[19]

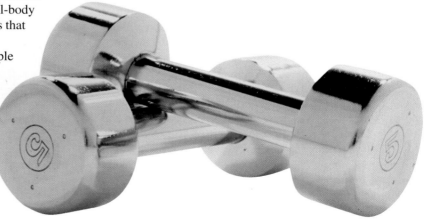

Strength training can be a safe and effective form of exercise if appropriate guidelines are followed:

- Warm up by gently stretching, jogging, or lifting light weights.

- Do not hold your breath or hyperventilate. As you are lifting, breathe rhythmically.

- To protect your back, hold weights close to your body. Do not arch your back. Weight belts may prevent arching.

- When using resistance training machines, always check to make sure the pins holding weights are in place. When using free weights, make sure collars are tight.

- Lift weights with a slow, steady cadence through a full range of motion. Do not jerk the weight to complete a repetition.

- Always use a spotter when working out with free weights.

- Allow at least 48 hours between training sessions if you will be exercising the same muscle groups.

Breathing and Safety Oxygen flow is vital for preventing muscle fatigue and injury during resistance training. Inhale when your muscles are relaxed, and exhale when you initiate the lifting or push-off action. Never hold your breath while performing resistance exercises.

Flexibility

Another important component of musculoskeletal fitness is **flexibility**, the ability of joints to move through their full range of motion. Good flexibility helps you maintain posture and balance, makes movement easier and more fluid, and lowers your risk of injury. It is a key factor in preventing low back pain and injury.

Your flexibility is affected by factors that you cannot change, such as genetic endowment, gender, and age, and by factors that you can change, such as physical activity patterns. A common misconception is that flexibility declines steadily once a person reaches adulthood. Flexibility does seem to be highest in the teenage years, and aging is accompanied by a shortening of tendons and an increased rigidity in muscles and joints. However, there is also strong evidence that much of the loss of flexibility that results from aging can be reduced by stretching programs.[27]

flexibility
Ability of joints to move through their full range of motion.

Types of Stretching Programs Medical and fitness experts agree that stretching the muscles attached to the joints is the single most important part of an exercise program because it promotes flexibility, reduces muscle tension, and prevents injuries. However, stretching done incorrectly can cause more harm than good. Thus, understanding the right stretching techniques and progressing gradually are keys to a successful program.

In *static stretching,* you stretch until you feel tightness in the muscle and then hold that position for a set period of time without bouncing or forcing movement. After you have held the stretch, the muscle tension will seem to decrease, and you can stretch farther without pain. Static stretching lengthens the muscle and surrounding tissue, reducing the risk of injury. Static stretching is the kind of stretching done in Hatha yoga and is the type recommended for general fitness purposes.

In *passive stretching,* a partner applies pressure to your muscles, typically producing a stretch beyond what you can do on your own. Passive stretching is often used by physical therapists. If you can totally relax your muscle fibers, the use of pressure by another person can help prevent the problem of partial contraction of muscle fibers. There is a danger, however, of forcing a stretch beyond the point of normal relaxation of the muscles and tendons, causing tearing and injury. For this reason, passive stretching should be limited to supervised medical situations and persons who cannot move by themselves.[27]

In *ballistic stretching,* the muscle is stretched in a series of bouncing movements designed to increase the range of motion. As you bounce, receptors in the muscles, called

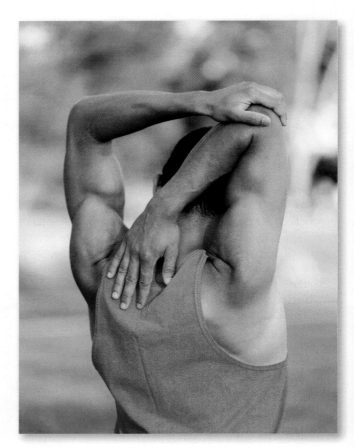

- Developing flexibility through stretching exercises should be part of a regular fitness program. Stretching is most beneficial and effective when the muscles are warm, as they are after a workout.

muscle spindles, are stretched. Ballistic stretching is used by experienced athletes, but because it can increase vulnerability to muscle pulls and tears, it is not recommended for most people.

Proprioceptive neuromuscular facilitation (PNF), a type of hold/relax stretching, is a therapeutic exercise that causes a stretch reflex in muscles. It is used primarily in the rehabilitation of injured muscles.[27]

Developing Your Own Flexibility Program The ACSM recommends that stretching exercise be done for all the major joints, including the neck, shoulders, upper back and trunk, hips, knees, and ankles. Stretching should be done two to three days a week or more. Stretch to a point of mild discomfort (not pain) and hold the stretch for 10 to 30 seconds. Do two to four repetitions of each stretch, to accumulate 60 seconds per stretch.

Stretching can be part of your warm-up for your cardiorespiratory or resistance training program as long as these stretches are gentle, slow, and steady. To prevent injury, warm up first with 5 to 10 minutes of brisk walking, marching in place, or calisthenics. This warm-up will increase your heart rate, raise your core body temperature, and lubricate your joints. You will experience the greatest improvement in flexibility, however, from stretching exercises after your other exercise, when your muscles are warm and less likely to be injured by stretching.

Body Composition

The final component of health-related fitness we consider here is **body composition**—the relative amounts of fat and fat-free mass in the body. Fat-free mass includes muscle, bone, water, body organs, and other body tissues. Body fat includes both fat that is essential for normal functioning, such as fat in the nerves, heart, and liver, and fat stored in fat cells, usually located under the skin and around organs. The recommended proportion of body fat to fat-free mass, expressed as *percent body fat,* is 21 to 35 percent for women and 8 to 24 percent for men.

The relative amount of body fat has an effect on overall health and fitness. Too much body fat is associated with overweight and obesity and with increased risk for chronic diseases like heart disease, diabetes, and many types of cancer. A greater amount of fat-free mass, on the other hand, gives the body a lean, healthy appearance. The heart and lungs function more efficiently without the burden of extra weight. Because muscle tissue uses energy at a higher metabolic rate than does fat tissue, the more muscle mass you have, the more calories you can consume without gaining weight.

We discuss body composition in more detail in Chapter 7, on body weight. Here, the basic message is that you can control body weight, trim body fat, and build muscle tissue by incorporating more physical activity into your daily life. Use the stairs rather than taking the elevator, walk or ride your bike rather than driving, and if you drive, park your car at the far end of the parking lot.

According to the *2008 Physical Activity Guidelines for Americans,* maintaining weight stability requires 150 to 300 minutes of moderate- to vigorous-intensity exercise per week. Strength training activities are helpful in maintaining weight stability but are not as effective as aerobic exercise. Losing a substantial amount of weight or maintaining substantial weight loss requires a high amount of physical activity unless calories are reduced. People who want to lose weight or prevent weight regain may need to do more than 300 minutes a week of moderate- to vigorous-intensity exercise.[18] If you work toward these goals, you will see improvements not only in your body composition but also in overall well-being.

Combining Fitness Activities

When you participate in one activity or sport to improve your performance in another, or when you use several different types of training for a specific fitness goal, you are **cross training**. For example, you might lift weights, run, and cycle on different days of the week. Two key advantages of cross training are that you avoid the boredom of participating in the same exercise every day and you reduce the risk of overuse injuries.

For a summary of physical activity recommendations for adults related to the various components of fitness, see Table 6.4.

IMPROVING YOUR HEALTH THROUGH MODERATE PHYSICAL ACTIVITY

As noted earlier, exercise does not have to be vigorous to provide health benefits. There are many simple, easy, and enjoyable ways to use physical activity to obtain health benefits.

Making Daily Activities More Active

How much time do you spend in sedentary activities in your day? How can you make these minutes more active? Try getting up to change the TV channel instead of using the remote, or walk around, stretch, or do sit-ups during commercials. Ride your bike to class instead of taking the bus, take the stairs instead of the elevator at the library, or walk around while checking your cell phone messages. These kinds of unstructured physical activities can actually make a difference. In one study, researchers found that obese people sat for an average of two hours longer a day than people who were not obese and that if the obese people were to mirror the unstructured physical activities of those who were not obese, they would burn an extra 350 calories a day.[28]

body composition
Relative amounts of fat and fat-free mass in the body.

cross training
Participation in one sport to improve performance in another, or use of several different types of training for a specific fitness goal.

Table 6.4   Summary of Physical Activity Recommendations for Adults

Aerobic (endurance) activity	150 minutes of moderate-intensity aerobic activity per week. OR 75 minutes of vigorous-intensity aerobic activity per week. OR A combination of moderate- and vigorous-intensity physical activity that meets the recommendation.
Muscle-strengthening activity	8 to 10 exercises that stress the major muscle groups on 2 or more nonconsecutive days per week. Do two to four sets of 8 to 12 repetitions for each exercise using sufficient resistance to fatigue the muscles.
Flexibility	Stretching exercise for all major joints, at least 2 to 3 days per week. Stretch to the point of tension, hold for 10 to 30 seconds, repeating 2 to 4 times, to accumulate 60 seconds per stretch.
Weight management	To prevent unhealthy weight gain, 150 to 300 minutes of moderate- to vigorous-intensity physical activity per week. For substantial weight loss or to sustain weight loss, 300 minutes or more of moderate- to vigorous-intensity exercise a week.

Sources: Adapted from *2008 Physical Activity Guidelines for Americans,* Department of Health and Human Services, 2009, www.health.gov/paguidelines; "Position Stand: Progression Models in Resistance Training for Healthy Adults," American College of Sports Medicine, 2009, *Medicine & Science in Sports & Exercise, 41* (3), pp. 687–708; *ACSM's Guidelines for Exercise Testing and Prescription,* American College of Sports Medicine, 2014, Baltimore: Lippincott Williams & Wilkins.

How helpful can it be to make your daily activities more active? Consider that an order of french fries contains about 400 calories. If you are sitting and watching television, it will take you 308 minutes, or more than 5 hours, to use up that many calories. If you are walking briskly or jogging slowly, it will take you about an hour. For more on the negative effects of inactivity, see the box, "Could You Spend Less Time Sitting?"

Walking for Fitness

Walking is the most popular physical activity in North America,[29] and it has many health benefits. As with other activities, increasing the pace and/or duration of walking results in greater health benefits.

Experts at the Shape Up America! program found that people could control their weight if they walked 10,000 steps each day.[30,31] Walking 10,000 steps (about 5 miles) expends between 300 and 400 calories, depending on body size and walking speed. Walking 10,000 steps a day five days a week expends the optimal 2,000 calories per week recommended for preventing premature death. This is good news for anyone who spends time on college campuses, which are usually designed to be pedestrian friendly. At a traditional university, college students walk between 9,000 and 11,000 steps a day.[32]

To set a walking goal for yourself, first determine how many steps you typically take each day. You can count your steps with a pedometer, a pager-sized device worn on the

belt or waistband centered over the hipbone. However, pedometers that convert activities into calories expended are not accurate because they do not factor in activity intensity.

Record the number of steps you take every day for seven days. Most inactive people take between 2,000 and 4,000 steps a day. Then increase this number by about 500 steps at a time. If you typically take 5,000 steps a day, set a goal of

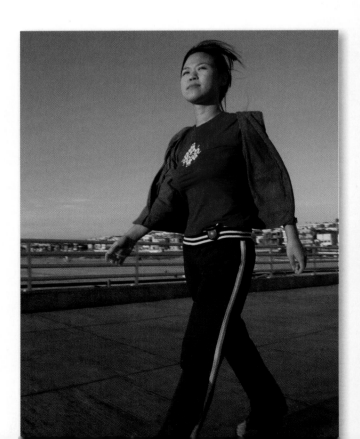

■ Counting steps with a pedometer is one way to move toward fitness. Walking 10,000 steps a day confers health benefits and helps people control their weight.

Starting the Conversation

Could You Spend Less Time Sitting?

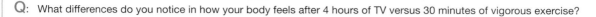

Q: What differences do you notice in how your body feels after 4 hours of TV versus 30 minutes of vigorous exercise?

Have you ever thought about how much time you spend sitting? Between classes, computer time, TV, movies, video games, and hanging out, your sitting time probably adds up to a significant portion of your day. Your sitting profile after graduation could look even worse, if you take a desk job. The average American spends more than 9 hours out of every 24 sitting. Some spend far more.

Research is now showing that prolonged sitting is bad for your health, even if you exercise regularly. Prolonged sitting sends the body into a kind of "shutdown" in which metabolism slows, electrical activity in the muscles drops, fat-burning enzymes turn off, and almost no energy is expended. People who sit for long periods of time have less healthy cholesterol and blood sugar profiles, as well as bigger waists and stiffer muscles. The "physiology of inactivity" puts people at higher risk for heart disease, obesity, diabetes, some cancers, chronic pain, and premature death. One study found that sitting for more than six hours a day for 10 to 20 years can shave off seven years of quality of life.

Experts recommend regularly interrupting sitting with a few minutes of physical activity—standing up, stretching, walking, or running in place. These short bouts of activity, along with smaller movements like fidgeting and bigger activities like doing daily tasks, all contribute to *non-exercise activity thermogenesis* (NEAT)—the expenditure of energy in activities other than exercise. Studies have found that burning calories in NEAT each day—standing, cooking, folding the laundry, and so on—can help counteract the effects of sitting. The more you can accumulate these short bouts of low-intensity activity throughout the day, the better.

Some researchers have begun designing environments that promote physical activity and NEAT. Dr. James Levine, the force behind the movement, created an "office of the future" with walking workstations, or "walkstations"—vertical desks where people walk at a slow pace on a treadmill while working on their computers. Levine sees offices becoming dynamic environments in the near future, with people using treadmill desks, bike desks, balance ball chairs, and more.

The bottom line is that getting regular exercise is not enough to keep you healthy if you spend most of your day sitting. Until every classroom, library, and office has options that promote physical activity, it's up to you to build movement into your day—the more the better!

Q: What changes can you make in your life right now to decrease your sitting time?

Q: As you think ahead to your working life, how will you build NEAT into your day? What will your work environment look like? What equipment helps motivate you to move?

Sources: "Just How Dangerous Is Sitting All Day?" (Infographic), by J. O'Dell, 2011, *Mashable Tech,* http://mashable.com/2011/05/09/sitting-down-infographic/; "Sitting All Day: Worse for You Than You Might Think," by P. Nieghmond, 2011, *NPR,* www.npr.org/2011/04/25/135575490/sitting-all-day-worse-for-you-than-you-might-think; "Is Sitting a Lethal Activity?" by J. Vlahos, April 14, 2011, *The New York Times Magazine,* www.nytimes.com/2011/04/17/magazine/mag-17sitting-t.html; Lifehacker, http://lifehacker.com/5879536/how-sitting-all-day-is-damaging-your-body-and-how-you-can-counteract-it.

5,500 steps. Once you achieve 5,500 steps, raise your goal by 500 steps, and continue until you reach 10,000 steps.[31] This is an easy and painless way to add physical activity to your day and to move from a light to a moderate activity level.

Taking the Stairs

Climbing stairs is an excellent activity for improving leg strength, balance, and fitness. Stair climbing is twice as taxing to your heart and lungs as brisk walking on a level surface. Walking upstairs burns about 5 times more calories than riding an elevator. A Harvard Health Alumni study found that men who climb an average of eight flights of stairs a day experience 33 percent lower mortality than men who are sedentary. Be sure the stairs are safe before taking them, though.[33] Architects are now designing staircases that encourage people to walk instead of using elevators.[34]

If you have access to stair-climbing machines at your fitness center, they also provide a good workout. Dual-action climbers exercise your legs, arms, and heart. This equipment provides a moderate- to high-intensity workout with low impact on your joints. If you don't have access to exercise machines, just take the stairs.

Exergaming: Replacing Sedentary Technology

The American College Health Association's Healthy Campus 2020 places emphasis on increasing regular physical activity for college students because research showed a decline in physical activity from secondary education to postsecondary education in moderate-to-vigorous physical activity. This document advocates ecological models for health that attempt to construct environments that support healthy behaviors and deter unhealthy behaviors. Efforts to reduce sedentary behaviors include replacing technology that encourages inactivity—watching television, using computers, playing traditional video games—with physical activity environments that are fun and engaging.

Exergaming does this by using video games to enhance physical activity.[35] Exergames, interactive activities that are safe, enjoyable, and inexpensive, can change people's attitudes about physical movement. This new generation of video games involving physical movement is marketed specifically as exercise and fitness games. You can bare-knuckle box with your PlayStation3 or learn and practice new dance moves with your Xbox360. New motion controllers and advanced sensors provide realistic simulations for tai chi, beach volleyball, golf, soccer, football, hockey, and many other activities. They track how many calories you burn as you play and can even analyze your body dynamics and track your progress over time. Amusement-park-like effects make exercising more fun. Some games, in which players do math problems by punching or kicking numbered targets, exercise the brain as well as the body.[36,37]

However, exergames do have their downsides. They can be expensive, they may limit social interaction, and they may send a message that being fit requires technology. In addition, research into the health benefits of these games has been inconclusive.[37] Fitness video games should not be considered a substitute for active outdoor play and physical activity. Real boxing, for example, expends 200 percent more energy than Wii boxing.[36] Video games can be a great addition to a regular workout routine, as well as part of an overall strategy to encourage children, teens, and adults to become more active.

Other kinds of interventions also focus on increasing physical activity by manipulating the environment. A more expensive option than exergaming is video-game exercise equipment, such as stationary bikes that provide virtual reality interaction. Although research on the benefits of virtual reality exercise equipment is in its infancy, outcomes to date are showing both physiological and psychological benefits.[38]

In addition, new software applications have been developed for cell phones to promote physical activity. Research suggests that high use of cell phones can disrupt leisure-time physical activity and promote sedentary behaviors such as Facebook, texting, tweeting, playing video games, or watching television. Cell phone fitness apps now can be used to count your steps or keep track of exercise routines from weight lifting to office yoga.[39] Examples of apps can be found at http://lifehacker.com/5607322/five-best-mobile-fitness-apps, and www.techradar.com/us/news/phone-and-communications/mobile-phones/10-best-fitness-apps-for-android-1145635.

SPECIAL CONSIDERATIONS IN EXERCISE AND PHYSICAL ACTIVITY

When you engage in exercise and physical activity, you need to warm up and cool down and pay attention to warning signs from your body. You also need to know how to accommodate the effects of heat and cold. In addition, physical activity is important for people with disabilities and chronic health problems; appropriate exercise opportunities need to be available to them.

Health and Safety Precautions

Injuries and illness associated with exercise and physical activity are usually the result of either excessive exercise or improper techniques. In this section, we look at several considerations related to health and safety.

Warm-Up and Cool-Down Proper warm-up before exercise helps to maximize the benefits of a workout and minimize the potential for injuries. Muscles contract more efficiently and more safely when they have been properly warmed up.

Suggested warm-up activities include light calisthenics, walking or slow jogging, and gentle stretching of the specific muscles to be used in the activity. You can also do a low-intensity version of the activity you are about to engage in, such as hitting tennis balls against a wall before a match. Your warm-up should last from 5 to 10 minutes.

A minimum of 5 to 10 minutes should also be devoted to cool-down, depending on environmental conditions and the intensity of the exercise program. Pooling of blood in the extremities may temporarily disrupt or reduce the return of blood to the heart, momentarily depriving your heart and brain of oxygen. Fainting or even a coronary abnormality may result. However, if you continue the activity at a lower intensity, the blood vessels gradually return to their normal smaller diameter.

Walking, mimicking the exercise at a slower pace, and stretching while walking are all excellent

■ Exergaming is the latest in consumer-oriented approaches to fitness.

cool-down activities. Never sit down, stand in a stationary position, or take a hot shower or sauna immediately after vigorous exercise.

Fatigue and Overexertion Fatigue is generally defined as an inability to continue exercising at a desired level of intensity. The cause of fatigue may be psychological—for example, depression can cause feelings of fatigue—or physiological, as when you work out too long or too hard, do an activity you're not used to, or become overheated or dehydrated. Or fatigue can occur because the body cannot produce enough energy to meet the demands of the activity. In this case, consuming enough complex carbohydrates to replenish the muscle stores of glycogen may solve the problem. Athletes need to eat a high-carbohydrate diet to make sure they have enough reserve energy for their sport.[26]

Overexertion occurs when an exercise session has been too intense. Warning signs of overexertion include (1) pain or pressure in the left or midchest area, jaw, neck, left shoulder, or left arm during or just after exercise; (2) sudden nausea, dizziness, cold sweat, fainting, or pallor (pale, ashen skin); and (3) abnormal heartbeats (such as fluttering), rapid heartbeats, or a rapid pulse rate immediately followed by a very slow pulse rate. These symptoms are similar to signs of a heart attack. If you experience any of these symptoms, consult a physician before exercising again.

Soft-Tissue and Overuse Injuries Injuries to soft tissue (muscles and joints) include tears, sprains, strains, and contusions; they usually result from a specific activity

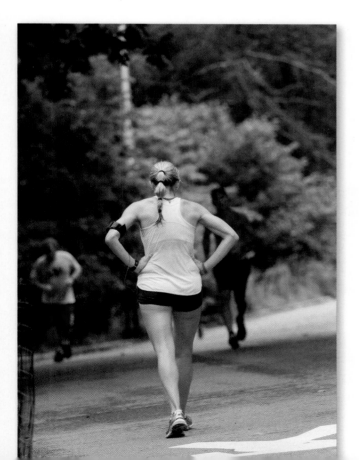

■ Cooling down after vigorous exercise gives the cardiovascular system time to return to normal. Cool down by walking or continuing your exercise activity at a much lower intensity.

incident, such as a bicycle crash. Some injuries, known as overuse injuries, are caused by the cumulative effects of motions repeated many times. Tendinitis and bursitis are examples of overuse injuries. (For tips on choosing the right shoe to prevent walking- and running-related injuries, see the box, "You and Your Shoes").

Both over-use injuries and soft tissue injuries should be treated according to the R-I-C-E principle: rest, ice, compression, and elevation. Immediately stop doing the activity, apply ice to the affected area to reduce swelling and pain, compress it with an elastic bandage to reduce swelling, and elevate it to reduce blood flow to the area. Do not apply heat until all swelling has disappeared. When you no longer feel pain in the area, you can gradually begin to exercise again. Don't return to your full exercise program until your injury is completely healed.

Effects of Heat and Cold on Exercise and Physical Activity

When it is very hot or very cold, you will need to adjust your physical activity and exercise workload.

Heat Heat disorders can be caused by impaired regulation of internal core temperature, loss of body fluids, and loss of electrolytes (Table 6.5).[26] Two strategies for preventing excessive increases in body temperature are skin wetting and hyperhydration. Skin wetting involves sponging or spraying the head or body with cold water. This strategy cools the skin but has not been shown to effectively decrease core body temperature.[26] Resting in a cool environment and hyperhydration are more effective strategies for reducing core body heat. Hyperhydration is taking in extra fluids shortly before participating in physical activity in a hot environment.[25] This practice is recommended by the ACSM and may improve cardiovascular function and temperature regulation during physical activity when it is very hot.[26]

If you are going to be exercising in very hot conditions, you can hyperhydrate by drinking a pint of water (16 ounces) when you get up in the morning, another pint 1 hour before your activity, and a final pint 15 to 30 minutes before exercising. Plan to consume from 4 to 8 ounces of fluid every 15 minutes during your exercise. After exercise, consume 24 ounces of water for every pint you lose.[26] The goal is to prevent excessive changes in electrolyte balance and body water loss of 2 percent or more.

hypothermia
Low body temperature, a life-threatening condition.

Cold Exercising in excessive cold also puts a strain on the body. Symptoms of **hypothermia**

Consumer Clipboard

You and Your Shoes

If walking or running are among your fitness activities, the right shoes are essential. In either case, to prevent injury, you should know the basic differences between walking shoes and running shoes.

In walking, your foot has a natural rolling motion from heel to toe, bending at the ball of the foot with each step. Your foot also rolls from the little toe to the big toe, and your toes bend upward fully. In running, you may strike the ground farther forward on the foot than when you're walking, and you strike the ground with more force than when you're walking. Running may create a force more than five times body weight on every foot strike, whereas walking creates a force about twice body weight.

For these reasons, running shoes need to provide more cushioning and stability than walking shoes. Both types need to be flexible, but in different places.

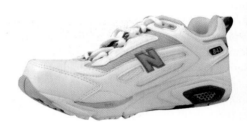

Walking shoe:

- **Heel:** Rounded or undercut, no more than 1 inch thicker than the rest of the sole
- **Mid-sole:** Bends at ball of foot
- **Toes:** Flexible toe area, twists horizontally and bends vertically

Running shoe:

- **Heel:** Flared or built-up heel for stability and cushioning
- **Mid-sole:** May bend at arch of foot
- **Toes:** More horizontal flex, less vertical flex than walking shoe

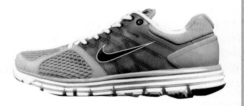

- **Mid-sole tests:** Place shoe on level surface; lift heel toward toe. Walking shoe should bend at ball of foot; running shoe may bend at arch. Then poke toe down; heel of walking shoe should rise off surface; this natural curvature helps you roll through step. Heel of running shoe should rise very little or not at all.
- **Toe tests:** Grasp shoe with both hands and twist toe area from side to side; then bend toes up and down. In walking shoe, there should be both horizontal flex and vertical flex. In running shoe, there should be more horizontal and less vertical flex.

Sources: "The Differences Between a Walking Shoe and a Running Shoe," by W. Bumgardner, 2006, http://walking.about.com/od/shoechoice/ss/runningshoe .htm; "Walking Shoe Guide: Test Your Shoe Flexibility," by W. Bumgardner, 2011, http://walking.about.com/cs/shoes/a/shoeflex.htm; "The Great Shoe Debate," by M. Spillner, 2011, *Prevention*, www.prevention.com/fitness/fitness-tips/differences-between-walking-and-running-sneakers.

(dangerously low body temperature) include shivering, feelings of euphoria, and disorientation.[26] Core body temperature influences how severe these symptoms are and whether the hypothermia is considered mild, moderate, or severe. To stay warm, dress in several thin layers of clothes and wear a hat and mittens. If cold air bothers your throat, breathe through a scarf.

Many people do not take in sufficient fluid when exercising outside during the winter. Fluid losses during the winter can be very high, because cold, dry air requires the body to humidify and warm the air, resulting in the loss of significant amounts of water. An effective strategy is to consume needed fluids 1.5 to 2 hours before exercising and to drink more fluids just before exercising.

Table 6.5   Heat-Related Disorders

Heat Disorder	Cause	Symptoms	Treatment
Heat cramps	Excessive loss of electrolytes in sweat; inadequate salt intake	Muscle cramps	Rest in cool environment; drink fluids; ingest salty food and drinks; get medical treatment if severe.
Heat exhaustion	Excessive loss of electrolytes in sweat; inadequate salt and/or fluid intake	Fatigue; nausea; dizziness; cool, pale skin; sweating; elevated temperature	Rest in cool environment; drink cool fluids; cool body with water; get medical treatment if severe.
Heat stroke	Excessive body temperature	Headache; vomiting; hot, flushed skin (dry or sweaty); elevated temperature; disorientation; unconsciousness	Cool body with ice or cold water; give cool drinks with sugar if conscious; get medical help immediately.

Source: Adapted from *Nutrition for Health, Fitness and Sport,* 7th ed., by M.H. Williams, 2007, New York: McGraw-Hill.

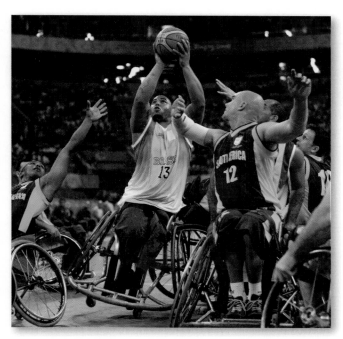

■ Having a disability does not mean a person can't exercise or be fit. Exercise counters the effects of immobility and inactivity, improves all body functions, and enhances self-esteem for individuals with disabilities as well as for people in the general population.

Exercise for People With Disabilities

Physical activity and exercise are especially beneficial for people with disabilities and chronic health problems. Immobility or inactivity may aggravate the original disability and increase the risk for secondary health problems, such as heart disease, osteoporosis, arthritis, and diabetes. The ACSM stresses the importance of physical activity for people with disabilities for two reasons: (1) to counteract the detrimental effects of bed rest and sedentary living patterns and (2) to maintain optimal functioning of body organs or systems.[40]

Not too long ago, regular physical activity was missing in the lives of many people with disabilities.[40] The reasons for this absence included lack of knowledge about the importance of physical activity, limited access to recreation sites and difficulty with transportation, a low level of interest, and the lack of exercise facilities and resources designed to accommodate people with disabilities.

Laws have strengthened the rights of people with disabilities and fostered their inclusion in programs and facilities providing physical activity opportunities. Increased visibility and positive images of people with disabilities engaging in physical activity, such as in the Special Olympics and wheelchair basketball, have also helped raise awareness.

PHYSICAL ACTIVITY FOR LIFE

The most significant drop in physical activity occurs in the last few years of high school and the first year of college.[41] The decline accelerates again after college graduation. However, people can make physical activity a lifetime pursuit. In this section, we consider two helpful factors—commitment to change and social and community support.

Making a Commitment to Change

Assess your physical activity status in terms of the Transtheoretical Model (described in Chapter 1). This model proposes six stages of change: precontemplation, contemplation, preparation, action, maintenance, and termination. In the precontemplation and contemplation stages, the biggest challenges for most people are barriers to exercise.[42] Common barriers to active lifestyles cited by adults are inconvenience, lack of self-motivation, lack of time, fear of injury, the perception that exercise is boring, lack of social support, and lack of confidence in one's ability to be physically active.[43] If you are in the precontemplation or contemplation stage and feel overwhelmed by these or other barriers, the box, "Identify and Overcome Barriers to Physical Activity," presents many helpful suggestions.

In the preparation stage, self-assessment is critical. Ask yourself these four questions: (1) What physical activities do I enjoy? (2) What are the best days and times for me to participate in physical activities? (3) Where is the best place to pursue these activities? (4) Do I have friends or family members who can join in my physical activities? In preparing to exercise, you also need to take into account your current level of fitness and your previous experiences in various physical activities. All this information will help you develop an exercise program that you can commit to and maintain.

In the action stage, goal setting is key. Your goals should be based on the benefits of physical activity, but they should also be specific and reasonable.

Action Skill-Builder

Identify and Overcome Barriers to Physical Activity

Lack of time

☐ Identify available time slots. Monitor your daily activities for one week. Identify at least three 30-minute time slots you could use for physical activity.

☐ Add physical activity to your daily routine. Walk or ride your bike to work or shopping, organize school activities around physical activity, walk the dog, or park farther away from your destination.

☐ Make time for physical activity. Walk, jog, or swim during your lunch hour; take fitness breaks instead of coffee breaks.

☐ Select activities requiring minimal time, such as walking, jogging, or stair climbing.

Social influence

☐ Explain your interest in physical activity to friends and family. Ask them to support your efforts.

☐ Invite friends and family members to exercise with you. Plan social activities involving exercise.

☐ Develop new friendships with physically active people. Join a group, such as the YMCA.

Lack of energy

☐ Schedule physical activity for times in the day or week when you feel energetic.

☐ Convince yourself that physical activity will increase your energy level; then try it.

Lack of willpower

☐ Plan ahead. Make physical activity a regular part of your schedule and write it on your calendar.

☐ Invite a friend to exercise with you on a regular basis, and write the dates on both your calendars.

☐ Join an exercise group or class.

☐ Sign up for a sport-based fund-raising event for a charity, such as an AIDS walk or a cycling challenge for cancer research. Many organizations provide training and mentoring, a training schedule, a team, and other kinds of support.

Fear of injury

☐ Learn how to warm up and cool down safely.

☐ Learn how to exercise appropriately considering your age, fitness level, skill level, and health status.

☐ Choose activities involving minimum risk.

Lack of skill

☐ Select activities requiring no new skills, such as walking, climbing stairs, or jogging.

☐ Exercise with friends who are at the same skill level as you.

☐ Find a friend who is willing to teach you new skills.

☐ Take a class to develop new skills.

Lack of resources

☐ Select activities that require minimal equipment, such as walking, jogging, or calisthenics.

☐ Identify inexpensive, convenient resources available in your community, such as park and recreation programs.

Weather conditions

☐ Develop a set of regular activities that are always available regardless of weather (indoor cycling, aerobic dance, indoor swimming, calisthenics, stair climbing, rope skipping, dancing).

☐ Think of outdoor activities that depend on weather conditions (cross-country skiing, outdoor swimming, outdoor tennis) as "bonuses"—extra activities possible when weather and circumstances permit.

Family obligations

☐ Trade babysitting time with a friend, neighbor, or family member who also has small children.

☐ Exercise with your children. Go for a walk together, play tag or other running games, or play active games and sports on your game machine or Wii.

☐ Hire a babysitter and look at the cost as an investment in your physical and mental health.

☐ Jump rope, do calisthenics, ride a stationary bicycle, or use other home gymnasium equipment while the kids are playing or sleeping.

☐ Try to exercise when the kids are not around (during school hours or their nap time).

☐ Encourage exercise facilities to provide child care.

Source: "Physical Activity for Everyone: Making Physical Activity Part of Your Life; Overcoming Barriers to Physical Activity," by Centers for Disease Control and Prevention, 2005, http://204.97.228.62/r85content/media/pictures/health/websites-pdfs/readings_on_health/physical_activity/overcome.pdf.

Achievable and sustainable goals are essential for exercise compliance. Include both short-term and long-term goals in your plan, and devise ways to measure your progress. Build in rewards along the way.

When you have been physically active almost every day for at least six months, you are in the maintenance stage. One key to maintaining an active lifestyle is believing that your commitment to physical activity can make a difference in your life. People who establish a personal stake in physical activity are more likely to maintain an active lifestyle. Being a mentor to friends and family members can also help you become or stay motivated to make exercise a lifelong habit. When exercise has become entrenched as a lifelong behavior—when it's as much a part of your day as eating and sleeping—you are in the termination stage. Remember, the more active you are, the more health benefits you will receive.

Using Social and Community Support

A network of friends, coworkers, and family members who understand the benefits of exercise and join you in your activities can make the difference between a sedentary and an active lifestyle. Family and friends are not enough, however; activity-friendly communities are also instrumental in promoting physical activity. Your health is a function of the interaction between your personal competencies and the environmental barriers and supports in your neighborhood. Many communities have paths, trails, sidewalks, and safe streets that encourage people to become physically active.[44] There are also community programs that encourage parents to walk their children to school, that promote "mall walking" (walking at shopping malls), and that sponsor biking and walking days. In addition, access ramps and adapted transportation help people with disabilities overcome barriers that discourage physical activity or make it difficult.[45]

What can you do to encourage community planning that promotes physical activity? You can advocate for new growth designed around public transportation hubs and for bicycle lanes incorporated into streets. As a citizen and taxpayer, you can vote on local growth measures and become active in local chapters of organizations such as New Urbanism and Smart Growth America.[44,46] You can support the National Physical Activity Plan's recommendation for rewarding regions that make progress toward active communities.[47]

When making personal choices about where to live and work, look at a map of the immediate area and think about how communities you're considering are planned. How

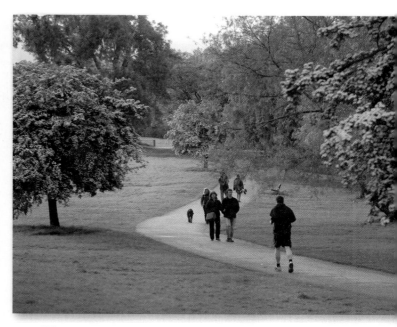

■ When communities provide spaces for physical activity and improve access to those spaces, people respond by becoming more active. Thus, public policy and community planning play important roles in the physical fitness of community members.

close are recreational areas? What types of places are within a 10-minute walking radius of home and work? Will living in this community help to make you more active and physically fit? Taking such questions into consideration will give you more opportunities to make physical activity and exercise a natural part of your life.

Accessibility, safety, aesthetics, and climate play key roles in determining levels of physical activity. Although new communities are being designed to incorporate these environmental factors, many existing communities lack resources to create more walkable environments. Awareness planning, or a design that encourage walkers to interact with the walking environment, such as identification of plants and landmarks and description of historic events, makes walking more appealing and engaging.[48,49]

The key message of this chapter is that physical activity is a natural, enjoyable, sometimes thrilling, frequently challenging part of human life. It is a part of life that children instinctively embrace but that adults may have lost touch with living in a fast-paced, sedentary culture. We encourage you to get up, get moving, and get back in touch with the lifelong pleasures of physical activity.

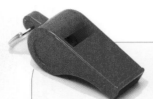

You Make the Call

Should Insurers and Employers Reward Healthy Behaviors and Punish Bad Ones?

There is no doubt that healthy lifestyles make for more vital individuals and more productive workers and citizens. When people increase their physical activity, they also bring economic benefits to themselves and society. The annual cost of inactivity is estimated at $24 to $76 billion and is a contributing factor in rapidly rising health care costs. Even if you are in good physical condition, some of the money you (or your parents) pay in insurance premiums goes toward treating other people's obesity- and inactivity-related health conditions.

The benefits of physical activity are clear, but getting people to live healthier lives has been difficult. Many health insurance companies have attempted to address this problem by offering incentives to people willing to adopt healthy behaviors such as not smoking. Corporations and other institutions have undertaken similar actions by offering incentives for employees who are physically active, maintain a healthy body weight, lower their blood pressure, have healthy cholesterol levels, wear their seat belts consistently, and so on. For example, employees at the University of Louisville receive a $20 credit on their monthly insurance premiums if they adopt good eating and physical activity habits. The university reports that for every $1 it has spent on the program, it has saved $5.

Some employers have gone even further, using disincentives to encourage their employees to make healthy behavior changes. For example, employees of Whirlpool who smoke are required to pay an extra $500 a year in insurance costs. Some employers have threatened smokers with termination of employment, and others will not hire a person who smokes. In 2005, Weyco, a health consulting firm, gave its employees 15 months to quit smoking and then fired all the employees who had not quit after the time had passed. At the end of the 15 months, 14 of the company's estimated 18 to 20 employees who were smokers had quit. One Cincinnati-based company fines employees an extra $15 to $75 a month in health care premiums if their body mass index is above what is considered healthy.

However, there has been a backlash against policies that either incentivize or penalize people for their good health and habits. About half of all states have passed laws prohibiting employers from firing or refusing to hire people who smoke during nonworking hours. These laws are intended to keep employers from discriminating against people who engage in a legal activity (smoking) on their own time. Some employees are reluctant to share personal data, such as their exercise, eating, and smoking habits, with their employer. Others point out that physical inactivity is only one of many factors that contribute to obesity and other health problems. Genetics play a factor, as do socioeconomic status and community resources. People should not be blamed for health conditions that are not entirely their fault, opponents argue.

The use of incentive programs, and especially disincentives, by employers and insurance companies to induce behavior change has been controversial. Should people who choose to take health risks be penalized? What do you think?

Pros

- Health care costs are skyrocketing, and sedentary lifestyles are a primary cause. Encouraging people to adopt healthy behaviors will decrease health care costs.
- The power to be more physically active is under the control of the individual.
- Empirical evidence supports the relationship between physical inactivity and preventable diseases.
- Insurance companies already use incentives and disincentives in their life insurance and automobile insurance plans.

Cons

- An overemphasis on individual health is part of a victim-blaming mentality that does not take into account the impact of genetics, culture, and racial inequalities on health.
- Use of incentives and disincentives is an invasion of privacy and a violation of personal rights.
- Some racial and ethnic groups, low-income people, and people with disabilities living in urban areas do not have adequate access to fitness or park and recreation facilities.

Sources: "Cost-Effectiveness of Community-Based Physical Activity Interventions," by L. Roux, M. Pratt, T.O. Teng, et al., 2008, *American Journal of Preventive Medicine, 35* (6), pp. 578–588; "Michigan Health Care Company Has Strict Anti-Tobacco Policy," Associated Press, 2005, www.msnbc.msn.com/id/6870458/; "Companies Penalizing Workers with High Health Risks," Associated Press, 2007, www.usatoday.com/money/industries/health/2007-09-09-risk-penalties_N.htm.

In Review

What is fitness?
Physical fitness is generally defined as the ability of the body to respond to the demands placed upon it, and good health depends on physical fitness. Skill-related fitness is the ability to perform specific skills associated with recreational activities and sports; health-related fitness is the ability to perform daily living activities with vigor.

What are the benefits of physical activity and exercise?
Physical activity is activity that requires any kind of movement; exercise is structured, planned physical activity. Physical activity and exercise confer benefits in every domain of wellness, including physical benefits to the cardiorespiratory, skeletal, and immune systems; improved cognitive functioning; relief from depression, anxiety, and stress; and benefits to LDL cholesterol and blood glucose. Inactivity is a leading preventable cause of premature death from such causes as cardiovascular disease and cancer. Of all the positive health-related behavior choices you can make, exercising may be the easiest, most effective, and most important.

How much should you exercise?
A widely accepted set of guidelines aimed at promoting and maintaining health and preventing chronic disease, issued by the U.S. Department of Health and Human Services, calls for 150 minutes of moderate-intensity aerobic activity or 75 minutes of vigorous-intensity aerobic activity each week. Activity should also be included each week for muscle strengthening, flexibility, and weight management.

What are the components of health-related fitness?
The components of health-related fitness are cardiorespiratory fitness, musculoskeletal fitness (muscular strength, muscular endurance, and flexibility) and body composition.

When you are designing an exercise program, consider the FITT dimensions of your sessions: frequency, intensity, time, and type. Cardio fitness, the center of any fitness program, is developed by activities that use the large muscles of the body in continuous movement. Muscular strength and endurance are developed by weight, or resistance, training. To gain muscle tissue, exercise is preferable to drugs and dietary supplements. Flexibility is developed by stretching. Body composition can be controlled by the amount of physical activity you engage in.

How can you improve your health through moderate physical activity?
To make your daily activities more active, try to lessen the time you spend sitting, try to walk 10,000 steps a day, take the stairs instead of the elevator, and try exergaming.

What special exercise-related considerations and precautions are important for health and safety?
It's important to warm up and cool down before and after exercise, to avoid fatigue and overexertion, to take proper care of injuries, wear shoes designed for your activity, and to take the temperature into account. Everyone can benefit from exercise, as long as they follow any relevant special guidelines, including people with disabilities.

What strategies can help you be physically active throughout your life?
Assess your commitment to physical activity by using the Transtheoretical, or Stages of Change, Model, and use the model to overcome obstacles to physical activity. Join with friends, coworkers, and family members in regular physical activity, and advocate for community planning that encourages physical activity.

7 Body Weight and Body Composition

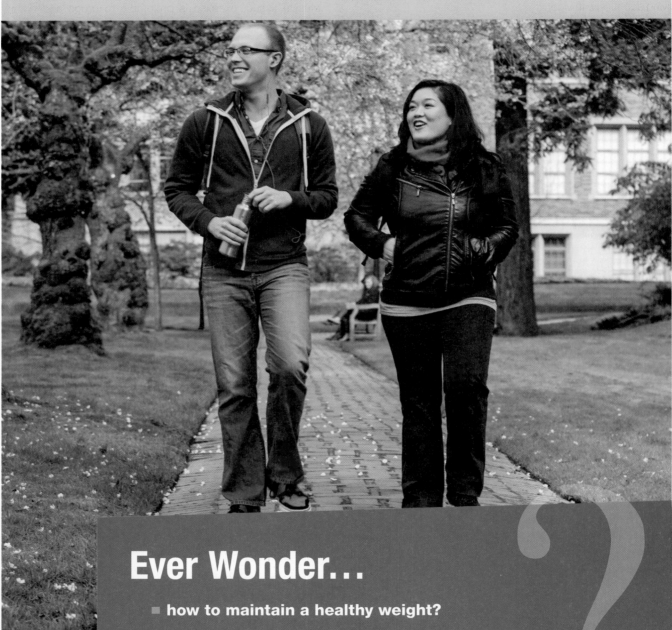

Ever Wonder...

- how to maintain a healthy weight?

- if being overweight can run in families?

- what normal portion sizes look like?

Overweight and obesity are increasingly worrisome problems in the United States and around the world. Among American adults, 33.6 percent meet the criteria for overweight and 34.9 percent meet the criteria for obesity.[1] **Overweight** is defined as body weight that exceeds the recommended guidelines for good health; **obesity** is body weight that greatly exceeds the recommended guidelines.

In 1990, 10 states reported a prevalence rate of obesity less than 10 percent, and no states reported prevalence greater than 15 percent. Twenty-two years later, in 2012, no state had a prevalence rate less than 20 percent, and 13 states had a prevalence rate greater than 30 percent (see the box, "State and Regional Variation in Prevalence of Obesity Among Adults in the United States").[2] There appears to be a slowing of the rate of increase or even a leveling off, which is critical because otherwise all Americans could be overweight within a few generations. Worldwide, an estimated 500 million people are obese; rates vary tremendously by country, ranging from less than 5 percent in parts of China, Japan, and certain African countries to more than 75 percent in urban Samoa.[3]

No sex, age, state, racial group, or educational level is spared from the problem of overweight, although the problem is worse for the young and the poor. Rates of obesity for children have almost tripled since 1980, and today an estimated 17 percent of children 2 to 19 years of age are obese.

Among low-income children ages 2 to 4, an estimated one in three are overweight or obese, although obesity among children aged 2 to 5 years old decreased recently for the first time.[1,4,5]

The number of overweight children is particularly worrisome because an elementary school child who is overweight has an 80 percent likelihood of being overweight at age 12; a person who is obese at age 18 faces odds 28 to 1 against maintaining a healthy adult weight.[5]

WHAT IS A HEALTHY BODY WEIGHT?

How much should you weigh? The answer to this question depends on who is asking and why. If you are a 16-year-old varsity wrestler getting ready for your competition weigh-in, your coach and the wrestling weight classes may influence your weight goals. If you are an 18-year-old girl comparing yourself with the fashion models you see in magazines, your goal may be determined by a media-generated cosmetic ideal. If you are a 50-year-old woman wondering whether

overweight
Body weight that exceeds the recommended guidelines for good health.

obesity
Body weight that greatly exceeds the recommended guidelines for good health, as indicated by a body mass index of 30 or more.

Who's at Risk?

State and Regional Variation in Prevalence of Obesity Among Adults in the United States

Rates of obesity have soared since 1990. Multiple factors—some known, some still to be identified—account for this trend. While no area is spared, there are significant state and regional variations in rates of obesity.

Prevalence of Self-Reported Obesity* Among U.S. Adults, 2012

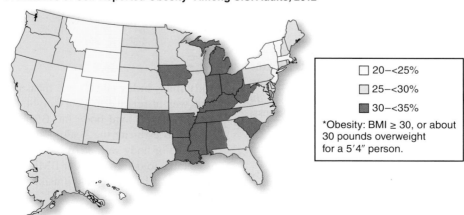

☐ 20–<25%
☐ 25–<30%
■ 30–<35%

*Obesity: BMI ≥ 30, or about 30 pounds overweight for a 5′4″ person.

connect
ACTIVITY

Source: "Adult Obesity Facts," from Behavioral Risk Factor Surveillance System, Centers for Disease Control and Prevention, 2013, www.cdc.gov/obesity/data/adult.html.

Table 7.1   Body Mass Index (BMI)

Find your height in the left-hand column and look across the row until you find the number that is closest to your weight. The number at the top of that column identifies your BMI. The darkest shaded area represents healthy weight ranges.

BMI	18	19	20	21	22	23	24	25	26	27	28	29	30	31	32	33	34
Height																	
4'10"	86	91	96	100	105	110	115	119	124	129	134	138	143	148	153	158	162
4'11"	89	94	99	104	109	114	119	124	128	133	138	143	148	153	158	163	168
5'0"	92	97	102	107	112	118	123	128	133	138	143	148	153	158	163	168	174
5'1"	95	100	106	111	116	122	127	132	137	143	148	153	158	164	169	174	180
5'2"	98	104	109	115	120	126	131	136	142	147	153	158	164	169	175	180	186
5'3"	102	107	113	118	124	130	135	141	146	152	158	163	169	175	180	186	191
5'4"	105	110	116	122	128	134	140	145	151	157	163	169	174	180	186	192	197
5'5"	108	114	120	126	132	138	144	150	156	162	168	174	180	186	192	198	204
5'6"	112	118	124	130	136	142	148	155	161	167	173	179	186	192	198	204	210
5'7"	115	121	127	134	140	146	153	159	166	172	178	185	191	198	204	211	217
5'8"	118	125	131	138	144	151	158	164	171	177	184	190	197	203	210	216	223
5'9"	122	128	135	142	149	155	162	169	176	182	189	196	203	209	216	223	230
5'10"	126	132	139	146	153	160	167	174	181	188	195	202	209	216	222	229	236
5'11"	129	136	143	150	157	165	172	179	186	193	200	208	215	222	229	236	243
6'0"	132	140	147	154	162	169	177	184	191	199	206	213	221	228	235	242	250
6'1"	136	144	151	159	166	174	182	189	197	204	212	219	227	235	242	250	257
6'2"	141	148	155	163	171	179	186	194	202	210	218	225	233	241	249	256	264
6'3"	144	152	160	168	176	184	192	200	208	216	224	232	240	248	256	264	272
6'4"	148	156	164	172	180	189	197	205	213	221	230	239	246	254	263	271	279
6'5"	151	160	168	176	185	193	202	210	218	227	235	244	252	261	269	277	286
6'6"	155	164	172	181	190	198	207	216	224	233	241	250	259	267	276	284	293

Underweight (≤18.5)		Healthy Weight (18.5–24.9)					Overweight (25–29.9)					Obese (≥30)				

Source: Adapted from "Body Mass Index Table," National Heart, Lung, and Blood Institute, retrieved from www.nhlbi.nih.gov/guidelines/obesity/bmi_tbl.htm.

---

body mass index (BMI)
Measure of body weight in relation to height.

you should be concerned about the 25 pounds you gained last year, you may be more interested in health goals for weight and fitness.

There is no ideal body weight for each person, but there are ranges for a healthy body weight. A healthy body weight is defined as (1) an acceptable body mass index (explained in the following sections), (2) body composition with an acceptable amount of body fat, (3) fat distribution that is not a risk factor for illness, and (4) the absence of any medical conditions (such as diabetes or hypertension) that would suggest a need for weight loss. If you currently meet these criteria, you will want to focus on maintaining your current weight. If you don't meet them, you may need to lose weight or gain weight.

Body Mass Index

Body mass index (BMI) is a measure of your weight relative to your height; it correlates with total body fat. BMI is used to estimate the health significance of body weight. You can use a table to determine your BMI (see Table 7.1) or calculate it using the following formula:

$$\text{BMI} = \frac{\text{weight in kg}}{(\text{height in meters})^2} \text{ OR } \frac{\text{weight in pounds}}{(\text{height in inches})^2} \times 703 \text{ (conversion factor)}$$

There appears to be a U-shaped relationship between BMI and risk of death. The lowest risk of death is in the 18.5 to 25 range. Consequently, the National Institutes of

Starting the Conversation

What's the Problem with the BMI?

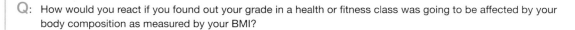

Q: How would you react if you found out your grade in a health or fitness class was going to be affected by your body composition as measured by your BMI?

In January 2011, a small group of parents in a Chicago suburb mounted a protest at their children's elementary school. They were angry about the use of BMI scores as part of their children's physical fitness grade on school progress reports. Some parents were concerned that their young children had become worried about their weight after receiving their BMI scores. Others argued that their children's weight and body composition were not something to be evaluated at school. School officials quickly announced that they would stop using BMI scores as part of children's progress reports, acknowledging that research does not support the use of BMI data for grading purposes.

Use of the BMI for inappropriate purposes is just one of several criticisms of this assessment tool. Another is that BMI is not an accurate measure of overweight and obesity because it doesn't measure body fat percentage, which is what matters for health purposes. BMI doesn't distinguish between body fat and lean body mass, and it also doesn't take into account the size of a person's body frame. It is unsuitable for older adults, children, and athletes, whom it frequently classifies as obese, and it often misses people in the healthy range who have a high body fat percentage.

Another criticism is that the distinctions among healthy weight, overweight, and obesity are arbitrary and that there is no scientific reason to set the thresholds for overweight and obesity at 25 and 30, respectively. Over the past several decades, the cutoff for overweight set by different health organizations has varied from 24.9 to 27.8. In 1998, the NIH lowered the cut-off for overweight from 27.8 to 25, to match international guidelines, and the media noted that overnight, millions of Americans became overweight.

Furthermore, there is little or no evidence that the BMI classification of overweight is correlated with an increased risk of disease or death. In fact, a 2005 study found that while there was a higher risk of death in the underweight and obese categories than in the normal weight category, there was no higher risk of death in the overweight category. A 2006 study found that for men, the lowest risk of death occurred in the overweight BMI range of 26 to 27.

Although research shows that the incidence of cardiovascular disease (CVD) and other diseases increases with overweight and obesity, BMI is not as good an indicator of risk of CVD and mortality as waist-to-height ratio, waist circumference, and waist-to-hip ratio. Some experts even speculate that overweight and obesity may not be causal factors in increased risk of CVD at all. Instead, poor diet and inactivity may be the causal factors, and overweight and obesity merely associated factors. In other words, a person who is sedentary and eats a high-fat, high-calorie diet is likely to be overweight and have health problems—but that doesn't mean that being overweight is the cause of the health problems.

Given all these problems, why does use of the BMI persist? Some point to the convenience and ease of administering the test. Others point to the simplicity of having a single number with which to make medical diagnoses and give weight-loss advice. Some cynics assert that it's good business for the pharmaceutical and diet industries if millions of people think they are overweight and should lose weight. No matter what the reason, with increasing dissatisfaction, the BMI may fall into disuse in the not-too-distant future.

Q: Given current public health efforts to combat childhood obesity, do you think schools have a role in educating parents about their children's weight-related health risks? If so, do you think measuring BMI is a way to do this?

Q: What factors do you think could account for findings that men in the slightly overweight BMI range of 26 to 27 have the lowest risk of death (lower than people in the "healthy" range of 20 to 25)?

Sources: "Excess Deaths Associated with Underweight, Overweight, and Obesity," by K.M. Flegel et al., 2005, *JAMA, 293* (15), pp. 1861–1867; "A Semiparametric Analysis of the Relationship of Body Mass Index to Mortality," by J.T. Groninger, 2006, *American Journal of Public Health, 96* (1), pp. 173–178; "The Predictive Value of Different Measures of Obesity for Incident Cardiovascular Events and Mortality," by H.J. Schneider et al., 2010, *Journal of Clinical Endocrinology and Metabolism, 95* (4), p. 1777; "Pathophysiology of Human Visceral Obesity: An Update," by A. Tchernof and J.P. Despres, 2013, *Physiology Review, 93* (1), pp. 359–404.

Health and the World Health Organization use the following guidelines for adult BMI categories:[2,3]

	BMI
Underweight	Less than 18.5
Healthy weight	18.5 to 24.9
Overweight	25 to 29.9
Obese	≥30

A comparative calculation is used to define overweight in children and adolescents. For these age groups, BMI is plotted using growth charts (for either boys or girls), and a percentile ranking is determined (percentile indicates the relative position of BMI compared to other children of the same sex and age).

There are some limitations to using the BMI to calculate risk of disease. BMI is only an estimate of body composition. For example, even if you and your friend have the same BMI, you may have different body compositions. BMI

149

may incorrectly estimate risk for some people. In athletes or others with a muscular build, BMI may overestimate body fat (and risk). In the elderly or others who have lost muscle mass, BMI may underestimate body fat (and risk). For more on the limitations of the BMI, see the box, "What's the Problem with the BMI?"

Body Fat Percentage

Body composition is measured in terms of percentage of body fat. There are no clear, accepted guidelines for healthy body fat ranges, although ranges of 8 to 24 percent have been used for men and 21 to 35 percent for women. Some body fat is essential to healthy function; the lower healthy range may be 5 to 10 percent for male athletes and 15 to 20 percent for female athletes. Below a certain body fat threshold, hormones cannot be produced and problems can occur, such as infertility, lack of menstruation, depression, lack of sex drive, hair loss, and loss of appetite.

At each level of BMI, there are differences in body fat percentage for different groups. Women on average have 10 to 12 percent more body fat than men. African American men average slightly less body fat than White men, and Asian men average slightly higher body fat percentage than White men. As people get older, body fat percentage increases at each level of BMI.[6-8]

Because body fat percentage is considered an important indicator of the need for weight reduction, it may be measured during a physical examination. Several methods exist to measure body fat percentage. The most accurate methods are expensive and require special equipment. They include weighing a person underwater (immersion), or using a special type of X-ray. Two simpler but slightly less reliable methods are measuring thickness of skin and fat in several locations of the body (skinfold measurement or caliper testing) and sending a weak electrical current through parts of the body that measures the electrical resistance of tissue and calculates body fat (bioelectrical impedance).[8]

Body Fat Distribution

Not only the amount but also where you carry your body fat is important in determining your health risk. Fat carried around and above the waist is abdominal fat and is considered more "active" than fat carried on the hips and thighs. Abdominal fat (also called *central obesity*) is a disadvantage because it breaks down more easily and enters the bloodstream more readily.

A large abdominal or waist circumference is associated with high cholesterol levels and higher risk for heart disease, stroke, diabetes, hypertension, and some types of cancer. If your BMI is in the healthy range, a large waist circumference may signify an independent risk for disease. If your BMI is in the overweight or obese range, measuring

your waist circumference can be an additional tool to determine your health risk. If your BMI is above 35, your health risk is already high.

To measure your waist circumference, use a tape measure. Measure your waist right above your hip bones, with the tape crossing your navel. Keep the tape level. It should be snug, but not tight. A high waist circumference is[9]

Greater than 40 inches (102 cm) for men
Greater than 35 inches (88 cm) for women

Obese men tend to accumulate abdominal fat, whereas obese women tend to accumulate fat on the hips and thighs. However, women have a change in body fat distribution at the onset of menopause with fat shifting to the abdomen. This shift coincides with an increased risk of heart disease for women.

Issues Related to Overweight and Obesity

If you are overweight or obese, you are at increased risk for serious health problems. Obese people are four times more likely than people with a healthy weight to die before reaching their expected lifespan. They have an increased risk for high blood pressure, diabetes, elevated cholesterol levels, coronary heart disease, stroke, gallbladder disease, osteoarthritis (a type of arthritis caused by excessive wear and tear on the joints), sleep apnea (interrupted breathing during sleep), lung problems, and certain cancers, such as uterine, prostate, and colorectal. Women who are obese may find it more difficult to become pregnant and, once pregnant, they have an increased risk for diabetes, high blood pressure, birth complications, and having a child with a birth defect.[10]

There has been some controversy over the number of annual deaths attributable to overweight and obesity; estimates range from 112,000 to 365,000. A recent study suggests that obesity may account for 18 percent of deaths

■ BMI can be an inaccurate indicator of healthy body weight and fat percentage in athletes with a high proportion of muscle tissue. For example, basketball player LeBron James, at 6 feet, 8 inches and 250 pounds, has a BMI of 27 and would be classified as overweight.

between ages 40 and 85. In addition, the earlier people become obese and thus the longer they live with obesity, the greater the risk of it contributing to poor health outcomes—a worrisome fact given the high rates of childhood obesity.[11,12]

Diabetes and Obesity Rates of obesity and diabetes in the United States have risen in parallel. Diabetes is a disease in which the levels of glucose circulating in the bloodstream are too high, setting the stage for such health complications as heart disease, kidney failure, blindness, and sexual dysfunction. (A detailed discussion of diabetes is in Chapter 15.) There are several types of diabetes, but 90 to 95 percent of people with diabetes have Type-2 diabetes, the form strongly associated with obesity. Not everyone who is obese will get diabetes, but it is the major risk factor. As more children and adolescents become overweight, Type-2 diabetes, which previously was rare in this age group, has become more common. Approximately 80 percent of American youth with Type-2 diabetes are obese. For people in any age group who are overweight or obese, a 7 percent reduction in body weight through diet and exercise will reduce the risk of developing diabetes by 58 percent.[13]

Discrimination and Obesity People who have been overweight or obese for most of their lives are likely to have suffered from childhood bullying or teasing. Weight-related bullying does not stop with adulthood; people who are overweight or obese may be faced by discrimination in hiring practices, lower wages, and social stigma. A recent study reported a significant wage difference between people of normal weight and those who are obese: the overall cost of obesity for a woman was $4,879 per year and for a man, $2,646.[14] The experience of weight discrimination increases the likelihood of engaging in behaviors that contribute to further weight gain—avoidance of physical activity, binge eating, low self-esteem—thus creating a vicious cycle.[14–16]

The Problem of Underweight

Although the problem of obesity receives more attention, the problem of underweight can be as serious. A sudden, unintentional weight loss without a change in diet or exercise level may signify an underlying illness and should prompt a visit to a physician. Depression, substance abuse, eating disorders (see Chapter 8), thyroid disease, infections, and cancer can all be associated with unexpected weight loss.

However, some people just have difficulty keeping on weight. For them, calorie intake is inadequate for energy output. To gain weight, they need to change the energy balance. Calories can be increased by eating more frequent meals (every three hours or so) and more energy-dense foods, such as nuts, fish, and yogurt. Adding protein powders or nutritional supplements to the diet is another option. The pattern of physical activity can also be changed to reduce aerobic exercise and increase weight training.

WHAT FACTORS INFLUENCE YOUR WEIGHT?

There is no simple answer to why Americans are gaining weight. Many factors contribute to this trend, both individual and environmental. You may look to other family members, for example, and think that it is your genes that make you overweight. Unless you are adopted, however, the people who gave you your genes also taught you how to eat, chose your neighborhood, and influenced your educational status and perhaps your occupation. It appears that for most people, obesity is a multifactorial condition; that is, your susceptibility to obesity is due to a complex interaction among multiple genes and your environment.[17]

Genetic and Hormonal Influences

If neither of your parents is obese, you have a 10 percent chance of becoming obese. The risk increases to 80 percent if both of your parents are obese. Adopted children also tend to be similar in weight to their biological parents, and twin studies support a genetic tendency toward obesity. These findings have led to the search for genes associated with obesity.

Nearly two dozen hormones identified thus far play a role in appetite and energy expenditure. They act in the brain to influence when to start or finish eating; to monitor external cues for food, such as smells, sights, texture, conditioned responses and advertising; to monitor internal cues, such as body fat stores, glucose level, free fatty acids, and stomach fullness; and to adjust metabolic rate. The food–brain pathways have some overlap with drug–brain pathways in that foods can trigger the release of dopamine and opioids in the brain. This release then contributes to our wanting and liking food (similar to addiction) and complicates our relationship with food, making it more than an energy source. It is not yet fully understood how our bodies regulate energy intake and output, but it is certainly complicated. If you are maintaining your current weight, the interaction of hormones controls your daily calorie intake to within 10 calories (a single potato chip) of balanced food intake and energy expenditure.[18–20]

The stress response also affects eating patterns. In response to stress, our bodies release several hormones, including adrenaline and cortisol. Fat cells release fatty acids and triglycerides in response to these hormones and increase the amount of circulating glucose. These responses are vital in enabling the body to handle acute stress, especially physical stress. But when stress is chronic, the constant presence of these hormones can influence fat deposits, increasing the amount of fat deposited in the abdomen. Adrenaline is an appetite suppressant, whereas cortisol stimulates the appetite. You may find that in high-stress situations, such as the transition to college or final exams week, you eat either more or less than usual. People respond differently to stress, but either pattern can affect your overall health and long-term weight.

Some medical conditions can be associated with weight gain. Thyroid disorders are a prime example. The thyroid gland, located in the neck, produces a hormone that is involved in metabolism. If the gland becomes less active, metabolism slows and weight is gained. If the gland is overactive, metabolism speeds up and weight can be inappropriately lost.

Except in rare cases of a single gene mutation, genetics alone does not fully explain obesity. The rapid rise in obesity since the 1980s is too sudden to be due to genetics. Genes are slow to change, requiring generations and hundreds of years. Environmental influences, such as abundant food, and behaviors, such as a sedentary lifestyle, can produce such effects in a much shorter period.[17–19,21]

Age and Gender

A life-course perspective is important to consider with regard to obesity because there are critical phases in your life when it is easier and harder to maintain a healthy weight. At birth, your susceptibility to obesity has already been programmed. Not only did you inherit half your genes from your mother, she gave you your first "environment"—in utero. If she experienced obesity, rapid weight gain, or starvation during pregnancy, your cells will maintain a memory (in the form of methylation of DNA—revisit the Chapter 1 discussion of epigenetics) of that, and it will increase your risk for future obesity.[21]

In early childhood, you develop your eating patterns from your family. Poor childhood eating habits are believed to be a major cause of the recent surge in overweight and obesity. There are several crucial times in your life when you may change these patterns, a critical one being the first time you leave home to attend college or to live independently. Take advantage of this opportunity to evaluate the eating habits you learned at home and make changes if they are needed.

The choices you make about what foods to eat are shaped as much by the social, cultural, and traditional influences in your life as they are by your biological need for nutrition. Your food preferences are largely shaped by what you have been exposed to in the past. For example, if the food your parents made for you as a child had lots of Indian spices and ingredients in it, you might find that you prefer Indian food when you want a treat or comfort. You can influence your taste preferences by trying new foods.

Adolescence is a critical period regarding body fat percentage. During puberty, boys and girls undergo significant hormonal changes that alter their body composition. Female hormones begin preparing girls for childbearing with increases in body fat,

especially on the hips, buttocks, and thighs. Before puberty, a girl of a healthy weight will have approximately 12 percent body fat. After puberty, the healthy range can increase to up to 25 percent body fat.[8] In contrast, a boy's hormones in late adolescence are geared more toward muscle development. Before puberty, a boy of healthy weight has approximately 12 percent body fat; after puberty, he levels out at approximately 15 percent body fat.

Puberty is also a time where the genders start to differ in activity level. Adolescent girls are on average less physically active than their male peers, an additional pressure toward increased body fat percentage. By high school, 6 percent of females and 18 percent of males meet the adolescent physical activity guidelines of 60 minutes of aerobic activity a day and strength training three times per week.[8,22]

Between the ages of 20 and 40, both men and women gain weight. With completion of high school comes a further decline in physical activity for men and women. The decline is steeper for men, in particular men who are going on to college or university. The transition to college is associated with weight gain for both sexes.[23,24] After college, married men weigh more than do men who have never been married or were previously married but are currently unmarried. For women, these are the years in which pregnancy typically occurs. Weight gain is a normal part of pregnancy. The majority of women will lose most of this weight within a year of delivery. However, about 15 to 20 percent of women

■ Family, social, cultural, and other environmental factors, as well as genes and hormones, play a role in weight. These can include favorite family and ethnic foods, mealtime rules and traditions, and the kinds of restaurants and grocery stores available in the community.

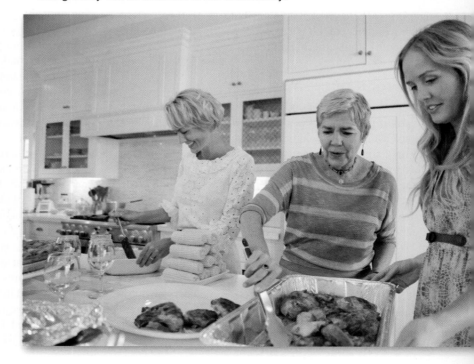

Life Stories

Grace: Trying to Make Healthy Changes

Grace, a sociology major at a state college, is the first member of her family to attend college. Her parents and two younger siblings live in a small industrial town about 200 miles from campus. Her father has worked in an automotive parts plant for the past two decades, and her mother works part-time as the school secretary at the central high school. Both of Grace's parents are overweight, and her maternal grandmother has diabetes. Because both adults work, the family tends to eat a lot of prepared and processed foods, like macaroni and cheese, beef stroganoff, pizza, and hot dogs. When her mom cooks, she tends to make "comfort meals" like meatloaf and mashed potatoes, fried chicken with biscuits and gravy, and pot roast. No one in the family exercises.

When Grace got to college she was about 20 pounds overweight, weighing in at about 160 pounds. She had heard about the "freshman 15" and was worried she would gain more weight that year. Instead, she did so much walking around campus that she actually started to lose weight. She became friends with two women in her residence hall who were much more conscious about food choices than she was, and they often ate dinner together. Following their lead, Grace found herself frequenting the salad bar more often than the taco bar. One of them was a vegetarian, and Grace started enjoying some vegetarian dishes as well. She still ate fast food when she was rushed during exam weeks, but her weight stabilized at just about 20 pounds less than what she had weighed when she arrived on campus.

Grace spent the summer after freshman year at home, working a summer job. Her mom served the same high-fat, high-calorie meals she always had. At first, Grace talked up her new eating patterns, trying to interest her parents in a healthier diet, but her mom seemed to be hurt by Grace's suggestions, and her dad got mad that her mom was hurt. Grace even offered to do the grocery shopping one week, thinking she would get some good fruits and veggies, at least for herself, if not for the whole family. She was disappointed to see there was not much choice in produce at the local supermarket, and what was there looked wilted and unappetizing. When she brought home strawberries for dessert, her younger brother and sister ignored them and went for the ice cream.

Grace slipped back into her old eating patterns and spent more and more time watching TV with her family in the evenings. Grace had hoped to continue walking, but her neighborhood wasn't very safe for walking, and there wasn't a fitness center or gym in town. She was unhappy with herself—and could feel her clothes getting tighter—but she felt guilty trying to be different from her family, and there was a certain comfort in doing the same old things.

When the summer was over, Grace felt both sad and relieved to be leaving her family and going back to school. She would be living in a campus apartment with her two friends, and she knew it would not be such a struggle to eat well and exercise. She worried about her family and wished they had the same resources she did.

- How did social or cultural factors influence Grace's food patterns at home and at school?

- Can you think of things she could have done differently with her family?

- What environmental factors made it harder for her to eat well while with her family?

In general, unhealthy foods are more available, more convenient, more heavily advertised, and less expensive than healthy foods, especially in low-income neighborhoods and urban areas. In these communities, fast-food outlets and small food markets dominate the retail food landscape, providing consumers with foods with high fat content and high sugar content. Obesity rates are highest among the poorest and least educated segments of the population.[25-27] In more affluent neighborhoods, where supermarkets predominate, low-fat and whole-grain foods are more readily available, along with diverse fruit and vegetable choices. On college campuses, all-you-can-eat, buffet-style dining has been associated with increased weight gain among students.[28,29]

Being aware of the factors influencing your food choices can help you attain and maintain a healthy diet. A little planning ahead can go a long way toward supporting healthy food choices (see the box, "Steps to Healthier Eating"). If you don't have healthy choices available on campus, consider packing a lunch or healthy snacks to take with you.

connect
ACTIVITY

---

maintain significant amount of weight a year after delivery, partly as a result of changes in lifestyle associated with childrearing.[30]

As people enter their 50s, both women and men can have potentially serious problems with weight gain. Men tend to see an increase in abdominal fat. Women in their late 40s and early 50s undergo significant hormonal changes associated with menopause and shifts in body fat distribution to a more central or abdominal location.

After age 60, weight tends to decline. This loss can be have a number of causes, including decreased calorie needs, less muscle tissue, and less body mass. These changes give older adults thinner limbs. During these years, weight-bearing exercise, such as walking, becomes critical to maintain body mass and bone strength.

Obesogenic Environments and Lifestyle

The term *obesogenic environment* has been coined to highlight the fact that components of our environment can make it easier for us to eat unhealthily and avoid physical activity—thus increasing the likelihood of obesity. The automobile, television, and the computer are three technological advances that have improved our lives in many ways, yet they have led to unhealthy habits. Before the mid-1900s, most people's daily lives involved regular physical activity. Our current lifestyle has become so mechanized and sedentary, however, that many of us can go through a day spending almost no energy on physical activity. For example, only 48.8 percent of college students, who often have access to recreational

Action Skill-Builder

Steps to Healthier Eating

If you are like many people, you'd like to have a healthier diet— but life gets in the way. You may be busy with school or work, you may be on a tight budget, or you just may not know much about cooking. Your environment may not help, either, especially if it's full of fast-food options. The following "three P's" can guide you to healthier choices. Try one or a few of these steps each week until you've acquired a good foundation for healthy eating.

Plan

☐ Plan to cook at home as often as possible—it's much less expensive than eating out, and you can make better choices.

☐ Plan and shop for a week so you don't have to think about what to cook when you're tired and hungry.

☐ Use leftovers creatively—used leftover rice to make fried rice, leftover chicken in a stir-fry, leftover veggies in a pita pocket with hummus—or pack them in a small plastic container for your lunch the next day.

☐ Avoid skipping meals or getting excessively hungry to prevent impulsive overeating later; if you aren't sure you'll have time for lunch, make sure you have a healthy snack with you.

Purchase

☐ Learn when fruits and vegetables are in season in your area—asparagus in April, strawberries in June, for example— to save money and enjoy fresh, locally grown produce.

☐ Buy healthy low-cost fruits and vegetables like carrots, potatoes, apples, bananas, and fresh greens.

☐ Add more beans to your diet in place of meat for a healthy and less expensive source of protein.

☐ Buy in bulk and prepare foods yourself, like rice and vegetables, macaroni and cheese, spaghetti with tomato sauce; prepackaged foods cost more and have added ingredients you don't need, like sugar, salt, and preservatives.

Prepare

☐ Prepare snacks ahead of time and carry them with you—a piece of fresh fruit, a small bag of nuts, some carrot sticks.

☐ Drink water instead of soda or juice; carry water with you—tap water is usually fine—in a reusable container.

☐ If you're a beginning cook, find quick and easy recipes and cooking tips online, learn from your family, or cook with friends.

☐ Prepare a meal in a slow cooker in the morning and have dinner ready when you get home later in the day.

☐ Cook up a large quantity of soup or stew when you have a slow day and freeze individual portions for days when you have less time.

Sources: "10 Tips Nutrition Education Series: Eating Better on a Budget," U.S. Department of Agriculture, 2012, www.choosemyplate.gov/food-groups/downloads/TenTips/DGTipsheet16EatingBetterOnABudget.pdf; "10 Tips Nutrition Education Series: Eating on a Budget: The Three P's," U.S. Department of Agriculture, 2012, www.choosemyplate.gov/downloads/PlanPurchasePrepare.pdf.

facilities and intramural sports, meet recommended aerobic physical activity guidelines for adults.[31] In addition, epigenetic research shows that prenatal and early childhood environments are particularly important in determining risk of adult obesity – excess food or starvation during early childhood makes people particularly susceptible to obesity later.[21]

Food Choices Your choice in foods is driven by availability—cost and convenience—as well as by your upbringing. As a college student, you are probably on a limited budget and have limited time to prepare food. This scenario will likely remain true after you leave college and enter the workforce. The ability to maintain a healthy diet depends on having sufficient knowledge about healthy food choices, the money to buy healthy foods, and the time to prepare a healthy meal[25] (see the box, "Grace: Trying to Make Healthy Changes").

Eating Out In the 1950s, eating out was a rare event; today, it has become a part of daily life. Twenty-one percent of households use some form of take-out food or food-delivery service daily.[27] The trend is likely related to the increased number of dual-career households and single-parent households and the convenience and accessibility of fast foods. The concern is that foods served in restaurants and fast-food outlets tend to be higher in fat and total calories and lower in fiber than foods prepared at home. Increased reliance on fast foods is associated with weight gain.[21,29]

Larger Portions Serving size has increased steadily both inside and outside the home. The largest increases in serving size have occurred in fast-food restaurants and may be due to "supersized" pricing strategies. The impact of supersizing on the caloric bottom line is dramatic. When given large servings in restaurants or prepackaged foods, people eat more. The larger the portion of food, the worse we become at estimating how much we are eating. (See Figure 7.1 for some visual images of portion sizes.) Paying attention to package labeling, dividing prepackaged food into smaller

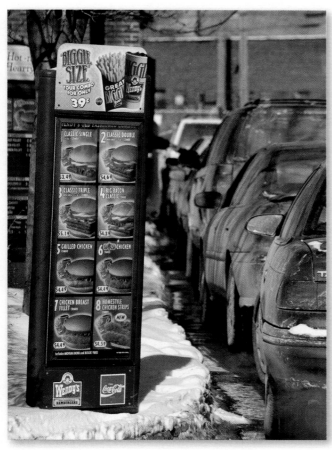

■ More and more Americans are eating out (or ordering in) on a daily basis, and many are getting their meals in the drive-through lane. This major cultural shift is one of the factors implicated in the current overweight and obesity phenomenon.

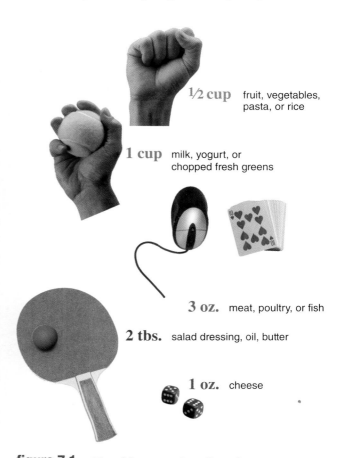

figure 7.1 **Visual images of portion sizes.**
Half a cup of fruit, vegetables, pasta, or rice is about the size of a small fist. One cup of milk, yogurt, or chopped fresh greens is about the size of a small hand holding a tennis ball. Three ounces of meat, poultry, or fish is about the size of a computer mouse or a deck of cards. Two tablespoons of salad dressing, oil, or butter is about the size of a ping pong ball. One ounce of cheese is about the size of a pair of dice.

serving sizes, and using visual cues can help with more appropriate serving sizes.[32] New federal regulations require restaurants and retail food establishments with 20 or more locations to list calorie counts on menus and menu boards.[33] See the box, "Get the Most Out of Your Menu," for more information on healthy eating when you're eating out.

Built Environment Because of our car-friendly, pedestrian-unfriendly community design, 25 percent of all trips in the United States are less than 1 mile, and yet 75 percent of these trips are taken by car.[34] Green space, safety considerations, and community structure significantly influence our method of transportation. If your neighborhood or campus is designed to favor walking or biking (with sidewalks, bike lanes, green space, and reliable public transportation), you are more likely to incorporate regular physical activity into your life and have a lower risk of obesity than if you live in a less walkable community.[35]

Sedentary Lifestyle Watching television continues to be the leading form of sedentary entertainment. Americans spend an average of 5 hours and 11 minutes a day watching television.[36] Computers and other technological advances have further altered the activity level of children and adults. Talking to friends, playing games, and shopping are just a few activities often done via computer that would previously have involved some physical activity. Whether at work, home, or play, sitting too long in front of a computer or television or in a car is bad for our health; for more on this topic, see the box, "Could You Spend Less Time Sitting?" in Chapter 6. Basically, if you sit or lie down for 23.5 hours a day, your 30 minutes of physical exercise is not going to reverse the negatives.[37,38]

Sleep How much you sleep may also put you at risk for gaining weight. Energy expenditure is less when you are sleeping, so it would seem that the less you sleep, the less likely you are to gain weight. However, studies have consistently shown the opposite—less sleep is associated with weight gain in young adults. The reason for this association is not clear—it could be that you eat more or exercise less if you are sleep deprived or that your hormones are affected.[39,40]

Consumer Clipboard

Get the Most Out of Your Menu

Restaurants with more than 20 outlets are required to list calories on their menus. Many restaurants have nutrition brochures available on request, and many post complete nutritional information on their websites.

Popular restaurant chains load up their menus with fat and salt. An order of 8 chicken nachos can have more than 1,000 calories and nearly 2,000 mg of sodium. Buffalo wings with blue cheese can have nearly 1,500 calories and more than 4,500 mg of sodium (twice the recommended daily limit).

If you can't tell from the menu, ask if a soup is cream based or broth based. Cream-based soups have more calories, fat, and saturated fat. Soups can also be laden with salt, so avoid them if you're trying to reduce sodium in your diet.

Calories and fat soar when you add a creamy or ranch dressing; most restaurants have a low-fat option, such as low-fat Italian or vinaigrette. Ask for dressing on the side so you can control the amount you consume.

If you need a sweet taste after a meal, order one dessert for the table with spoons for everyone. Instead of pie (300 to 500 calories per slice) or ice cream (270 calories per half-cup scoop), try a yogurt parfait (300 calories) at Starbucks, a fruit and yogurt parfait (130 calories) at McDonald's, or cup of fresh berries (about 50 calories).

Portion and plate sizes can be three or more times the amount considered a serving.

- Consider splitting an entrée or taking half home for lunch the next day. Notice when you feel full and stop eating!
- Grilled chicken and grilled fish are likely to be the healthiest items on the menu.
- Ask for any sauce on the side.

One fast-food meal can provide your entire recommended daily allowance of calories, fat, saturated fat, cholesterol, and sodium. A burger and fries from a restaurant can have 2,000 calories.

A large order of french fries from a fast-food restaurant can have 500 calories, with 200 or more of those calories from fat. Consider a side salad instead.

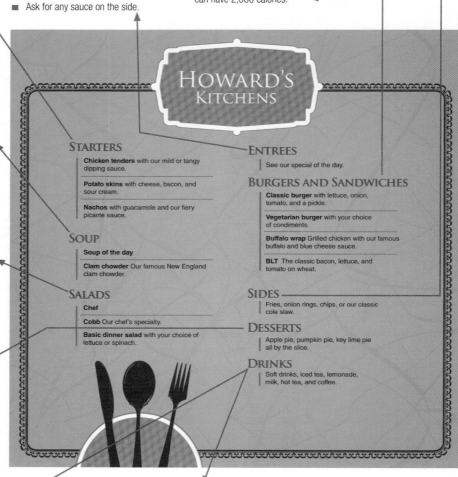

HOWARD'S KITCHENS

STARTERS

Chicken tenders with our mild or tangy dipping sauce.

Potato skins with cheese, bacon, and sour cream.

Nachos with guacamole and our fiery picante sauce.

SOUP

Soup of the day

Clam chowder Our famous New England clam chowder.

SALADS

Chef

Cobb Our chef's specialty.

Basic dinner salad with your choice of lettuce or spinach.

ENTREES

See our special of the day.

BURGERS AND SANDWICHES

Classic burger with lettuce, onion, tomato, and a pickle.

Vegetarian burger with your choice of condiments.

Buffalo wrap Grilled chicken with our famous buffalo and blue cheese sauce.

BLT The classic bacon, lettuce, and tomato on wheat.

SIDES

Fries, onion rings, chips, or our classic cole slaw.

DESSERTS

Apple pie, pumpkin pie, key lime pie all by the slice.

DRINKS

Soft drinks, iced tea, lemonade, milk, hot tea, and coffee.

Regular soda is loaded with sugar and calories. A large (32-ounce) cola drink has 86 grams of sugar, the equivalent of about 21 teaspoons, and 310 calories, virtually all from sugar (4 grams of sugar = 1 teaspoon = 16 calories). Water is free and has 0 calories.

Calculate calories from fat by multiplying grams of fat by 9 (fat supplies 9 calories per gram). Calories from fat should not exceed 30 percent of total calories. For example, if an item has 300 calories and 15 grams of fat, it has 135 calories from fat (15 × 9), which equals 45 percent of the total calories (135/300). Calculate calories from saturated fat the same way. Calories from saturated fat should not exceed 10 percent of total calories.

Coffee drinks can be very high in calories, especially if they include whipped cream or ice cream.

- A 16-ounce Starbucks Mocha Frappuccino with whipped cream has 400 calories, 15 grams of fat, and 60 grams of sugar (15 teaspoons). Ask for nonfat milk and skip the whipped cream—that reduces calories to 260 and fat to 1 gram, but sugar stays high (58 grams).
- Starbucks "Trente" size for iced drinks is 31 ounces, a volume of 916 milliliters. The capacity of the average adult stomach is about 900 milliliters. Ask for a smaller size.
- Coffee and tea have 0 calories (but not if you add milk and sugar!).
- A medium smoothie has about 250 calories, whether at McDonald's or at Jamba Juice. A medium vanilla shake at McDonald's has 680 calories.
- A glass of wine has about 100 calories; a 12-ounce beer has between about 150 and 180 calories; a light beer usually has fewer than 100 calories. Because of added sugar and other ingredients, a mixed drink can soar to hundreds of calories. Alcohol itself supplies 7 calories per gram.

Social Networks Friends and social networks also appear to influence weight. If your friends gain weight, you are more likely to gain weight. The more strongly you identify a person as a friend, the more likely you are to match his or her weight gain. This effect may relate to social norms and how comfortable you are with overweight and obesity. The good news is that recruiting friends in your efforts to maintain a healthy weight or lose weight may make you more successful.[41,42]

Dieting and Obesity Contributing to the obesity trend is the "yo-yo dieting" effect, or **weight cycling**. People frustrated with their weight often turn to fad diets in hopes of finding a solution. Fad diets do not consist of realistic food plans that can be maintained for a lifetime. People may lose weight initially, but most find it difficult to maintain the harsh restrictions, returning to their previous patterns. With rapid weight loss on a highly restrictive diet, the body can enter starvation mode, with decreased basal metabolism. When the person goes off the restrictive diet, he or she rapidly gains back the weight lost and sometimes gains even more before the body's metabolism readjusts.

THE KEY TO WEIGHT CONTROL: ENERGY BALANCE

The relationship between the calories you take in and the calories you expend is known as **energy balance**. If you take in more calories than you use through metabolism and movement (a positive energy balance), you store these extra calories in the form of body fat. If you take in fewer calories than you need (a negative energy balance), you draw on body fat stores to provide energy. Energy in must equal energy out in order to maintain your current weight. If you adjust one or the other side of the equation, you will gain or lose weight.

Estimating Your Daily Energy Requirements

In Chapter 5, we discussed energy intake, the calories-in side of the energy equation. Here, we are more interested in energy expenditure, the calories-out side. Components of energy expenditure include the energy required to process food and respond to environmental and physiological changes, the basal metabolic rate, and physical activity. These components are influenced by genetics, age, sex, body size, fat-free mass, and intensity and duration of activity.

The **thermic effect of food** is an estimate of the energy required to process the food you eat—chewing, digesting, metabolizing, and so on. The

thermic effect of food is generally estimated at 10 percent of energy intake. If, for example, you ingested 2,500 calories of food during a day, you would burn approximately 250 calories processing what you ate. Your baseline energy expenditure also varies with changes in the environment, such as in response to cold, and with physiological events, such as trauma, overeating, and changes in hormonal status; this is called *adaptive thermogenesis.*

The **basal metabolic rate (BMR)** is the rate at which the body uses energy at rest to maintain the function of the vital organs, such as the heart, lungs, nervous system, liver, intestines, muscles and skin. About 60 to 70 percent of energy consumed is used for these basic metabolic functions. BMR is affected by several factors, including age, gender, and weight.

Between 10 and 30 percent of the calories consumed each day are used for physical activity, depending on level and duration of activity. Physical activity influences the energy balance in two ways: exercise itself burns calories, and exercise increases muscle mass, which is associated with a higher BMR.

You can estimate your daily energy expenditure by considering (1) the thermic effect of food, (2) the energy spent on basal metabolic rate, and (3) the energy spent on physical activities. The effects of adaptive thermogenesis on basal metabolic rate are not usually taken into account except in extreme situations, such as severe injury or prolonged illness. To estimate your daily energy expenditure, complete the Personal Health Portfolio activity for Chapter 7 at the end of the book.

Adjusting Your Caloric Intake

If you are trying to lose weight, 1 pound to 2 pounds per week is a healthy goal. Because a pound of body fat stores about 3,500 calories, you need to decrease your total calorie intake for the week by about 3,500 calories in order to lose 1 pound per week. If you lose weight at a faster rate, you are likely to lose lean tissue like muscle and decrease your basal metabolic rate. Additionally, diets too low in calories may not provide enough nutrients. If you are trying to increase your weight, you will need to increase your total calorie intake for the week by 3,500 calories in order to gain 1 pound per week. (Note that these are estimates.)

weight cycling
Repeated cycles of weight loss and weight gain as a result of dieting; sometimes called yo-yo dieting.

energy balance
Relationship between caloric intake (in the form of food) and caloric output (in the form of metabolism and activity).

thermic effect of food
Estimate of the energy required to process the food you eat.

basal metabolic rate (BMR)
Rate at which your body uses energy for basic life functions, such as breathing, circulation, and temperature regulation.

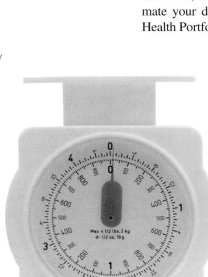

Table 7.2   A Comparison of Selected Diets and Weight Management Organizations

Diet/Organization	Theory	Pros and Cons
Volumetrics (self-help book)	Focus on low-energy-dense foods (vegetables, soup broth, nonfat milk) in place of high-energy-dense foods (chips, cookies, candy, nuts, oils)	Includes physical activity Emphasis on lifelong eating patterns Low drop-out rate* Recipes may be time-consuming to prepare
Weight Watchers (commercial organization)	Point exchange system (calorie counting equivalent) Earn or spend points with exercise and food Weekly behavioral component (group support), weigh-ins, and physical activity recommendations	Low drop-out rate* 4.6-pound weight loss at 1 year**
Jenny Craig (commercial organization)	Restrict calorie intake Prepackaged meals only Individual behavioral counseling and exercise recommendations	Expensive due to meals Minimal time for food prep Average drop-out rate* 14-pound weight loss at 1 year***
Slim-Fast (commercial products)	Meal replacement system—1 to 2 meals a day are replaced with 400-calorie drink or bar	Convenient, minimal time involvement High drop-out rate* Reported "as effective as calorie-control diet"
Atkins (self-help book)	Low-carbohydrate diet No restriction on proteins or fats	Requires total calorie restriction for weight loss Average drop-out rate* 4.6-pound weight loss at 1 year**
Ornish (self-help book)	Low-fat diet Bans on meat, fish, oils, alcohol, sugar, white flour	Drastic diet change for most people Average drop-out rate* 3.3-pound weight loss at 1 year**
TOPS (nonprofit organization)	Group-format weekly sessions teaching skills for healthy eating and exercise Low-calorie diet emphasis Encourages exercise	Nonprofit No recent published data on weight loss or retention
Overeaters Anonymous (self-help organization)	12-step program Weekly sessions emphasizing healthy eating and physical, emotional, and spiritual recovery Assigned sponsor	May be beneficial for binge eaters or others with emotional issues attached to eating No published data on weight loss or retention

*Drop-out rate: low drop out = more than 50% continue at 1 year; average drop out = approximately 50% continue at 1 year; high dropout = less than 50% continue at 1 year.
**Independent study trials confirm weight loss amounts listed.
***Recent small randomized trial evaluating Jenny Craig versus control.

Sources: "Comparison of Atkins, Ornish, Weight Watchers and Zone Diets for Weight Loss and Heart Disease Risk Reduction: A Randomized Trial," by M. L. Daninger, J. A. Gleason, J. L. Griffith, et al., 2006, *Journal of the American Medical Association, 293* (1), pp. 43–53; "Systematic Review: An Evaluation of Major Commercial Weight Loss Programs in the United States," by A. G. Tsai and T. A. Wadden, 2005, *Annals of Internal Medicine, 142* (1), pp. 56–67; "Randomized Trial of a Multifaceted Commercial Weight Loss Program," by C. L. Rock, B. Pakiz, S. W. Flat, et al., 2007, *Obesity, 15,* pp. 939–949.

Reducing your intake of fat is also important. High-fat foods are energy-dense, meaning they have many calories per ounce of food. Intake of high-fat foods usually leads to higher total caloric intake and is linked with obesity. Foods high in complex carbohydrates have a greater thermic effect than do high-fat foods. Thus, it takes more energy to process a high-carbohydrate diet, and less of the food's energy is available for storage as fat.

ARE THERE QUICK FIXES FOR OVERWEIGHT AND OBESITY?

Most of us would love a quick and easy way to stay at a healthy body weight. But how healthy are fad diets? Are they worth the money? And do they work?

The Diet Industry

Americans pay an estimated $61 billion for the diet industry's quick fixes.[43] This money goes mainly to promoters of fad diets and weight management organizations. You need to be skeptical of unrealistic promises and to use your critical thinking skills when considering a diet or weight loss program. Some programs have been around for years, while others seem to come and go. For a comparison of several programs, see Table 7.2.

Fad Diets   Every year, "new and improved" fad diets seduce consumers despite the fact that their safety and effectiveness are often unproven. No matter what the latest title, fad diets follow a pattern of altering the balance of carbohydrates, protein, and fat with the goal of promoting weight

teaching. Overeaters Anonymous may be more suitable for binge eaters or others with emotional issues related to weight.[45] (See Table 7.2.)

The Medical Approach

Because obesity is a major risk factor for many health conditions, health centers are involved in helping people find solutions. We consider here three medical strategies used to treat obesity: very-low-calorie diets (VLCDs), diet drugs, and surgical procedures.

Very-Low-Calorie Diets An aggressive option for patients with high health risks because of obesity, VLCDs require a physician's supervision. These diets provide a daily intake of 800 calories or less and *must* be monitored closely.

VLCDs are used for moderately to severely obese patients (people with BMIs greater than 30) who are highly motivated but have not had success with more conservative plans. Patients with BMIs of 27 to 30 with medical conditions that could improve with rapid weight loss are also candidates. Weight loss after a 26-week program averages 20 percent of the patient's initial weight. However, maintaining weight loss is challenging.

Prescription Drugs Because of the expense, potential for side effects, and need for medical supervision, the use of weight loss drugs is not recommended for everyone. Before beginning a medication regimen, one must consider whether the health risks of being obese outweigh the risks of medication side effects. The history of medications for weight loss is a sordid one with multiple medications being approved and then removed from the market due to serious side effects.

There are two types of weight loss drugs—those that act in the brain to reduce food intake and those that act elsewhere in the body to reduce food absorption. The Food and Drug Administration (FDA) has recently approved two medications that reduce appetite. Lorcaserin leads to an average 5 percent loss of baseline weight at 12 weeks but should be continued for a year. Side effects of headache, dizziness, nausea, and fatigue are low. Phentermine-topiramate is a combination of an amphetamine analogue (phentermine) and an anti-seizure medication (topiramate) that leads to an average weight loss of 3 to 8 percent after 12 weeks, but it too should be continued for a year. Side effects of rapid heart rate, increase blood pressure, and mood changes are low. As with all newly released medication, these will be watched closely to ensure safety.

Orlistat works in the intestines to block the absorption of fat; its use results in an average weight loss of 6 to 8 percent. Digestion of fat is reduced by approximately 30 percent, and the undigested fat passes through the body; as such, Orlistat has minimal effectiveness in someone with a low-fat diet. Orlistat has some potential side effects: stomach cramps, gas, and fecal incontinence (leaking stool). In addition, the

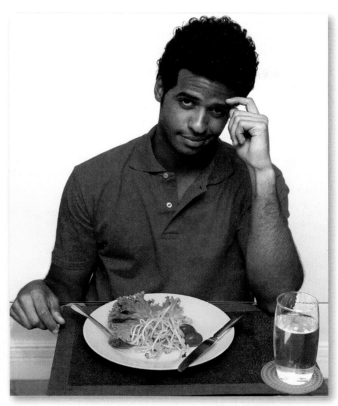

■ Any diet plan that requires you to eat only certain foods or to stop eating entire food groups is not a recipe for long-term success.

loss. Many will label certain foods as "good" or "bad," require the elimination of one of the five food groups, or prescribe certain "fat-burning foods." Be wary of diets with these features because no scientific data exist to support these claims.

Most dietitians and physicians encourage people to monitor energy balance and eat a diet that emphasizes complex carbohydrates rather than trying fad diets. When evaluating a diet, consider if the food plan is something you can live with for the long haul. Remember, the factors that influence our food choices most are taste, cost, and convenience. You are unlikely to stick with a diet if it is too drastically different from your current eating patterns, if it calls for complete elimination of certain foods (especially ones you really like), if it requires hours of preparation, or if it requires the purchase of expensive prepackaged foods.[44]

Weight Management Organizations Weight management organizations offer group support, nutrition education, dietary advice, exercise counseling, and other services. Weight Watchers, Take Off Pounds Sensibly (TOPS), and Overeaters Anonymous are three well-known weight management organizations. TOPS and Overeaters Anonymous are free and provide group support. Weight Watchers is a commercial program. TOPS focuses on

reduction in fat absorption leads to a decrease in the absorption of certain fat-soluble vitamins (vitamins A, D, E, and K). An over-the-counter version of Orlistat, called Alli, is now available. It is a reduced-strength version with the same potential side effects.[46,47]

Another combination medication is currently under review by the FDA. It is a combination of naltrexone (a centrally acting medication used in opioid addiction) and bupropion (a centrally acting medication used in depression and tobacco cessation) that appears to be effective in reducing calorie intake and increasing physical activity.[48]

Other drugs and medications are sometimes used in an attempt to help with weight loss, but they are not currently approved for such use by the FDA. The antidepressant fluoxetine (Prozac) has been shown to have some potential weight loss benefits. Caffeine, a stimulant available in many over-the-counter forms, is sometimes used to increase basal metabolic rate and produce weight loss. Caffeine can cause side effects such as shakiness, dizziness, and sleep problems.

Surgical Options Gastric surgery is never a first-line approach to obesity. The National Institutes of Health has determined that surgical therapy should be considered for patients with a BMI of 40 or greater and a history of failed medical treatments for obesity, or for patients with a BMI of 35 or greater with illnesses or risk factors. Recommending surgery for people with a BMI 30 or higher and poorly controlled diabetes is being considered, but surgery is not recommended for anyone with a BMI less than 30. Typical weight loss after gastric surgery ranges from 48 to 66 percent of excess weight. Most people have significant improvement in or resolution of diabetes, hypertension, and other obesity-related conditions. As with any surgical procedure, side effects can occur at the time of surgery or after surgery.[49]

Nonprescription Diet Drugs and Dietary Supplements Popular over-the-counter diet drugs and dietary supplements include diet teas, bulking products, starch blockers, diet candies, sugar blockers, and benzocaine. A range of herbal supplements, including ginseng, CQ (Cissus quadrangularis), bittermelon, and zingiber, may have modest benefits for weight loss, but the studies of them are limited in regard to long-term benefits or risk.[50]

Safety concerns have arisen over the use of some of these drugs and supplements. One example is ephedra, a stimulant formerly found in many over-the-counter weight loss supplements. Ephedra can cause cardiac arrhythmia (abnormal heart rhythm) and even death by constricting blood vessels while increasing the heart rate and speeding up the nervous system. In February 2004, the FDA banned dietary supplements containing ephedra because of the association of this drug with heart attack, stroke, hypertension, and heat stroke.

Manufacturers of dietary supplements do not have to submit proof of their efficacy or safety to the Food and Drug Administration prior to sale. Use your critical thinking skills when considering the use of any product, including herbal and dietary supplements, to help in weight loss. All medications, supplements, and herbal treatments have the potential for side effects and risks. Ask yourself the following questions prior to use:

- Is there evidence to support the claims that this product works? Look for peer-reviewed research in mainstream publications and be wary of small, unpublished studies conducted by the product's manufacturer.

- What are the potential risks and side effects of the product? Do the proven benefits (if any) outweigh the risk and side effects?

If you cannot find the answers to these questions, it is best to avoid the product!

The Size Acceptance Movement

The size acceptance movement started in response to the frustration felt by many people in attempting to lose weight and in response to the discrimination faced by those who are overweight or obese. The approach seeks to decrease negative body image, encourage self-acceptance, and end discrimination. The focus is on how people can be healthy at any size. The movement also aims to draw attention to the fact that good health is a state of physical, mental, and social well-being. Self-esteem and body image are strongly linked, and helping people respect themselves improves their overall health. Size acceptance also emphasizes that people of any size can become more fit and benefit from healthier food choices.[51,52]

The size acceptance movement has made strides in changing health approaches from weight loss to weight management and improving fitness at any size—sometimes being referred to as the "fit and fat movement." However, pleas by the size acceptance movement should not obscure the fact that obesity is associated with serious medical problems. The goal is to find a balanced approach that combines personal acceptance with promotion of a healthy body composition.[53]

ACHIEVING A HEALTHY BODY WEIGHT AND BODY COMPOSITION FOR LIFE

Overweight and obesity are long-term problems and require long-term solutions. Both individuals and society have roles to play in reversing this trend.

Tasks for Individuals

If your genetics or behavioral history predisposes you to being overweight or underweight, you can improve your overall health through moderate lifestyle changes. The emphasis should be on a healthier lifestyle, with these components:

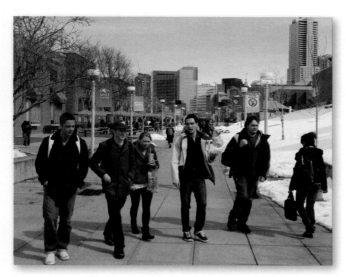

■ Building physical activity into your routine in small ways every day is one key to weight management and weight loss maintenance.

■ A balanced diet emphasizing fruits, vegetables, and whole grains in appropriate portion sizes.

■ A goal of 150 minutes of moderate-intensity physical activity every week. This should be divided into smaller sections of time throughout the week (more physical activity may be necessary if you are aiming to lose weight, less if you are aiming to gain weight).

■ Reduced time spent in sedentary activities, such as watching TV, working or playing on a computer, and riding in a car.

■ A goal of overall health improvement through targeted improvement in selected areas, such as blood pressure, cholesterol level, and blood sugar level.

■ Peer support for your health goals.

■ Self-acceptance of body size.

■ Follow-up evaluation by a health professional, as needed.

Set Realistic Goals Drastic diet changes and quick-fix solutions are unlikely to last for long. The key to long-term weight management is making reasonable, moderate changes that fit in with your life, culture, and tastes. You are also more likely to be successful if you set a goal. Let's revisit SMART goals, which were presented in Chapter 1, and apply them to weight management:

■ *Is the goal* specific? Deciding to eat fresh fruit as a late night snack instead of candy is a specific goal. So

is deciding to go to the gym to run on the treadmill for 30 minutes on Monday, Wednesday, and Friday after chemistry class. Specific goals are easier to accomplish.

■ *Is the goal* measurable? You can track how often you actually eat fresh fruit as a snack instead of candy or how often you make it to the gym after chemistry class. A measurable goal allows you to track your progress and see how close you are to reaching it.

■ *Is the goal* attainable? Your goal should be something that you are able to do rather than something that happens to you. There should be an action on your part.

■ *Is the goal* realistic? Small, gradual changes, such as deciding to change from regular soda to diet soda or from whole milk to low fat milk, are realistic. Once you accomplish the first change, you can then add another small change. With small steps, you are more likely to be successful.

■ *Is the goal* timely? When you make a decision to change behavior, set a time line for when you will reach your goal. You might, for example, give yourself an entire semester to reach your goal of getting 150 minutes of exercise a week.

Manage Behavior Many behavior management tools are available to help you learn new eating and activity patterns. The following strategies may help get you started:

■ *Stimulus control.* Identify environmental cues associated with unhealthy eating habits. Become conscious of when, where, and why you are eating. For example, if you eat a pastry for breakfast because you stop at a coffee shop on the way to class, consider changing your routine—brew coffee at home and make your own fruit-and-yogurt parfait to take with you.

■ *Self-supervision.* Keep a log of the foods you eat and the physical activity you do. Schedule time for exercise and plan meals to preempt urges and cravings.

■ *Social support and positive reinforcement.* Recruit others to join you in your healthier eating and exercising habits. Exercise together, encourage each other, and plan nonfood rewards for reaching goals.

■ *Stress management.* Use relaxation techniques, exercise, and problem-solving strategies to handle stresses in your life, instead of overeating or skipping meals.

■ *Cognitive restructuring.* Moderate self-defeating thoughts and emotions, redefine your body image by thinking about what your body can do (rather than how it looks), and be realistic about weight loss or gain.

Public Health Is Personal

Getting Involved in a Community Garden

Does your campus have a community garden? Many colleges do:

- College of the Atlantic in Bar Harbor, Maine, owns and operates several small community gardens as well as a 70-acre farm that sells produce to community members. Students are encouraged to volunteer at the farm and its farm stand.

- The University of Delaware runs a community garden that supplies fresh organic produce to a local food bank. Students can volunteer in the garden.

- Evergreen State College in Olympia, Washington, has several community gardens where students can learn farming as interns or volunteers. The farm stocks the school's salad bar with fresh produce.

Thousands of communities and cities across the country have community gardens as well, from Seattle to New York City. The United States has a long history of community gardens, dating back to World Wars I and II, when people came together to grow food for the war effort in "victory gardens." The 1970s saw a resurgence of interest in community gardening in response to environmental concerns. Today, a growing movement is taking shape in response to several trends: concern about obesity and diet-related diseases; concern about inequities in access to healthy foods among low-income and urban populations; a desire for organic, locally grown produce; and interest in sustainable agricultural practices that don't deplete the earth's resources.

How does community gardening support healthy weight management? Data show that people who have garden plots eat more fruits and vegetables than those who don't have them.

Gardening offers leisure-time, recreational physical activity and gets people moving. These two benefits alone—more fruits and veggies and more physical activity—make community gardening a healthy pursuit. In addition, communal gardening may help reduce feelings of isolation and stress as people get to know their neighbors, develop a sense of community, and gain access to nutritious foods. Following a tradition dating back to the early 19th century, the University of Delaware has developed a "therapeutic" community garden to help students who are depressed or struggling with other mental health problems. The garden promotes contemplation, collaboration, recreation, and contact with nature.

Although community gardens tend to spring from grassroots efforts, it's easy to see why public health officials support them. Michelle Obama's "Let's Move!" campaign encourages community and religious leaders to get people involved in community gardening. The states of New York and Tennessee have laws in place to protect and encourage the conversion of vacant land to vegetable gardens. The USDA National Agricultural Library provides a wealth of resources and guides to planning and starting a community garden. The USDA Community Food Projects Grant provides funds to set up community gardens in low-income neighborhoods to promote food security. The National Park Service even provides land inside parks for groups that want to start community gardens.

Community gardening builds connections among people and between people and their food; at the same time, it produces a delicious harvest for all to share. If your campus has a community garden, think about getting involved. If it doesn't, think about starting one!

connect ACTIVITY

Sources: "4 Notable Campus Community Gardens and Farms," by S. Frydenlund, 2011, *Organic on the Green,* http://organiconthegreen.wordpress.com/2011/01/07/4-notable-campus-community-gardens-and-farms; "Farms and Community: Community Gardening," USDA National Agricultural Library, 2011, http://afsic.nal.usda.gov/nal_display/index.php?info_center=2&tax_level=2&tax_subject=301&topic_id=1444; "Therapeutic Community Gardens Offer Natural Relief," *University of Delaware Daily,* 2010, www.udel.edu/udaily/2011/dec/garden-natural-relief-120310.html.

Tasks for Society

Changes in social policies are also needed to combat the obesity epidemic.

Promote Healthy Foods The U.S. surgeon general has asked that all schools reduce junk food and promote healthy, balanced meals. Schools can limit access to candy and soda, and municipalities can provide better access to healthy foods through community gardens and equitable supermarket distribution. Federal, state, and local governments can provide financial incentives, such as loan guarantees and reduced property taxes, for supermarkets and small stores that provide healthy foods.

Food subsidies and pricing strategies are a broad-based intervention that can alter eating patterns. Lowering the price of low-fat, nutritious food would increase the rates at which people would buy them. However, in the 15-year period from 1985 to 2000, the cost of fruits and vegetables increased 117 percent, while the cost of soft drinks increased just 20 percent.

Look around your campus to see what is being done to promote healthy foods. Do dining halls and food courts offer nutritious choices? Is food labeling available to tell you what meals contain or which are healthier choices? Do healthy food choices, such as fresh fruits, vegetables, and salads, cost more than the fried foods or sweets?

Support Active Lifestyles Through Community Planning Suburbanization and a cultural focus on cars play a major role in Americans' decreased physical activity. As a society, we need to consider ways to encourage a more active lifestyle (see the box, "Getting Involved in a Community Garden"). Community planning can incorporate ideas to encourage physical activity, such as walking areas and parks in all communities, increased public transportation, showering and changing room facilities in workplaces to encourage biking or walking to work, and flexible work hours to reduce stress and encourage activity.

Support Consumer Awareness In a free society, we avoid restricting the media and advertising, but consumers can become more conscious of their effects on eating patterns. Advertising is a supply-and-demand industry. If consumers don't buy the products depicted in ads, or if they complain about the content of ads, food manufacturers will eventually respond.

What types of food advertising are present on your campus? How does the campus encourage or limit exposure to media? If a promotional event is occurring on campus, is it clear to students who the sponsor is and what, if anything, is being marketed?

Encourage Health Insurers to Cover Obesity Prevention Programs Health insurance companies have been slow to cover all preventive health care, and prevention of obesity is no exception. Although conclusive evidence shows that obesity is associated with risks of multiple medical conditions, few insurance plans currently cover health visits for obesity education or treatment. With concern about health care and health care costs rising, we may see changes in the future. Employers and educational institutions can push legislators to make preventive medicine a priority for insurance companies.

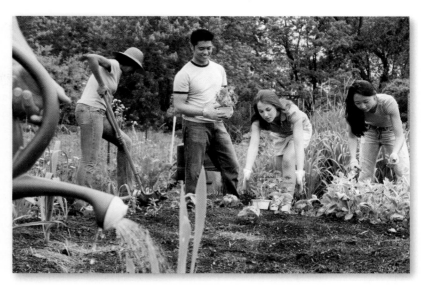

■ Community gardens have been promoted as a way to support physically active lifestyles as well as social involvement and healthy eating.

Obesity is considered a chronic degenerative condition, which may help individuals, insurers, and health care providers move away from the "quick fix" mentality. As with any chronic condition, the focus has to be on sustainable changes. Programs that combine nutritional education, exercise education, and lifestyle modification may help promote healthier, more sustainable weight loss.

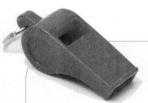

You Make the Call

Does *The Biggest Loser* Support Health Changes or Promote Stigma?

Television has long played a role in health education with news shows releasing results of health studies and updates on health policy. Fictional characters on prime-time sitcoms and dramas and real people on reality television showcase interpersonal relationships and values about alcohol, sexual behaviors, and communication. Television shows help shape societal views of acceptable attitudes and behaviors.

On the reality show *The Biggest Loser,* obese contestants compete to lose the most weight. For 18 weeks they live at *The Biggest Loser* camp and work with trainers, nutritionists, and physicians. Reporting a combined weight loss of 26,600 pounds among contestants in the first 14 seasons, *The Biggest Loser* promotes itself as helping people reclaim their lives and rewrite their futures. In its 15th season, to start addressing rising rates

of obesity among youth, children from 13 to 17 years old were included on the teams.

While *The Biggest Loser* is primarily providing entertainment, the show does provide important information on dietary changes and exercise as necessary components of weight loss. The workouts are extreme, with contestants often cheering each other on and sometimes complaining about how hard they are. The foods provided at camp are quite different from what regular people eat.

Although the environment is tightly controlled, there is little acknowledgment about the role of environment, context, food access, or policies in weight management. The emphasis is on individual behavior change and success (or failure) of contestants is based on their personal responsibility. Research shows that viewers watching *The Biggest Loser* are more likely to perceive weight control as an individual responsibility and in turn this increases their anti-fat attitudes and perpetuates societal stigma around obesity. One only has to consider the double entendre of

Continued…

Concluded...

the title of this show—*The Biggest Loser*—to see the conflict. In addition, viewers are more likely to internalize a negative attitude about exercise after watching the show—likely because exercise is consistently depicted as hard work. Despite these negative views, illustrating how reality TV can transform culture, "Biggest Loser" competitions are now common in work sites, on college campuses, and among other groups of people across the country.

Is the show increasing negative perceptions of obesity by saying that obese people are the biggest losers, or is it encouraging a movement toward healthy life change by supporting people in their weight loss goals?

Pros

- Some of the life stories provide inspirational examples of how contestants can take control of their bodies, and team members support one another's success.
- The show can be educational and provide useful weight-loss tips to viewers.

- *The Biggest Loser* is motivational and has inspired similar contests on college campuses, work sites, and among friends encouraging people to become active and engaged with weight loss.

Cons

- The focus on individual behavior change with minimal acknowledgment of the role of the environment, policy, and circumstances beyond an individual's control leads viewers to assign personal responsibility to contestants and increases anti-fat attitudes and stigma against obese people.
- Contestants participate in unrealistic weight-loss and exercise regimes that would not be maintainable by the average person. The focus on extreme exercise creates negative attitudes in viewers about exercise in general.
- The show promotes meanness and competition, which are not values we should aspire to as a culture.

connect
ACTIVITY

Sources: "Effects of Biggest Loser Exercise Depictions on Exercise-Related Attitudes." by T. R. Berry, N. C. McLeod, M. Pankratow, and J. Walker, 2013, *American Journal of Health Behavior, 37* (1), pp. 96–103; "The Reality of Health: Reality Television and the Public Health," by P. Christenson and M. Ivancin, October 2006, The Henry J. Kaiser Family Foundation, http://kaiserfamilyfoundation.files.wordpress .com/2013/01/7567.pdf; "No Clear Winner: Effects of *The Biggest Loser* on the Stigmatization of Obese Persons," by J. H. Yoo, 2013, *Health Communication, 28* (3), pp. 294–303; *The Biggest Loser,* on NBC, www.nbc.com/the-biggest-loser/about/.

In Review

How is healthy body weight defined?
Overweight and obesity, defined respectively as body weight that exceeds or greatly exceeds the guidelines for good health, have been increasing in the United States. Healthy body weight can be defined as an acceptable body mass index (a measure of weight relative to height), an acceptable percentage of body fat, a pattern of body fat distribution that is not a risk factor for illness, or the absence of a medical condition that suggests a need for weight loss (e.g., diabetes or hypertension). People who don't meet these criteria could probably avoid some health problems by losing weight. Unexpected weight loss can be the sign of an illness.

What factors influence weight?
Influences on weight include genetic and hormonal factors (including the stress response), gender, age, and obesogenic environments and lifestyle (e.g., eating out, sedentary living, inadequate sleep, "yo-yo dieting").

What is the best way to manage body weight?
The key to weight control is balancing energy intake (calories) with energy output (physical activity and exercise).

Are there quick fixes for overweight and obesity?
Quick fixes such as fad diets usually don't work, and consumers who join weight management organizations often regain the weight they lose. Medical approaches, including surgery and prescription drugs, have potentially serious side effects, but they are available for people with serious health risks due to obesity. The size acceptance movement is an alternative that focuses on self-esteem.

How can individuals and society promote healthy weight throughout life?
The best approach for individuals is long-term, moderate lifestyle changes that include a balanced diet, daily physical activity, specific health-related goals, social support, and self-acceptance. Goals that are specific, measurable, attainable, realistic, and timely are key to long-term weight management. Behavior management strategies can also help. Communities can support healthy weight by promoting healthy foods, planning activity-friendly environments, supporting consumer awareness, and encouraging insurance coverage of obesity prevention programs.

Body Image

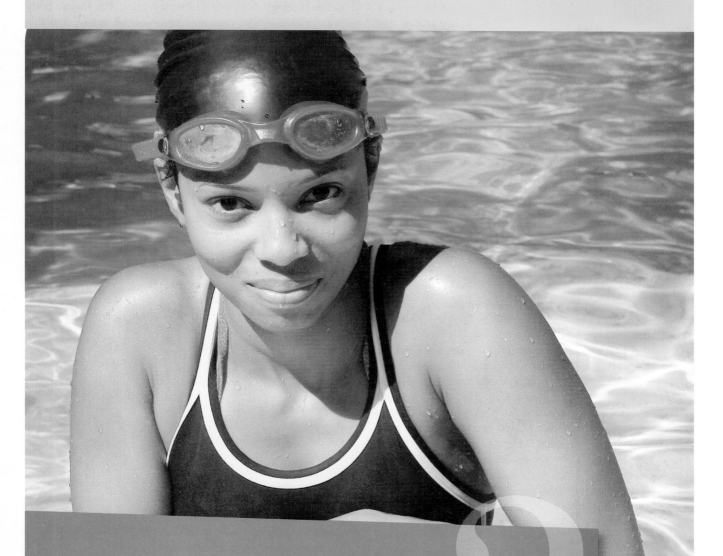

Ever Wonder. . .

- if men stress about their bodies as much as women do?
- how to know if your dieting crosses the line to an eating disorder?
- if you're ever going to change your mind about your tattoo, and what you can do about it?

re you satisfied with your body? If so, you are in the significant minority among college students. Ninety percent of women and 70 percent of men report body dissatisfaction![1] Why is this? How you evaluate your appearance usually reflects societal and cultural values and ideals conveyed by family, peers, language, advertising, and the media. Very often, cultural ideals are far removed from people's natural appearance, and for some, the discrepancy can produce feelings of inadequacy, dissatisfaction, and self-criticism. For others, it can lead to a resolve to reach the ideal, no matter how unrealistic the goal or unhealthy the means. And for a few, it leads to a quest for perfection that results in psychological illness.

Chapter 7 focused on the current problem of overweight and obesity, and we explored ways to achieve and maintain a healthy body weight and body composition. This chapter considers the other side of the coin—our society's obsession with thinness and dieting and the corresponding prevalence of disordered eating and eating disorders. The message about attaining a healthy body weight has to be balanced with a message about developing a healthy body image, setting realistic goals, and maintaining emotional well-being.

WHAT SHAPES BODY IMAGE?

Like all beliefs, **body image**—the mental representation that a person has of his or her own body, including perceptions, attitudes, thoughts, and emotions—is strongly influenced by culture. American culture places a premium on appearance, especially for women but increasingly for men. Every day we see hundreds of images and messages about how we should look and about the newest great diet, whether we are reading a magazine, seeing a movie, noticing ads in public places or on the Internet, or watching television in the privacy of our homes. The advertising industry and the media are relentless in selling the American consumer an image of the ideal body, and many of us buy into what they are selling. The message of the media is powerful. For some tips on critically evaluating media messages, see the box, "Media Literacy."

body image
Mental representation that a person has of his or her own body, including perceptions, attitudes, thoughts, and emotions.

Women and Body Image

For girls and women, beauty has long been held up as a desirable trait. Pioneering English feminist Mary Wollstonecraft pointed out back in 1792 that women would submit to anything to reach the ideal of beauty, even giving up the right to think for themselves. Repeated cycles of feminist thinking and activism over the past two centuries have attempted to change the message society sends to women and to free women from their obsession with the body.

Current Cultural Messages Today, women have more educational and occupational opportunities than ever before, and they fulfill a broad range of valued roles in society. Despite progress in women's rights, however, our culture still tells women that their most important job is to be beautiful. From infancy onward, when baby girls are described as "delicate," "soft," and "pretty," females are encouraged to define themselves in terms of their bodies. The female body is portrayed by the media as an object of desire, and this objectification reinforces women's focus on their appearance. The media place a heavy emphasis on women's physical attributes rather than on their abilities, performance, or accomplishments.

Since the 1950s, what is held to be the ideal female body in U.S. culture has been getting thinner. Actresses and beauty queens of the 1940s and 1950s had much more ample proportions, as exemplified by the curvaceous Marilyn Monroe. The 1960s brought a trend toward thin, boyish figures that persists to this day. Many girls and women aspire to the weight and shape of the super-thin fashion model. Unfortunately, the average fashion model is thinner than 98 percent of all American women. Models represent a tiny subset of the population but provide an unattainable goal for millions of women.[2]

It is not surprising, then, that women experience high levels of dissatisfaction with their bodies. Internalizing media messages about body image—whether in the form of magazines, television, gaming, or movies—creates a form of social comparison. Studies show that after women view media images of thin women, they are less satisfied with their own bodies than they are after viewing images of average-sized women.[1–6] The overwhelming number of unrealistic images can leave women feeling inadequate, preoccupied with a desire to be thin, unhappy with their own bodies, and afraid of becoming fat.

Belief in the thin ideal and body dissatisfaction can lead to dieting. This combination increases the risk for disordered eating behaviors,

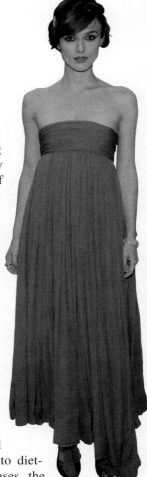

■ Standards of beauty change with the times. Kiera Knightly's waif-like proportions match today's thin ideal.

Consumer Clipboard

Media Literacy

Media images and advertisements for consumer products— from clothes to cosmetics to food to cars—are everywhere. These images and ads are a form of communication created by an industry with something to sell. They have been carefully crafted to convey values, reflect a point of view, and sell a product or an idea. They are designed to make you feel a certain way when you view them. What "reality" do the messages ask you to believe? How accurate is this reality? What message is being left out or goes untold? These are some of the important factors to consider in developing media literacy.

Once you become conscious of all the images around you and what they are designed to make you think and feel, you can gain control over whether you want to buy into the image or message being sold. To protect your self-esteem and body image, it's important to carefully filter media images and understand what the advertiser wants you to believe. Then decide if you want to believe the message.

Answer the following questions about the two advertisements in this box:

- What is the product or service being advertised?
- Who created the advertisement? Who paid for it? Who profits from it?
- What does the advertisement imply the product will do? What is its message?
- What persuasive techniques are being used? Commonly used persuasive techniques include symbols, flattery, perfection, fear, humor, power, and sex.
- Do you think the image has been altered or enhanced? Has it been edited, colored, airbrushed, lightened, or darkened? To what end?
- What values are being promoted? What meaning do they have for you? How might they mean something different to people of another age, race, ethnicity, or religion?
- What does the ad make you think or feel about yourself? Does it make you feel good about yourself, or does it make you feel inadequate and somehow lacking? The latter is an indicator that the message is designed to manipulate your feelings and induce you to buy the product.

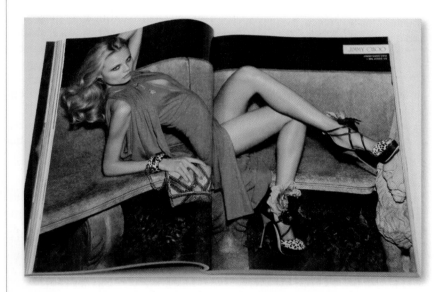 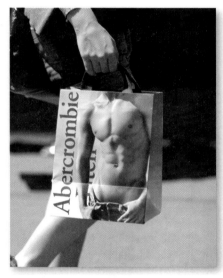

such as severe **calorie restriction** or getting rid of calories by **purging**. Disordered eating can progress further into an eating disorder. Eating disorders occur most often in cultures in which female attractiveness is linked with being thin, and frequent exposure to media messages about thinness can increase the risk for eating disorders. However, not all women develop eating disorders. Other factors to be considered are genetics, self-esteem, and cultural support.[5,7]

Effects of Puberty Eating disorders and many other mental health disorders are most likely to develop during adolescence. This is a time of transition and change— physically, emotionally and socially. As noted in Chapter 7,

hormonal changes cause increases in body fat in girls, especially on the hips, buttocks, and thighs. The percentage of body fat in healthy girls increases from about 12 percent to about 25 percent during puberty. Given the cultural emphasis on thinness, many girls become concerned about their bodies at this time.

However, girls are concerned with their body image even before puberty. By sixth grade, twice as many girls as boys consider themselves fat, even though they are not overweight by objective standards.

calorie restriction
A reduction in calorie intake below daily needs.

purging
Using self-induced vomiting, laxatives, or diuretics to get rid of excess calories that have been consumed.

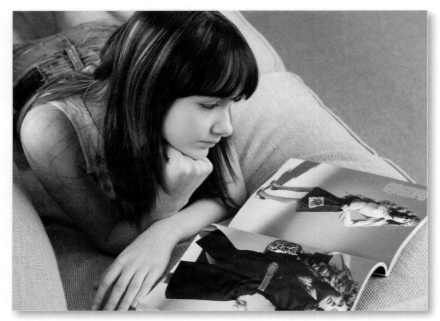

■ Girls get many of their ideas about what our society considers beautiful and desirable in a woman from the media, especially fashion magazines. Unrealistic hopes and dreams set some girls on a course toward disordered eating.

Sixth-grade girls are more likely to want to lose weight to become thin, whereas boys are more likely to want to gain weight, especially in the upper body, to become more muscular.[5]

Men and Body Image

Male body image has been less affected by cultural expectations and the media than female body image has. Historically, men have been judged more by achievement and strength than by looks. Media and advertising have tended to promote a masculine image that emphasizes power, performance, and choice for men, focusing on action and achievement rather than on appearance. Correspondingly, men are generally more satisfied with their body size and appearance than women are.

However, men are not immune to body image concerns. They are increasingly drawn into the world of beauty and appearance. Hair, skin, and grooming products directed toward men are making male use of beauty

products acceptable, although they are given a manly aura. Words like *musk, wood, spice,* and *surf* are used to describe scents, and product names are chosen to suggest power ("Brut," "The Baron").

The marketing of the male body image has also started to make a man's physique as important as his possessions and accomplishments. As with women, the ideal male body shape has become more unrealistic, distorted, and extreme. Men's magazines publish more advertisements and articles about how to change body shape than about weight loss. Men are increasingly displayed as sexual objects.

Today's male models have trimmer waists and bulkier biceps than in the past. The evolution of G.I. Joe action figures mirrors society's changing male image. In 1964 G.I. Joe had the physique of an average man in reasonably good shape. By 1992 he had a build that most men could not attain without the use of anabolic steroids. The exposure to muscular male images leads men to feel worse about their bodies and to have increased feelings of depression. The response appears to be strongest among college-aged men.[1,2,8,9]

For some men, this unrealistic message about supersized bodies can lead to a condition known as **muscle dysmorphia**

■ The marketing of the male body image has made physique an increasingly important part of male attractiveness in our society. Boys and men are coming under pressure to attain the kind of muscle development seen in actors and athletes like David Beckham.

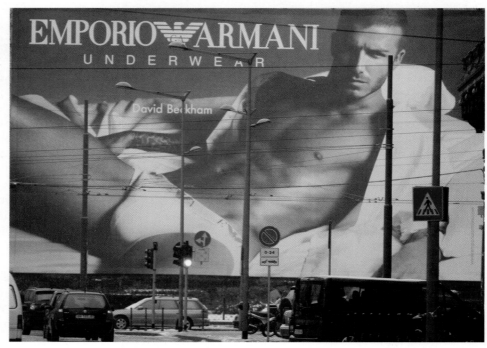

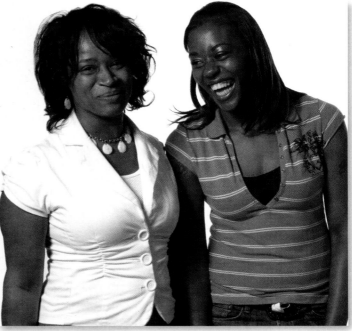

(a disorder in which one's muscles are perceived as too small regardless of their size; sometimes referred to as "bigorexia"). Men with this condition perceive themselves as being insufficiently massive or muscular in appearance, no matter how bulked up they really are. (Muscle dysmorphia is discussed in more detail later in this chapter.) Some observers suggest that supermuscularity may be one way men believe they can distinguish themselves in a world of increasing gender equality.[10]

About 10 percent of eating disorders are diagnosed in men. However, recent studies show more men reporting patterns of disordered eating (such as binge eating or self-induced vomiting) as well as anorexia nervosa and bulimia nervosa, accounting for nearly one in four cases.[11,12] As men buy into the cultural quest for physical perfection and pursue unrealistic goals, they may have increasing feelings of inadequacy and body dissatisfaction. This may lead to further increases in dieting and body-building. Men appear to report dieting for different reasons than those of women. Men are shape oriented rather than weight oriented; they focus on the upper body rather than the lower body; and they usually diet for a specific reason, such as sports performance.

Much speculation exists about why eating disorders occur less often among men. Perhaps the earlier societal focus on male accomplishments rather than physique is protective. However, eating disorders among men may also have been underdiagnosed because they have been considered a female problem. Until 2013, the criteria for diagnosing anorexia nervosa included the cessation of menstrual periods. Obviously, this excluded men from the diagnosis. With the increasing recognition of disordered eating among men, the criteria have changed to more accurately include all affected people.[13] Another factor thought to be important in the lack of recognition of eating disorders among men is that it remains

■ African American women are more likely than White, Asian, and Latina women to be satisfied with their bodies and less likely to experience eating disorders.

a social taboo for men to publicly discuss anxiety about their bodies. Thus, men are secretive about their body dissatisfaction and their drive to bulk up.[12]

Ethnicity and Body Image

Body satisfaction is also affected by one's ethnicity or cultural group. Historically, White women have been reported as experiencing greater body dissatisfaction and eating disturbance than women in other ethnic groups. Ethnic minorities were believed to have less cultural pressure to be thin. However, among women, differences between some ethnic groups regarding fear of fatness, body dissatisfaction, dieting, and pressure to be thin appear to be decreasing. White, Asian, and Hispanic women report similar concerns. A greater degree of acculturation to mainstream culture is associated with higher levels of body dissatisfaction among Mexican American and Cuban American women. Black women, however, continue to report higher body satisfaction and higher self-esteem than White women.[14–16]

Among men, Blacks report a greater preference for larger body size and more positive body image than Whites. Hispanics' body satisfaction level is similar to Whites but may be affected by degree of acculturation. Native American men report slightly greater body image concerns than White men. Among Asian men, findings have been inconsistent, perhaps because of the range of cultural groups considered "Asian." Interestingly, when non-White males engage in disordered patterns, they appear to engage in more extreme weight loss strategies and binge eating than do White males. As patterns of disordered eating change, education and treatment programs

muscle dysmorphia Disorder in which a person perceives his body to be underdeveloped no matter how highly developed his muscles really are.

will also have to change to respond to the needs, perceptions, and values of diverse ethnic and cultural groups.[17,18]

Sports and Body Image

Participation in sports confers many health and fitness benefits, including higher levels of self-esteem in both boys and girls. Sports may provide protection against eating disorders by promoting a focus on performance rather than on appearance. However, participation in sports also carries pressure both from oneself and from coaches, teammates, and parents. High-level athletes often succeed because they have high expectations of themselves, accompanied by varying degrees of perfectionism and compulsiveness. Athletes often learn to disregard signals from their bodies, including pain, during training. Parents and coaches can directly and indirectly encourage disordered eating by commenting on appearance or performance when an athlete has lost weight. They can also indirectly foster disordered eating by not recognizing patterns of rapid weight loss.

Certain types of sports have higher rates of disordered eating or eating disorders among athletes. This is especially true of some high-intensity sports in which leanness is a competitive advantage, such as wrestling, dance, gymnastics, swimming, cycling, distance running, and horse racing. The risk for eating disorders appears to be greatest for athletes competing at elite levels, such as college teams. Women who compete in nonelite sports that do not emphasize leanness have the least risk of developing eating disorders.[19]

DISORDERED EATING AND EATING DISORDERS

Disordered eating behaviors include restrictive dieting, skipping meals, binge eating and purging, laxative abuse, and other behaviors that are unhealthy but not severe enough to reach the level of an eating disorder. These behaviors may occur in response to emotional stress, an upcoming athletic event, concern about personal appearance, a new diet recommendation, or any of innumerable other stressors. Disordered eating behaviors may or may not develop into a full-blown eating disorder. The rates of disordered eating are higher in college populations than in the general population, with studies showing 50 to 60 percent of college women and 10 percent of college men reporting disordered eating.[20]

Eating disorders are chronic illnesses that jeopardize physical and mental health; they can be life threatening. The key characteristic of eating disorders is a severe disturbance in eating behavior. A second characteristic is a distorted body image and often associated low self-esteem. What begins as a diet turns into self-induced starvation or repeated cycles of binge eating and purging. The frequency of eating disorders appears to be directly related to rates of dieting, although of course not all people who diet have eating disorders.

Anorexia nervosa, bulimia nervosa, and binge eating disorder are classified as psychiatric disorders in the American Psychiatric Association's *Diagnostic and Statistical Manual of Mental Disorders* (DSM-5). Using the strict criteria proposed by the DSM-5, about 0.4 percent of women have anorexia and 1.0 to 1.5 percent of women have bulimia; the rate in men is about 10 percent of that in women. There is less gender difference in binge eating disorder with an estimated 1.6 percent of women and 0.8 percent of men suffering from it.[13] In the past 30 years, the number of diagnosed cases of eating disorders in the United States has doubled.

Eating disorders occur primarily among people in Western industrialized countries. They occur in every ethnic, cultural, and socioeconomic group. They appear to become more prevalent when food is abundant and has taken on symbolic meanings, such as comfort, love, belonging, fun, and control. They are also more common where being attractive is related to being thin.

Contributing Factors

Many factors contribute to the development of disordered eating and eating disorders, and much about the process remains unknown. Why the widespread cultural ideals and beliefs promoting thinness and dieting for women and extreme muscularity for men become an overvalued, ruling passion for some is not totally clear. Exposure to the thin ideal, social pressure to conform, and recognition of a discrepancy between the ideal and one's own body can certainly lead to body dissatisfaction and have been shown to increase risk for eating disorders. However, this can't be the entire story, because the social pressures to be thin (or muscular) are pervasive and spreading globally and yet only a fraction of women and men go on to develop eating disorders. Other factors play a role (see the box, "Eating Disorders"). Eating disorders and other associated traits run in families. A family history of eating disorders, depression, substance abuse, anxiety, obsessive-compulsive disorder, or obesity increases the risk for anorexia and bulimia. Most likely, genes predispose an individual, and then certain experiences or characteristics further contribute to the development of eating disorders.[5,7,21]

Gender is clearly a risk factor for eating disorders, with female gender increasing risk. Sexual orientation may alter risk for males, with gay and bisexual men at greater risk than heterosexual men. Gay and bisexual men report higher rates of body dissatisfaction and disordered eating. They aim to attract men and thus may be subject to the same pressures as heterosexual women. They may place greater value on physical appearance than do heterosexual men. Lesbians

disordered eating behaviors Abnormal eating patterns (e.g., vomiting, use of laxatives, extreme dieting) that may not fit the rigid diagnostic rules for anorexia or bulimia but affect quality of life.

eating disorders Conditions characterized by severely disturbed eating behaviors and distorted body image; eating disorders jeopardize physical and psychological health.

Who's at Risk?

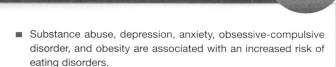

Eating Disorders

No one seems to be immune to eating disorders. They affect women and men; they affect people of all different ages, races, ethnicities, and backgrounds; they affect people who grew up with loving families and those who had difficult childhoods. Still, a few trends can be observed.

- Eating disorders are most common during the teens and early 20s.

- Eating disorders are more likely to occur during life transitions because they can trigger emotional stress and a sense of loss of control.

- Although the incidence is increasing among men, especially gay men, eating disorders remain more common in heterosexual women and lesbians.

- Substance abuse, depression, anxiety, obsessive-compulsive disorder, and obesity are associated with an increased risk of eating disorders.

- Frequent dieting is associated with the onset of eating disorders.

- Overly controlling or critical family relationships can increase the risk for eating disorders.

- Frequent exposure to media messages promoting a thin body size and shape can increase the risk for eating disorders.

- Sports that emphasize thin body type or weight restrictions may increase the risk for eating disorders.

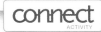

---

appear to have the same rates of eating disorders as heterosexual women.[22–24]

The connection between eating disorders and depression and anxiety disorders is complicated. People with anorexia and bulimia frequently report symptoms of depression and anxiety. A history of depression appears to increase risk for eating disorders, but it can be difficult to diagnose depression in a person with anorexia because the starvation process produces similar symptoms, including changes in sleep patterns, a decline in energy level, and decreased interest in activities.

Certain characteristics or thought patterns are associated with eating disorders, including the following:

- Low self-esteem.
- Self-critical attitude.

- Belief in the importance of thinness.
- Black-and-white thinking.
- Feelings of emptiness.
- Need for power and control.
- Difficulty expressing feelings.
- Lack of coping skills.
- Lack of trust in self or others.
- Perfectionism.

Not all of these patterns must be present, and many of these are found in people with anxiety disorders or depression but not eating disorders. Factors thought to increase risk for eating disorders are shown in Figure 8.1.

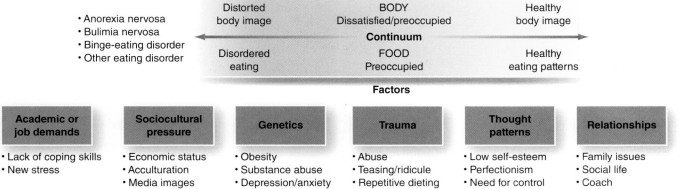

figure 8.1   Eating disorder continuum and factors contributing to eating disorders.
Body image and eating patterns fall along a continuum. Multiple factors interact and contribute to movement along the continuum and eventual development of eating disorders.

Diagnosing Eating Disorders

As recently as the 1980s the terms *anorexia nervosa* and *bulimia nervosa* were unknown to the general public. Today, many people are familiar with the concept of disturbed eating patterns. Detecting when someone with disordered eating makes the transition to having an eating disorder is difficult, however. Guidelines have been developed, but disordered eating and eating disorders occur on a continuum, as shown in Figure 8.1. In this section, we review the most common eating disorders and their diagnostic criteria.

anorexia nervosa
Eating disorder marked by distortion of body image and refusal to maintain a minimally normal body weight.

bulimia nervosa
Eating disorder marked by distortion of body image and repeated episodes of binge eating, usually followed by purging in the form of self-induced vomiting, misuse of diuretics or laxatives, excessive exercising, or fasting.

binge-eating disorder
Eating disorder marked by binge-eating behavior without the vomiting or purging of bulimia.

Anorexia Nervosa The word *anorexia* is of Greek origin: *an,* which means "lack of," and *orexis,* which means "appetite." However, most people with **anorexia nervosa** do not have a lack of appetite; they are more likely to be obsessed with food. At the same time, they are starving themselves and appear ultrathin or emaciated.

Criteria for anorexia nervosa are as follows:[13]

■ Restriction of energy intake relative to requirements leading to significantly low body weight, which is defined as weight that is less than minimally normal (generally, BMI < 18.5).

■ Intense fear of gaining weight or becoming fat even though significantly underweight or engaging in persistent behavior that interferes with weight gain.

■ Disturbance in the way in which one's body weight or shape is experienced, undue influence of body weight or shape on self-evaluation, or persistent lack of recognition of the seriousness of the current low body weight.

People with anorexia control their weight by severely restricting calories or excessively exercising. To get a sense of how anorexia plays out in a person's life, see the box, "Alexis: The Gradual Onset of an Eating Disorder."

Bulimia Nervosa The word *bulimia* is of Latin origin and means "hunger of an ox." People with **bulimia nervosa** consume a huge amount of food at one sitting and then use an inappropriate method to get rid of the calories they have consumed, either by purging or through excessive exercise. People with bulimia are usually neither underweight nor overweight, but they have a disturbed perception of body size and image. Binge-eating and purging behaviors are usually socially isolating.

Criteria for bulimia nervosa are as follows:[13]

■ Recurrent episodes of binge eating, characterized by both (1) eating, in a discrete period of time (e.g., 2 hours), an amount of food that is definitely larger than most people would eat in that period of time and (2) a sense of lack of control during the episode—a feeling of being unable to stop eating or control what or how much one is eating.

■ Recurrent inappropriate compensatory behavior to prevent weight gain, such as self-induced vomiting; misuse of laxatives, diuretics, or other medications; fasting; or excessive exercise.

■ The episodes occur, on average, at least once a week for three months.

■ Self-evaluation is unduly influenced by body shape and weight.

Binge-Eating Disorder Disordered eating patterns can also cause obesity. **Binge-eating disorder** has increasingly been recognized as a psychological disturbance that is associated with weight fluctuation and obesity. This disorder involves binge-eating behaviors without vomiting or purging.[13]

People with binge-eating disorder can be normal weight or overweight, but if the disorder goes unrecognized, they often eventually become obese. They have body weight and shape concerns, emotional distress (possibly including depression), and disordered eating patterns similar to those of people with anorexia or bulimia.[13,25]

Criteria for binge-eating disorder are as follows:[13]

■ Recurrent episodes of binge eating, as defined for bulimia.

■ The episodes are associated with (1) eating much more rapidly than usual; (2) eating to the point of feeling uncomfortably full; (3) eating large amounts of food when not feeling physically hungry; (4) eating alone because of being embarrassed by how much one is eating; and (5) feeling disgusted with oneself, depressed, or guilty about overeating.

■ Marked distress about binge eating.

■ Paula Abdul suffered from bulimia in high school. Today, she is the spokesperson for the National Eating Disorders Association.

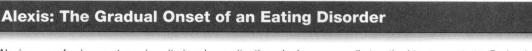
Alexis: The Gradual Onset of an Eating Disorder

Alexis was a freshman at a university in a large city, though she had grown up in a small town in the same state. When she first arrived on campus, she was assigned to a dorm room with Leah, a student from out of state. Leah was tall and thin and made friends easily, and she quickly became popular in the residence hall. Alexis was introverted and not used to making friends quickly. Most of the people she knew at school were friends from her hometown, people she had known her entire life. She began to avoid the room because she felt self-conscious about her lack of friends.

Classes were also harder than she had expected, and she began to question her ability to succeed. She wanted to talk to her parents, but they had always told her how much fun college was going to be, and she feared they would not understand why she was struggling.

Alexis had never been overweight, but she had never really been happy with her body either. She often compared herself to slim, svelte Leah and concluded that if she lost weight, it might be easier to fit in. She decided she would start eating a healthier diet by cutting out saturated fat, which meant most meat and dairy products. This made it hard to eat in the dining hall, so she started eating foods that she could prepare herself in her room. She tried to be in the room as little as possible to avoid Leah, so she ended up eating only twice a day, in the morning and at night. She also started walking a lot around campus. She found that she felt better if she could keep moving, and pretty soon she was walking several hours a day. When she tried to sit and study, she was usually too tired to concentrate. During lectures, her mind would wander to how much she had eaten the day before and when she could eat today.

Alexis did not think she had lost much weight, but when she went home for winter break, her parents were shocked to see her. When they asked her about it, she denied intentionally trying to lose weight and said she was just trying to be healthier. They took her to see the family doctor, who observed that Alexis's weight and BMI had plummeted. The doctor was concerned by her weight loss as well as by her lack of insight into her condition and appearance. Alexis wanted to return to school, but her parents were reluctant to allow it. Her doctor and parents finally agreed to let her go back on the condition that she see a nutritionist at the student health center who could monitor her weight while she worked to get it back into a healthy range. They also wanted her to see a counselor to address the emotional and interpersonal issues that were affecting her self-esteem and body image. Reluctantly, she agreed.

- How has your transition to college been going? Are you outgoing like Leah and make friends easily, or are you more introverted like Alexis and find it more challenging? What do you think about these different styles of interacting with others?

- Are there any foods that you have eliminated from your diet? If so, why? Are these changes in your diet truly making you healthier, or do they limit your calorie intake or nutrient intake to an unhealthy degree?

connect ACTIVITY

- The binge eating occurs, on average, at least once a week for three months.

- The binge eating is not associated with the regular use of inappropriate compensatory behaviors (purging, fasting, excessive exercise) and does not occur exclusively during the course of anorexia or bulimia.

Health Consequences of Eating Disorders

Eating disorders have serious health implications. Some short-term problems, such as heart rate abnormalities, can lead to death. Long-term problems can cause significant disability. Although anorexia and bulimia often overlap, they are associated with slightly different medical problems.

Health Effects of Anorexia Anorexia nervosa carries the highest death rate of all psychiatric diagnoses and all eating disorders.[26] Death is usually due to cardiac arrest, electrolyte imbalance, or suicide. The signs and symptoms of anorexia are due to starvation and are shown in Figure 8.2. Most of the complications are reversible if the person receives enough calorie replacement. However, some complications—most notably, bone loss—do not appear to be reversible. Decreased bone calcium (osteoporosis) is one of the most serious long-term effects of severe calorie restriction. Peak bone density is reached during the adolescent years. After that it remains relatively stable until the middle 30s, when it starts a slow decline. Children and adolescents with anorexia do not reach the same peak bone density as those without the disease and thus have a lifelong increased risk of bone fracture.[27]

Health Effects of Bulimia Bulimia is associated more with electrolyte imbalance than with starvation. Electrolytes, such as sodium, potassium, calcium, phosphate, and magnesium, are essential components of body fluids and required for cell function. The body attempts to maintain the correct amount in different areas. Repetitive vomiting causes the loss of certain electrolytes—in particular, potassium—and makes it difficult for the body to maintain electrolyte balance. Bulimia can also be deadly due to low potassium because heart cells and the cardiac electrical conduction system can malfunction and lead to cardiac arrest. The signs and symptoms of bulimia are shown in Figure 8.3.

Health Effects of Binge-Eating Disorder The health consequences of binge-eating disorder are related primarily to obesity. As discussed in Chapter 7, obesity is a

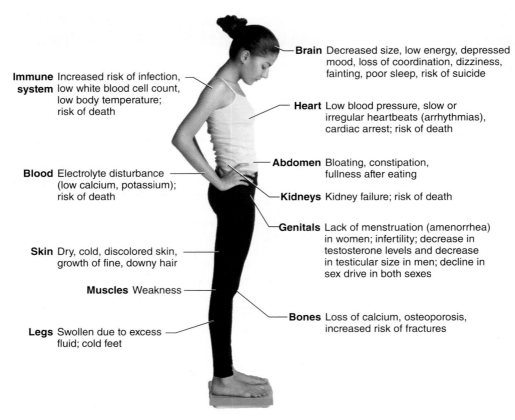

Immune system Increased risk of infection, low white blood cell count, low body temperature; risk of death

Blood Electrolyte disturbance (low calcium, potassium); risk of death

Skin Dry, cold, discolored skin, growth of fine, downy hair

Muscles Weakness

Legs Swollen due to excess fluid; cold feet

Brain Decreased size, low energy, depressed mood, loss of coordination, dizziness, fainting, poor sleep, risk of suicide

Heart Low blood pressure, slow or irregular heartbeats (arrhythmias), cardiac arrest; risk of death

Abdomen Bloating, constipation, fullness after eating

Kidneys Kidney failure; risk of death

Genitals Lack of menstruation (amenorrhea) in women; infertility; decrease in testosterone levels and decrease in testicular size in men; decline in sex drive in both sexes

Bones Loss of calcium, osteoporosis, increased risk of fractures

figure 8.2 **Anorexia can cause changes throughout the body.**
Not all of these will be present in all people with the disease.

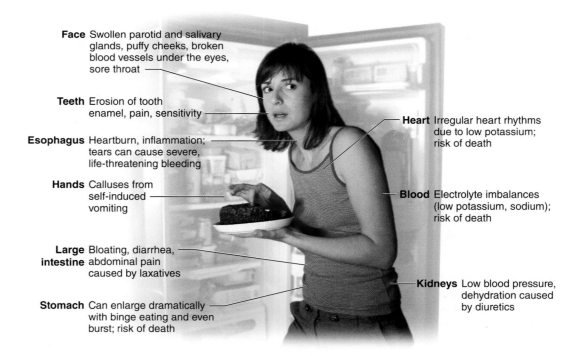

Face Swollen parotid and salivary glands, puffy cheeks, broken blood vessels under the eyes, sore throat

Teeth Erosion of tooth enamel, pain, sensitivity

Esophagus Heartburn, inflammation; tears can cause severe, life-threatening bleeding

Hands Calluses from self-induced vomiting

Large intestine Bloating, diarrhea, abdominal pain caused by laxatives

Stomach Can enlarge dramatically with binge eating and even burst; risk of death

Heart Irregular heart rhythms due to low potassium; risk of death

Blood Electrolyte imbalances (low potassium, sodium); risk of death

Kidneys Low blood pressure, dehydration caused by diuretics

figure 8.3 **Bulimia can cause changes throughout the body.**
Not all of these will be present in all people with the disease.

Starting the Conversation

Social Media and Health Apps

Q: Have you downloaded an app to assist you in monitoring calories, daily weight, and physical activity? Is it helpful or harmful?

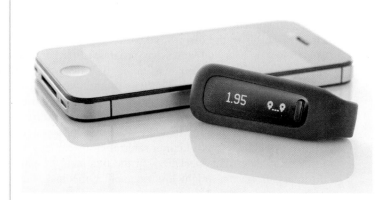

Your new health app gives you points for entering daily weights, keeps accurate calorie counts for each meal, and monitors your physical activity level. You open your Facebook account, and in your news feed, an article pops up called "Five Foods Never to Eat." Social media is the new advertising front focusing on raising awareness about health and energy balance. However, much of the language may promote unhealthy thinking about food. When does calorie counting cross the line between healthy focus on energy equations to an obsession or an unhealthy task? We are in conflict as a society. We have rising rates of obesity and an increasing need for people to maintain energy balance, and yet we have unhealthy relationships with food and the potential for disordered eating. The constant messaging and positive reinforcement for weight loss and calorie counting may be detrimental to some of the population.

FitBit, MyFitnessPal, Livestrong, and DailyBurn are just a few of the applications available for download. Each is designed to assist in daily monitoring of activity, calorie intake, and weight. The goal is to motivate behavior change by raising awareness and educating people. However, meticulous daily calorie counting can become an obsession and move people further away from "intuitive eating"—listening to the body's cues and learning to recognize when one is hungry. Advertisements of forbidden foods promote food being seen as good or bad; reward or punishment. With intuitive eating, the goal is to learn how to actually listen to your body and eat when the body is in need of energy. This counters the primary triggers for much eating—such as boredom, stress, sadness, celebration, or other sources of emotional eating. Social media and apps that focus on counting calories, measuring activity level, weight, and forbidden categories of food may create added stress and distraction. How do these factors influence your life?

Q: What social media tools do you use to track nutrition and physical activity?

Q: When is tracking calories unhealthy? How do you decide?

---

degenerative chronic health condition that often significantly shortens the lifespan. Diseases associated with overweight and obesity include cardiorespiratory disease, diabetes, high blood pressure, gallbladder disease, osteoarthritis, sleep apnea, and certain cancers.

Treating Eating Disorders

Aside from osteoporosis, most medical conditions associated with anorexia and bulimia are reversible. Keys to recovery appear to be early intervention, lower incidence of purging behavior, the support and participation of family members and loved ones, and lack of other diagnosed psychological problems. Nearly 80 percent of people with anorexia or bulimia achieve full or partial recovery with treatment, while approximately 20 percent go on to have a more protracted course of illness.[28,29] A person is considered to have recovered when weight is restored to within 15 percent of recommended weight and eating patterns normalize. The earlier you recognize an eating disorder, the more successful treatment will be.

Recognizing the Problem The first step toward treatment is the recognition that there is a problem. People with eating disorders often deny that they are ill and refuse treatment. At the heart of many eating disorders is a desire to have a sense of control over one's life, and treatment involves both weight gain and a perceived loss of this control. Health care providers may face the dilemma of wanting to respect a patient's autonomy and wishes and at the same time wanting to provide effective treatment for a potentially life-threatening illness.

Friends, roommates, parents, and others who are close to those with eating disorders may also deny that there is a problem or fail to recognize it because dieting, exercise, and preoccupation with food are so much an accepted part of our culture. The box, "Social Media and Health Apps," looks at the fine line between monitoring and obsessing about your diet and exercise regimen. Treatment is most effective when the patient and family members all recognize the problem and are involved in treatment decisions.

Action Skill-Builder

Take Action to Prevent Eating Disorders

Disordered eating and eating disorders are associated with the internalization of society's idealizations of thinness. Low self-esteem and a distorted self-image can start you down the road of unhealthy habits. Do you ever have disordered eating habits? Do you or your friends talk negatively about yourselves or others? If you are concerned about slipping into disordered eating, or even if you maintain a positive perspective on your body, try taking these actions as early steps.

☐ Avoid skipping meals or restricting types of foods. Regular meals facilitate healthier nutrition. Notice if you are starting to alter your eating patterns, and think about why.

☐ Exercise for fitness, not to compensate for eating too much or to punish yourself. Exercise is good for you, but if you sense that it is becoming a compulsion, it may no longer be healthy. Find ways to exercise that you enjoy.

☐ Avoid sudden weight loss or gain in a short period of time. Healthy weight loss or gain is gradual—1 to 2 pounds per week. Sudden loss or gain may be a sign that you are not using healthy methods to manage your weight.

☐ Use positive language about what your body can do for you. Do you find yourself or friends talking about "being fat" or not liking the look of a body part? Try to be aware of the language you use when you talk about your body. Focus on what your body does for you rather than on how it looks. Try going a week without making any critical remarks about your body—or anyone else's.

☐ Recognize discrepancies between real bodies and the images of bodies in the media. When you see the human body represented in ads, television, and other media, step back and contrast it with your life experience.

☐ Give yourself a break! Do you find yourself focusing on areas you consider your weaknesses? Try focusing on your strengths instead. Think of "weaknesses" as "areas for growth." Even here, distinguish between what is within your control and what isn't. For things within your control, think about small steps you can take. For things not in your control, keep a sense of perspective or try to let go of them as best you can. Remember that no one is perfect and that differences among people are what make life interesting.

because, as with any habit, the more firmly entrenched disordered eating patterns become, the more difficult it is to reestablish healthy eating patterns.[30]

Local campus resources may be sufficient to address unhealthy thought patterns, identify sources of stress, and teach healthier coping mechanisms. For some suggestions, see the box, "Take Action to Prevent Eating Disorders." Many campuses have a health center, counseling facilities, food and nutritional services, recreational facilities, and student groups that may be of sufficient help in an early phase on the disordered eating continuum.

However, if an individual has progressed farther along the continuum to a full-blown eating disorder, treatment often involves a multidisciplinary or multimodality team. This group of health care providers with different expertise—physician, psychiatrist, psychologist, social worker, nutritionist, nurses—work together to address all areas of a patient's health. Sometimes this requires referral from campus services to a center that specializes in the treatment of eating disorders. If severe weight loss or another medical abnormality has occurred, hospitalization may be required while adequate nutrition is restored. While patients are in a physical crisis, they may find it hard to work on long-term change.

Once weight is stabilized, the second phase of treatment—including psychotherapy, behavioral relearning and modification, and nutritional rehabilitation and education—can be initiated. Because eating disorders are psychiatric illnesses, the most important part of treatment (aside from weight gain for severely anorexic patients) is psychotherapy. A goal of treatment is to teach the person to recognize self-destructive patterns of behavior and to develop better coping skills. Therapy focuses on learning how to maintain a positive body image, high self-esteem, and healthy eating patterns for life. Nutritional education includes information about healthy eating patterns, normal weight, and nutritional needs. Treatment for eating disorders often involves the entire family.

In some cases, medications, particularly antidepressants, may be used as a component of treatment. During the weight gain phases of anorexia treatment, antidepressants do not appear to be beneficial, but they do seem to be somewhat helpful in reducing relapses during the weight maintenance phase. In the treatment of bulimia, the use of antidepressants leads to a rapid decrease in the binge-purge cycle.[31] Treatment for binge-eating disorder may differ from other obesity treatment programs; emphasizing patterns of eating and putting less emphasis on dieting can be important.

BODY DYSMORPHIC DISORDER

Many of us look at our bodies and see things we'd like to change. For an estimated 1 to 2 percent of the general population (and 2 to 13 percent of college students), however, the pattern of seeing faults becomes an obsession that significantly interferes with their lives.[32,33] A key feature of **body dysmorphic disorder** is a preoccupation with a

body dysmorphic disorder
Preoccupation with an imagined or exaggerated defect in appearance.

Components of Treatment
Ideally, a pattern of food obsession or body image preoccupation can be detected by the individual or by friends and family at an early point. When identified early, restricting or binge-purge patterns of eating are not as firmly established. This is key

defect in appearance. The preoccupation can be about a wholly imagined defect or exaggerated concern about a slight defect.

Criteria for body dysmorphic disorder are as follows:[13]

- One or more perceived defects or flaws in physical appearance that are not observable or appear slight to others.

- Repetitive behaviors (mirror checking, excessive grooming, skin picking) or mental acts (comparing with others) in response to appearance concerns.

- The preoccupation causes significant distress or impairment in social, occupational, or other important areas of functioning.

- The preoccupation is not better accounted for by another mental disorder (such as anorexia).

The perceived fault can be any part of the body. For men, the preoccupation tends to be about the genitals, muscle mass, and hair. For women, it tends to be about breasts, thighs, and legs. Concern about the perceived defect can lead to low self-esteem, social isolation, and impairment of daily life.[30]

Muscle Dysmorphia

In the discussion of body image, we mentioned muscle dysmorphia, which is a subcategory of body dysmorphic disorder. This condition occurs predominantly in men who are focused on increasing muscle size.[10,13] These men are ashamed of their bodies and obsessed with working out with weights to develop muscular strength and bulk. They may avoid social contact because they believe other people are contemptuous of their bodies. They may also become isolated because of the time demands of maintaining a meticulous diet and excessive workout schedule.

If they turn to anabolic steroids to increase muscle size, they run mental and physical health risks. Side effects of steroids include extreme mood swings, aggression, impaired judgment, acne, shrinking of the testicles, liver damage, and increases in blood pressure.[32,34]

It is unclear why some people develop muscle dysmorphia. The condition may be related to obsessive-compulsive disorder, which is marked by recurring thoughts that people can't get out of their heads. The disorder may originate in childhood experiences that undermine self-esteem, such as taunting by peers, and it may be aggravated by media images that glorify bulging muscles and present them as a realistic goal. Still, most men who are exposed to these experiences and images do not develop muscle dysmorphia.

Cosmetic Surgery

Some people with body dysmorphic disorder turn to cosmetic surgery to correct the supposed flaw in their appearance. However, not everyone who turns to cosmetic surgery

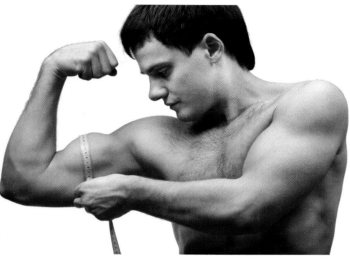

- Like eating disorders, muscle dysmorphia involves a distorted body image and compulsive behaviors. People with this disorder exercise to feel in control and to manage uncomfortable emotions rather than to improve their fitness and health.

has this disorder. In fact, cosmetic surgery and makeovers of every kind have become commonplace in the past few decades. The increase is most likely related to the ever-growing emphasis on appearance. By definition, cosmetic surgery is elective; it is not done to treat a medical condition.

In the United States, more than 10 million cosmetic procedures were performed in 2012, at a cost of nearly $11 billion. Women have the majority of procedures, but rates have increased for men. The most common cosmetic surgical procedures in 2012 were breast augmentation, liposuction, tummy tucks, eyelid surgery, and nose reshaping. The most commonly performed nonsurgical procedures were Botox injections (for wrinkles), skin fillers (such as for lip enlargement), hair removal, and skin resurfacing.[35]

As with any surgery or medical procedure, there are risks. A key risk is psychological: if a person is unhappy with her appearance because she has a distorted body image or is comparing herself to an unrealistic ideal, it is unlikely that a single operation is going to make her significantly happier. There are also physical risks, both at the time of surgery (e.g., reactions to anesthesia, blood loss, infection) and later (e.g., reactions to the silicone in breast implants).

Cosmetic surgery can also have psychological and physical benefits. Some people are happy with the results of cosmetic surgery. Some become more confident about their appearance and more successful socially or professionally. Surgeries such as otoplasty (cosmetic ear surgery) and rhinoplasty (nose reshaping) can change a physical characteristic that has caused a person emotional distress for years; breast reduction can enable a woman to feel less self-conscious about her appearance or engage in sports or activities that were previously uncomfortable.

Body Art

Some people choose to use body art to express themselves and present a certain image. Like other forms of self-expression, body art is closely tied to an individual's sense of self. The tattoos, eyebrow rings, and nose piercing you see on campus may seem like a recent trend, but their roots go far back in history. Many cultures have used piercing or tattoos to mark tribal origin or status. Ancient Egyptians used navel piercing as a sign of royalty. Crusaders in the Middle Ages were tattooed with crosses so that they would be given a Christian burial.

In the United States, approximately one in three 18- to 25-year-olds and one in two 26- to 40-year-olds report having a tattoo. Rates among men and women are now about even. Most tattoos are obtained by people aged 16 to 23; reasons for getting them include expressing individuality or independence, conforming to fashion or flouting fashion, saying something about a significant life experience, and just wanting to look good.

Among those with a tattoo, about one in five is dissatisfied with his or her tattoo and 6 percent seek removal—about twice as many women as men seek removal. The most common reasons for wanting a tattoo removed are embarrassment, negative comments from others, difficulty covering the tattoo with clothing, and decreased need to feel unique.[36,37]

Permanent tattooing involves making a puncture wound in the skin and injecting ink deep into the second layer of skin (called the dermis) to make the tattoo long-lasting. There is some pain, minor bleeding, and possible risk of infection. Some people may also develop an allergic reaction to the dye. If a decision is made to remove the tattoo at a later date, it can be done with laser treatment, but the process is painful, time-consuming, and expensive, and it can leave scars.[37]

Body piercing involves some of the same risks as tattooing. Certain body sites are more likely than others to result in problems. Piercing of the mouth and nose is often associated with infection, and tongue piercing can damage teeth. The longer a piercing is left in place, the more likely it is that scarring or a residual opening will occur should the jewelry be removed.

Tattoos and piercing should be approached with caution and considered permanent alterations of the body. If you decide to proceed with either, give yourself a waiting period to make sure that the location, design, and type of tattoo or piercing are what you really want. Consider how it will look 5, 10, or 20 years from now and how you might feel about it in a different phase of your life.

female athlete triad Interrelated conditions of disordered eating, amenorrhea, and osteoporosis.

activity disorder Excessive or addictive exercising, undertaken to address psychological needs rather than to improve fitness.

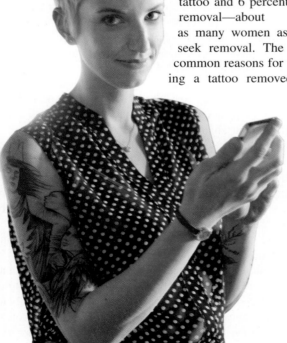

■ Tattoos and piercings are a popular form of self-expression. Over time, however, social norms around body art may shift, leaving some with regrets about these relatively permanent alterations.

EXERCISE DISORDERS

Like eating disorders, exercise disorders are on the rise, and researchers are beginning to look into exercise patterns that may be abnormal. Such patterns may exist in conjunction with eating disorders or by themselves.[13]

Female Athlete Triad

Female athletes are susceptible to a condition called the **female athlete triad**, a set of three interrelated conditions: disordered eating patterns (often accompanied by excessive exercising), amenorrhea (cessation of menstruation), and premature osteoporosis (reduced bone density). The triad often begins when a female athlete engages in unhealthy eating patterns (restrictive or purging) and excessive exercise to lose weight or to attain a lean body appearance to fit a specific athletic image or improve performance. This then may lead to amenorrhea due to alterations in hormone levels (low estrogen and progesterone). Low estrogen leads to reduced calcium absorption and bone thinning.

This disorder overlaps with anorexia and bulimia, and risk factors are similar. Often, a first sign of a problem is a decrease in performance, a muscle injury, or an exercise-related stress fracture. Amenorrhea is another important sign. Female athletes need to understand the importance of good eating habits and moderation in exercise and recognize the patterns and dangers of eating disorders.

Activity Disorder

People with **activity disorder** control their bodies or alter their moods by being overly involved in exercise or addicted to exercise. People who are addicted to exercise continue to exercise strenuously even when the activity causes such problems as illness, injury, or the breakdown of relationships. At the heart of activity disorder is the use of exercise to gain a sense of control and accomplishment, to maintain self-esteem, and to soothe emotions rather than to increase fitness, relaxation, or pleasure. The disorder is not about exercise itself but about meeting psychological needs through exercise. The hallmark of activity disorder is a pattern of exercise that becomes detrimental to health rather than beneficial.

Some of the signs and symptoms of activity disorder resemble those of anorexia and bulimia. Physical symptoms include fatigue, reduction in performance, decreased focus, increased compulsion to exercise, decreased heart rate response to exercise, and muscle degeneration. Cycles of repetitive overuse injuries are common.

Activity disorder is more common among men than among women, a difference that may be related to childhood experiences and cultural values. Males tend to be more active than females during childhood, and our culture supports male independence and physical achievement. The association between activity and achievement may influence active people with perfectionist tendencies to become addicted to exercise.

Treatment for activity disorder is similar to that for eating disorders, although most cases of pure activity disorder can be handled in an outpatient setting. Unfortunately, activity disorder often occurs in conjunction with an eating disorder; the combination can rapidly increase the physical problems of both disorders.

PROMOTING HEALTHY EATING AND A HEALTHY BODY IMAGE

Promotion of healthy eating and a healthy body image involves many components and coordinated efforts by individuals and institutions.

Individual Attitudes

As an individual, you can begin to challenge the way you interact with the world. Value yourself based on your goals, talents, and strengths rather than your body shape or weight. Start to look critically at the images and messages you receive from people and the media. Develop skills to handle stress in a healthy way, and avoid judging yourself or others. Complete the Personal Health Portfolio activity for Chapter 8 to take a closer look at your self-esteem and body image.

College Initiatives

Colleges have a role in ensuring that students learn how to transition successfully to new environments, new relationships, and different sociocultural pressures. These are skills that will translate well into future environments and relationships. Ideally, efforts to prevent eating disorders will include both individual measures and campuswide activities. Campus life typically affords many opportunities for people to recognize individuals who are at increased risk for disordered eating patterns and psychological distress. Residence advisors, professors, coaches, trainers, and other college staff can be trained to watch for signs that students are having problems with the transition to college life. Health and counseling services can be visible and accessible so that students feel comfortable accessing help early if they are feeling distressed.

Public Health Approaches

Public health approaches focus on raising awareness about eating disorders and changing widely accepted social norms. The "Love Your Body Day" campaign is one example of a public health campaign aimed at promoting healthy body images. Its goal is to encourage acceptance of physical differences, including different body shapes and sizes and the normal changes of healthy aging (see the box, "Love Your Body Day").

National youth organizations have also developed programs to promote healthy body image and lifestyle patterns for young people. For example, the new Girl Scouts' "Free Being Me" program emphasizes inner strength and healthy differences instead of outer appearances. It encourages girls to think about who they really are and what they like to do, to understand and resist peer pressure, to learn about eating disorders and substance abuse, and to celebrate diversity.[38]

Girls Inc. is a nationwide educational and advocacy organization that encourages girls to be "strong, smart, and bold." Its programs focus on building girls' interest and skills in math, science, and technology; on developing media literacy, emotional literacy, strategies for self-defense, and leadership; and on helping girls participate in sports and take healthy risks in life.

College students can enroll in an eight-week online course called Student Bodies, where multimedia and self-exploration modules guide them through the process of building self-esteem and a healthy body image. Developed by researchers from Stanford University and Washington University in St. Louis, the program can be tailored to the needs of any institution that wishes to administer it.[39]

In short, to counteract unhealthy attitudes, we can begin to resist current cultural messages and become active in changing them. The media and advertising industry spends millions of dollars every year finding out what consumers want and selling products. It conducts research on consumer attitudes, holds focus groups, monitors sales, and pays attention to consumer reactions. By supporting healthy body images and buying products that reflect diversity, we can move our society in the direction of realistic, accepting, and healthy attitudes toward the body.

Public Health Is Personal

Love Your Body Day

A healthy lifestyle, regardless of body type, should be the ideal, *ideally*. Every body is built differently. Too big for one person may be too small for another; one size typically never fits all. The standards to which people have been subconsciously primed by television, movies, music videos, magazines, toys, clothing, and advertisements are unfortunately engrained, leading to mental distortions and unrealistic ideals.

Since 1998, the National Organization for Women (NOW) has sponsored a public health intervention against negative media influence, "Love Your Body Day." The day is a fun but serious way to help people fight back against unrealistic body images promoted by Hollywood and the fashion, cosmetics, and diet industries. NOW encourages colleges and schools across the country to host events that draw attention to body-image issues and highlight the importance of healthy diversity in body shape, size, and function.

Events have included picketing the headquarters of publications that promote offensive images of women and girls, creating T-shirts with slogans that initiate discussions (such as "This is what Barbie OUGHT to look like"), and hosting forums to discuss and highlight body image issues. Every year there is a "Love Your Body" poster contest; the winner receives a monetary prize and distribution of his or her design as the official poster for the upcoming year's event. The poster positively highlights a healthy body image.

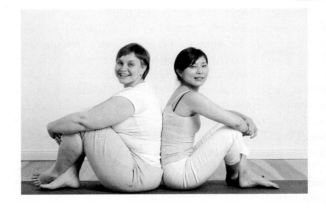

On the Love Your Body website, NOW provides other resources to help the public become active in confronting the media. For example, it posts "Offensive Ads" and "Positive Ads" with explanations of how ads affect body image, thus enhancing media literacy. It also promote advocacy by asking visitors to nominate ads for posting. For further information and to find out when the next annual Love Your Body Day is scheduled, visit the website at loveyourbody.nowfoundation.org.

connect ACTIVITY

Source: "Love Your Body: What's It All About?" NOW Foundation, November 24, 2013, http://loveyourbody.nowfoundation.org/ whatsitallabout.html.

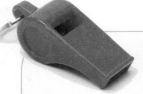

You Make the Call

Should "Warning" Labels Be Added to Digitally Enhanced Photos?

Magazine cover and ad photos are routinely altered to create idealized versions of models and celebrities. Standard graphics software (e.g., Photoshop) is all that a skilled photo editor needs to enlarge busts, reduce waists, remove cellulite, whiten teeth, lighten dark skin, darken light skin, erase lines and wrinkles, increase biceps, and modify a host of other human "flaws." The alterations are often hard to recognize, but sometimes they are hard to miss.

In June 2013, for example, Beyoncé released a digitally enhanced promotional photo for her upcoming tour. Her body proportions were not physically possible, and her designers stated it was intended as an artistic vision. When *Men's Fitness* enlarged his biceps next to the headline "How to Build Big Arms in 5 Easy Steps," tennis star Andy Roddick joked on his blog about his "22-inch guns." Actor Kate Winslet publicly objected to the slimmed-down version of herself on the cover of *British GQ,*

saying, "I don't look like that and I don't desire to look like that." Supermodel Cindy Crawford, commenting on digitally altered images of herself, remarked, "I wish I looked like Cindy Crawford."

What difference does enhancement make? It is not exactly clear, but we do know that men and women experience feelings of inadequacy, lower self-esteem, and increased dissatisfaction with their bodies after viewing fashion magazines. Models and actors already represent a look shared by only 2 percent of the population, and photo enhancement sometimes gives them body proportions that are physically unattainable. Men and women take the images of models and celebrities at face value and either aspire to achieve the same look or compare themselves unfavorably to them, or both. False representation raises questions about responsibility and transparency.

Members of the fashion and advertising industries discount objections, asserting that photo enhancement and "post-production corrections" are well-known standards of their industries. Cover photos aren't meant to convey reality, they say; rather they demonstrate artistry and creativity and are meant to

Continued…

Concluded...

inspire and please. Photographers have manipulated their images since the beginning of the technology in the 19th century, and digital enhancement is commonplace today among the general population. With photo enhancement part of everyday life, only the very naïve would take a magazine cover or ad at face value, according to fashion and advertising spokespeople.

In response to concerns about the effects of false and unattainable images, advocates have begun to promote the attachment of health warnings ("Warning: Trying to look as thin as this model may be dangerous to your health") or disclaimers ("These images have been digitally altered") to digitally enhanced photos. They feel clearly stating when the physical appearance of an individual has been altered will allow consumers to be more informed—and thus less likely to internalize unrealistic (and unreal) representations as a cultural ideal. Studies about the effectiveness of warnings, however, have not been conclusive. Initial studies showed a possible decrease in body dissatisfaction among women viewing fashion spreads with warning labels. An accumulating collection of subsequent studies have shown no difference in body satisfaction after exposure to labeled or unlabeled images. And one study has even shown that college women increase their comparison of self against images labeled as digitally altered, leading researchers to hypothesize that perhaps labeling creates a perception that a digitally altered image may be more socially desirable than an unaltered image.

Media literacy encourages consumers to think critically and to assess sociocultural ideals portrayed in the media. Should all digitally altered photographs be required to have a disclaimer or warning attached? What do you think?

Pros

- Alteration of media images can be difficult to identify, and the practice is becoming increasingly common.
- Models and actors already represent an unrealistic ideal, so further alteration of their photographs makes the ideal even less attainable for the general public.
- Media literacy training reduces body dissatisfaction, and identification of false messaging can improve critical thinking skills.

Cons

- Advocating for change in a system can take a tremendous amount of effort.
- Research suggests that warning labels may not have the intended consequences and may actually increase body dissatisfaction for some viewers.
- Labeling is not realistic given the prevalence of digital alteration, and drawing the line between acceptable and unacceptable alterations would be difficult.

connect
ACTIVITY

Sources: "Effects of Exposure to Thin-Ideal Media Images on Body Satisfaction: Testing the Inclusion of a Disclaimer Versus Warning Label," by R. N. Ata, J. K. Thompson, and B. J. Small, 2013, *Body Image, 10* (4), pp. 472–480; "Disclaimer Labels on Fashion Magazine Advertisements: Effects On Social Comparison and Body Dissatisfaction," by M. Tiggemann, A. Slater, B. Bury, et al., 2013, *Body Image, 10* (1), pp. 45–53; "Photo Tampering Throughout History," *Four and Six,* 2012, www.fourandsix.com/photo-tampering-history/?currentPage=2.

IN REVIEW

What is body image, and how is it determined?

Body image is our mental representation of our body—our perceptions, attitudes, thoughts, and emotions about it. Body image is strongly influenced by culture. Via advertising, fashion, and language, our culture sends messages about appearance, beauty, and acceptable body size and shape, especially for women but increasingly for men. The media typically promotes unrealistic thinness for women and muscularity for men.

What is disordered eating, and what are eating disorders?

To meet society's standards, many people practice disordered eating behaviors like dieting or binging and purging on occasion, but some people develop full-blown eating disorders. These disorders are characterized by severe disturbances in eating behavior and by a distorted body image. They are serious, chronic illnesses and are classified as mental disorders. Anorexia nervosa, characterized by self-starvation, is the most severe eating disorder. Bulimia nervosa, characterized by binge eating and purging, is more difficult to identify because people with bulimia are of normal weight. Binge-eating disorder leads to obesity, but only a small percentage of obese

people have this disorder. All eating disorders have serious health consequences.

Why do people develop eating disorders?

Aside from social pressures and cultural messages, which affect everyone, some people may be vulnerable to eating disorders because of a genetic predisposition, family factors, or other underlying emotional problems and characteristics, such as low self-esteem, a sense of powerlessness, perfectionism, and lack of coping skills. Eating disorders are more common among women than men and among gay men than heterosexual men. They are most common during the teens and early 20s and likely to occur during life transitions at any age. Frequent dieting, obesity, substance abuse, depression, anxiety, and obsessive-compulsive disorder are all associated with an increased risk of eating disorders.

How are eating disorders treated?

The first step is recognition of the problem, and early recognition makes successful treatment more likely. Because they are mental disorders, treatment usually includes psychotherapy to address psychological issues, along with weight stabilization, behavior modification, nutritional rehabilitation and education, and, in some cases, medication, especially antidepressants. For anorexia, hospitalization may be required at first to prevent starvation. Treatment usually involves the whole family, and recovery can be lifelong.

What is body dysmorphic disorder?

Body dysmorphic disorder is an acute preoccupation with a perceived flaw in one's physical appearance. A subcategory, which affects mainly men, is muscle dysphoria, an obsessive need to bulk up one's body regardless of one's physique. People with body dysmorphic disorder who undergo cosmetic surgery are likely not to be satisfied with the results, but opting to alter one's appearance with cosmetic surgery or body art does not indicate a body dysmorphic disorder. Dissatisfaction with a tattoo or other body art is usually due to changing life circumstances that make body art less desirable.

What are exercise disorders?

Exercise disorders, or abnormal exercise patterns, include the female athlete triad (disordered eating patterns, amenorrhea, and premature osteoporosis) and activity disorder (extremely time-consuming and strenuous exercise for emotional rather than physical reasons). Both share some symptoms with eating disorders, and treatments are also similar.

What are individual and public ways to promote healthy eating and healthy body images?

Individuals can learn to think critically about social pressures for a particular body shape or weight and be supportive of healthy body images. Colleges can train staff to look for signs of eating disorders. Organizations can mount campaigns supporting acceptance of physical diversity.

Alcohol and Tobacco

9

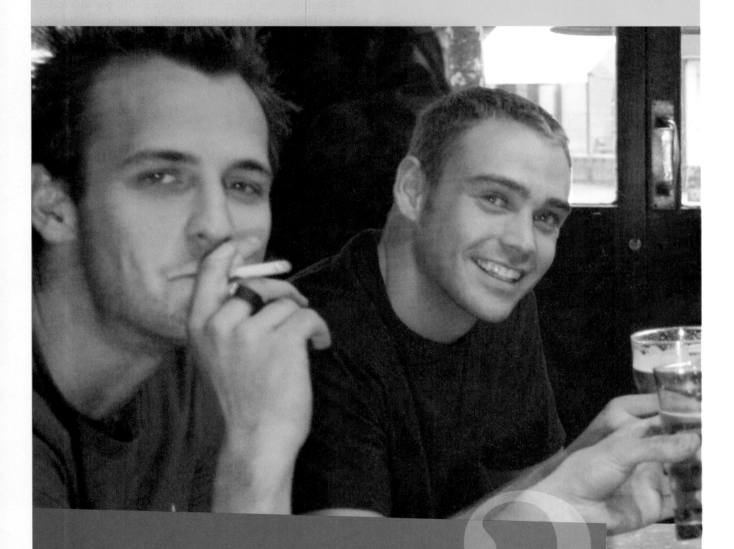

Ever Wonder...

- what counts as having "too much to drink"?
- what to do for someone who has passed out?
- if electronic cigarettes are safer than regular cigarettes?

Alcohol and tobacco are the most commonplace—and the most problematic—addictive substances in our society. Both can have profound effects on individuals, families, communities, and society in general. The use of both also illustrates the tension between personal choice and the common good. For these reasons, making responsible choices about alcohol and tobacco is particularly important.

UNDERSTANDING ALCOHOL USE

psychoactive drug
A substance that causes changes in brain chemistry and alters consciousness.

intoxication
Altered state of consciousness as a result of drinking alcohol or ingesting other substances.

low-risk drinking
Fourteen drinks a week for men and no more than four on one day; seven drinks a week for women and no more than three on one day.

The alcohol culture permeates many college campuses, in tailgate parties, bar crawls, 21-shot birthday celebrations, and an endless variety of rituals marking the end of classes, the first snowfall, or spring break. For decades, college administrators ignored or condoned this culture. But recently, chilling statistics have brought alcohol-related problems to the forefront. High-risk alcohol drinking kills 1,825 students between the ages of 18 and 24 every year and causes injury to 599,000. Sexual assaults, physical violence, vandalism, and academic casualties are additional problems associated with the campus alcohol culture.[1–3]

Because alcohol is a **psychoactive drug**—it causes changes in brain chemistry and alters consciousness, a state referred to as **intoxication**—it can have wide-ranging effects on all aspects of our thinking, emotions, and behavior. It is in society's interest to regulate the use of such a powerful substance, but it is up to individuals to determine what role they want alcohol to play in their lives.[4]

Who Drinks? Patterns of Alcohol Use

About 65 percent of American adults drink, at least occasionally. About 35 percent of the adult U.S. population label themselves *abstainers.* They do not drink at all, or they do so less often than once a year. Of the 65 percent who do drink, 28 percent are considered *at-risk drinkers,* and the remainder are *low-risk drinkers.*[1]

The National Institute on Alcohol Abuse and Alcoholism (NIAAA) has set parameters for low-risk and high-risk drinking. For men, **low-risk drinking** means no more than 14 drinks per week and no more than 4 drinks on any one day. For women, it means no more than 7 drinks per week and no more than 3 drinks on any one day. Alcohol consumption above these levels is considered heavy or at-risk drinking. Another way to think about the guidelines is that *moderate drinking* is 2 drinks a day for men and 1 for women. Regardless of these specific guidelines,

alcohol should not be consumed at any level in a situation that would put you or others at risk.[5] The Personal Health Portfolio Activity for Chapter 9 at the back of your book will help you determine if you are a low-risk or at-risk drinker.

"One drink" is defined by the NIAAA as 0.5 ounce (or 15 grams) of alcohol, the amount contained in about 12 ounces of beer, 5 ounces of wine, a 1.5-ounce shot of 80-proof distilled liquor, or 1.5 ounces of liquor in a mixed drink (Figure 9.1). The term *proof* refers to the alcohol content of hard liquor, defined as twice the actual percentage of alcohol in the beverage; for example, 80-proof liquor is 40 percent alcohol by volume.

Drinking patterns are established by the adolescent years. In general, people are more likely to drink at certain stages in the lifespan, such as adolescence and early adulthood, the threshold of middle age, and following retirement. Older adults drink significantly less than younger adults do. Women of all ages drink less than men do and start later.

Alcohol consumption is higher among Whites than among African Americans across most of the lifespan.[6] Alcohol consumption is high among Hispanic/Latino men, but it is very low among Hispanic/Latina women. Consumption of alcoholic beverages is highest between the ages of 18 and 25 for Whites and then begins a steady descent. The peak period for heavy drinking among Hispanic and African American men occurs between the ages of 26 and 30, and the decline tends to be less marked than that for White men.[5,6]

Differences in alcohol consumption among ethnic groups are strongly influenced by sociocultural or environmental factors, including poverty, discrimination, feelings of powerlessness, immigration status, and degree of acculturation.[7] Economic factors, such as the heavy marketing of alcoholic beverages in minority neighborhoods, play a considerable role. For example, the number of liquor stores located in African American communities is proportionately much higher than the number in White communities.[6] Given these pressures, it is notable that alcohol consumption is generally lower among African Americans than among other groups.

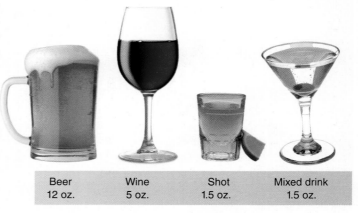

| Beer 12 oz. | Wine 5 oz. | Shot 1.5 oz. | Mixed drink 1.5 oz. |

figure 9.1   **What is "one drink"?**
Each drink contains about 0.5 ounce of alcohol.

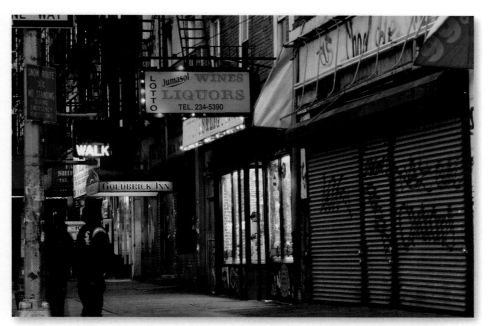

■ An oversupply of liquor stores in poor and minority neighborhoods plays a role in both the availability of alcohol and the social acceptability of alcohol use.

Among Native Americans, alcoholism is recognized as the number one health problem.[6] The death rate from alcoholism for Native Americans is more than five times greater than that for other groups.[8] Numerous factors contribute to these disparities, most notably sociocultural factors such as poverty and discrimination. Scientists have also suggested that genetic factors may contribute to patterns of alcohol use by Native Americans.

Among Asian Americans, alcohol consumption overall is lower than among White Americans. Approximately half of all Asian Americans have a gene that impairs the metabolism of alcohol, causing a set of unpleasant reactions (facial flushing, sweating, nausea) referred to as the *flushing effect*.[7,8]

Why Do Some People have Problems with Alcohol?

Why do some people develop problems with alcohol while others do not? This question has no simple answers. Instead, a complex interaction of many factors—individual, psychological, and sociocultural—is at work.

A family history of alcoholism is a risk factor for the development of alcoholism. Family dysfunction in general, even without an alcoholic parent, increases the likelihood that children will grow up to have alcohol problems. However, most children who grow up in dysfunctional family environments do not develop problems with alcohol. Sociocultural or environmental factors also play an enormous role in how alcohol is used and misused. Some cultures have higher acceptance of alcohol use, more tolerant attitudes toward drinking and drunkenness, and/or higher levels of alcohol consumption than others do. Economic factors, such as the availability and cost of alcohol and the ease of access, also play a role, as do laws governing drinking age and the sale of alcoholic beverages.

Drinking on the College Campus

Drinking rates at most colleges are very high; surveys indicate that up to 79 percent of college students drink alcoholic beverages.[9,10] College students under the age of 21 drink less frequently than older students do, but they are more likely to binge drink during these episodes and to drink simply to get drunk.[11] They are also more likely to be injured or encounter trouble with law enforcement than are older students who binge drink.[11,12] Although college students binge drink, 70 percent of binge drinking episodes involve adults age 26 years or older.[11]

Binge Drinking and Extreme Drinking Binge drinking, also called **heavy episodic drinking**, is generally defined as the consumption of five or more drinks within two hours for men and four or more drinks within two hours for women, at least once in the previous two-week period. When people have that many drinks in a two-hour period, their blood alcohol content rises to 0.08 percent or more.

> **heavy episodic drinking**
> Consumption of five or more drinks in a row by a man or four or more drinks in a row by a woman.

The Harvard School of Public Health College Alcohol Study (CAS) found that 44 percent of college students binge drank in the 30 days prior to the survey and 23 percent were *frequent binge drinkers,* meaning they had binged three or more times in the previous two weeks or more than once a week on average.[1,11]

Some health experts believe the current definition of binge drinking (five or more drinks in two hours for a man, four or more for a woman) is too broad and classifies a large number of people as binge drinkers who may not have a problem.[13] Other terms, such as *heavy drinking* or *high-risk drinking,* may be preferable to describe the drinking currently labeled *binge drinking.* The latter term could be reserved for a prolonged period of intoxication (two days or more). This definition would direct attention to the minority of students who have real problems with alcohol consumption. The term *extreme drinking* is now being used to describe alcohol consumption that goes well beyond binge drinking, to double or triple the amounts in the current definition—10 to 15 drinks a day for men and 8 to 12 drinks a day for women. Many colleges and universities are now targeting such extreme drinking on campus.

Consequences of Binge Drinking in College

Binge drinking can have serious physical, academic, social, and legal consequences. Individuals who have been drinking heavily are more likely to be injured, to commit a crime or fall victim to violence, and to be involved with the law. Half to two-thirds of campus homicides and serious assaults are believed to involve drinking by the offender, the victim, or both.[14] Women who binge drink are nearly 150 percent more likely to be victims of date rape, sexual battering, and unplanned sexual activity than are women who do not drink alcohol.[14] According to the College Alcohol Survey, about one in four students reported that their drinking caused them to miss class, turn in mediocre work, fail exams, or earn failing grades.[11]

Binge drinkers also cause problems for other students. About 9 out of 10 students reported experiencing at least one adverse consequence of another student's drinking during the school year.[11] These "secondhand effects" of binge drinking include serious arguments, physical assault, damaged property, interrupted sleep or studying, unwanted sexual advances, sexual assault, and having to take care of a drunk student.[14]

Binge drinkers are more likely to meet the *Diagnostic and Statistical Manual of Mental Disorders* criteria for alcohol abuse and alcohol dependence 10 years after college and are less likely to work in prestigious occupations, compared with non–binge drinkers. Alcohol-related convictions for crimes like driving under the influence, vandalism, assaults, and providing alcohol to a minor may jeopardize ambitions in many careers, especially engineering, medicine, law enforcement, and teaching.

Why Do College Students Binge Drink?

Students may drink to ease social inhibitions, fit in with peers, imitate role models, reduce stress, soothe negative emotions, or cope with academic pressure—or for a variety of other reasons. The mistaken belief that alcohol increases sexual arousal and performance (heavy drinking actually suppresses sexual arousal) may also account for some binge drinking.[1]

Binge drinking is also promoted by easy access to alcohol and cheap prices. Thus, social norms and the campus culture contribute to patterns of drinking.[2] For example, tailgating before sporting events and "pre-gaming" (consuming alcohol prior to going out for a social occasion) often involve drinking large quantities of alcohol in a compressed time period. Research on tailgating and pre-gaming is scant, but students are more likely to binge drink on campuses where heavy drinking is the norm and less likely to do so where drinking is discouraged.[15]

Pre-Gaming Drinking

Pre-gaming is the excessive consumption of alcohol prior to attending an event or activity in which alcohol will be consumed. It is also referred to as pre-partying, pre-bar, and front-loading. Pre-gaming is considered high risk since it usually involves a heavy consumption of alcoholic drinks in a short period of time. One study found that students who pre-game consumed more than three drinks in about an hour and usually consumed hard alcohol. Although college men and women consume similar levels of alcohol in pre-gaming, men typically drink more during events following pre-gaming. One study found that about 40 percent of underage college students pre-gamed on more days per month and had more drinks on pre-gaming days than of-age students. Freshmen were more likely to pre-game than non-freshmen. The first weeks of college appear to be the highest-risk period for pre-gaming.[15,16]

Spring Break Drinking

Thousands of college students descend on spring break locales every year to celebrate. Beaches, bikinis, bands, and free or cheap alcohol beverages marketed by the alcohol industry and bars create an environment conducive to excessive drinking. Males average 18 drinks per day and females 10 drinks per day. Forty percent of men and 33 percent of women reported being drunk daily during spring break.[17] Collapse, sexual assaults, and unprotected sex are common. One study found that more than 50 percent of all men and 40 percent of all women drank until they became sick or passed out. Another study on frequent binge drinkers reported 50 percent engaged in unplanned sex, 52 percent engaged in unprotected sex, 58 percent had trouble with law enforcement, and 59 percent were injured. The American Medical Association concluded

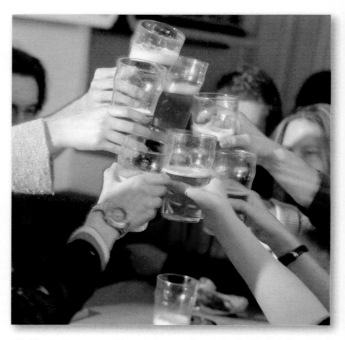

■ Alcohol consumption among college students is influenced by the social norms around drinking on their campus. In some cases, there is a gap between student-perceived levels of alcohol consumption and actual consumption by most students.

that spring break is no longer an innocent respite from college academic rigors, it is life threatening. Some colleges and universities have responded by banning spring break marketing and promotion on campus.[18]

Addressing the Problem The problem of excessive drinking by college students requires an integrated response at several levels. At the level of the individual student, the focus is on reducing the amount of drinking by students and identifying and helping high-risk students. Screening tools used during health care visits can also help students compare their drinking behaviors with those of other students. Other student-level measures include enforcing college alcohol policies consistently and punishing students who violate policies or break the law, mandating treatment for substance-related offenses, educating students to resist peer pressure, helping students cope with stress and time management difficulties, and issuing prevention messages during high-risk times and events, such as freshman year, athletic events, and spring break.

Colleges can also implement strategies aimed at changing the campus drinking culture. Some schools sponsor alcohol-free social and cultural events, while others have gone further by prohibiting alcohol at all college-sponsored events and maintaining alcohol-free residence halls and fraternity and sorority houses. Some colleges have also focused on restricting alcohol advertising and promotion on campus, but this can be tricky because the alcohol industry provides significant financial support to athletic programs at many colleges.

Finally, colleges can work cooperatively with their communities to support such strategies as increased enforcement of drinking-age laws, provision of "safe rides" programs, and limits on the density of alcohol retailers near campus.

EFFECTS OF ALCOHOL ON THE BODY

Within minutes of ingestion, alcohol is distributed to all the cells of the body (Figure 9.2). In the brain, alcohol alters brain chemistry and changes neurotransmitter functions. It particularly affects the cerebellum—the center for balance and motor functions—and the prefrontal cortex—the center for executive functions, such as rational thinking and problem solving.[19]

Alcohol is a **central nervous system depressant**. While your body is absorbing alcohol and alcohol levels in the blood and brain are rising, you experience feelings of relaxation and well-being and a lowering of social inhibitions. At higher levels, and especially when blood levels are

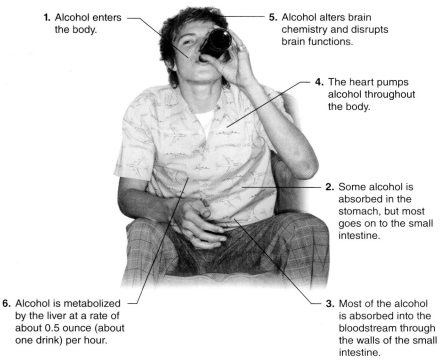

1. Alcohol enters the body.

5. Alcohol alters brain chemistry and disrupts brain functions.

4. The heart pumps alcohol throughout the body.

2. Some alcohol is absorbed in the stomach, but most goes on to the small intestine.

6. Alcohol is metabolized by the liver at a rate of about 0.5 ounce (about one drink) per hour.

3. Most of the alcohol is absorbed into the bloodstream through the walls of the small intestine.

figure 9.2 **The path of alcohol in the body.**

falling, you are more likely to feel depressed and withdrawn and to experience impairments in thinking, balance, and motor coordination. These effects last until all the alcohol is metabolized (broken down into energy and wastes) and excreted from the body.

central nervous system depressant Chemical substance that slows down the activity of the brain and spinal cord.

Alcohol Absorption

The faster absorption of alcohol into the blood results in a quicker increase in blood alcohol concentration than when alcohol is absorbed more slowly. Many factors affect the rate of alcohol absorption.

- *Food in the stomach.* Alcohol consumed on an empty stomach can reach the brain in less than one minute. Food slows down the movement of alcohol into the small intestine.

- *Gender.* Women absorb alcohol into the bloodstream more quickly than men do.

- *Age.* Older adults do not tolerate alcohol as well as younger people.

- *Body fat.* The more body fat a person has, the less alcohol is absorbed by body tissues and the more there is to circulate in the bloodstream and reach the brain. In other words, higher body fat results in a quicker intoxication than lower body fat.

- *Drug interaction.* Interactions with many prescription and over-the-counter drugs can intensify a drinker's reaction to alcohol, leading to more rapid intoxication.

- *Cigarette smoke.* Nicotine extends the time alcohol stays in the stomach, increasing time for absorption into the bloodstream. This means smoking slows the increase in blood alcohol concentration.

- *Mood and physical condition.* Fear and anger tend to speed up alcohol absorption. The stomach empties more rapidly than normal, allowing the alcohol to be absorbed more easily. People who are stressed, tired, or ill may also feel alcohol's effects sooner.

- *Alcohol concentration.* The more concentrated the alcohol, the more quickly it is absorbed. Hard liquor is absorbed faster than are beer and wine.

- *Carbonation.* The carbon dioxide in champagne, cola, and ginger ale speeds the absorption of alcohol. On the other hand, drinks that contain water, juice, or milk are absorbed more slowly.

- *Diet soda.* The artificial sugars cause alcohol to empty more rapidly from the stomach into the small intestine and thus speed up absorption in the bloodstream. Health scientists believe that, in contrast, the body may treat the sugar in regular mixers like food, which slows the release of alcohol into the small intestine.

- *Tolerance.* The body adapts to a given alcohol level. Each time a person drinks to the point of impairment, the body attempts to minimize impairment by adapting to that level. More alcohol is needed to overcome the body's adaptation and achieve the desired effect. This means an experienced drinker has a slower absorption of alcohol into the blood than a less experienced drinker.

Alcohol Metabolism

A small amount of alcohol is metabolized in the stomach, but about 90 percent is metabolized in the liver. Between 2 and 10 percent is not metabolized at all; instead, it is excreted unchanged in the breath and urine and through the pores of the skin. This is why you can smell alcohol on the breath of someone who has been drinking.

In the liver, alcohol is converted to acetaldehyde, an organic chemical compound, by the enzyme *alcohol dehydrogenase (ADH)*. The ability to metabolize alcohol depends on the amount and kind of ADH enzymes available in the liver. If more alcohol molecules arrive in the liver cells than the enzymes can process, the extra molecules circulate through the brain, liver, and other organs until enzymes are available to degrade them. Slower degrading of alcohol molecules means a high blood alcohol concentration until they are metabolized.

blood alcohol concentration (BAC) The amount of alcohol in grams in 100 milliliters of blood, expressed as a percentage.

Blood Alcohol Concentration Blood alcohol concentration (BAC) is a measure of the amount of alcohol in grams in 100 milliliters of blood, expressed as a percentage. For example, for 100 milligrams of alcohol in 100 milliliters of blood, the BAC is 0.10 percent.

BAC is influenced by the amount of alcohol consumed and the rate at which the alcohol is metabolized by the body (see Figure 9.3). Because alcohol is soluble in water and somewhat less soluble in fat, it does not distribute to all body tissues equally.[19] The more body water a person has—in body tissues and fluids that contain water, such as muscle tissue and blood—the more the alcohol is diluted and the lower the person's BAC will be. The more body fat a person has, the less alcohol is absorbed by body tissue and the more there is to circulate in the bloodstream and reach the brain. Thus, a person with high body fat will have a higher BAC than will a person of the same weight but more lean body tissue who drinks the same amount. Body size alone influences BAC as well; a larger, heavier person has more body surface to diffuse the alcohol (as well as a higher body water content to dilute the alcohol).

BAC provides a good estimate of the alcohol concentration in the brain, which is why it is used as a measure of intoxication by state motor vehicle laws. The alcohol concentration in the blood corresponds well with alcohol concentration in the breath, so breath samples are accurate

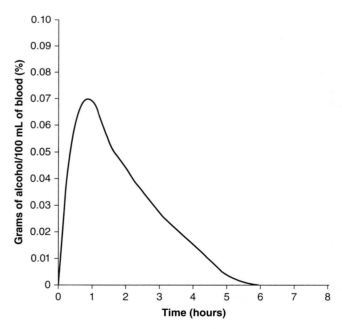

figure 9.3   **Blood alcohol concentration over time.**
The shape of this BAC curve is affected by variables such as gender, body size and build, amount and type of alcohol, duration of drinking, and presence or absence of food in the digestive tract.
Source: Figure 8, "Teacher's Guide: Information about Alcohol," *Understanding Alcohol: Investigations into Biology and Behavior,* NIH and NIAAA, 2003, http://science.education.nih.gov/supplements/nih3/Alcohol/guide/info-alcohol.htm.

indicators of BAC. For this reason, breath analyzers are legal in most states for identifying and prosecuting drunk drivers, which will be discussed later in the chapter.

Gender Differences in Alcohol Absorption and Metabolism

Both body size and body fat percentage play a role in gender differences in the effects of alcohol. Women are generally more susceptible to alcohol's effects and have a higher BAC than men do after drinking the same amount, because women are generally smaller than men and have a higher body fat percentage. Women also absorb more of the alcohol they drink because they metabolize alcohol less efficiently than men do. Women generally have less alcohol dehydrogenase (ADH) than men. ADH is an enzyme that breaks down alcohol metabolites in the liver.

These differences make women more vulnerable to the health consequences of alcohol, including alcohol-related liver disease, heart disease, and brain damage.[19] The risk for cirrhosis starts at two and a half drinks to four drinks a day for men, but for women this risk starts to increase at less than two drinks a day.[19] Women are more susceptible to every cause of death associated with alcohol and die at higher rates than men do from them.[20]

Rates and Effects of Alcohol Metabolism

Alcohol is metabolized more slowly than it is absorbed. This means that the concentration of alcohol builds when additional drinks are consumed before previous drinks have been metabolized. As a rule of thumb, people who have normal liver function metabolize about 0.5 ounce of alcohol (about one drink) per hour.[19]

The behavioral effects of alcohol, based on studies of moderate drinkers, are summarized in Table 9.1. A person with a BAC of 0.08 percent is considered legally drunk in all states. Because of individual differences in sensitivity to alcohol, people experience impairment at different BAC levels. The National Highway Traffic Safety Administration reports that driving function can be impaired by BAC levels as low as 0.02 to 0.04 percent.[6] For more on the public debate about the legal limit, see the box at the end of the chapter, "Should the Legal Limit for Driving Under the Influence Be Lowered to 0.05 BAC?"

Visible Effects

Deeper wrinkles, red cheeks, and weight gain are just a few of the visible effects of regular heavy drinking. DrinkSmarter has

Table 9.1   Stages of Effects of Alcohol

Blood Alcohol Concentration (grams/100 ml)	Physiological and Psychological Effects	Impaired Functions
0.01–0.05	Relaxation Sense of well being Loss of inhibition	Decreased alertness Impaired concentration Impaired judgment Impaired coordination (especially fine motor skills)
0.06–0.10	Euphoria Blunted feelings Nausea Sleepiness	Slower reflexes Impaired reasoning Impaired visual tracking Reduced depth perception
0.11–0.20	Emotional arousal Mood swings Anger or sadness Boisterousness	Slowed reaction time Staggering gait Slurred speech Impaired balance
0.21–0.30	Aggression Reduced sensations Depression Stupor	Lethargy Increased pain threshold Severe motor impairment Memory blackout
0.31–0.40	Unconsciousness Coma Death possible	Loss of bladder control Impaired temperature regulation Slowed breathing Slowed heart rate
0.41 and greater	Death	Respiratory arrest

Source: Adapted from "Information About Alcohol," Biological Sciences Curriculum Study, 2003, retrieved from http://science.education.nih.gov/supplements/nih3/alcohol/guide/info-alcohol.htm.

created a "Drinking Mirror" app to show the visible effects of heavy alcohol consumption. You upload a picture of yourself and enter your drinking behavior to see how you might look after 10 years at your current rate of alcohol consumption.

Alcohol's calories are empty, providing almost no nutrients while contributing to weight gain. A regular beer has about 144 calories; a glass of wine, 100 to 105 calories; and a shot of gin or whiskey, 96 calories. Mixers add more calories, as do *alcopops* or *malternatives*—sugary, fizzy, fruit-flavored drinks popular among younger drinkers. The National Institute on Alcoholism and Alcohol Abuse has an Alcohol Calorie Calculator you can use to total your weekly alcohol calories. These calories have a tendency to be deposited in the abdomen, giving drinkers the characteristic "beer belly."

On the other hand, long-term heavy drinkers who substitute the calories in alcohol for those in food are at risk for weight loss and malnutrition. They are also vulnerable to mental disorders caused by vitamin deficiencies.

Acute Alcohol Intoxication

People who drink heavily in a relatively short time are vulnerable to **acute alcohol intoxication** (also called *acute alcohol shock* or *alcohol poisoning*), a potentially life-threatening BAC level of about 0.35 or greater. Acute alcohol intoxication can produce collapse of vital body functions, notably respiration and heart function, leading to coma and/or death (see the box, "Alcohol Poisoning: Know the Signs, Know What to Do"). Vomit can also be inhaled leading to death by asphyxiation. Dehydration caused by vomiting can cause seizures, which can permanently damage the brain.

Slow, steady drinking suppresses the vomiting reflex, and BAC can increase to dangerously high levels. The gag reflex is also slower or nonexistent when a person experiences alcohol poisoning. At very high alcohol concentrations, 0.35 or greater, a person can become comatose, sustain irreversible brain damage, or die. Some colleges have instituted "good Samaritan" rules that provide amnesty for students who seek help for themselves or others in a medical emergency due to drinking that occurred in a residence hall room or where underage drinkers were present.

acute alcohol intoxication
A life-threatening blood alcohol concentration.

blackout
Period of time during which a drinker is conscious but has partial or complete amnesia for events.

Blackouts

A **blackout** is a period of time during which a drinker is conscious but has impaired memory function; later, he or she has amnesia about events that occurred during this time. The impairment is associated with changes in the hippocampus, a brain structure essential for memory and learning.[19] These changes may be temporary or permanent. Either way, a blackout is a warning sign that fundamental changes have

Action Skill-Builder

Alcohol Poisoning: Know the Signs, Know What to Do

Do you know the symptoms of alcohol poisoning? Do you know what you should do and when you should seek help? People who have passed out from heavy drinking should be watched closely. All too often they are carried to bed and forgotten. For their safety, follow these measures:

☐ Know and recognize the symptoms of acute alcohol intoxication:

- Lack of response when spoken to or shaken.
- Inability to wake up.
- Inability to stand up without help.
- Rapid or irregular pulse (100 beats per minute or more).
- Rapid, irregular respiration or difficulty breathing (one breath every three to four seconds).
- Cool, clammy, bluish skin.
- Bluish fingernails or lips.

☐ Call 911. An intoxicated person who cannot be roused or wakened or has other symptoms listed here requires emergency medical treatment.

☐ Do not leave the person to "sleep it off." He or she may never wake up. BAC can continue to rise even after a person has passed out.

☐ Roll an unconscious drinker onto his or her side to minimize the chance of airway obstruction from vomit.

☐ If the person vomits, make certain his or her head is positioned lower than the rest of the body. You may need to reach into the person's mouth to clear the airway.

☐ Try to find out if the person has taken other drugs or medications that might interact with alcohol.

☐ Stay with the person until medical help arrives.

occurred in the structure of the brain.[19,21] Alcohol-induced blackouts are a common experience among nonalcoholics who binge drink. Some people may be genetically predisposed to experience blackouts.

Effects of Alcohol Ingestion Fads

Up to 28 percent of college students reportedly mix alcohol and energy drinks, despite evidence that doing so is dangerous.[22] Alcohol acts as a depressant, which sedates the body and causes a drinker to become sleepy. The stimulants in energy drinks keep the body awake. When alcohol and stimulants are combined, the alcohol intoxicates the drinker, but the stimulants keep the drinker awake, tricking the body into believing it is sober. College students who mix alcohol and energy drinks are three times more likely to leave a bar drunk and four times more likely to drive drunk. There is also an increased risk for sexual assaults.[22]

Some college students who are bored with the liquid form of alcohol, want to get drunk faster, or think they can limit alcohol's calories have turned to vaporizing alcohol with dry ice, carbon dioxide pills, asthma nebulizers, pressurized air pumps, or a device called a Vaportini and inhaling, or "smoking," the alcohol vapor. A Vaportini is a glass ball containing a small amount of alcohol, which is heated over a small candle; the resulting vapors are sucked through a straw. Inhaling alcohol is extremely dangerous because it bypasses the buffering effects of the digestive system and delivers alcohol vapors directly into the lungs, where the chemicals are absorbed into the bloodstream and sent directly to the brain. At a minimum, the inhaled vapors can dry out nasal passages and the mouth, which increases the risk for infections. Of greater concern—because the alcohol is absorbed into the bloodstream so quickly and the gag reflex cannot be triggered—inhaling alcohol makes alcohol poisoning more likely. Liver failure, brain damage, and blindness are additional health concerns.[23,24]

Another dangerous fad is the alcohol enema. A beer enema involves inserting a full beer bottle into the anus or pouring beer through a funnel and tube or a drip bag into the anus. Alcohol enemas can make the user very drunk in a very short period of time. They bypass the stomach so the alcohol is absorbed directly into the intestines. Risks include rectal damage and alcohol poisoning.[25]

Hangovers

Hangovers are characterized by headache, stomach upset, thirst, and fatigue. Health experts speculate that alcohol disrupts the body's water balance, causing excessive urination and thirst the day after excessive drinking. The stomach lining may be irritated by increased production of hydrochloric acid, resulting in nausea. Alcohol also reduces the water content of brain cells. When the brain cells rehydrate and swell the next day, nerve pain occurs. The only known remedy for a hangover is pain medication, rest, and time.

HEALTH RISKS OF ALCOHOL USE

Alcohol is toxic and has an effect on virtually all body organs and systems as well as all aspects of a person's functioning, as indicated in Table 9.1.

Medical Problems Associated with Alcohol Use

The major organs and systems damaged by alcohol use are the cardiovascular system, the liver, the brain, the immune system, and the reproductive system (Figure 9.4). When pregnant women drink, alcohol can cause a set of fetal birth defects known as **fetal alcohol syndrome (FAS)** (discussed in Chapter 12). Children born with FAS have permanent physical and mental impairments.

Heart Disease and Stroke   Chronic heavy drinking is a major cause of degenerative disease of the heart muscle, a condition called alcoholic **cardiomyopathy**, and of heart arrhythmias (irregular heartbeat). Abnormal heart rhythm is a cause of sudden death in alcoholics, whether or not they already had heart disease. Heavy drinking also causes coronary heart disease (disease of the arteries serving the heart). In addition, long-term heavy drinking can elevate blood pressure and increase the severity of high blood pressure, which increases the risk for stroke (an interruption in the blood supply to the brain).[19]

Liver Disease   The liver enables the body to digest food, absorb nutrients, control infections, and rid itself of toxins. Excessive alcohol consumption interferes with these functions. Alcohol-related liver disease occurs in three phases. The first, called **fatty liver**, occurs when the liver is flooded with more alcohol than it can metabolize, causing it to swell with fat globules. This condition can literally develop overnight as a result of binge drinking. It makes the liver more vulnerable to inflammation, such as alcoholic hepatitis. Fatty liver can be reversed with abstinence (usually about 30 days or so).

The second phase of liver disease is called **alcoholic hepatitis**, which includes liver inflammation and liver function impairment. This condition can occur in the absence of fatty liver, which suggests that direct toxic effects of alcohol may be the cause.[19] Inflammation causes fibrous tissue, called collagen, to develop, which interferes with blood flow to liver cells.

The third phase of liver disease is **cirrhosis**, scarring of the liver tissue. Although other diseases can cause cirrhosis (such as viral hepatitis), between 40 and 90 percent of people with cirrhosis have a history of alcohol abuse.[19] The risk rises sharply with higher levels of consumption. It usually takes at least 10 years of steady, heavy drinking for cirrhosis to develop.[19]

As cirrhosis sets in, liver cells are replaced by collagen, which changes the structure of the liver and decreases blood flow to the organ. Liver cells die and liver function is impaired, leading to fluid accumulation in the body, jaundice (yellowing of the skin), and an opportunity for infections or cancers to establish themselves. Cirrhosis can also lead to a fatal brain disorder called hepatic encephalopathy.[19] The prognosis for people with alcoholic hepatitis or cirrhosis is poor.

Cancer   Alcohol accounts for about 3.5 percent of all cancer deaths in the United States. It is associated with several types of cancer, particularly cancers of the head and neck

fetal alcohol syndrome (FAS) Set of birth defects associated with use of alcohol during pregnancy.

cardiomyopathy Disease of the heart muscle.

fatty liver Condition in which the liver swells with fat globules as a result of alcohol consumption.

alcoholic hepatitis Inflammation of the liver as a result of alcohol consumption.

cirrhosis Scarring of the liver as a result of alcohol consumption.

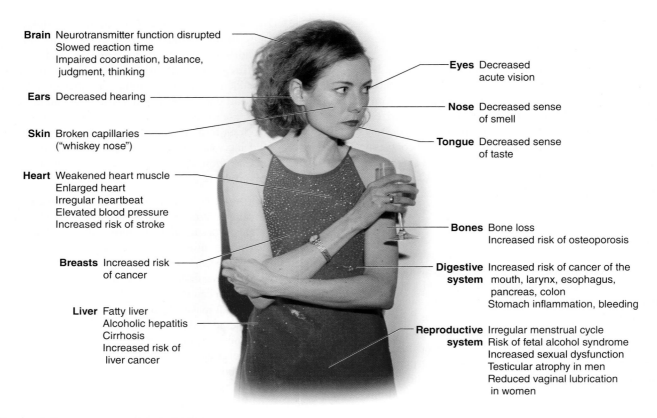

Brain Neurotransmitter function disrupted
Slowed reaction time
Impaired coordination, balance,
judgment, thinking

Ears Decreased hearing

Skin Broken capillaries
("whiskey nose")

Heart Weakened heart muscle
Enlarged heart
Irregular heartbeat
Elevated blood pressure
Increased risk of stroke

Breasts Increased risk
of cancer

Liver Fatty liver
Alcoholic hepatitis
Cirrhosis
Increased risk of
liver cancer

Eyes Decreased
acute vision

Nose Decreased sense
of smell

Tongue Decreased sense
of taste

Bones Bone loss
Increased risk of osteoporosis

**Digestive
system** Increased risk of cancer of the
mouth, larynx, esophagus,
pancreas, colon
Stomach inflammation, bleeding

**Reproductive
system** Irregular menstrual cycle
Risk of fetal alcohol syndrome
Increased sexual dysfunction
Testicular atrophy in men
Reduced vaginal lubrication
in women

figure 9.4 **Effects of alcohol on the body.**

(mouth, pharynx, larynx, and esophagus), and cancers of the digestive tract.[27] In 2011, researchers reported finding that low levels of alcohol consumption, three to six drinks per week, may moderately increase the risk for breast cancer. Binge drinking also appears to increase the risk for breast cancer. These results remain consistent regardless of the type of alcohol consumed. Why alcohol increases the risk for breast cancer is not known, but scientists believe it may be due to its effects on estrogen levels.[26–28]

Brain Damage Heavy alcohol consumption causes anatomical changes in the brain and directly damages brain cells. Alcohol can cause a loss of brain tissue, inflammation of the brain, and a widening of fissures in the cortex (covering) of the brain.[21] Heavy drinking, especially binge drinking, has been shown to disrupt short-term memory and the ability to analyze complex problems.[21] Although women are more sensitive to alcohol, research suggests that men and women are equally vulnerable to alcohol-induced brain damage.[21]

Because the brain continues to grow and mature until the early 20s, heavy alcohol use during the teen years can be harmful to the developing brain. Studies have revealed that the hippocampus (a center for learning and memory) is 10 percent smaller in teenagers who drink heavily than in those who don't. Research has also found differences in the prefrontal cortex, the center for executive functions (rational thinking, planning).

In long-term alcohol abuse, loss of brain tissue results in a mental disorder called alcohol-induced persisting dementia, an overall decline in intellect. Some of this loss may be reversible if the person abstains from alcohol use for a few months, but after age 40, improvement is less likely, even with abstinence.[21]

Lung Damage Recent studies suggest that alcohol abuse causes dysfunction in lung cells that can increase the risk of severe lung injury or impairment following a major trauma, such as a car crash, a gunshot wound, or an acute illness. This disruption in lung function also makes a person more susceptible to lung infections.[19,24]

Drunkorexia As the name suggests, drunkorexia is the combination of three dangerous behaviors: excessive alcohol consumption, excessive exercise, and disordered eating. In fact, between 20 and 33 percent of people with eating disorders also struggle with alcohol and drug problems.[29,30] People with drunkorexia avoid consuming calories from food so that they can drink more alcohol. They may drink alcohol on an empty stomach, binge on foods such as pizza and hamburgers, and then purge. Motivations for drunkorexia include staying slim, getting intoxicated quickly, and saving money on food. Women are three times more likely than men to have drunkorexia.[30] One study found that about 16 percent of college women restricted food calories in

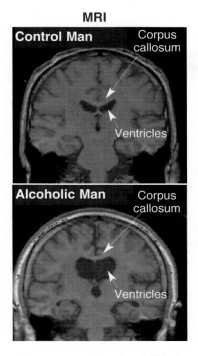

MRI

Control Man — Corpus callosum

Ventricles

Alcoholic Man — Corpus callosum

Ventricles

■ This magnetic resonance imaging (MRI) shows how chronic alcohol use can damage the frontal lobes of the brain, increase the size of the ventricles, and cause an overall reduction in brain size (shrinkage).

order to offset calories from alcohol. Potential consequences of drunkorexia include risk for sexual assault, alcohol poisoning, substance abuse, chronic diseases, malnutrition, and cognitive difficulties.

Social Problems Associated with Alcohol Use

As shown in the box, "Drinking-Related Problems for College Students," alcohol can lead to many kinds of difficulties. Alcohol reduces social inhibitions, and reduced inhibition may lead to high-risk sexual activity and a lowered likelihood of practicing safe sex (such as using a condom). Heavy drinkers are more likely to have multiple sex partners and to engage in other risky sexual behaviors. These behaviors are associated with increased risk of sexually transmitted disease and unplanned pregnancy.[3]

Violence is another problem associated with alcohol use. The National Crime Victimization Survey (NCVS) has consistently found that alcohol is more likely than any other drug to be associated with all forms of violence, including robbery, assault, rape, domestic violence, and homicide. Women who binge drink or date men who binge drink are at increased risk for sexual exploitation (rape and other forms of nonconsensual sex).[3]

The relationship between alcohol and risk of injury has been established for a variety of circumstances, including automobile crashes, falls, and fires. Reduced cognitive function, impaired physical coordination, and increased risk-taking behavior (impulsivity) are the alcohol-related factors that lead to injury.[31]

Alcohol use is also a factor in about one-third of suicides, and it is second only to depression as a predictor of suicide attempts by youth.[32] The relationship between alcohol and depression is very strong. Estimates are that 20 to 36 percent of people who commit suicide were drinking shortly before their suicide or had a history of alcohol abuse.[32] Alcohol-associated suicides tend to be impulsive rather than premeditated acts.

Another View: Health Benefits

Scientists speculate that moderate alcohol consumption can have some health benefits. Alcohol has an anticlotting effect on the blood, and it enhances the body's sensitivity to insulin, which may lower the risk of developing Type-2 diabetes. Because alcohol is a depressant, it may help reduce stress. The high water content in beer and its diuretic effect may also help prevent the forming of kidney stones.[33]

Moderate alcohol consumption also appears to be associated with a lowered risk of heart disease because it increases high-density lipoproteins (HDL, also called "good cholesterol"). The beneficial effects of alcohol on HDL levels and blood clotting may be only temporary, lasting perhaps 24 hours, so that optimal protection against heart disease requires drinking moderately every day.

It is apparently the pattern of drinking, not the type of alcoholic beverage, that confers benefits. People who drink wine, for example, tend to do so in small amounts every day rather than in large amounts. Binge drinking does not serve as a protective factor and can actually increase the risk for heart disease.[33]

The *Dietary Guidelines for Americans* advises that moderate alcohol consumption—one drink a day for women and two drinks a day for men—can be beneficial for middle-aged and older adults, the age groups most susceptible to coronary heart disease. In younger adults, however, alcohol appears to have fewer, if any, health benefits, and it is associated with more deaths from injuries and accidents. It is not recommended that anyone begin drinking or drink more frequently because of anticipated health benefits.

Alcohol Misuse, Abuse, and Dependence

Alcohol misuse refers to the consumption of alcohol to the point where it causes physical, social, and moral harm to the drinker. **Problem drinking** is a pattern of alcohol use that impairs the drinker's life, causing personal difficulties and difficulties for other people. For college students, such difficulties might be missed classes or poor academic

problem drinking
Pattern of alcohol use that impairs the drinker's life, causing difficulties for the drinker and for others.

Who's at Risk?

What are the more common problems resulting from drinking according to this graph? What differences do you see between men's and women's experiences?

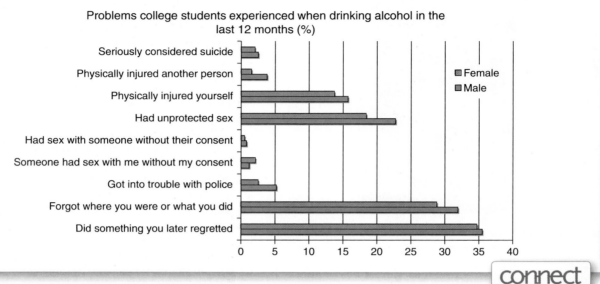

Problems college students experienced when drinking alcohol in the last 12 months (%)

	Female	Male

- Seriously considered suicide
- Physically injured another person
- Physically injured yourself
- Had unprotected sex
- Had sex with someone without their consent
- Someone had sex with me without my consent
- Got into trouble with police
- Forgot where you were or what you did
- Did something you later regretted

Source: American College Health Association–National College Health Assessment II: Reference Group Executive Summary, by American College Health Association, Spring 2013, Hanover, MD: ACHA, www.acha-ncha.org/docs/ACHA-NCHA-II_ReferenceGroup_ExecutiveSummary_Spring2013.pdf.

connect
ACTIVITY

---

performance. **Alcohol abuse** is defined as the continued use of alcohol despite negative consequences. It is a pattern of drinking that not only impairs the person's ability to fulfill major obligations at home, work, or school, but also often causes legal or social problems.[6]

Alcohol dependence is characterized by a strong craving for alcohol. People who are dependent on alcohol use it compulsively, and most will eventually experience physiological changes in brain and body chemistry as a result of alcohol use. As described in Chapter 2, one indicator of dependence is the development of *tolerance,* reduced sensitivity to the effects of a drug so that larger and larger amounts are needed to produce the same effects.[19,34] Another indicator is experiencing *withdrawal,* a state of acute physical and psychological discomfort when alcohol consumption stops abruptly.

Alcohol dependence is also known as **alcoholism,** defined as a chronic disease with genetic, psychosocial, and environmental causes.[6] It is often progressive and fatal. About one in four heavy drinkers or at-risk drinkers can be defined as an alcoholic or alcohol abuser. The manifestations of alcoholism include lack of control over drinking, preoccupation with alcohol, use of alcohol despite adverse consequences, and distortions in thinking (most notably denial).

Are you a problem drinker—or an alcoholic? It may not matter because the new edition of the *Diagnostic and Statistical Manual of Mental Disorders* (DSM-5) eliminated the medical distinction between problem drinking and alcoholism. Many health experts are critical of this change. They are concerned that college binge drinkers could be wrongly labeled as lifelong alcoholics. Previous editions of the DSM included the less severe "alcohol abuse" classification for people with less-entrenched problems, such as college binge drinkers. The new edition combines abuse and dependence into a single condition with varying levels of severity. College binge drinkers are likely to be diagnosed as "mild alcoholics." The stigma of this diagnosis could limit employment and insurance opportunities even if the alcohol problem is resolved. The Health Affordability Act increases screening for alcohol problems so that even temporary abuse will go into the patient's electronic medical record.[35]

alcohol abuse
Pattern of alcohol use that leads to distress or impairment, increases the risk of health and/or social problems, and continues despite awareness of these effects.

alcohol dependence
Disorder characterized by a strong craving for alcohol, the development of tolerance for alcohol, and symptoms of withdrawal if alcohol consumption stops abruptly.

alcoholism
A primary chronic disease characterized by excessive, compulsive drinking.

TREATMENT OPTIONS

Treatment options for alcohol-related disorders include brief interventions, inpatient treatment programs, outpatient treatment programs, self-help, and harm reduction approaches.

Brief Interventions

Many colleges and universities focus their intervention efforts on high-risk groups such as freshmen, athletes, fraternity members, and, more recently, gay men, lesbians, and transgender individuals. Programs are also directed at high-risk times and events such as spring break, fraternity rushing, homecoming, and pre-graduation events for seniors.

The Alcohol Skills Training Program is a model brief intervention program adapted by many colleges and community-based organizations around the country. It is designed for college students and other young adults considered at risk for alcohol-related problems, such as poor class attendance and grades, accidents, sexual assault, and violence. It consists of a series of group sessions (usually six to eight) focusing on skills and knowledge development through lectures, discussion, and role-plays.

The Brief Alcohol Screening and Intervention for College Students (BASICS) program is another brief intervention model for college students who drink heavily and have experienced or are at risk for alcohol-related problems. BASICS is conducted in two 50-minute interviews and includes personalized feedback on the effects and consequences of alcohol use, strategies for reducing risks and making better decisions, and options that can help students make changes. Students who receive BASICS report fewer consequences and more rapid changes in their alcohol-related behavior and consequences than at-risk drinkers who do not receive the intervention.[36]

Some colleges have introduced Internet-based programs that educate students about alcohol use on and around campus. For example, AlcoholEdu is a two- to three-hour online course that provides students with personalized information and feedback about alcohol. It offers information about the physical, social, and behavioral effects of alcohol abuse, as well as strategies for finding alcohol-free activities and drinking responsibly. Sites like e-CHUG and MyStudentBody target students who have recently engaged in heavy drinking.

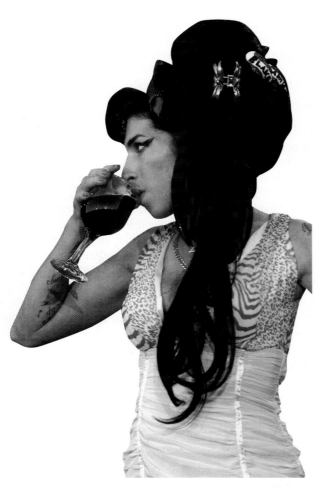

■ Alcohol is believed to have caused the death of Amy Winehouse in 2011, ending the Grammy-award-winning singer's very public battle with alcohol and drugs.

■ Brief intervention programs for high-risk young adult drinkers include counseling sessions that help individuals see the consequences of alcohol use and develop strategies for change.

These sites engage students with personalized interactive exercises and normative feedback, which help them to correct misperceptions about heavy drinking on campus and equip them with skills needed to avoid situations that will put them at risk of drinking heavily.[37]

Inpatient and Outpatient Treatment

When alcohol-related problems are severe, individuals benefit from placement in a residential facility specializing in alcohol recovery. The first stage of treatment is detoxification, the gradual withdrawal of alcohol from the body. During this time, the patient usually experiences withdrawal symptoms. This phase may include medications, such as antidepressants and anti-anxiety drugs. Treatment programs typically also include group and individual counseling, education, and skills training. Because recovery from alcoholism is a lifelong process, relapse prevention strategies are emphasized. In outpatient programs, patients participate in treatment programs during the day and return home in the evening. In both types of programs, family members are encouraged to participate in the recovery process.

Self-Help Programs

The best-known self-help program is Alcoholics Anonymous (AA). The goal of AA is total abstinence from alcohol. A basic premise of AA is that alcoholics are biologically different from nonalcoholics and consequently can never safely drink any alcohol at all. Key components of AA are progression through a 12-step path to recovery and group support.

Other self-help programs include Rational Recovery and Women for Sobriety. Programs for family members of alcoholics include Al-Anon and Alateen. Adult Children of Alcoholics is a program that provides support for people recovering from the effects of growing up in an alcoholic household.

Harm Reduction: Approach, Policies, and Laws

The harm reduction approach to treatment focuses on reducing the harm associated with drinking, both to the individual and to society. An example of harm reduction is **controlled drinking**, which emphasizes moderation rather than abstinence.[13] Controlled drinking is considered appropriate for early-stage problem drinkers.[36] Most mental health experts agree that total abstinence is the most effective approach for recovery from alcoholism.[13]

controlled drinking
Approach to drinking that emphasizes moderation rather than abstinence.

A variety of public policies and laws are aimed at reducing the harm caused by alcohol consumption. A prime example is the minimum drinking age. Since 1984, all states have had laws prohibiting the purchase and public possession of alcohol by people under the age of 21. Despite inconsistent compliance with these laws, research suggests that they result in less underage drinking than occurred when the drinking age was 18.[13] Evidence also suggests that these laws result in less drinking after age 21.[6]

Some leaders in the higher education community would like the drinking-age laws revisited. In 2008, a collection of college and university presidents and chancellors joined to form the Amethyst Initiative (AI), which seeks to spark a national debate about whether the current legal drinking age of 21 actually keeps teens from drinking. Members of AI believe that lowering the drinking age is a practical and sensible way to confront binge drinking among young people. The signatories of AI argue that the principal problem is no longer drunk driving but clandestine binge drinking, particularly by college students. Opponents of AI believe that lowering the age would undercut efforts by colleges and universities to curb binge drinking.[38,39] To date, the Amethyst Initiative has not received strong support from the higher education community.

Drunk driving laws are another form of harm reduction, and sobriety checkpoints are a tool that substantially increases compliance with these laws. Law enforcement agents check drivers for intoxication with alcohol sensors and breath analyzer tests. Alcohol sensors are noninvasive tests that can detect the presence of alcohol on the breath when held in the vicinity of a driver. Breath analyzer tests measure the amount of alcohol exhaled in the breath. The box, "Driver Alcohol Detection System for Safety," describes new technologies that are being developed to measure BAC in all drivers.

People convicted of alcohol-related offenses might be required to wear ankle bracelet breathalyzers as part of their sentences. The ankle bracelet monitors whether the person has been consuming alcohol by periodically sampling the perspiration on the skin. A small amount of consumed alcohol is expelled through the skin, and the bracelet can detect the presence of alcohol. If the device's reading indicates alcohol is detected at 0.02 or higher BAC, the court or probation officer is notified.

Another harm reduction approach to alcohol use involves restrictions on liquor sales and outlets. The more places there are to purchase alcohol within a certain geographical area, the higher the rates of alcohol consumption and alcohol-related harm.[6] Some communities have worked for a more even distribution of alcohol outlets throughout their area to curb this problem. Although underage drinkers usually get their alcohol from parents and other adults, they also buy alcoholic beverages at convenience stores, liquor stores, and bars.[6,39] Most states have passed laws holding such establishments liable for harm caused by intoxicated patrons (referred to as "dram shop liability"). Recently, the Internet has become a source for underage purchase of alcoholic beverages, although regulations are being put in place to curb this practice.

Starting the Conversation

Driver Alcohol Detection System for Safety

The National Highway Traffic Safety Administration (NHSTA) collaborated with the automobile manufacturers on a five-year research project to develop in-vehicle technology that can be used to prevent alcohol-impaired driving in the United States. The Driver Alcohol Detection System for Safety (DADSS) project is researching accurate technologies that measure a driver's blood alcohol content (BAC) in a noninvasive manner. If the driver's BAC is at or above 0.08 percent, the legal limit in all states, the vehicle will be disabled and cannot be driven. Many states already mandate installation of an ignition interlock device (IID) for drivers convicted of a DUI, especially repeat offenders and first-time offenders with a BAC above 0.20; however, the IIDs used today rely on an ethanol-specific fuel cell sensor that is not as accurate or reliable as the infrared spectroscopy technology used in evidentiary breathalyzers by law enforcement officers.

Two technologies are being developed by the DADSS: tissue spectrometry (TS) and distant spectrometry (DS). TS is a touch-based technology that estimates BAC in tissue through detection of light absorption. DS uses part of the infrared light spectrum to detect alcohol concentration in the driver's breath. Phase I, proof-of-concept, was completed in 2013. Phase II, a practical demonstration of alcohol detection subsystems, will last for about two years. The actual integration of the recommended DADSS technology is projected for 2021 to 2023. The cost for the DADSS system has not been determined. Ignition interlock systems today can cost more than $1,000.

The DADSS maintains a log that can printed out or downloaded each time the detection system is calibrated, usually at 30-, 60-, or 90-day intervals. Law enforcement and insurance companies may require periodic reviews of the log. Violations above the 0.08 BAC may result in legal and insurance sanctions. After the vehicle is started, the IID will require random breath samples to prevent someone other than the driver to provide a breath sample. If the breath sample is not provided, or if the sample exceeds the set IID BAC level, the sensor device will log the event, warn the driver, and then initiate an alarm (flashing lights, horn honking) until the engine is turned off or the driver provides a clean breath sample. Data from the IID can be sent directly to state law enforcement.

So, what do you think? Should the DADSS be mandated to be in every vehicle? Should all drivers under the age of 18 be required to have a DADSS installed in their vehicle? Should federal law mandate the DADDS for first-time offenders who have a BAC above 0.20?

Source: Driver Alcohol Detection System for Safety: Fact Sheet, Interlockfacts.com/downloads/DADSS_NHTSA_inAllCars_1_31_11_HL.pdf.

Another way to control alcohol consumption is by increasing the tax on alcohol. Research suggests that an increase in the price of alcohol reduces consumption by underage and moderate drinkers but not by heavy drinkers. College students tend to be price sensitive, and increased taxes have been shown to decrease student drinking, making abstainers less likely to become moderate drinkers and moderate drinkers less likely to become heavy drinkers. On the other hand, raising prices too high has the potential to create a black market for alcoholic beverages.[6,40]

Finally, local communities have a variety of other harm reduction measures at their disposal, including limiting drink specials at local bars, prohibiting out-of-sight sales (purchases made by one person for several others), imposing a minimum drink price, enforcing fines, revoking liquor licenses, and controlling house parties.[40] Research suggests that comprehensive community programs that unite city agencies and private citizens are effective in reducing drunk driving, related driving risks, and traffic deaths and injuries.[6,41]

■ Breath analysis and sobriety checkpoints are public health measures designed to reduce the harm to self and others associated with alcohol use.

TAKING ACTION

Is alcohol a problem in your life? Do you wonder what you can do to reduce or prevent harm from alcohol-related activities? In this section, we provide some suggestions for individual actions.

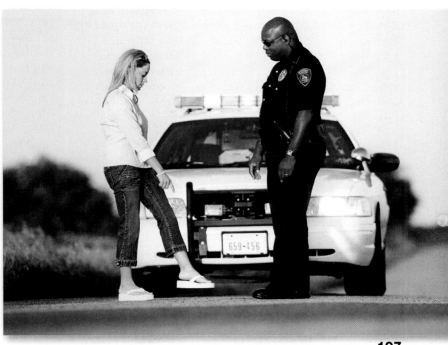

Are You at Risk?

Physicians sometimes use the CAGE questionnaire to identify individuals at risk for alcohol problems:

C: Have you ever tried to *cut down* on your drinking?

A: Have you ever been *annoyed* by criticism of your drinking?

G: Have you ever felt *guilty* about your drinking?

E: Have you ever had a morning *"eye-opener"?*

A yes answer to one or more of these questions suggests that you may be at risk for alcohol dependence.

Developing a Behavior Change Plan

If you decide you would like to change your behavior around alcohol, you can develop a behavior change plan to do so. First, keep track of when, how much, and with whom you drink for 2 weeks, and then analyze your record to discover your drinking patterns. Do you drink mostly on weekends, or do you drink every day? Do you drink mostly with certain people, or do you drink alone? Do you drink when you're under stress? Information like this can help you get a sense of the role alcohol plays in your life.

If you decide you want to change your drinking behavior, set goals for yourself. Goals should be specific, motivating, achievable, and rewarding. "I'm going to drink less" is too vague a goal. "I'm going to drink only once a week and have no more than four drinks" is a more specific, measurable goal.

Then develop specific strategies to attain your goals. For example, if you drink in social situations or with certain people, learn to say no to some drinks. Tell people you feel better when you don't drink, and avoid people who can't accept that. Plan ahead what you will do when you're tempted to have a drink. Ask family and friends for their support. After a few weeks, evaluate the outcome of your behavior change plan. Did you achieve your goals? If not, what obstacles prevented you from succeeding? How can you overcome these obstacles? Periodically assessing your progress allows you to devise alternative strategies for reaching your goals.

Be an Advocate

Boost Alcohol Consciousness Concerning the Health of University Students (BACCHUS Network) is a non-profit organization with hundreds of chapters across North America. It is run by student volunteers and promotes both abstinence and responsible drinking. Some BACCHUS chapters have joined with Greeks Advocating Mature Management of Alcohol (GAMMA) to provide a peer education network. This network program may be called BACCHUS or GAMMA on your college campus. The merging of BACCHUS and GAMMA has led to a broadening of approaches to health issues that affect college students.

UNDERSTANDING TOBACCO USE

Like alcohol, tobacco poses a problem of individual rights versus social good. Adults are free to use it, but such use causes an array of health problems, both for users and for those around them. Tobacco use is the leading preventable cause of death in the United States, implicated in a host of diseases and debilitating conditions. The health hazards of tobacco use are well known, yet almost one in five adult Americans smokes, and nearly 4,000 young people under the age of 18 start smoking every day.[42]

Who Smokes? Patterns of Tobacco Use

About 19 percent of people 18 years old or over in the United States are smokers. The percentage of Americans who smoke is down from a high of nearly 42 percent in 1965. The decline since then has occurred largely as a result of public health campaigns about the hazards of smoking. Although the prevalence of smoking in the United States continues to decline, the rate of decline has slowed since 1990.[42]

More men than women smoke, and rates of smoking are higher among young people than among older people. Most smokers get hooked in adolescence—more than 90 percent of smokers began smoking before the age of 21.[42] Forty percent of men and 34 percent of women with mental illness smoke.[43]

Currently, college students are more likely than the general population to smoke. Overall, however, cigarette smoking is negatively correlated with educational attainment. Adults with less than a high school education are three times as likely to smoke as those who graduate from college.[44]

Other psychosocial factors that increase the likelihood that a person will smoke include having a parent or sibling who smokes, associating with peers who smoke, being from a lower socioeconomic status family, doing poorly in school, and having positive attitudes about tobacco. Evidence also suggests that tobacco companies directly market their products to people with mental illness. Stressful living and lack of access to health insurance and health care make it more difficult for people with mental illness to stop smoking.[43]

Smoking is more prevalent among the White population than among African Americans, Hispanics, or Asian Americans and Pacific Islanders. As Figure 9.5 shows, the highest rates of smoking occur among American Indians and Alaska Natives.[45]

Smoking rates can vary tremendously within the broad ethnic categories in Figure 9.5. For example, despite low rates of smoking overall among Asian Americans and Pacific Islanders, rates are very high among some of the 50 distinct ethnic groups that fall under this umbrella label. Among Cambodian American men, for example, the smoking rate is 71 percent.[45] Clearly, behaviors like smoking are influenced by sociocultural factors, including acculturation and access to health information and health care.

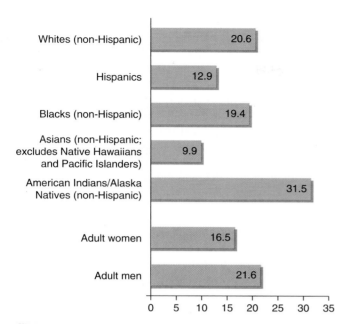

figure 9.5 **Percentages of U.S. adults who were smokers in 2011.**

Source: "Adult Cigarette Smoking in the United States Current Estimate," Centers for Disease Control and Prevention, www.cdc.gov/tobacco/data_statistics/fact_sheets/adult_data/cig_smoking/index.htm.

Tobacco Products

Tobacco is a broad-leafed plant that grows in tropical and temperate climates. Tobacco leaves are harvested, dried, and processed in different ways for the variety of tobacco products—rolled into cigars, shredded for cigarettes, ground into a fine powder for inhalation as snuff, or ground into a chewable form and used as smokeless tobacco.

Substances in Tobacco When tobacco leaves are burned, thousands of substances are produced, and nearly 70 of them have been identified as carcinogenic (cancer causing). The most harmful substances are tar, carbon monoxide, and nicotine.

Tar is a thick, sticky residue that contains many of the carcinogenic substances in tobacco smoke. Tar coats the smoker's lungs and creates an environment conducive to the growth of cancerous cells. Tar is responsible for many of the changes in the respiratory system that cause the hacking "smoker's cough."

One of the most hazardous gaseous compounds in burning tobacco is carbon monoxide, the same toxic gas emitted from the exhaust pipe of a car. Carbon monoxide interferes with the ability of red blood cells to carry oxygen, so that vital body organs, such as the heart, are deprived of oxygen. Many of the other gases produced when tobacco burns are carcinogens, irritants, and toxic chemicals that damage the lungs.

Nicotine is the primary addictive ingredient in tobacco. It is carried into the body in the form of thousands of droplets suspended in solid particles of partially burned tobacco.

These droplets are so tiny that they penetrate the alveoli (small air sacs in the lungs) and enter the bloodstream, reaching body cells within seconds.

Nicotine is both a poison (it is used as a pesticide) and a powerful psychoactive drug. The first time it is used, it usually produces dizziness, light-headedness, and nausea, signs of mild nicotine poisoning. These effects diminish as tolerance grows. Nicotine causes a cascade of stimulant effects throughout the body by triggering the release of adrenaline, which increases arousal, alertness, and concentration. Nicotine also stimulates the release of endorphins, the body's "natural opiates" that block pain and produce mild sensations of pleasure. (The effects of nicotine are discussed in greater detail later in the chapter.)

Cigarettes By far the most popular tobacco product is cigarettes, followed by cigars and chewing tobacco. Cigarettes account for nearly 95 percent of the tobacco market in the United States.[42] Nicotine from a cigarette reaches peak concentration in the blood in about 10 minutes and is reduced by half within about 20 minutes, as the drug is distributed to body tissues. Rapid absorption and distribution of

tar
Thick, sticky residue formed when tobacco leaves burn, containing hundreds of chemical compounds and carcinogenic substances.

nicotine
Primary addictive ingredient in tobacco; a poison and a psychoactive drug.

■ Tobacco use originated in the Americas, where it was used ceremonially and medicinally by native populations. By 1600, it was being exported to Europe and Asia. Today, tobacco is still an important crop in Virginia, Kentucky, North and South Carolina, and other southeastern states.

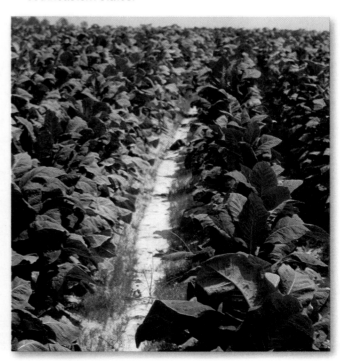

nicotine enable the smoker to control the peaks and valleys of nicotine absorption and effect. This process of control—absorption, distribution, elimination—makes cigarettes an effective drug-delivery system for nicotine.

In 2009, the U.S. Congress passed the Family Smoking Prevention and Tobacco Control Act, which gave the Food and Drug Administration (FDA) the power to regulate tobacco and banned a variety of once-legal cigarettes. Fruit- and candy-flavored cigarettes are now prohibited due to concerns that they appealed particularly to children. Also banned are clove cigarettes, which contain higher levels of tar and nicotine than regular cigarettes, and bidis, small cigarettes made from unprocessed tobacco that also contain higher levels of tar and nicotine than regular cigarettes.

E-Cigarettes The electronic cigarette (e-cigarette) was introduced in the U.S. market in 2007. Because e-cigarettes contain no tobacco, they can be purchased without proof of age. Although they are marketed as a safe cigarette, they still contain nicotine and have other health risks. (To evaluate the advertising claims, see the box, "Are E-Cigarettes Safer Than Regular Cigarettes?") Smoking e-cigarettes with drags longer than three to five seconds can cause liquid nicotine to be released in the mouth. Accidental breakage of the e-cigarette may expose users to diethylene glycol, an anti-freeze component, and cancer-causing compounds like nitrosamines. In addition to disease concerns, there have been anecdotal reports of e-cigarettes exploding, particularly during recharging. E-cigarettes are now coming under the scrutiny of the FDA.[46,47]

If the potential health effects of e-cigarettes are not enough to alarm you, consider "smart packs," a new type of e-cigarette that can alert (with a light flash or vibrator) the user to anyone else using the same device within 50 feet. Smart pack devices can connect to each other and share information about their respective owner's social networking profiles.

Should e-cigarettes be banned in public places? Manufacturers claim the water vapor emitted does not harm people who are subjected to these vapors. This claim has not been verified by the FDA.

Hookahs Hookahs, or water pipes, have become popular as a supposedly safe alternative to cigarettes. Groups of smokers pass the mouthpiece around, inhaling *shisha,* a mixture of tobacco, molasses, and fruit flavors. The aromatic flavors of hookah tobacco and the smooth smoke produced by the water pipe, which is less irritating to the throat than cigarette smoke, have driven the perception that hookah use is safe. Hookah tobacco is also known as narghile and arghile. Steam stones and hookah pens are new forms of hookah smoking. They are battery-powered devices that convert liquid nicotine, flavorings, and other chemicals into a vapor that is inhaled.

The American College Health Association reports that about 33 percent of college students use hookahs.[48] The popularity of hookah is expected to grow due to hookah cafés being located near college campuses and "hookah rooms" in fraternity houses.

The World Health Organization and the CDC warn that hookah use can pose even greater dangers than cigarette smoking. The average cigarette provides 20 puffs, whereas a one-hour session of hookah results in about 200 puffs. The depth of inhalation and frequency of puffs may cause hookah smokers to absorb high concentrations of carbon monoxide, heavy metals, and cancer-causing chemicals. Risks for lung, bladder, and oral cancers are of particular concern. The smoke from the tobacco and heat source also poses a secondhand smoke risk for non-smokers.[49,50]

Cigars Cigars have more tobacco and nicotine per unit than cigarettes do, take longer to smoke, and generate more smoke and more harmful combustion products than cigarettes do. The tobacco mix used in cigars makes it easier for cigar smoke to be absorbed through the mucous membranes of the oral cavity than is the case with cigarettes. Nicotine absorbed via this route takes longer to reach the brain than nicotine absorbed in the lungs and has a less intense but longer-lasting effect.

Cigar smokers who do not inhale have lower mortality rates than cigar smokers who do.[51,52] Inhalation substantially increases the cigar smoker's exposure to carcinogenic chemicals and increases the risk for lung cancer and chronic respiratory disease.[51] Whether or not smoke is inhaled, cigar smoking exposes the oral mucosa to large amounts of carcinogenic chemicals; consequently, cigar smokers have a higher risk than cigarette smokers for oral cancers.[52]

Black & Mild cigarillos, or "little cigars," are popular among teens and young adults. Black & Milds are long and thin like a cigarette but wrapped in tobacco leaf rather than paper, like a cigar. The difference in wrapping means they are not subject to certain cigarette regulations and taxes. They contain more tobacco and more nicotine than cigarettes and are addictive if inhaled. Use of Black & Mild cigarillos is much higher among African Americans (54 percent) than any other ethnic group.[52]

Pipes Pipe smoke has more toxins than cigarette smoke does and is more irritating to the respiratory system. Pipe smokers who do not inhale are at less risk for lung cancer and heart disease than are cigarette smokers. Like cigar smokers, however, pipe smokers are exposed to more toxins than cigarette smokers. Pipe smokers are just as likely as cigarette smokers to develop cancer of the mouth, larynx, throat, and esophagus.[52]

Smokeless Tobacco *Snuff* is a powdered form of tobacco that can be inhaled through the nose or placed between the bottom teeth and lower lip. *Chewing tobacco* is available as loose leaf or as a plug (a compressed, flavored bar of processed tobacco); a cud or pinch is lodged between the

Consumer Clipboard

Are E-Cigarettes Safer Than Regular Cigarettes?

If the claim made by a product sounds too good to be true, it probably is. The following is a list of some questions you can ask when you want to evaluate the validity of a product's claim. Here, the questions are applied to e-cigarettes.

How does the product work in comparison to other products on the market?
A battery-powered device provides inhaled doses of nicotine by heating a nicotine chemical solution into a vapor. The vapor provides flavor and a physical sensation similar to that of inhaled smoke.

What claims does the manufacturer make about the product in ads and on product packaging?
E-cigarettes are marketed as a safer alternative to regular cigarettes because they produce no tar or smoke, do not pollute the air, and are odorless. Target markets include young people and people who have never smoked, and e-cigarettes come in flavors that may especially appeal to young people.

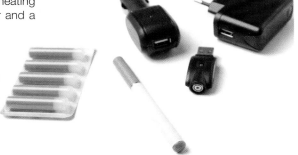

What doubts might a reasonable person have about these claims?
E-cigarettes contain tobacco-specific organic compounds and other potentially carcinogenic chemicals, so they can't really be safe. They deliver nicotine, so they must be addictive. They replicate the rituals, actions, and flavor of lighting up a real cigarette, which would reinforce their addictive potential. E-cigarettes appear to be another way to recruit new customers for the tobacco industry.

How is the product regulated?
Initially, the FDA sought to regulate e-cigarettes as a drug delivery device. This would have meant that manufacturers would have to prove their products are safe. The courts struck down the FDA's request, so there are no legal age restrictions on their sale and no health warnings on the packages. Several states have banned the use of e-cigarettes in public places, however.

Does independent research suggest that the product is safe to use?
Clinical studies have not been submitted to the FDA, so consumers have no way of knowing whether e-cigarettes are safe or exactly what an e-cigarette contains. The FDA discourages the use of these products and warns parents to caution their children about them.

Sources: "FDA Cracks Down on E-Cigarettes," by C. Hutchinson, *ABC News,* 2011, http://abcnews.go.com/print?id=11594556; "Do Stop-Smoking Products Really Work?" by Lifescript, 2011, www.lifescript.com/Health/centers/Smoking_Cessation/Articles/Do_Stope-Smoking; "FDA Warns of Health Risks of E-Cigarettes," U.S. Food and Drug Administration, 2009, www.fda.gov/ForConsumers/ConsumerUpdates/ucm173401.htm; "Electronic Cigarette Dangers and Side Effects," www.primehealthchannel.com/electronic-cigarette-dangers-and-side-effects.html.

cheek and gum. Smokeless tobacco is sometimes called *spit tobacco* because users spit out the tobacco juices and saliva that accumulate in the mouth.

Spit tobacco is believed to cause about 10 to 15 percent of oral cancers, leading to about 6,000 deaths each year. When spit tobacco is kept in contact with the oral mucosa, it can cause *dysplasia,* an abnormal change in cells, and *oral lesions,* whitish patches on the tongue or inside the mouth that may become cancerous. Spit tobacco also causes gum disease, tooth decay and discoloration, and bad breath.[53] The amount of nicotine absorbed from smokeless tobacco is two to three times greater than that delivered by cigarettes.

Snus is a smokeless tobacco that is marketed as a safer alternative to cigarettes. It is made from tobacco mixed with water, salt, sodium carbonate, and aroma and is often packaged in small bags resembling teabags. It is produced and sold mainly in Sweden and Norway but is being test-marketed in the United States. Snus contains more nicotine than cigarettes but lower levels of other dangerous compounds, and because it isn't burned, there is no secondhand smoke. The risk of certain cancers is lower with snus than with other types of smokeless tobacco, but snus may cause oral lesions, hypertension, and complications of pregnancy.[51,52]

Dissolvable Tobacco Products Dissolvable tobacco products are small pellets, sticks, or strips that consist of finely ground and pressed tobacco; they dissolve on the tongue

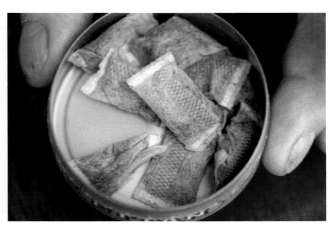

■ Snus is a form of smokeless tobacco produced in Sweden and Norway, where it is marketed as a safe way to enjoy tobacco. Users place one of the small, prepackaged bags under the upper lip and leave it there for an extended period of time.

Ramiro: An Occasional Smoker

Ramiro tried a cigarette when he was 15 and a sophomore in high school. A group of friends he was hanging out with after a basketball game were smoking, and he asked to take a hit off his friend's cigarette, just out of curiosity. He was embarrassed that he started coughing as he inhaled the first drag, but he tried a few more puffs and felt dizzy and a little bit high—kind of good. However, Ramiro's parents were vehemently opposed to smoking. Ramiro respected them and knew that it would be impossible to get away with smoking behind their backs, so he didn't try cigarettes again.

About two months into his freshman year at a college in another state, Ramiro was at a party and started talking to a friend from one of his classes. His friend pulled out a pack of cigarettes and lit up. The smell of the smoke distracted Ramiro and reminded him of his first time smoking. His friend noticed him staring at her cigarette and offered him one. He hesitated, but he was opening up to a lot of new experiences, and his parents' rules seemed part of his distant past. He didn't see the harm of having just one, so he accepted the cigarette and lit up. He felt the same dizzy and high feelings he had with his first cigarette. Later in the evening he had a second cigarette, and the following Saturday he bummed a few cigarettes from someone at a party.

On Sunday, feeling independent, he bought a pack of cigarettes of his own. He told himself he would have only a few, maybe one or two, and would smoke only occasionally, in social situations. But later that day, after finding out on Facebook that a friend was dating a girl he was interested in, he went downstairs and smoked a cigarette outside his dorm. It helped him calm down and not think about his troubles.

Over the next two months, Ramiro gradually started smoking more. He allowed himself a cigarette to celebrate a good grade on a paper or to get over a disagreement with a roommate. He no longer felt high when he smoked, but he still enjoyed it. He knew he was smoking more, but he knew several other people with smoking patterns similar to his. None of them really considered themselves smokers—they just smoked occasionally and could quit at any time.

When he went home for winter vacation, Ramiro thought it would be a good idea to take a break from cigarettes, and he didn't want his parents to know he was smoking. After being at home for two days, he felt unusually irritable and unfocused. He wanted a cigarette to calm down and clear his mind, and the more he tried not to think about it, the more he wanted one. That night after everyone had gone to bed, he pulled out his cigarettes from where he had hidden them in his backpack, sneaked out of the house, and lit up. He instantly felt better. At the same time, he realized that what he had just gone through was an indication that he had gotten hooked. Although he enjoyed smoking, he didn't want to be addicted. He decided that he had to quit and find better ways to reward himself, deal with stress, and socialize.

- What has your experience with smoking been so far in your life? Do any of Ramiro's experiences ring true for you?

- Why do you think some people seem to be able to smoke only on occasion and others become regular smokers?

- What are some healthy ways that Ramiro could relieve stress without smoking?

connect
ACTIVITY

---

like a breath mint. They are marketed as forms of tobacco to use when you can't smoke. These products can contain a potent level of nicotine, and the health risks are similar to those associated with other oral tobacco products, particularly oral cancer.

WHY DO PEOPLE SMOKE?

Tobacco use and its relationship to health are complex issues that involve nicotine addiction, behavioral dependence, and aggressive marketing by tobacco companies, among other factors.

Nicotine Addiction

Nicotine is a highly addictive psychoactive drug—some health experts believe it is the most addictive of all the psychoactive drugs—and tobacco products are very efficient delivery devices for this drug. Once in the brain, nicotine follows the same pleasure and reward pathway that other psychoactive drugs follow (see Chapter 10). Increases in release of the neurotransmitter dopamine produce feelings

of pleasure and a desire to repeat the experience. As noted earlier, nicotine also affects alertness, energy, and mood by increasing levels of endorphins and other neurotransmitters, including serotonin and norepinephrine.

With continued smoking, neurons first become more sensitive and responsive to nicotine, causing *addiction*, or dependence on a steady supply of the drug; over time, they become less responsive to nicotine, developing *tolerance*. Smokers experience *withdrawal* symptoms if nicotine is not present (see the box, "Ramiro: An Occasional Smoker"). Nicotine withdrawal symptoms include irritability, anxiety, depressed mood, difficulty concentrating, restlessness, decreased heart rate, increased appetite, and increased craving for nicotine.[54]

More than two-thirds of cigarette smokers who attempt to quit relapse within two days, unable to tolerate the period when withdrawal symptoms are at their peak. It takes about two weeks for a person's brain chemistry to return to normal. Withdrawal symptoms decrease and become more subtle with prolonged abstinence, but some smokers continue to experience intermittent cravings for years. Smoking tobacco may cause permanent changes in the nervous

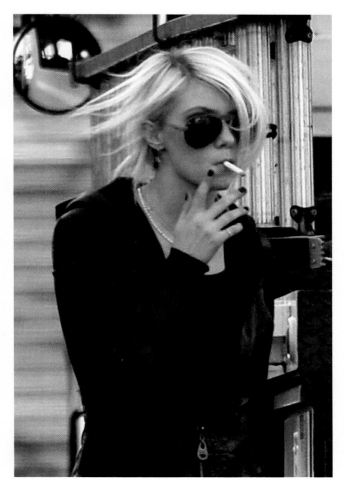

■ The vast majority of smokers start when they are teenagers, like actress Taylor Momsen, who was 16 years old when this photo was taken. Many young smokers don't realize they are addicted to nicotine until they try to quit.

system, which may explain why some people who haven't smoked in years can become addicted again after smoking a single cigarette.[54]

Behavioral Dependence

People who smoke are not just physiologically dependent on a substance; they also become psychologically dependent on the habit of smoking. Through repeated paired associations, the effects of nicotine on the brain are linked to places, people, and events. Tobacco companies design their advertising to take advantage of these associations. Many smokers have a harder time imagining their future life without cigarettes than they do dealing with the physiological symptoms of withdrawal.[54]

Weight Control

Nicotine suppresses appetite and slightly increases basal metabolic rate (rate of metabolic activity at rest). People who start smoking often lose weight, and continuing smokers gain weight less rapidly than nonsmokers. Weight control is one of the major reasons young women give for smoking, and weight gain can be a deterrent to quitting. People who quit smoking initially consume about 300 to 400 additional calories a day but only expend an additional 100 to 150 calories a day. Gaining 7 to 10 pounds is typical before the body adjusts to the absence of nicotine.[55] Once a person has successfully quit, this small amount of weight can be lost through exercise and sensible eating.

Tobacco Marketing and Advertising

Every day, the tobacco industry loses 4,600 smokers, either to quitting or to death.[54] These users have to be replaced if tobacco companies are to stay in business. Because most smokers get hooked in adolescence, children and teenagers are prime targets of tobacco advertising. Tobacco advertising aimed at children associates smoking with cartoon characters, and advertising aimed at teenagers associates smoking with alcohol, sex, and independence. Judging by the number of people who take up tobacco use every year, tobacco advertising and marketing are extremely effective. Although the industry continues to claim that it does not market its products to children, research suggests otherwise.[54]

EFFECTS OF TOBACCO USE ON HEALTH

Besides its role in cancer, tobacco use is also a causal factor in heart disease, respiratory diseases, and numerous other debilitating conditions. Overwhelming evidence confirms that smoking is the single greatest preventable cause of illness and premature death in North America. The CDC reports that 443,000 Americans die of smoking or exposure to secondhand smoke each year. For every smoking death, another 20 people suffer from smoking-related illnesses.[56,57] Even people who are only occasional smokers, or "chippers," face health risks.[58,59]

Short-Term Effects

Smoking affects virtually every system in the body (Figure 9.6). When a smoker lights up, nicotine reaches the brain within 7 to 10 seconds, producing both sedating and stimulating effects. Adrenaline causes heart rate to increase by 10 to 20 beats per minute, blood pressure to rise by 5 to 10 points, and body temperature in the fingertips to decrease by a few degrees.[54]

The tar and toxins in tobacco smoke damage cilia, the hairlike structures in the bronchial passages that prevent toxins and debris from reaching delicate lung tissue. Researchers believe that chemicals in tar, such as benzopyrene, switch on a gene in lung cells that causes cell mutations that can lead to cancerous growth.[54,56] These chemicals may also damage a gene with a role in killing cancer cells.[54]

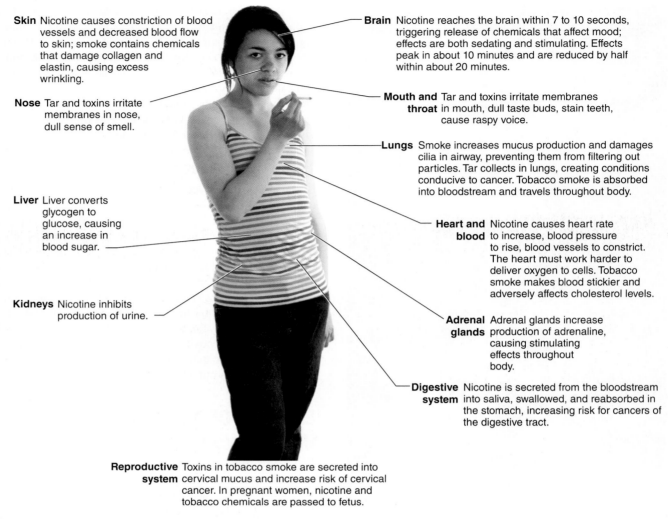

Skin Nicotine causes constriction of blood vessels and decreased blood flow to skin; smoke contains chemicals that damage collagen and elastin, causing excess wrinkling.

Nose Tar and toxins irritate membranes in nose, dull sense of smell.

Liver Liver converts glycogen to glucose, causing an increase in blood sugar.

Kidneys Nicotine inhibits production of urine.

Brain Nicotine reaches the brain within 7 to 10 seconds, triggering release of chemicals that affect mood; effects are both sedating and stimulating. Effects peak in about 10 minutes and are reduced by half within about 20 minutes.

Mouth and throat Tar and toxins irritate membranes in mouth, dull taste buds, stain teeth, cause raspy voice.

Lungs Smoke increases mucus production and damages cilia in airway, preventing them from filtering out particles. Tar collects in lungs, creating conditions conducive to cancer. Tobacco smoke is absorbed into bloodstream and travels throughout body.

Heart and blood Nicotine causes heart rate to increase, blood pressure to rise, blood vessels to constrict. The heart must work harder to deliver oxygen to cells. Tobacco smoke makes blood stickier and adversely affects cholesterol levels.

Adrenal glands Adrenal glands increase production of adrenaline, causing stimulating effects throughout body.

Digestive system Nicotine is secreted from the bloodstream into saliva, swallowed, and reabsorbed in the stomach, increasing risk for cancers of the digestive tract.

Reproductive system Toxins in tobacco smoke are secreted into cervical mucus and increase risk of cervical cancer. In pregnant women, nicotine and tobacco chemicals are passed to fetus.

figure 9.6 **Short-term effects of smoking on the body.**

Carbon monoxide in tobacco smoke affects the way smokers process the air they breathe. Normally, oxygen is carried through the bloodstream by hemoglobin, a protein in red blood cells. When carbon monoxide is present, it binds with hemoglobin and prevents red blood cells from carrying a full load of oxygen. Heavy smokers quickly become winded during physical activity because the cardiovascular system cannot effectively deliver oxygen to muscle cells.[54]

Athletes who smoke have to work harder than nonsmokers in the same physical activity. Respiration is immediately affected by smoking because of the increased carbon monoxide in the blood and decreased oxygen absorption. Nicotine constricts bronchial tubes, and lung function is compromised further by phlegm production. The smoker has less oxygen available for exercise as well as for recovery.

Long-Term Effects

The greatest health concerns associated with smoking are cardiovascular disease, cancer, and chronic lower respiratory diseases.

Cardiovascular Disease The increased heart rate, increased tension in the heart muscle, and constricted blood vessels caused by nicotine lead to hypertension (high blood pressure), which is both a disease in itself and a risk factor for other forms of heart disease, including coronary artery disease, heart attack, stroke, and peripheral vascular disease. Nicotine also makes blood platelets stickier, increasing the tendency of blood clots to form. It raises blood levels of low-density lipoproteins ("bad cholesterol") and decreases levels of high-density lipoproteins ("good cholesterol").[52,58–59] People who smoke more than one pack of cigarettes per day have three times the risk of nonsmokers for heart disease and congestive heart failure.[54] People who smoke only one to four cigarettes a day still double their risk of heart disease.[52]

Cancer Smoking is implicated in about 30 percent of all cancer deaths. It is the cause of 87 percent of deaths from lung cancer, and it is associated with cancers of the pancreas, kidney, bladder, breast, and cervix. Smoking and using smokeless tobacco play a major role in cancers of the mouth, throat, and esophagus. Oral cancers caused by smokeless tobacco tend to occur early in adulthood. The use of alcohol in combination with tobacco increases the risk of oral cancers.[60]

Why does smoking cause cancer? Usually, the immune system sends tumor-fighting white blood cells to attack and kill cancer cells. However, research suggests that poisons in cigarette smoke weaken the immune system's tumor-fighting cells, so cancer cells are able to multiply. Therefore, smoking not only causes cancer, it can block the immune system from effectively battling cancer.[52]

Chronic Obstructive Pulmonary Disease Smoking is a key factor in causing the diseases encompassed by the category *chronic obstructive pulmonary disease* (COPD, also called chronic lower respiratory disease). These are emphysema, chronic bronchitis, and asthma.

Emphysema is an abnormal condition of the lungs in which the alveoli (air sacs) become enlarged and their walls lose their elasticity. Late in the disease, it becomes increasingly difficult to breathe. Bronchitis is irritation and inflammation of the bronchi, the airway passages leading to the lungs. **Chronic bronchitis** is characterized by mucus secretion, cough, and increasing difficulty in breathing. **Asthma** is a respiratory disorder characterized by recurrent episodes of difficulty in breathing, wheezing, coughing, and thick mucus production.[57]

Almost as many people die from COPD today as from lung cancer.[52] Thousands more people live with COPD complications and discomfort that seriously compromise their quality of life.[58,59]

Other Health Effects Tobacco is associated with a variety of physical and health risks, including changes in the skin (wrinkling), increased risk during surgery, infertility and sexual dysfunction, periodontal disease, duodenal ulcers, osteoporosis, and cataracts. Smoking also reduces the effectiveness of some medications, particularly anti-anxiety drugs and penicillin.

Special Health Risks for Women

Increased smoking among women since the 1970s has led to an increase in rates of lung cancer, heart disease, and respiratory disease in women; deaths from lung cancer in women, for example, have increased by 400 percent. Women are also more vulnerable than men to the addictive properties of nicotine.[61] Scientists conjecture that this may be due to estrogen receptors.

In addition, smoking is associated with fertility problems in women, menstrual disorders, early menopause, and problems in pregnancy. Women who smoke during pregnancy are at increased risk for miscarriage, stillbirths, pre-term delivery, low birth weight in their infants, and perinatal death (infant death a few months before or after birth). Research indicates that infants are at three times higher risk for sudden infant death syndrome (SIDS) if their mother smoked during pregnancy.[52] Their risk continues to be higher after birth if they are exposed to environmental tobacco smoke.[61]

Special Health Risks for Men

The overall drop in smoking rates for men in the past three decades has led to a reduction of lung cancer deaths in men, but the greater use by men of other forms of tobacco—cigars, pipes, and smokeless tobacco—places them at higher risk for cancers of the mouth, throat, esophagus, and stomach. Like women, men who smoke experience problems with sexual function and fertility. Smoking adversely affects blood flow to the erectile tissue, leading to a higher incidence of erectile dysfunction (impotence); it also alters sperm shape, reduces sperm motility, and decreases the overall number of viable sperm.[52]

Special Health Risks for Ethnic Minority Groups

Mortality rates from several diseases associated with tobacco use, including cardiovascular disease, cancer, and SIDS, are higher for ethnic minority groups than for Whites.[7,54] For

emphysema
Abnormal condition of the lungs characterized by decreased respiratory function and increased shortness of breath.

chronic bronchitis
Respiratory disorder characterized by mucus secretion, cough, and increasing difficulty in breathing.

asthma
Respiratory disorder characterized by recurrent episodes of difficulty in breathing, wheezing, coughing, and thick mucus production.

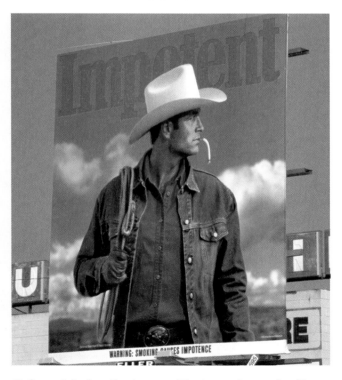

■ Sexual dysfunction is one of the lesser-known health effects of tobacco use for both men and women. This billboard is part of an antismoking campaign warning that "smoking causes impotence."

environmental
tobacco smoke (ETS)
Smoke from other people's tobacco products;
also called secondhand
smoke or passive
smoking.

example, African American men and women are more likely to die from lung cancer, heart disease, and stroke than are members of other ethnic groups, despite lower rates of tobacco use. The reasons for these disparities are conjectured to include genetics, access to health care, workplace exposures, smoking behaviors, and stress. Reductions in smoking among African Americans since the mid-1980s have led to a decline in lung cancer for African American men and a leveling off in African American women. Reduced smoking rates have also led to a decrease in lung cancer deaths in Hispanic men.[52]

Benefits of Quitting

Smokers greatly reduce their risk of many health problems when they quit. Health benefits begin immediately and become more significant the longer the individual stays smoke free. Respiratory symptoms associated with COPD, such as smoker's cough and excess mucus production, decrease quickly after quitting. Recovery from illnesses like colds and flu is more rapid, taste and smell return, and circulation improves.

In addition to reducing risk of diseases, quitting also increases longevity. Individuals who quit before the age of 50 cut their risk of dying within the next 15 years in half. Men who quit between ages 35 and 39 add an average of five years to their lifespan, and women who quit add three years. Even quitting after the age of 70 substantially lowers the risk of dying and improves the quality of life[62] (see Table 9.2).

Effects of Environmental Tobacco Smoke

You don't have to be a smoker to experience adverse health effects from tobacco smoke. Abundant evidence shows that inhaling the smoke from other people's tobacco products—called **environmental tobacco smoke (ETS)**, secondhand smoke, or passive smoking—has serious health consequences. Even 30 minutes of daily secondhand smoke exposure causes heart damage similar to that experienced by a habitual smoker. People who are exposed daily to secondhand smoke have a 30 percent higher rate of death and disease than nonsmokers.[59] About 4 in 10 nonsmokers are exposed to secondhand smoke. This exposure is higher for children than adults and higher for African Americans than for other groups. Nonsmoking Mexican Americans have the lowest secondhand exposure.[57,59] Nonsmokers are exposed to about 1 percent of the smoke that active smokers inhale.[57,59]

In 1993, the Environmental Protection Agency designated ETS a Class A carcinogen—an agent known to cause cancer in humans. In 2000, the U.S. Department of Health and Human Services added ETS to its list of known human

Table 9.2   When You Quit Smoking: Health Benefits Timeline

Immediately	You stop polluting the air with secondhand smoke; the air around you is no longer dangerous to children and adults.
20 minutes	Blood pressure decreases; pulse rate decreases; temperature of hands and feet increases.
12 hours	Carbon monoxide level in blood drops; oxygen level in blood increases to normal.
24 hours	Chance of heart attack decreases.
48 hours	Nerve endings start to regrow; exercise gets easier; senses of smell and taste improve.
72 hours	Bronchial tubes relax, making breathing easier; lung capacity increases.
2–12 weeks	Circulation improves; lung functioning increases up to 30 percent.
1–9 months	Fewer coughs, colds, and flu episodes; fatigue and shortness of breath decrease; lung function continues to improve.
1 year	Risk of smoking-related heart attack is cut by half.
5 years	Risk of dying from heart disease and stroke approaches that of a nonsmoker; risk of oral and esophageal cancers is cut by half.
10 years	Risk of dying from lung cancer is cut by half.
10–15 years	Life expectancy reaches that of a person who never smoked.

Source: Health Canada: On the Road to Quitting, www.hc-sc.gc.ca. Health Canada, 2008.

carcinogens. In 2006, the U.S. surgeon general stated that there is *no* safe level of ETS exposure.

Because of their smaller body size, infants and children are especially vulnerable to the effects of ETS. Children exposed to ETS experience 10 percent more colds, flu, and other acute respiratory infections than do those not exposed. ETS aggravates asthma symptoms and increases the risk of SIDS.[59] Some city governments have enacted local laws to protect children from secondhand smoke by banning smoking in apartment buildings and public housing projects, where rates of smoking tend to be much higher than they are among the general population. Some states, including California, Arkansas, and Louisiana, have moved to ban smoking in cars when children under the age of 6 are present.

QUITTING AND TREATMENT OPTIONS

Once a person becomes an established smoker, quitting is exceptionally difficult. Nearly four of every five smokers want to quit smoking. Only about 7 percent of smokers who quit are successfully abstaining a year later. Even among smokers who have lost a lung or undergone major heart surgery, only about 50 percent stop smoking for more than a few weeks.[62]

The good news is that smokers who quit for a year have an 85 percent chance of maintaining their abstinence. Those who make it to five years have a 97 percent chance of continued success. Most people don't succeed the first time they try to quit—in fact, the average number of attempts required for successful smoking cessation is seven—but many succeed on subsequent attempts.[62]

Treatment Programs to Quit Smoking

Treatment programs can be quite effective; 20 to 40 percent of smokers who enter good treatment programs are able to quit smoking for at least a year.[62] In some cases, smokers choose an intensive residential program; such a program might include daily group and individual therapy, stress reduction techniques, nutrition information, exercise, and a 12-step program similar to Alcoholics Anonymous.

Many programs encourage smokers to limit or eliminate their consumption of alcohol while they are quitting because alcohol interacts with nicotine in complex ways and can make quitting more difficult. Dieting is not recommended while trying to quit, despite the potential for weight gain. Combining exercise with smoking cessation appears to be the most effective approach to managing the potential for weight gain. Another element is social support and encouragement from important people in the smoker's life.

Medications to Quit Smoking

In **nicotine replacement therapy (NRT)**, a controlled amount of nicotine is administered, which gradually reduces daily nicotine use with minimal withdrawal symptoms.

Over-the-counter nicotine replacement products include the transdermal patch, lozenges, nicotine hand gel, and nicotine gum. Prescription-only products are sold under the brand name Nicotrol and include a nasal spray and an oral inhaler. The nicotine gel, sold under the name Nicogel, is marketed as a product for tobacco users who find themselves in situations where they can't smoke. A quick-evaporating hand gel made from tobacco extracts, Nicogel can reduce nicotine cravings for up to four hours.[63]

Although nicotine is addictive no matter how it is administered, NRT products contain none of the carcinogens or toxic gases found in cigarette smoke, so they are a safer form of nicotine delivery.[1] Using one or more of the NRT products doubles a person's chances of success in quitting. NRT is beneficial when used as part of a comprehensive physician-promoted cessation program. It can help control withdrawal symptoms and craving while the individual is learning new behavioral patterns.[63] Before taking a NRT product, you should consult your health care professional.

nicotine replacement therapy (NRT) Treatment for nicotine addiction in which a controlled amount of nicotine is administered to gradually reduce daily nicotine use with minimal withdrawal symptoms.

Other smoking cessation aids work not by replacing nicotine but by acting on the neurotransmitter receptors in the brain that are affected by nicotine. Bupropion is a prescription smoking cessation drug that acts in this way. It was approved in 2001 by the FDA and a low-dose version is marketed under the trade name Zyban. Bupropion is also prescribed at a higher dose as an antidepressant under the name Wellbutrin; Zyban and Wellbutrin should not be taken together. Bupropion is not approved by the FDA for use by people under the age of 18.

Varenicline (marketed in the United States as Chantix) is another smoking cessation drug that acts on neurotransmitter receptors. It was approved by the FDA in 2006. Clinical studies found that more than one in five people using varenicline quit smoking for at least one year, a significant improvement over rates for other smoking cessation drugs. This medication is not recommended for people under the age of 18.

Both Chantix and Zyban now carry black-box warnings due to the potential risks of psychiatric problems associated with their use, particularly depression and suicidal thinking. Black-box is the strictest drug warning imposed by the FDA. Additionally, the FDA mandated that these drugs include more prescription information on the drug label and new information for patients that explains the potential mental health risks and their symptoms.[64]

NicVax is an experimental nicotine vaccine that blocks the pleasurable effects of smoking. It works by eliciting the production of antibodies that bind with nicotine molecules in the bloodstream, preventing them from entering nicotine receptors in the brain. NicVax has not been approved by the FDA, but early studies have been encouraging.

■ Zyban and Chantix belong to a category of smoking cessation aids that work by acting on neurotransmitter receptors in the brain rather than replacing nicotine. However, both carry black-box warnings about potential side effects, such as depression and suicidal thinking.

Quitting on Your Own: Developing a Behavior Change Plan

Despite the hardships of withdrawal and the challenges of behavior change, quitting smoking is worth it, and the majority of people who quit do so on their own.

One approach is to develop a behavior change plan similar to the one described for cutting back on alcohol consumption. The first step is determining your readiness to quit. As discussed in Chapter 1, trying to change a behavior when you are not ready to change is pointless and counterproductive. It will only lead to failure and discouragement. Refer to the box, "Change to a New Behavior," in Chapter 1 (p. 12) for a quick evaluation of your own stage of change in regard to quitting smoking. If you are in the contemplation or action stage, you can develop a behavior change plan by following the steps described next.

Record and Analyze Your Smoking Patterns First, keep track of your smoking for two weeks, noting when, where, and with whom you smoke. Note the triggers or cues for smoking and your thoughts and feelings at the time. Then analyze your record to get a sense of your smoking patterns. Understanding these patterns can help you develop strategies for avoiding or dealing with the most challenging times and situations.

Establish Goals Set a specific date to quit. Choose a time when you will be relatively stress free—not during exams, for example—so that you will have the needed energy, attention, and focus. Experts recommend aiming for some time within two weeks of when you begin to plan. Plan to quit completely on that date; tapering off rarely works because it only prolongs withdrawal.

Prepare to Quit Your most important asset in quitting is your firm commitment to do so. At the same time, you can take specific, concrete steps to increase your chances of success. Consider these questions:

■ Why do you want to quit? Make a list of your reasons and post them in a prominent place.

■ If you tried to quit in the past, what helped and what didn't? Learn from your mistakes.

■ What situations are going to be the most difficult? How can you plan ahead to handle them? To the extent you can, reorganize your life to avoid situations in which you were accustomed to smoking.

■ What pleasures do you get from smoking? How can you get those pleasures from life-enhancing activities instead of smoking?

■ Who can help you? Tell your family and friends you are planning to quit and ask for their support. Find out the number of your state's telephone quitline.

Implement Your Plan Be prepared to experience symptoms of withdrawal and have a plan for handling them, even if it's just "toughing it out." Exercise will help ease cravings for nicotine and elevate your mood, so make sure you exercise daily. Exercise will also improve sleep and help limit weight gain. Drink plenty of fluids; they help flush nicotine from your body.[62]

Prevent Relapse Symptoms of nicotine withdrawal last from two to four weeks, although the most acute symptoms may last only a few days. See Table 9.3 for a summary of symptoms, their causes, and suggested relief strategies.

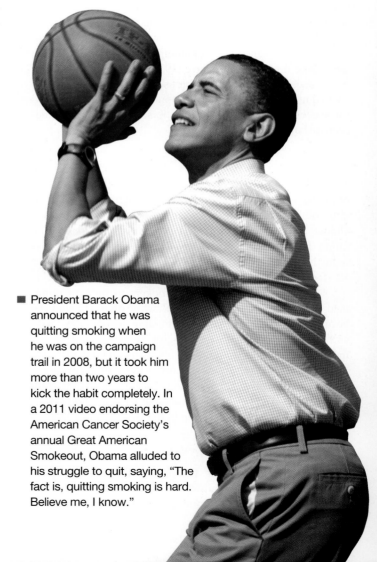

■ President Barack Obama announced that he was quitting smoking when he was on the campaign trail in 2008, but it took him more than two years to kick the habit completely. In a 2011 video endorsing the American Cancer Society's annual Great American Smokeout, Obama alluded to his struggle to quit, saying, "The fact is, quitting smoking is hard. Believe me, I know."

Table 9.3   What to Expect When You Quit

Symptom	Reason	Duration	Relief
Irritability	Body craves nicotine.	2–4 weeks	Take walks, hot baths; use relaxation techniques.
Fatigue	Nicotine is a stimulant.	2–4 weeks	Take naps; don't push yourself.
Insomnia	Nicotine affects brain waves.	2–4 weeks	Avoid caffeine after 6:00 p.m.; use relaxation techniques.
Coughing, dry throat, nasal drip	Body is getting rid of excess mucus.	A few days	Drink fluids; try cough drops.
Poor concentration	Nicotine is a stimulant, boosts concentration.	1–2 weeks	Get enough sleep; exercise; eat well.
Tightness in chest	Muscles are tense from nicotine craving or sore from coughing.	A few days	Use relaxation techniques, especially deep breathing; take hot baths.
Constipation, gas, stomach pain	Intestinal movement decreases for brief time.	1–2 weeks	Drink fluids; add fiber to diet (fruits, vegetables, whole grains).
Hunger	Nicotine craving can feel like hunger.	Up to several weeks	Drink water or low-calorie drinks; have low-calorie snacks on hand.
Headaches	Brain is getting more oxygen.	1–2 weeks	Drink water; use relaxation techniques.
Craving for a cigarette	Withdrawal from nicotine.	Most acute first few days; can recur for months	Wait it out; distract yourself; exercise; use relaxation techniques.

Source: www.quitnet.com.

Abstinence becomes easier with time, although it can still be difficult. Most relapses occur within the first three months.[62] There are two main lines of defense for maintaining prolonged abstinence. First, avoid high-risk situations, and second, develop coping mechanisms. Relapses are prompted by stress, anger, frustration, and depression.[62] Make sure you have strategies to deal with these feelings, whether relaxation techniques, exercise, social support, or cognitive techniques. Examples of cognitive techniques are reminding yourself of why you quit, thinking about the people you know who have quit, adjusting your self-image so that you think of yourself as an ex-smoker or a nonsmoker rather than a smoker, and congratulating yourself every time you beat an urge to smoke.

CONFRONTING THE TOBACCO CHALLENGE

Given the cost of tobacco use, why are the manufacture and sale of tobacco products legal in this country? The answer to this question is complex. Tobacco has been part of the economy of the country since colonial times, and today it is a multibillion-dollar industry with tremendous lobbying power and a huge impact on the nation's economic health. Many state economies depend on tobacco, and elected representatives from those states make sure tobacco interests are protected at the federal level. Because smoking is viewed as a personal decision, there are many constraints on the government's ability to protect citizens and consumers from the hazards of tobacco use. Still, significant inroads have been made in confronting the challenge posed by tobacco, and the tobacco industry is facing tremendous pressure on many fronts. Successes in the United States, however, have caused tobacco companies to turn to foreign markets to sell their products.

The Nonsmokers' Rights Movement and Legislative Battles

Beginning in the 1970s, a nonsmokers' rights movement took shape as a result of growing public awareness of the damage inflicted by tobacco. Smoking came to be seen as both a public health problem and a problematic behavior.[65]

By 2003, thousands of local laws and ordinances were in place across the country, creating smoke-free workplaces, restaurants, bars, and public places. Some tobacco control laws have also been passed at the state level. California banned smoking in workplaces in 1994 and smoking in bars in 1998. Since then, 28 states have banned smoking in all enclosed public places, but 10 states have no statewide smoking bans.[66] The federal government also has tobacco control measures in place, such as the ban on smoking on domestic airline flights.

Lawsuits and Court Settlements

In the 1990s, tobacco companies began to face class action suits, cases representing claims of injury by hundreds or thousands of smokers. In addition, states began suing tobacco companies for losses incurred by state health insurance funds used to pay for tobacco-related diseases.

These pressures led to the 1998 Master Settlement Agreement (MSA), in which the tobacco industry agreed to pay $206 billion to 46 states over a 25-year period in exchange for protection from future lawsuits by the states and other public entities. Other provisions of the MSA included a ban on billboard advertising and restrictions on advertising aimed at children. The settlement money from the MSA was to be used by the states primarily to fund tobacco education and prevention programs.[67]

Limiting Access to Tobacco

Access to tobacco can be limited by increasing cost, reducing physical availability, and regulating tobacco-marketing campaigns. When taxes on tobacco products are increased, raising their price, sales and use decline. Cigarette tax increases have been particularly effective in discouraging people from starting smoking.[67]

Physical availability of tobacco products is reduced when the laws restricting sales to minors are enforced. States are required to conduct random, unannounced inspections of places where tobacco is sold, and reports detailing results of these inspections must be submitted to the federal government each year.

FDA Regulation of Tobacco

The Family Smoking Prevention and Tobacco Control Act of 2009 (also known as the Tobacco Control Act) granted authority to the FDA to regulate tobacco products specifically for the protection of the public. Congress's goal was to decrease the number of Americans who die or who are harmed by tobacco products. As the box, "Product Warnings Versus Free Speech," describes, cigarette manufacturers have so far successfully challenged its requirement for larger and stronger warning labels on cigarette packs. Other key provisions include the following:[68–70]

- The advertising descriptors "light," "low," or "mild" can no longer be placed on tobacco packaging.

- Reinforcing state laws that already existed, federal law now officially prohibits cigarettes and smokeless tobacco products from being sold to anyone under 18 years of age.

- Cigarettes and smokeless tobacco can be sold in vending machines only in venues that prohibit entry to persons under 18 years.

- Retailers may not sell single cigarettes or packages containing fewer than 20 cigarettes, except in vending machines in venues that prohibit entry to persons under 18 years.

- Free samples of tobacco products are no longer permitted. Free samples of smokeless tobacco products are allowed only in adult-owned facilities in certain restricted situations.

- Free branded product tie-ins, such as T-shirts, and branded sponsorships of athletic or cultural events are prohibited.

Tobacco-Free College Campuses

A very important cultural issue is whether college campuses should become tobacco free unless there is a way to enforce that. Of the more than 6,000 college campuses in the United States, 1,182 college campuses are smoke-free or tobacco-free, according to Americans for Nonsmoker Rights.[71] The enforcement policies for tobacco-free campuses in many cases receive only lip-service attention. Policy that cannot be enforced has minimal impact. A growing number of colleges are considering issuing warnings and then fining repeat violators; money from fines would be used to support smoking cessation initiatives.[72]

Public Health Is Personal

Product Warnings Versus Free Speech

Would you buy a product if the packaging was designed to scare you, disgust you, or otherwise turn you off? Tobacco companies are crying foul over new cigarette labeling requirements that give more prominence to graphic antismoking images than to their brand name. The FDA says that's exactly the point.

Although cigarette smoking has declined from its peak in the 1960s and about half of all Americans who ever smoked have quit, about one in five Americans still smokes. So Congress passed the Family Smoking and Tobacco Control Act of 2009, authorizing the FDA to develop new warning labels that would convey the health risks of tobacco use in more graphic form.

In June 2011, the FDA released nine proposed graphic images selected from a field of 36 through public comment and feedback. The images have been described as disturbing, if not gruesome, and deliberately so, because upsetting images have been shown to be more likely to cause behavior change. They include images of a man smoking through a tracheotomy hole in his throat ("Warning: Cigarettes are addictive"), a cadaver with a heart surgery scar ("Warning: Smoking can kill you"), diseased lungs next to healthy lungs ("Warning: Cigarettes cause fatal lung disease"), and stained teeth and a cancerous mouth sore ("Warning: Cigarettes cause cancer"), among others. The law required that, beginning in the fall of 2012, one of the images appear on the top half of the front and rear of the cigarette package, effectively making the image more prominent than the cigarette brand itself.

In response, four of the top five U.S. tobacco manufacturers successfully sued the federal government, claiming the labels violated their first amendment rights to free speech. They asserted that as manufacturers of a lawful product, they should not have to use their own packaging to convey a message urging consumers to avoid their product. They said the images go beyond providing information to unfairly appeal to buyers' emotions, and they claimed the law would cost them millions in new equipment to print and rotate the messages.

A federal judge hearing the case in August 2011 upheld the labeling requirements, but in November 2011 and August 2012, appellate courts ruled that the images unconstitutionally compel speech and that there was little evidence that they would reduce smoking rates. The case may ultimately go to the Supreme Court.

The FDA estimated that the labels would reduce the number of smokers by 213,000 in 2013, with smaller reductions through 2031. If true, there would be enormous savings—tobacco addiction costs the U.S. economy nearly $200 billion each year in health care costs and lost productivity.

But changing a person's health behavior is difficult and complex. Studies of warning labels on alcohol and tobacco products have produced conflicting results, showing marginal effectiveness at best. Critics of the new labels say the government is ignoring the obvious conclusion that warning labels, no matter how graphic, simply don't deter people from smoking if they want to smoke. Advocates of the labels say that every law, regulation, and educational campaign contribute to the ultimate goal of a tobacco-free nation. In the meantime, the battle between the government and the tobacco industry over this formidable public health challenge rages on.

Canada introduced pictured-based health warnings on cigarette packages in 2001. Since 2001, warning labels have become more graphic and extensive on the front and back of cigarette packages; see www.tobaccolabels.ca/countries/canada for examples. Research of graphic exterior warnings led to a sharp decrease in smoking rates in Canada. The U.S. Food and Drug Administration's 2011 study of graphic warning labels, however, conceded that there was no evidence to support a reduction of smoking rates from graphic labels in the United States. The FDA impact model study was a key factor in the 2012 decision by a federal district court to strike down mandated graphic health warning labels on cigarette packages. One study published after the district court decision, however, suggested that the 2011 FDA study model significantly underestimated the potential impact of graphic smoking health warning labels in the United States. This study estimated that the potential smoking rate reduction would be 33 to 53 times higher than the estimated FDA model projections. Results from this new analysis may lead to appeals within the federal district courts or the Supreme Court to re-implement graphic health warning labels on cigarette packages. More than 60 countries have implemented graphic warning or passed legislation to do so.

What do you think? Would the larger warnings with photos change American attitudes about smoking, motivate smokers to quit, and discourage youth from smoking?

connect
ACTIVITY

Sources: "Do Warning Labels on Alcoholic Beverages Deter Alcohol Abuse," by R. C. Engs, 2011, www.indiana.edu~engs/articles/warn.html; "Big Tobacco Sues Feds Over Graphic Warnings on Cigarette Labels," by J. Collins, 2011, www.msnbc.msn.com/id/44171861/ns/health-cancer/t/big-tobacco-sues-feds-over-graphic-warnings-cigarette-labels/#.Tw; "US Judge Blocks Graphic Warnings on Cigarettes," Medicalxpress, 2011, http://medicalxpress.com/news/2011-11-blocks-graphic-cigarettes.html; "Graphic Warning Labels on Cigarette Packs Could Lead to 8.6 Million Fewer Smokers in US," summary of study from University of Waterloo, November 25, 2013, *Science Daily,* www.sciencedaily.com/releases/2013/11/131125121904.htm.

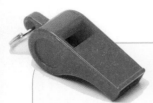

You Make the Call

Should the Legal Limit for Driving Under the Influence Be Lowered to 0.05 BAC?

The National Transportation Safety Board (NSTB) in 2013 proposed that the legal driving-under-the influence (DUI) threshold for blood alcohol content (BAC) should be lowered from 0.08 to 0.05 in the United States. This recommendation was announced on the 25th anniversary of one of the deadliest traffic accidents in the United States: on May 14, 1988, an intoxicated driver drove on the wrong side of the road in Kentucky crashing into a bus, killing 27 people, and injuring more than 30. Twenty-four of the victims were children returning from a church outing at an amusement park.

According to the NSTB, about 10,000 people die each year from alcohol-related crashes, so lowering the legal threshold to 0.05 may save 500 to 800 lives each year. More than 100 countries have legal threshold laws for DUI of 0.05 or lower. The NSTB emphasizes that these countries have experienced a significant decrease in alcohol-related traffic deaths.

However, the NTSB does not have the power to implement its recommendation. Congressional, as well as federal and state agency, action is needed. Passage of a 0.05 legal threshold for DUI will not be easy. In essence, a 0.05 threshold would make driving after moderate consumption of alcohol illegal for many people. A 180-pound man will usually reach 0.05 BAC after four drinks in an hour, but a 120-pound woman reaches this level after one drink, and a 160-pound man after two drinks. Critics of the NSTB 0.05 proposal have referred to it as the "one drink limit."

Not surprisingly, the National Restaurant Association (NRA) and the American Beverage Institute (ABI) argue that federal and state efforts should be directed at offenders with higher BAC levels and with multiple convictions. Both organizations consider the NSTB 0.05 recommendation as "ludicrous" and the needless criminalization of a perfectly responsible behavior. Surprisingly, Mothers Against Drunk Driving (MADD) does not support it either. MADD emphasizes that it took years to reduce the legal threshold from 0.10 to 0.08 and argues that a 0.05 BAC threshold would not be as effective as the further use of technologies such as ignition interlock devices.

The NSTB has not been deterred by the torrent of criticism over its 0.05 BAC legal threshold. The Insurance Institute for Highway Safety, for example, estimates that lowering the BAC from 0.08 would save over 7,000 lives each year. This estimate is drawn from research on motor behavior at different BAC levels. According to one study, even a BAC of 0.01 is capable of producing a "buzz" that can increase the odds of a deadly accident. (A BAC of 0.01 for many adults is about half a beer in an hour.) Drivers who are buzzed are more likely to speed and less likely to use a seat belt. The bottom line is that alcohol in any amount is dangerous for the driver.

So, what do you think? Should the legal threshold for BAC and driving be lowered to 0.05?

Pros

- Studies have found that accidents are about 37 percent more severe even when alcohol is barely detectable in a driver's blood.
- NTSB studies suggest that a driver with a BAC of 0.05 is 38 percent more likely to be in a crash than a driver who had not consumed alcohol. In contrast, a driver with a BAC of 0.08 percent is 169 percent more likely to be involved in a vehicle crash than a sober driver.
- Most people begin to feel the effects of alcohol when their BAC is between 0.03 and 0.59. The brain's ability to handle multiple tasks is impaired and severely compromises safe driving.
- The idea is prevention. If reducing the BAC from 0.08 to 0.05 saves only one life, then this change will be worth it.

Cons

- Prevention efforts should be on hard-core offenders. Lowering the BAC limit is nothing more than government intrusion on social drinkers.
- Having two glasses of wine or two beers at dinner should not make someone a criminal when they drive home. This amounts to law enforcement harassment.
- The focus should be on a comprehensive plan to prevent drunk driving. Increasing law enforcement visibility, driver education, and incarceration for hard-core offenders is needed and should not be overshadowed by an effort to lower the BAC that will experience stiff state opposition.
- Many states already have zero-tolerance laws that prohibit alcohol at any level for drivers under the age of 21 or people convicted of a DUI.

connect ACTIVITY

Sources: "Proposal to Reduce Legal Driving Limit to 0.05% Attracts Wide-Ranging Opposition," from *Shanken News Daily,* May 16, 2013, www.shankennewsdaily.com/index.php/2013/05/16/5867/proposal-to-reduce-legal-driving-limit-to-0-05-bac-attracts-wide-ranging-opposition/; "Blood Alcohol Concentration," from In the Know Zone,. n.d., http://inthe knowzone.com/substance-abuse-topics/alcohol/bac.html.

In Review

Why do people drink, and why do some people develop problems with alcohol?

People ingest psychoactive substances like alcohol for a wide range of reasons, from wanting to enhance positive feelings to wanting to numb negative feelings. A complex interplay of individual and environmental factors leads some people who drink to develop problems with alcohol, including alcohol dependence. Binge drinking, or heavy episodic drinking, is common on college campuses because of easy access to alcohol and social norms.

What are alcohol's effects on the body?

After alcohol is drunk, it goes to the stomach, where a small amount is absorbed. The rest goes into the small intestine, where it is absorbed into the bloodstream. The heart pumps the alcohol in the blood throughout the body. In the liver, it is metabolized at the rate of about one drink an hour. In the brain, it impairs cognitive and motor functioning. Acute alcohol intoxication can lead to death.

What are the health risks of alcohol consumption?

Over the long term, alcohol consumption can cause cardiovascular disease, liver disease, cancer, brain damage, and unhealthy changes in body weight and food absorption. Alcohol use is also associated with high-risk sexual activity, violence, injury, and suicide. On the other hand, scientists have found some health benefits to moderate alcohol consumption for middle-aged and older adults.

What are treatment approaches for problem drinking?

Treatment options for alcohol-related disorders include brief interventions, inpatient and outpatient treatment programs, self-help programs such as AA, and harm reduction approaches, which range from controlled drinking to laws regulating the drinking age and driving while drunk.

What kinds of actions can one take to reduce harm caused by alcohol?

You can assess your personal risk for alcohol dependence and develop a behavior change plan if you are at risk. You can also be an advocate for abstinence and responsible drinking on your campus.

Who smokes, and why is it a problem?

About 19 percent of the U.S. adult population are smokers, with higher rates of smoking among men than women and among college students than the general population. Tobacco use is the leading preventable cause of death in the United States.

What are the main tobacco products?

Cigarettes are by far the most commonly used tobacco products, trailed by cigars and cigarillos, pipes, and smokeless (chewing) tobacco. Other products (e.g., tobacco for water pipes, e-cigarettes) are marketed as safer alternatives, but nearly all contain nicotine, and, when burned, produce thousands of toxic substances. Electronic cigarettes deliver nicotine through inhaled vapor but still contain potentially harmful chemicals.

What are tobacco's effects on health?

Smoking affects every system in the body from the brain to the reproductive system. Tobacco is a causal factor in cancer, heart disease, respiratory diseases, and numerous other debilitating conditions. Smoking is the single greatest preventable cause of illness and premature death in the United States. Secondhand smoke, or environmental tobacco smoke, has serious health consequences for the people around the smoker. Smokers greatly reduce their risk of many health problems when they quit.

What treatment options are available for quitting tobacco?

Quitting smoking is very difficult, and smokers try an average of seven times before they succeed. Aids for quitting include treatment programs, medications, and behavior change plans. Some withdrawal symptoms last for only a day or two; others can last for a month.

What are various governmental and public health approaches to the tobacco challenge?

Over the last four decades, the nonsmokers' rights movement has encouraged the passage of laws to limit the use of tobacco in public places. Lawsuits have been won against tobacco companies. Cigarette taxes have been increased, and bans on selling cigarettes to minors have become stricter.

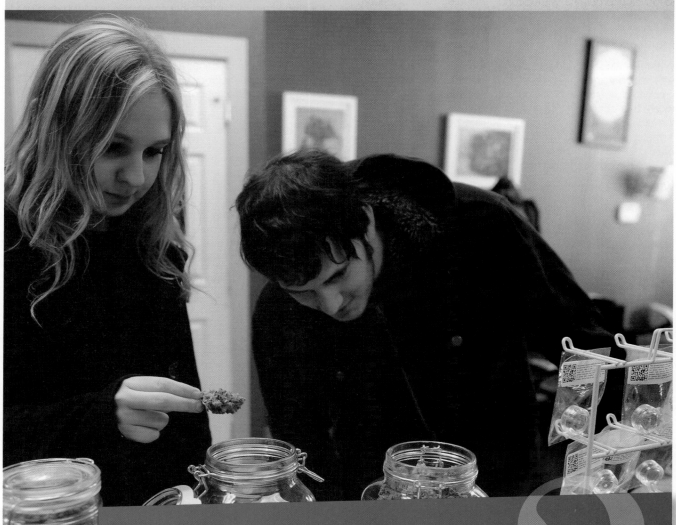

10 Drugs

Ever Wonder...

- which drugs have the highest potential for physical and psychological dependence?

- why some people can't seem to stop using drugs?

- how to know if someone is starting to have a problem with drugs?

ike alcohol, drugs have a pervasive presence in American life. We use them for headaches, insomnia, anxiety, stress—and some of us use them for fun. In 2012, an estimated 23.9 million Americans aged 12 or older were current users of illicit (illegal) drugs, representing 9.2 percent of the population aged 12 or older (Figure 10.1). Illicit drugs include marijuana, hashish, cocaine, heroin, hallucinogens, and prescription medications used for non-medical reasons.

Drugs are used by different people for different reasons. Many people take drugs as a recreational activity—to alter their state of consciousness, to relax and feel more sociable, to experience euphoria, to get high. Some people take drugs to rebel, and others take them to fit in. For some people, drug use is a way to cope with stress, pain, or adversity, and for some, it is a way of life, a behavior they can no longer control.

WHO USES? PATTERNS OF ILLICIT DRUG USE

Rates of illicit drug use vary by age, gender, race and ethnicity, education, employment status, and geographical region (see Figure 10.2 and the box, "Rates of Current (Past Month) Illicit Drug Use by Geographical Region and Urban and Rural Areas, 2012"). Among Americans aged 12 or older, more than 47 percent report having used an illicit drug in their lifetime.

The most commonly used drug is marijuana, with more than 18.9 million current users among Americans aged 12 or older, up from 14.5 million in 2007. The number of people using marijuana daily or almost daily increased from

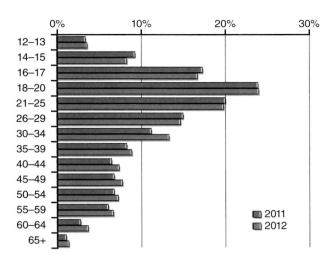

figure 10.2 **Illicit drug use by age, 2011 and 2012.**
These statistics represent people aged 12 and older who reported using drugs within the last month at the time of being surveyed.
Source: Substance Abuse and Mental Health Services Administration, *Results from the 2012 National Survey on Drug Use and Health: Summary of National Findings,* NSDUH Series H-46, HHS Publication No. (SMA) 13-4795, Figure 2.5, Rockville, MD: SAMHSA, 2013.

5.1 million in 2007 to 7.6 million in 2012. There is also a substantial misuse of psychotherapeutics (prescription-type drugs)—including pain relievers, tranquilizers, stimulants, and sedatives—by an estimated 5 million Americans. It appears illicit drug use often starts with marijuana, but pain relievers are the drug of first use for a substantial number of individuals.

Among young adults aged 18 to 25, the most commonly used drugs are marijuana, prescription-type drugs used nonmedically, hallucinogens, and cocaine. Over a longer time frame, prescription drug abuse stands out as a relatively recent phenomenon among college students. One survey found that the percentage of college students who abuse the following types of prescription drugs increased dramatically over the 12-year period from 1993 to 2005:[1]

- Pain relievers (e.g., OxyContin, Vicodin, Percocet): use increased by 343 percent.

- Stimulants (e.g., Ritalin, Adderall): use increased by 93 percent.

- Tranquilizers (e.g., Xanax, Valium): use increased by 450 percent.

- Sedatives (e.g., Nembutal, Seconal): use increased by 225 percent.

It appears that most individuals get their prescription drugs from a friend or relative for free and that this friend or relative had obtained the drugs from a single doctor (Figure 10.3).[2]

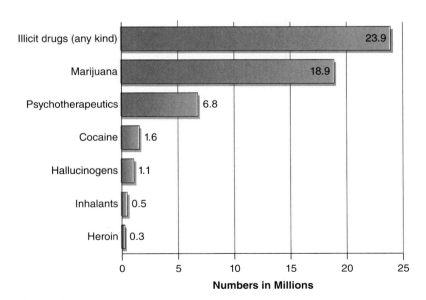

figure 10.1 **Illicit drug use in past month among persons aged 12 or older: percentages, 2012.**
Source: Substance Abuse and Mental Health Services Administration, *Results from the 2012 National Survey on Drug Use and Health: Summary of National Findings,* NSDUH Series H-46, HHS Publication No. (SMA) 13-4795, Figure 2.1, Rockville, MD: SAMHSA, 2013.

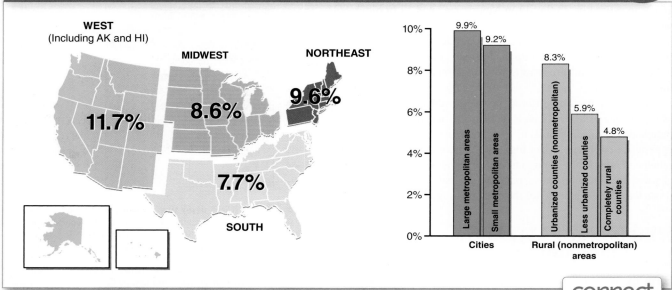

Rates of Current (Past Month) Illicit Drug Use, by Geographical Region and Urban and Rural Areas, 2012

WEST (Including AK and HI)

MIDWEST

NORTHEAST

11.7%

8.6%

9.6%

7.7%

SOUTH

10%
9.9%
9.2%
8%
8.3%
6%
5.9%
4.8%
4%
2%
0%

Large metropolitan areas
Small metropolitan areas
Urbanized counties (nonmetropolitan)
Less urbanized counties
Completely rural counties

Cities   **Rural (nonmetropolitan) areas**

Source: Substance Abuse and Mental Health Services Administration, *Results from the 2012 National Survey on Drug Use and Health: Summary of National Findings,* NSDUH Series H-46, HHS Publication No. (SMA) 13-4795, pp. 26, 27, Rockville, MD: SAMHSA, 2013.

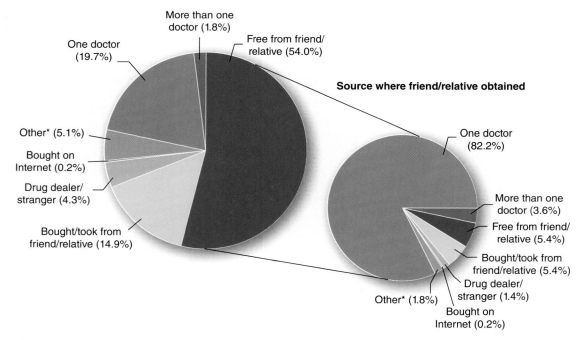

Source where user obtained

More than one doctor (1.8%)

One doctor (19.7%)

Free from friend/ relative (54.0%)

Source where friend/relative obtained

Other* (5.1%)

Bought on Internet (0.2%)

Drug dealer/ stranger (4.3%)

Bought/took from friend/relative (14.9%)

One doctor (82.2%)

More than one doctor (3.6%)

Free from friend/ relative (5.4%)

Bought/took from friend/relative (5.4%)

Drug dealer/ stranger (1.4%)

Other* (1.8%)

Bought on Internet (0.2%)

figure 10.3 **Source of pain relievers for most recent nonmedical use among past-year users aged 12 and older, 2011–2012.**

*The "Other" category includes the sources "Wrote Fake Prescription," "Stole from Doctor's Office/Clinic/Hospital/Pharmacy," and "Some Other Way."

Source: Substance Abuse and Mental Health Services Administration, *Results from the 2012 National Survey on Drug Use and Health: Summary of National Findings,* NSDUH Series H-46, HHS Publication No. (SMA) 13-4795, Figure 2.16, Rockville, MD: SAMHSA, 2013.

Consumer Clipboard

Understanding Drug Side Effects and Interactions

A side effect is an undesirable or unexpected secondary effect of a particular drug, whether prescription or over the counter (OTC). Some side effects are common and mild (such as constipation or an upset stomach), and others are severe and require immediate medical attention (such as chest pain or blurred vision). If you aren't expecting a side effect, or if a side effect is unpleasant, it may cause you to stop taking the medication before it's had a chance to work, so it is important to be aware of side effects at the outset.

Medications can also have unwanted interactions with foods or other medications, amplifying the effects of another drug or interfering with them.

Prescription drugs include a required patient insert that includes information about side effects, and OTC drugs carry a "Drug Facts" label. The FDA sets the format for OTC labels. You can get information about potential side effects and drug interactions from several parts of the label. Use the following tips to make sure you are using your OTC medications safely.

- Note the active ingredients, and don't take more than one medication with the same active ingredient; doing so could cause you to consume too much of that ingredient.

- Ask if it's safe to consume food or beverages containing grapefruit juice with the medication; grapefruit juice contains an enzyme that can raise levels of some medications in the blood.

- Ask a doctor or pharmacist before use if you are taking tranquilizers or sedatives.

- Talk with your doctor and pharmacist about all the drugs you take, whether prescription, OTC, or dietary supplement (vitamins, herbals).

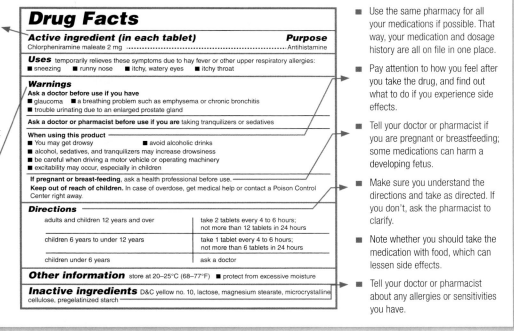

- Use the same pharmacy for all your medications if possible. That way, your medication and dosage history are all on file in one place.

- Pay attention to how you feel after you take the drug, and find out what to do if you experience side effects.

- Tell your doctor or pharmacist if you are pregnant or breastfeeding; some medications can harm a developing fetus.

- Make sure you understand the directions and take as directed. If you don't, ask the pharmacist to clarify.

- Note whether you should take the medication with food, which can lessen side effects.

- Tell your doctor or pharmacist about any allergies or sensitivities you have.

Source: "OTC Drug Facts Label," U.S. Food and Drug Administration, 2009, www.fda.gov/Drugs/ResourcesForYou/Consumers/ucm143551.htm.

WHAT IS A DRUG?

A **drug** is a substance other than food that affects the structure or the function of the body through its chemical action. Alcohol, caffeine, aspirin, and nicotine are all drugs, as are amphetamines, cocaine, hallucinogens, sedatives, and inhalants. The drugs discussed here are *psychoactive drugs*—substances that cause changes in brain chemistry and alter consciousness, perception, mood, and thought. This state is known as *intoxication.*

Psychoactive drugs are used for both medical and non-medical (recreational) purposes. For example, Ritalin, a central nervous system (CNS) stimulant with effects similar to those of amphetamine, is prescribed to treat hyperactivity in children—a medical use. Cocaine, another CNS stimulant, is used recreationally to cause a burst of pleasurable sensations and to increase energy and endurance—a

nonmedical use. When a medical drug is used for nonmedical (recreational) purposes, or when a drug has no medical uses, it is referred to as a *drug of abuse.*

All drugs have the potential to be toxic, that is, poisonous, dangerous, or deadly. Central nervous system depressants, such as alcohol, barbiturates, tranquilizers, and opium-derived drugs such as morphine and heroin can cause death if used in sufficient amounts to suppress vital functions like respiration. At the other extreme, CNS stimulants such as cocaine can cause sudden death by speeding up heart rate, elevating blood pressure, and accelerating other body functions to the point that systems are overwhelmed and collapse. Also see the box, "Understanding Drug Side Effects and Interactions."

drug
Substance other than food that affects the structure or function of the body through its chemical action.

The American Psychiatric Association (APA) uses the term **substance** to refer to a drug of abuse, a medication, or a toxin.[3] In this chapter, we use the terms *drug* and *substance* interchangeably.

Types of Drugs

Drugs are classified in several different ways. A basic distinction is between legal drugs and illicit (illegal) drugs. *Legal drugs* include medications prescribed by physicians, over-the-counter (OTC) medications, and herbal remedies.

Drugs developed for medical purposes, whether OTC or prescription, are referred to as **pharmaceutical drugs**. Prescription drugs can be ordered only by a specific health care provider. They must undergo a rigorous testing and approval process by the Food and Drug Administration (FDA). Today, the pharmaceutical industry is one of the largest and most profitable industries in the United States, with sales well over $100 billion a year. Despite these astronomical sales, however, more than half of all prescriptions are filled with only 200 drugs.

OTC medications include common remedies for headache, pain, colds, coughs, allergies, stomach upset, and other mild symptoms and complaints. Herbal remedies are usually botanical in origin; there are hundreds of substances in this group. At this time, the federal government's Food and Drug Administration does not regulate herbal remedies the way it regulates the development and approval of pharmaceutical drugs. The FDA does have the power to remove an herbal remedy from the market if it has proven harmful. This was the case with the dietary supplement ephedra, a stimulant used for weight loss and body building, which the FDA banned after it was linked with more than 100 deaths from heart attack and stroke.

Illicit drugs are generally viewed as harmful, and it is illegal to possess, manufacture, sell, or use them. Many prescription drugs are legal when obtained through a physician but illicit when manufactured or sold outside of the regulated medical system. Tobacco and alcohol are illegal drugs in the hands of minors, but they are usually not considered illicit because of their widespread availability to adults.

substance
Drug of abuse, a medication, or a toxin; the term is used interchangeably with *drug*.

pharmaceutical drugs
Drugs developed for medical purposes, whether over the counter or prescription.

illicit drugs
Drugs that are unlawful to possess, manufacture, sell, or use.

drug misuse
Use of prescription drugs for purposes other than those for which they were prescribed or in greater amounts than prescribed, or the use of nonprescription drugs or chemicals for purposes other than those intended by the manufacturer.

drug abuse
Use of a substance in amounts, situations, or a manner such that it causes problems, or greatly increases the risk of problems, for the user or for others.

Drug Misuse and Abuse

There are different ways to define problematic use of drugs. The term **drug misuse** generally refers to the use of prescription drugs for purposes other than those for which they were prescribed or in greater amounts than prescribed. The term can also refer to the use of nonprescription drugs such as Tylenol or chemicals such as glues, paints, or solvents for any purpose other than that intended by the manufacturer.

The term **drug abuse** generally means the use of a substance in an amount, a situation, or a manner that causes problems, or greatly increases the risk of problems, for the user or for others. The APA's most recent version of the *Diagnostic and Statistical Manual of Mental Disorders,* DSM-5,[3] defines *substance use disorders* as a number of cognitive, behavioral and physiological symptoms that persist even as the individual experiences a number of significant life-changing substance-related problems. These include changes in brain circuitry that may continue after detoxification and can cause repeated relapses and drug cravings. Unlike the DSM-IV-TR, the DSM-5 does not separate substance use disorders and dependence and includes a description of criteria for a diagnosis of substance use disorder with criteria for intoxication and withdrawal, while adding new criteria such as craving drugs. For professionals, these distinctions are important for diagnostic and treatment purposes, but many individuals will continue to talk about drug addiction, withdrawal symptoms, and tolerance.

For professionals, these distinctions are important for diagnostic and treatment purposes, but many organizations and individuals will continue to view substance use problems in terms of drug abuse, addiction, dependence, withdrawal symptoms, and tolerance. The federal National Institute of Drug Abuse (NIDA) defines any use of an illicit drug as *drug abuse* and defines *addiction* as a chronic, relapsing brain disease characterized by compulsive drug seeking and use, despite harmful consequences.[4] Significant adverse consequences is a key component of many definitions of abuse, addiction, and substance abuse disorders.

As described in Chapter 2, the main two indicators of physiological dependence are the development of *tolerance,* or reduced sensitivity to the effects of the drug, and *withdrawal,* or uncomfortable feelings when drug use stops. Withdrawal symptoms are different for different drugs. For example, withdrawal from amphetamines is marked by intense feelings of fatigue and depression, increased appetite and weight gain, and sometimes suicidal thinking. Withdrawal from heroin causes nausea, vomiting, sweating, diarrhea, yawning, and insomnia.

EFFECTS OF DRUGS ON THE BODY

All psychoactive drugs have an effect on the brain, and they reach the brain by way of the bloodstream. Like alcohol, some psychoactive drugs are consumed by mouth, but other routes of administration are used as well.

Routes of Administration

Psychoactive drugs can be taken by several methods: orally (by mouth), injection, inhalation, application to the mucous membranes, or application to the skin. The speed and efficiency with which a drug acts are strongly influenced by the route of administration (Table 10.1 shows these routes in the order of their speed).

Oral Most drugs are taken orally. Although this is the simplest way to take a drug, it is the most complicated way for the drug to enter the bloodstream. A drug in the digestive tract must be able to withstand stomach acid and digestive enzymes and not be deactivated by food before it is absorbed. Drugs taken orally are absorbed into the bloodstream in the small intestine.

Injection The injection route uses a hypodermic syringe to deliver the drug directly into the bloodstream (intravenous injection), to deposit it in a muscle mass (intramuscular injection), or to deposit it under the upper layer of skin (subcutaneous injection). With an intravenous (IV) injection ("mainlining"), the drug enters the bloodstream directly; onset of action is more rapid than with oral administration or other means of injection.

Inhalation The inhalation route is used for smoking tobacco, marijuana, and crack cocaine and for "huffing" gasoline, paints, and other inhalants. An inhaled drug enters the bloodstream quickly because capillary walls are very accessible in the lungs.

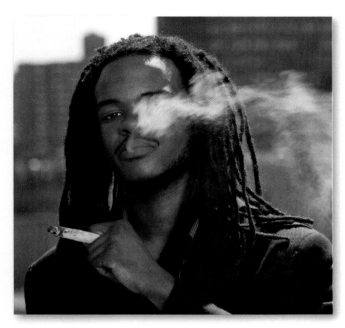

■ The most commonly used illicit drug in the United States is marijuana. More than 14 million Americans are current users.

Application to Mucous Membranes Application of a drug to the mucous membranes results in rapid absorption because the mucous membranes are moist and have a rich blood supply. People who snort cocaine absorb the

Table 10.1 Routes of Administration

Route	Time to Reach Brain	Drug Example	Potential Adverse Effects

Inhalation
  Smoking
  Huffing
	7–10 seconds	Marijuana
		Crack cocaine
		Tobacco
		Inhalants
			Irritation of lungs

Injection
  Intravenous
  Intramuscular
  Subcutaneous
	
	15–30 seconds
	3–5 minutes
	5–7 minutes
		Heroin
		Cocaine
		Methamphetamine
			Danger of overdose
			Collapsed veins
			Infection at injection site
			Blood infection
			Transmission of HIV, hepatitis C, and other pathogens

Mucous membranes Snorting	3–15 minutes	Cocaine Methamphetamine Heroin	Irritation or destruction of tissue Difficulty controlling dose
Oral ingestion Eating, drinking	20–30 minutes	Alcohol Pills	Vomiting

Skin contact
  Dermal
  Transdermal
	1–7 days	Oils, ointments
		Nicotine patch
			Irritation of skin

drug quickly into the bloodstream through the mucous membranes of the nose. People who chew tobacco absorb nicotine through the mucous membranes lining the mouth. Rectal and vaginal suppositories are also absorbed quickly, although these methods are less commonly used.

Application to the Skin Application to the skin is a less common method of drug administration. Most drugs are not well absorbed through the skin. *Dermal absorption* occurs when an oil or ointment is rubbed on the skin, producing a topical, or local, effect. *Transdermal absorption* occurs when a longer-lasting application produces a systemic effect, such as when a patch delivers estrogen or nicotine. The advantage of the transdermal route is that it affords slow, steady absorption over many hours, producing stable levels of the drug in the blood.

Factors Influencing the Effects of Drugs

The effect a drug has on a person depends on a number of variables, including the characteristics of the drug, the characteristics of the person, and the characteristics of the situation.

The drug's chemical composition may speed up body processes or slow them down, produce a mild high or acute anxiety, or cause disorientation or hallucinations. These effects also depend on how much of the drug is taken, how often it is taken, and how recently it was taken. In addition, if a person has taken other drugs, the interactions of the chemicals can influence outcomes, such as when one CNS depressant intensifies the effect of another.

Characteristics of the person include age, gender, body weight and mass, physical condition, mood, experience with the drug, and expectations. Generally speaking, the same amount of a drug has less effect on a 180-pound man than on a 120-pound woman.

The effects of drugs are also influenced by the characteristics of the situation or the environment. Taking a drug at home while relaxing with friends may produce a different experience than will taking the same drug at a crowded, noisy bar or club, surrounded by strangers.

pleasure and reward circuit
Pathway in the brain involving three structures—the ventral tegmental area, the nucleus accumbens, and the prefrontal cortex—associated with drug dependence.

endorphins
Natural chemicals in the brain that block pain during stressful or painful experiences.

Effects of Drugs on the Brain

What accounts for the phenomenon of drug dependence? Scientists studying the effects of drugs on the brain have found that many addictive drugs, including cocaine, marijuana, opioids, alcohol, and nicotine, act on neurons in three brain structures—the ventral tegmental area (VTA) in the midbrain, the nucleus accumbens, and the prefrontal cortex.[5] Neurons in these

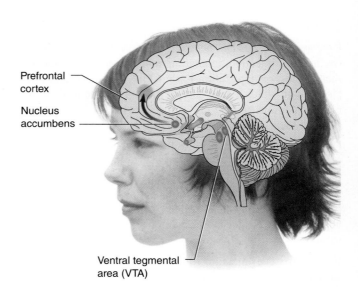

Prefrontal cortex

Nucleus accumbens

Ventral tegmental area (VTA)

figure 10.4   The pleasure and reward circuit in the brain.

three structures form a pathway referred to as the **pleasure and reward circuit** (Figure 10.4).

Under normal circumstances, this network of neurons is responsible for the feelings of satisfaction and pleasure when a physical, emotional, or survival need is met (e.g., hunger, thirst, bonding, and sexual desire). When it is activated, the circuit powerfully reinforces the behavior that satisfied the need (e.g., eating), sending the message to "do it again." Neurons in the VTA increase production of dopamine, a neurotransmitter associated with feelings of pleasure. The VTA neurons pass messages to clusters of neurons in the nucleus accumbens, where the release of dopamine produces intense pleasure, and to the prefrontal cortex, where thinking, motivation, and behavior are affected.

Addictive psychoactive drugs activate this same pathway, causing an enormous surge in levels of dopamine and the associated feelings of pleasure. The nucleus accumbens sends the message to repeat the behavior that produced these feelings, and using an addictive drug begins to take on as much importance as normal survival behaviors. Because the drug produces such huge surges of dopamine, the brain responds by reducing normal dopamine production. Eventually, the person is unable to experience any pleasure, even from the drug, due to the disrupted dopamine system. Parts of the brain involved in rational thought and judgment are also disrupted, leading to loss of control and powerlessness over drug use. The very parts of the brain needed to make good life decisions are "hijacked" by addiction. Nonaddictive drugs do not cause these changes.

All or nearly all addictive drugs, whether "uppers" or "downers," operate via the pleasure and reward circuit, but some also operate via additional mechanisms. An example is the opioids (opium and its derivatives, morphine, codeine, and heroin). The brain has neurons with receptors for its own "natural opiates," **endorphins**—brain chemicals that block pain when the body undergoes stress, such as during extreme exercise or childbirth. The structure of drugs in the opium family is similar to the structure of endorphins, so opioids readily bind to endorphin receptors, reducing pain and increasing pleasure. These effects occur in addition to the dopamine-related changes in the pleasure and reward circuit.

Individuals trying to recover from addiction are disadvantaged by their altered brain chemistry, drug-related memories, and impaired impulse control. Recovery is not simply a matter of willpower, nor does it involve abstinence from substances alone. Rather, multiple areas of the person's life have to be addressed—emotional, psychological, social, occupational, and so on. As a chronic, recurring disease, addiction typically involves repeated relapses and treatments before the person achieves recovery and returns to a healthy life.

DRUGS OF ABUSE

Drugs of abuse are usually classified as

- Stimulants
- Depressants
- Opioids
- Hallucinogens
- Inhalants
- Cannabinoids

For an overview of commonly abused drugs, their trade and street names, their intoxication effects, their potential for physical and psychological dependence, their potential health consequences, and their withdrawal effects, see Table 10.2.

Central Nervous System Stimulants

Drugs that speed up activity in the brain and sympathetic nervous system are known as **stimulants**. Their effects are similar to the response evoked during the fight-or-flight reaction (see Chapter 2). Heart rate accelerates, breathing deepens, muscle tension increases, the senses are heightened, and attention and alertness increase. These drugs can keep people going, mentally and physically, when they would otherwise be fatigued. The drugs may stimulate movement, fidgeting, and talking, and they may produce intense feelings of euphoria and create a sense of energy and well-being. Although stimulants do not meet the strict definition for physical dependence, users can develop tolerance and experience serious withdrawal effects.

Cocaine A powerful CNS stimulant, cocaine heightens alertness, inhibits appetite and the need for sleep, and provides intense feelings of pleasure. Pure cocaine was first extracted from the leaves of the coca plant in the mid-19th century; it was introduced as a remedy for a number of ailments and used medically as an anesthetic. Cocaine has high potential for abuse.

The most common form of pure cocaine is cocaine hydrochloride powder, made from coca paste. The intensity and duration of cocaine's effects—which include increased energy, reduced fatigue, and mental alertness—depend on the route of administration. Injecting or smoking produces a quicker, stronger high than snorting. Snorting produces a relatively quick effect that lasts from 15 to 30 minutes, but the high from smoking may last only 5 to 10 minutes.[6]

Crack is a form of cocaine that has been processed to make a rock crystal. It can be freebased or smoked. Freebasing involves heating cocaine hydrochloride with a volatile solvent such as ether or ammonia and smoking it. This practice is dangerous because the solvent can ignite and burn the user. It appeared in the mid-1980s and led to an epidemic of cocaine use in the United States. When smoked, crack cocaine produces the highest rate of dependence. Cocaine mixed with heroin produces a drug called a "speedball."

Cocaine is still used as a local anesthetic, often for nose and throat surgeries. Most uses, however, are recreational. Like other CNS stimulants, cocaine causes acceleration of the heart rate, elevation of blood pressure, dilation of the pupils, and an increase in alertness, muscle tension, and motor activity. It produces feelings of euphoria, often accompanied by talkativeness, sociability, and a sense of grandiosity. A person high on cocaine will have dilated pupils and will be uninterested in food or sleep. When the effects wear off, the user typically wants to repeat the experience. Dependence can occur after only a few uses. Withdrawal after prolonged use is characterized by a depressed mood, fatigue, sleep disturbances, unpleasant dreams, and increased appetite.

At higher doses, cocaine use can lead to cardiac arrhythmias, respiratory distress, bizarre or violent behavior, psychosis, convulsions, seizures, coma, and even death. Regular snorting can irritate the nasal passage and result in a chronic runny nose. Some users may become malnourished because the drug suppresses appetite.

Amphetamines For centuries, practitioners of Chinese medicine have made a medicinal tea from herbs called Ma-huang. In the 1920s, a chemist working for the Eli Lilly Company identified the active ingredient in Ma-huang as the compound ephedrine. The actions of this compound include opening the nasal and bronchial passages, allowing people to breathe more easily. The drug quickly became an important treatment for asthma, allergies, and stuffy noses. Researchers worked to develop synthetic forms of this botanical product, and a few years later, amphetamine was synthesized. Nasal amphetamine inhalers quickly grew in popularity; consumers found that they not only cleared the bronchioles but also produced elation.

stimulants
Drugs that speed up activity in the brain and the sympathetic nervous system.

Table 10.2   Commonly Abused Drugs

Category and Name	Trade Names/ Street Names	DEA Schedule*/ How Administered	General and Specific Intoxication Effects/ Acute Effects**	General and Specific Health Risks and Consequences**
CNS Stimulants			**Exhilaration, increased mental alertness, energy; tremors; irritability; anxiety; panic; paranoia; violent behavior; psychosis.**	**Increased heart rate, blood pressure, metabolism; reduced appetite; weight loss; nervousness; insomnia; seizures; heart attack, stroke; tolerance and withdrawal.**
Cocaine	*Cocaine hydrochloride;* blow, bump, C, candy, Charlie, coke, crack, flake, rock, snow, toot	II/Snorted, smoked, injected		Abdominal pain, nausea. In rare cases, sudden death on the first use of cocaine or afterward. Nasal damage from snorting.
Amphetamine	*Biphetamine, Dexedrine, Ritalin, Adderall;* bennies, black beauties, crosses, hearts, LA turnaround, speed, truck drivers, uppers	II/Injected, swallowed, smoked, snorted		Rapid breathing, loss of coordination, delirium, hallucinations, impulsive behavior, aggressiveness, tolerance, addiction.
Methamphetamine	*Desoxyn;* speed, meth, ice, chalk, crank, crystal, fire, glass, go fast	II/Swallowed, snorted, smoked, injected		Mood disturbances, confusion, severe dental problems. Injection adds the risk of infectious diseases such as HIV/AIDS and hepatitis.
Club Drugs				
MDMA	Ecstasy, Adam, clarity, Eve, lover's speed, peace, uppers	I/Swallowed, snorted, injected	Mild hallucinogenic effects, increased tactile sensitivity, empathic feelings, lowered inhibition, anxiety, chills, sweating, teeth clenching, muscle cramping.	Sleep disturbances, depression, impaired memory, hyperthermia, addiction.
Flunitrazepam	*Rohypnol;* forget-me pill, Mexican Valium, R2, roach, Roche, roofies, roofinol, rope, rophies	IV/Swallowed, snorted	Sedation, muscle relaxation, confusion, memory loss, dizziness, impaired coordination.	Addiction. Associated with sexual assault.
GHB	*Gamma-hydroxybutyrate;* G, Georgia home boy, grievous bodily harm, liquid ecstasy, soap, scoop, goop, liquid X	I/Swallowed	Drowsiness/nausea, headache, disorientation, loss of coordination, memory loss.	Unconsciousness, seizures, coma. Associated with sexual assault.
CNS Depressants			**Sedation/drowsiness, reduced anxiety, feelings of well-being; lowered inhibitions; slurred speech; poor concentration, confusion; dizziness; impaired coordination, memory.**	**Slowed pulse, lowered blood pressure, slowed breathing; tolerance, withdrawal, addiction; increased risk of respiratory distress and death when combined with alcohol.**
Barbiturates (sedatives)	*Amytal, Nembutal, Seconal, Phenobarbital;* barbs, reds, red birds, phennies, yellows, yellow jackets, sticks	II, III, V/Injected, swallowed	Euphoria	Unusual excitement; fever; irritability; life-threatening withdrawal in chronic users.

(continued)

Table 10.2   Commonly Abused Drugs *(continued)*

Category and Name	Trade Names/ Street Names	DEA Schedule*/ How Administered	General and Specific Intoxication Effects/ Acute Effects**	General and Specific Health Risks and Consequences**
Benzodiazepines (tranquilizers)	*Ativan, Halcion, Librium, Valium, Xanax, Klonopin*: candy, downers, sleeping pill, tranks	IV/Swallowed		
Sleep medications	*Ambien* (zolpidem), *Sonata* (zaleplon), *Lunesta* (eszopiclone)	IV/Swallowed		
Opioids and Morphine Derivatives			**Pain relief, euphoria, drowsiness, sedation; weakness, dizziness, nausea, impaired coordination, confusion, dry mouth, itching, sweating, clammy skin, constipation.**	**Slowed or arrested breathing; constipation, lowered pulse, blood pressure; tolerance, addiction; unconsciousness, coma; death especially when combined with alcohol or other CNS depressant.**
Heroin	*Diacetylmorphine;* smack, horse, brown sugar, dope, H, skag, junk	I/Injected, snorted, smoked	Euphoria followed by alternately wakeful and drowsy states/dizziness; feeling of heaviness in body.	Endocarditis; hepatitis; HIV. Depresses breathing so overdose can be fatal.
Codeine	*Empirin with Codeine, Fiorinal with Codeine, Robitussin A-C, Tylenol with Codeine;* Captain Cody, Cody, schoolboy; (with glutethimide: doors and fours, loads, pancakes and syrup)	II, III, IV/Injected, swallowed		Less analgesia, sedation, and respiratory depression than morphine.
Morphine	*Roxanol, Duramorph;* M, Miss Emma, monkey, white stuff	II, III/Injected, swallowed, smoked		
Methadone	*Methadose, Dolophine;* fizzies, amidone (with MDMA: chocolate chip cookies)	II/Swallowed, injected. Used to treat opioid addiction and pain		Significant overdose risk when used improperly.
Fentanyl and analogs	*Actiq, Duragesic, Sublimaze;* Apache, China girl, China white, dance fever, friend, goodfella, jackpot, murder 8, TNT, Tango and Cash	II/Injected, smoked, snorted		For fentanyl: 80–100 times more potent analgesic than morphine.
Other opioid pain relievers: Oxycodone HCL Hydrocodone Bitartrate Hydromorphone Oxymorphone Meperidine Propoxyphene	*Tylox, Oxycontin, Percodan, Percocet:* Oxy, O.C., oxycotton, oxycet, hillbilly heroin, percs. *Vicodin, Lortab, Lorcet;* Vike, Watson-387. *Dilaudid;* juice, smack, D, footballs, dillies. *Opana, Numorphan, Numorphone;* biscuits, blue heaven, blues, Mrs. O, octagons, stop signs, O bomb. *Demerol;* demmies, pain killer. *Darvon, Darvocet.*	II, III, V/Chewed, swallowed, snorted, injected, suppositories		For oxycodone: Muscle relaxation, twice as potent an analgesic as morphine; high abuse potential.

(continued)

Table 10.2 Commonly Abused Drugs (continued)

Category and Name	Trade Names/ Street Names	DEA Schedule*/ How Administered	General and Specific Intoxication Effects/ Acute Effects**	General and Specific Health Risks and Consequences**
Hallucinogens			Increased body temperature, heart rate, blood pressure; sleeplessness; loss of appetite, nausea; numbness, dizziness, weakness, tremors.	
LSD	*Lysergic acid diethylamide;* acid, blotter, boomers, cubes, microdot yellow sunshine, blue heaven.	I/Swallowed. Sold in capsules, tablets, liquid or absorbent paper.	Altered states of perception and feelings, with "trips" lasting about 12 hours; impulsive behavior; rapid shifts in emotion.	Flashbacks; delusions; Hallucinogen Persisting Perception Disorder
PCP	*Phencyclidine;* angel dust, ozone, wack, rocket fuel	I/Smoked, snorted, eaten. Sold as tablets, capsules, white or colored powder.	Slurred speech; loss of coordination.	Anxiety, memory loss; symptoms mimicking schizophrenia (delusions, hallucinations, disordered thinking, extreme anxiety).
Inhalants				
Solvents (paint thinner, gasoline, glue); gases (butane, propane)	Laughing gas, whippets, poppers, snappers	Inhaled through nose or mouth	Varies by chemical: stimulation; loss of inhibition; headache; nausea or vomiting; slurred speech; loss of motor coordination; wheezing	Hearing loss; limb spasms; CNS, brain, bone marrow damage. Death from heart failure or suffocation (inhalants displace oxygen in the lungs).
Cannabinoids				
Marijuana	Pot, weed, ganja, grass, Mary Jane, reefer, herb, joint, bud, sinsemilla	I/Smoked, eaten	Euphoria, relaxation; slowed reaction time, distorted sensory perceptions; impaired balance and coordination; increased heart rate and appetite.	Cough, frequent respiratory infections, chronic bronchitis; impaired learning, memory; panic attacks; psychosis; possible mental health decline; addiction.

*DEA Schedule: *Schedule I* drugs have a high potential for abuse; they are available for research only and have no approved medical use. *Schedule II* drugs have a high potential for abuse; they are available only by unrefillable prescription. *Schedule III* drugs have a lower potential for abuse than Schedule II drugs and are available by refillable prescription. *Schedule IV* drugs have a lower potential for abuse than Schedule III drugs and are available by refillable prescription. Some *Schedule V* drugs are available over the counter.

**Effects and consequences in the Substance Category row apply to all substances listed in the category.

Note: Taking drugs by injection, especially common with opioids, can increase the risk of infection through needle contamination with staphylococci, HIV, hepatitis, and other organisms.

Source: "Commonly Abused Drugs," National Institute on Drug Abuse, revised March 2011, www.drugabuse.gov/drugs-abuse/commonly-abused-drugs/commonly-abused-drugs-chart.; "Commonly Abused Prescription Drugs," National Institute on Drug Abuse, revised October 2011, www.drugabuse.gov/drugs-abuse/commonly-abused-drugs/commonly-abused-prescription-drugs-chart.

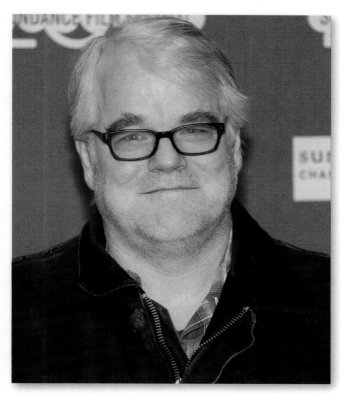

■ Actor Philip Seymour Hoffman died in 2014 at age 46 from acute drug intoxication; substances found in his system included drugs from the categories of stimulants, depressants, and opioids—cocaine, amphetamines, benzodiazepines, and heroin. He relapsed after 23 drug-free years.

In the 1930s, amphetamines were put to additional uses: helping patients with narcolepsy stay awake, suppressing appetite in people who wanted to lose weight, and treating depression. In the 1940s, soldiers fighting in World War II took amphetamines to stay alert and combat drowsiness. By the 1960s, amphetamines were so widely available that they were quickly swept up into the drug culture of that period.

Amphetamines are no longer recommended for depression or weight control. Particularly in the case of depression, a host of newer, more effective drugs are available. Amphetamines are still used to treat *attention deficit/hyperactivity disorder* (*ADHD*) in children and adults. Although they are stimulants, they have a paradoxical effect in individuals with ADHD, helping them gain control of their behavior. More than 3 million children and adolescents in the United States now take medication for ADHD.[28]

Concerns about the use of amphetamines involve their effects on the heart, lungs, and many other organs. At low levels, they may cause loss of appetite, rapid breathing, high blood pressure, and dilated pupils. Decision making can be impaired even at moderate dosage levels. At higher levels, amphetamines can cause paranoia, panic, fever, sweating, headaches, blurred vision, dizziness, and sometimes aggressiveness and violence. Very high doses may cause flushing, rapid or irregular heartbeat, tremors, and even collapse. Deaths due to heart failure and burst blood vessels in the brain have also been reported. Withdrawal symptoms after continued amphetamine use include a drop in energy, feelings of helplessness, and thoughts of suicide. The person may "crash" into depression or sleep for 24 hours. Some symptoms can continue for days or weeks.

Methamphetamine ("speed") has a chemical structure similar to that of amphetamine and produces similar but more intense effects. It is usually snorted. A very pure form of methamphetamine, called "ice" or "crystal meth," can be smoked, producing an intense rush of pleasure lasting a few minutes. A person high on meth will be energetic, talkative, and possibly argumentative or irritable.

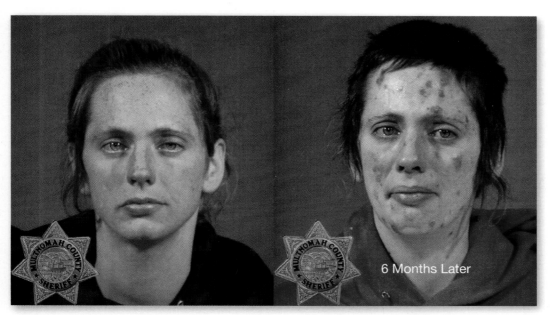

6 Months Later

■ Faces of Meth is a project initiated by an Oregon sheriff to combat methamphetamine addiction in his county. The before-and-after photographs he compiled of methamphetamine users are shown in presentations to high school students. To see more photographs, go to www.facesofmeth.us.

Meth is more addictive and dangerous than most other forms of amphetamine because it contains so many toxic chemicals. Aside from addiction and brain damage, health effects of meth use include severe weight loss, cardiovascular damage, increased risk of heart attack and stroke, extensive tooth decay and tooth loss ("meth mouth"), and oily skin. Users are also at risk for paranoia and violent behavior. Although methamphetamine can be prescribed by a physician, its medical uses are limited. There is a high potential for abuse, and repeated use can lead to addiction.[7] The popular body-building supplement Craze contains a chemical that is similar to methamphetamine and is marketed as a performance fuel. Its effectiveness and danger are not clearly known.

Meth can be manufactured from relatively inexpensive and commonly available drugs and chemicals. One such drug is pseudoephedrine, a nasal decongestant used in some cold and allergy medications. In 2005, Congress passed the Combat Methamphetamine Epidemic Act requiring that over-the-counter drugs like pseudoephedrine be sold from behind the counter and subjected to additional regulations.

MDMA Also known as Ecstasy, MDMA has chemical similarities to both stimulants (such as methamphetamine) and hallucinogens (such as mescaline).[7] Thus, it produces both types of effects. MDMA appears to elevate levels of the neurotransmitter serotonin, the body's primary regulator of mood, perhaps in a manner similar to the action of antidepressants. Users experience increased energy, feelings of euphoria, and a heightened sense of empathy with and closeness to those around them. Some users report enhanced hearing, vision, and sense of touch, but only a few report actual visual hallucinations.

In addition to the drug's euphoric effects, MDMA can cause increased heart rate, elevated body temperature (sometimes to dangerous levels), profuse sweating, dry mouth, muscle tension, blurred vision, dilated pupils, and involuntary teeth clenching. Serious risks include dehydration, hypertension, and heart or kidney failure.[8] MDMA use can lead to psychological problems, such as depression, anxiety, confusion, paranoia, and sleep disturbances. Findings from several studies show that long-term users of MDMA can suffer cognitive defects, including problems with memory. However, more research on the long-term effects of this drug is needed.

Molly is the powder or crystal form of MDMA and is especially popular at music festivals. Short for *molecule,* Molly is pure MDMA and is a Schedule I controlled substance. Between 2005 and 2011 there has been a 128 percent increase in ER visits due to MDMA and Molly, and a number of deaths have been the result of its use.

Bath Salts A relatively recent development is the use of "bath salts" to get high. The term *bath salts* refers to an emerging group of drugs containing an amphetamine-like stimulant found in the khat plant, which has been chewed for centuries by people living in the Horn of Africa and the Arabian Peninsula. Bath salts appear to have effects on the brain similar to those produced by amphetamines, although they are chemically different. They come in a powder form and can be taken by mouth, snorted, or injected. They are marketed under names like Ivory Wave, Vanilla Sky, Cloud Nine, and Red Dove. Because of the risk of serious side effects and the potential for overdose, the U.S. Drug Enforcement Agency and some local governments have banned these products.[9]

Caffeine The mild stimulant caffeine is probably the most popular psychoactive drug. Common sources of caffeine include coffee, tea, soft drinks, headache and pain remedies

■ MDPV and mephedrone are synthetic stimulants that are not approved for human consumption in the United States. However, they are sold as "bath salts" at headshops and convenience stores and are used as a recreational drug. Due to the potential side effects and health risks that bath salts pose when consumed— paranoia, violent aggression, seizures, irregular heartbeat, and even death—it is likely that future drug laws will tighten restrictions on such substances in an effort to prevent misuse and abuse.

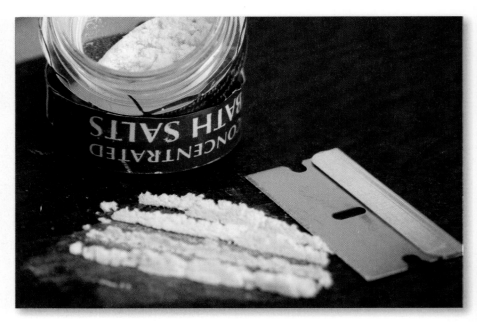

like Excedrin, stay-awake products like No-Doz, and weight loss aids. Chocolate contains caffeine but at much lower levels than these sources.

At low doses, caffeine increases alertness; at higher doses, it can cause restlessness, nervousness, excitement, frequent urination, and gastrointestinal distress. At very high levels of consumption (1 gram a day, or 8 to 10 cups of coffee), symptoms of intoxication can include muscle twitching, irregular heartbeat, insomnia, flushed face, excessive sweating, rambling thoughts or speech, or excessive pacing or movement. People can develop tolerance to caffeine and experience withdrawal symptoms (usually irritability, headache, and fatigue) when cutting back on or eliminating it.

Central Nervous System Depressants

Central nervous system **depressants** slow down activity in the brain and sympathetic nervous system. This category of drugs includes sedatives (e.g., barbiturates), hypnotics (sleeping medications), and most anti-anxiety drugs. They can be deadly if misused, especially when mixed with one another or with alcohol (another CNS depressant). CNS depressants carry a high risk for dependence.

Barbiturates and Hypnotics Barbiturates ("downers") are powerful sedatives that produce pleasant feelings of relaxation when first ingested, usually followed by lethargy, drowsiness, and sleep. Users experience impairments in judgment, decision making, and problem solving, as well as slow, slurred speech and lack of coordination. Dependence is common among middle-aged and older adults who use barbiturates as sleep aids. Withdrawal is difficult, and symptoms, including insomnia, anxiety, tremors, and nausea, can last for weeks; they can be mitigated by gradually tapering off the drug.

Hypnotics are prescribed for people with insomnia and other sleep disorders. They are also used to control epilepsy and to calm people before surgery or dental procedures.

Anti-Anxiety Drugs The most widely prescribed CNS depressants fall into the group of anti-anxiety drugs known as the *benzodiazepines*; examples are Xanax, Valium, and Ativan. Also known as *tranquilizers*, the benzodiazepines are used to control panic attacks and anxiety disorders. Users are at risk for dependence and for increasing dose levels as they become tolerant.

Another concern is the **rebound effect**, which occurs when a person stops using a drug and experiences symptoms that are worse than those experienced before taking the drug. The rebound effect can make it difficult to stop taking a particular medication.

Rohypnol A relatively new CNS depressant is flunitrazepam (Rohypnol); it started appearing in the United States in the 1990s. This powerful sedative has depressive effects and causes relaxation, lowered inhibitions, confusion, loss of memory, and sometimes loss of consciousness. It is especially dangerous when mixed with alcohol. Rohypnol

is known as a "date rape drug" because men have slipped it into women's drinks in order to sexually assault them later. As of this writing, the drug's manufacturer has changed the formulation of this drug so that it will not remain colorless when dissolving in a drink.[10]

GHB Another so-called date rape drug is gamma hydroxybutyrate (GHB). This CNS depressant produces feelings of pleasure along with sedation and is a drug of choice among young people at bars, clubs, and parties. It can be produced in several forms, including a clear, tasteless, odorless liquid and a powder that readily dissolves in liquid. Like Rohypnol, it has been slipped into the drinks of women who later did not remember being sexually assaulted. It usually takes effect within 15 to 30 minutes and lasts from three to six hours. Besides sedation and amnesia, GHB can cause nausea, hallucinations, respiratory distress, slowed heart rate, loss of consciousness, and coma. Users are at risk for dependence with sustained use.

GHB, Rohypnol, and MDMA are sometimes referred to as *club drugs* because of their widespread use at clubs and parties. Their use is particularly dangerous because of the unpredictable setting in which they are usually taken. When GHB and Rohypnol are consumed with alcohol, the combined sedative effects can lead to life-threatening conditions. Additionally, all of these drugs are typically produced in basement labs, so dose and purity are uncertain.[11]

Opioids

Natural and synthetic derivatives of opium, a product harvested from a gummy substance in the seed pod of the opium poppy, are known as **opioids**. Opium originated in the Middle East and has a long history of medical use for pain relief and treatment of diarrhea and dehydration. Currently, opioids are prescribed as pain relievers, anesthetics, antidiarrheal agents, and cough suppressants.

Drugs in this category include morphine, heroin, codeine, and oxycodone. Also known as *narcotics*, opioids are commonly misused and abused. They produce a pleasant, drowsy state in which cares are forgotten, the senses are dulled, and pain is reduced. They act by altering the neurotransmitters that control movement, moods, and a number of body functions, including body temperature regulation, digestion, and breathing.

With low doses, opioid users experience euphoria, followed by drowsiness, constriction of the pupils, slurred speech, slowed movement, and impaired coordination, attention, and memory. With higher doses, users can experience depressed respiration, loss of consciousness, coma, and death. When first used, opioids often cause nausea,

depressants
Drugs that slow down activity in the brain and sympathetic nervous system.

rebound effect
Phenomenon that occurs when a person stops using a drug and experiences symptoms that are worse than those experienced before taking the drug.

opioids
Natural and synthetic derivatives of opium.

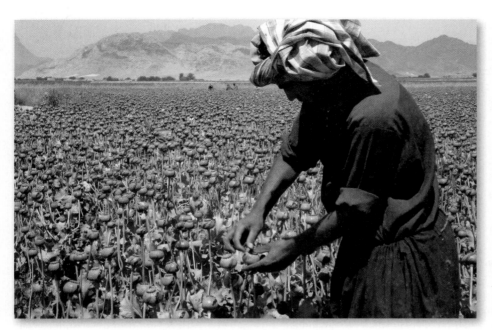

■ Opium poppies are an important cash crop for subsistence farmers in developing countries around the world. Although there are legal medical uses for opium, virtually all of Afghanistan's opium poppy harvest is sold on the international market as heroin.

vomiting, and a negative mood rather than euphoria. Chronic users usually experience dry mouth, dry, itchy skin, constipation, and vision problems. Opioids have a high potential for dependence.

Morphine The primary active chemical in opium, morphine is a powerful pain reliever. Its first widespread use, facilitated by the development of the hypodermic syringe in the 1850s, was during the Civil War. So many soldiers became addicted that after the war, morphine addiction was called "the soldier's disease."[11] Because of the high risk of dependence, physicians prescribing morphine today do so conservatively.

Heroin Heroin is three times more potent than morphine. It was developed in the late 19th century as a supposedly nonaddictive substitute for codeine (another derivative of morphine, useful for suppressing coughs). Just as Civil War veterans suffered from morphine addiction, many soldiers came home from the war in Vietnam addicted to heroin.

Whereas morphine has medical uses, heroin is almost exclusively a drug of abuse. Its use is associated with unemployment, divorce, and drug-related crimes. Heroin abuse is associated with a variety of health conditions, particularly for those who inject it and do not practice safe use by using clean syringes. Among health conditions for which heroin users are at high risk are infectious diseases

hallucinogens
Drugs that alter perceptions and thinking, intensifying and distorting visual and auditory perceptions and producing hallucinations; also called psychedelics.

(including hepatitis, tuberculosis, and HIV/AIDS), various types of pneumonia, collapsed veins, liver and kidney disease, and permanent damage to various vital organs. Among individuals who use heroin, about 23 percent become dependent on it.[12] Babies born to women who used heroin during pregnancy are often drug dependent at birth.

Synthetic Opioids Some of the most widely prescribed drugs in the United States are synthetic opioids, made from oxycodone hydrochloride. Brand names include OxyContin, Vicodin, Demerol, Dilaudid, Percocet, and Percodan. Some people who start using these drugs for pain become addicted and misuse or abuse them (see the box, "Diana: Pain, Stress, and Painkillers").

OxyContin, for example, provides long-lasting, timed-release relief for moderate to severe chronic pain when taken in tablet form. If the tablets are chewed, crushed and snorted, or dissolved in water and injected, they provide an immediate, intense rush similar to that of heroin. A person high on OxyContin may be energetic and talkative at first, before becoming relaxed and drowsy. One group particularly susceptible to opioid misuse is medical personnel with access to controlled substances.

The nonmedical use and abuse of prescription drugs, particularly opioids and benzodiazepines (drugs used to treat anxiety) is a serious public health problem, which some believe is out of control. There has been a dramatic increase in the number of prescriptions written for pain killers because chronic pain affects approximately 100 million adults and is the most common reason people see a medical provider. Abuse of these drugs has resulted in an increase in emergency room visits and fatal drug overdoses.[13]

Hallucinogens

LSD, psilocybin, and peyote are a few of the so-called **hallucinogens** (also called *psychedelics*). They differ chemically, but their effects are similar: they alter perceptions and thinking in characteristic ways. They produce intensification and distortion of visual and auditory perceptions as well as hallucinations. Some hallucinogens are synthetic (e.g., LSD), and others are derived from plants (e.g., mescaline, from peyote, and psilocybin, from psilocybin mushrooms).[14]

LSD Lysergic acid diethylamide (LSD) is a synthetic hallucinogen that alters perceptual processes, producing visual

Life Stories

Diana: Pain, Stress, and Painkillers

Diana was a junior with dreams of becoming an athletic trainer after college. In high school she was overweight, but since coming to college she had taken up running and become healthy and fit. She had run two half-marathons and was training for a third. One day while she and her friend Ravi were out running, she landed wrong on her left foot and twisted her ankle. She collapsed in pain and with Ravi's help eventually got up and limped back to her car. Ravi drove her home and left to go to class, promising to return afterward. Diana called the health clinic and made an appointment for the next morning. Ravi returned and brought her a bottle of Percocet with a few pills left in it. He had been prescribed the drug last year after he had injured his back and hadn't finished the whole bottle. Diana's pain was intense, so she took one right away. Soon the pain vanished, and Diana began to feel blissful.

The next day she woke up in pain and took another Percocet. With crutches borrowed from a friend, she hobbled to her appointment. The nurse-practitioner who examined her took an X-ray of her foot to make sure she hadn't fractured her ankle. She hadn't, so he wrapped her ankle in an Ace bandage and told her to keep her weight off the foot, ice it, elevate it, and take ibuprofen for the pain. Diana lied that she had taken ibuprofen yesterday and that it hadn't helped. She asked him to prescribe something stronger. The nurse-practitioner agreed to write a five-day prescription for Vicodin—after a few days her pain should subside, he said.

Diana went through the Vicodin in three days. She was stressed about gaining weight now that she wouldn't be able to run for a while, and the high from the Vicodin, like that of the Percocet, helped her not think about it. On the fourth day, she had to take ibuprofen because her Vicodin had run out. It helped some with the pain, but not as much as the Vicodin had, and it didn't give her the same buzz. She returned to the health clinic the day after and met again with the nurse-practitioner. He examined her ankle and said that the swelling had gone down and that she was on the path to recovery. She told him that she needed more Vicodin because she was still in a lot of pain. He explained that for her type of injury—a simple sprain—Vicodin was not necessary and that the school also had specific guidelines for when synthetic opioids could be prescribed. He told her that prescription-strength ibuprofen should be sufficient.

Diana was upset and a little panicked as she left the appointment. She had been expecting to get more Vicodin. She called Ravi on her cell phone and asked if he could get a refill on his Percocet prescription. Ravi was surprised and concerned. He couldn't get a refill on a prescription that had expired a year ago. Was she okay? Diana said she was and that she was sorry for having asked him. After she hung up, Diana felt embarrassed that she had asked Ravi to get her more pills. She realized that she was not acting like herself and was becoming someone she didn't want to be.

- Based on Diana's experience, how would you describe the process of becoming dependent on prescription painkillers? What role do you think is played by psychological mechanisms like denial, wishful thinking, and rationalization?

- What steps do you think Diana needs to take at this point to overcome her growing dependence on painkillers?

- What are some cautions you would give about the best ways to educate teens and young adults about the possibilities of dependence on prescription drugs?

connect ACTIVITY

---

distortions and fantastic imagery. Use of LSD peaked in the late 1960s and then declined, as reports circulated of "bad trips," prolonged psychotic reactions, "flashbacks," self-injurious behavior, and possible chromosomal damage.

LSD is one of the most potent psychoactive drugs known. It is odorless, colorless, and tasteless, and a dose as small as a single grain of salt (about 0.01 mg) can produce mild effects. At higher doses (0.05 mg to 0.10 mg), hallucinogenic effects are produced. Most users take LSD orally; absorption is rapid. Effects last for several hours and vary depending on the user's mood and expectations, the setting, and the dose and potency of the drug. It usually takes hours or days to recover from an LSD trip. Although LSD is thought to stimulate serotonin receptors in the brain, its exact neural pathway is not completely understood.

Besides visual distortion, LSD can produce auditory changes, a distorted sense of time, changes in the perception of one's own body, and *synesthesia*—a "mixing of senses" in which

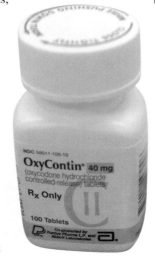

sounds may appear as visual images or a visual image changes in rhythm to music. Feelings of euphoria may alternate with waves of anxiety. A person on LSD may be disoriented or delusional. In a bad trip, the user may experience acute anxiety or panic. LSD does not produce compulsive drug-seeking behaviors, and physiological withdrawal symptoms do not occur when use is stopped.

Phencyclidine (PCP) First developed in the 1950s as an anesthetic, PCP was found to produce such serious side effects—agitation, delusions, irrational behavior—that its use was discontinued. Since the 1960s, it has been manufactured illegally and sold on the street, often under the

- Abuse of prescription painkillers has soared in the past 10 to 15 years, especially among teenagers and young adults. Overdoses from these central nervous system depressants now kill more people than overdoses from either heroin or cocaine.

name "angel dust." It has fewer hallucinogenic effects than LSD and more disturbances in body perception. A drug with similar effects is ketamine.

PCP is a white crystalline powder that is readily soluble in water or alcohol. It can be smoked, snorted, or injected intravenously. At low doses, it produces euphoria, dizziness, nausea, slurred speech, rapid heartbeat, high blood pressure, numbness, and slowed reaction time. At higher doses, it causes disorganized thinking and feelings of unreality, and at very high doses it can cause amnesia, seizures, and coma. A person who has taken PCP is anesthetized enough to undergo surgery.

The drug is particularly associated with aggressive behavior, probably as a result of impaired judgment and disorganized thinking. Combined with insensitivity to pain, these effects can produce dangerous or deadly results.

Inhalants

The drugs called **inhalants** are breathable chemical vapors that alter consciousness, typically producing a state of intoxication that resembles drunkenness. The vapors come from substances like paint thinners, gasoline, glue, and spray can propellant. The active ingredients in these products are chemicals like toluene, benzene, acetone, and tetrachlorethylene—all dangerously powerful toxins and carcinogens.[15]

inhalants
Breathable chemical vapors that alter consciousness, producing a state resembling drunkenness.

At low doses, inhalants cause light-headedness, dizziness, blurred vision, slurred speech, lack of coordination, and feelings of euphoria. At higher doses, they can cause lethargy, muscle weakness, confusion, apathy, and stupor. An overdose of an inhalant can result in a loss of consciousness, coma, or death. Inhalants can also cause behavioral and psychological changes, including belligerence, confusion, apathy, and impaired social and occupational functioning. Perhaps the most significant negative effect for chronic users is widespread and long-lasting brain damage. There was a steady decline in inhalant use by young adults through 2013.[16]

Cannabinoids

The most widely used illicit drug in the United States is marijuana. In 2009, it was reported that 42 percent of 12th graders had tried marijuana at least once.[17]

Marijuana is derived from the hemp plant, *Cannabis sativa*, thus the name *cannabinoids*. The leaves of the plant are usually dried and smoked, but they can also be mixed in tea or food. Hashish is a resin that seeps from the leaves; it is usually smoked. The active ingredient in marijuana is delta-9-tetrahydrocannabinol (THC). The potency of the drug is determined by the amount of THC in the plant, which in turn is affected by the growing conditions. Since the 1960s, the amount of THC in marijuana sold on the street has increased from 1 to 5 percent to as much as 10 to 15 percent.

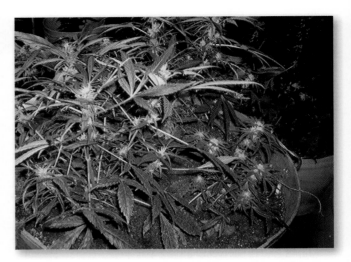

■ The *Cannabis* plant has a variety of uses, including as fiber (hemp), food, medications, and for its psychedelic effects. From its probable origin in China or central Asia, the plant spread to India, ancient Rome, Africa, Europe, and the Americas.

Marijuana use produces mild euphoria and talkativeness, sedation, lethargy, short-term memory impairment, an increase in appetite, distorted sensory perceptions, a distorted sense of time, impaired motor coordination, and an increase in heart rate. A person high on marijuana has bloodshot eyes and dilated pupils. Effects typically begin within a few minutes and last from three to four hours. Sometimes the drug causes anxiety or a negative mood. At high doses, marijuana can have hallucinogenic effects, accompanied by acute anxiety and paranoid thinking. Chronic, heavy users of marijuana may develop tolerance to its effects and experience some withdrawal symptoms if they stop using it, but most dependence seems to be psychological.

Researchers have found that THC has a variety of effects on the brain. One effect is the suppression of activity in the information processing system of the hippocampus, perhaps accounting for some impairment in problem solving and decision making associated with being high on marijuana. Marijuana smoke has negative effects on the respiratory system; it contains more carcinogens than tobacco smoke and is highly irritating to the lining of the bronchioles and lungs. In addition to coughs and chest colds, frequent marijuana users who do not smoke cigarettes report more health problems and miss more days of work than non-cigarette smokers.[17]

Many people claim that marijuana does have medical uses, especially as a treatment for glaucoma, for the pain and nausea associated with cancer and chemotherapy, and for the weight loss associated with AIDS. Research suggests that smoking marijuana is no more effective than taking THC in pill form for these purposes, but the use of marijuana for medical reasons has become a matter of political debate. Proponents of its use assert that it makes life livable for many people with painful and debilitating medical conditions and that there is no reason not to legalize it. Supporters of medical marijuana suggest that cannabidiol (CBD) may stop the spread of many aggressive cancers. Currently 21 states and the District of Columbia have laws legalizing marijuana in some form. Colorado and Washington have legalized marijuana for recreational use, and both are beginning to develop the framework for legal sales. Opponents argue that legalizing marijuana would imply approval of its use for recreational purposes and open the floodgates to abuse of all drugs.

Like alcohol, marijuana affects the skills required to drive a car safely, including concentration, attention, coordination, reaction time, and the ability to judge distance. Because it also clouds judgment, people who are high may not realize their driving skills are impaired.

A recently recognized drug with effects similar to those of marijuana is *spice,* a diverse family of herbal mixtures containing shredded plant material and possibly chemical additives. Spice can be smoked or prepared as a drink. No large-scale studies on the health effects of this drug have yet been conducted.[18]

Emerging Drugs of Abuse

New drugs appear quickly and are often accompanied by rumor, inaccurate information about effects, and minimization of toxicity. The newest set of drugs being experimented with include the following:

- "Krokodil," a homemade synthetic form of a heroin-like drug called desmorphine that is made by combining codeine with other chemicals such as lighter fluid and industrial cleaners. This dangerous mixture gets its name from the scaly, gray-green dead skin that forms at the site of the injection. The high lasts 90 minutes to two hours. Withdrawal is difficult, and individuals who are able to stop may be left with speech impediments, a vacant gaze, and erratic movements.

- "N-Bomb," a synthetic hallucinogen that is more powerful than LSD. Extremely small amounts can cause seizures, heart attacks, and possibly death. At least 14 young people were reported to have died between March 2012 and April 2013 due to its use.

- "Syrup," "Purple Drank," "Sizzurp," and "Lean," all names for prescription-strength cough syrup containing codeine and promethazine mixed with soda. This combination of an opioid and an antihistamine presents a risk of fatal overdose by slowing or stopping the heart and lungs.

- "Devils Breath," a drug considered similar to Rohypnol because it can be used to take advantage of people. The drug used in Devils Breath is scopolamine, which comes from plants and has a number of medical uses. It has hallucinogenic properties and has been described as hypnotizing people, making them powerless to resist while still seeming to be completely articulate.

APPROACHES TO THE DRUG PROBLEM

Drug abuse and dependence have negative consequences affecting individuals, communities, and society. In addition to the human costs, illicit drug use and addiction cause considerable economic damage. An estimated $193 billion is drained from the U.S. economy by drug use annually, most of which is spent on health care and justice system costs.[19] Only a very small percentage goes toward prevention and treatment.[20] In 2009, an estimated 4.6 million drug-related hospital emergency room visits were reported in the United States. Between 2004 and 2009, the total number of drug-related ER visits increased by 81 percent, and the number of ER visits related to the nonmedical use of prescription drugs increased by more than 98 percent. The largest increases were associated with oxycodone products, hydrocodone products, and alprazolam (Xanax, an anti-anxiety drug).[21] For more on this misuse of prescription drugs, see the box, "Should We Hold Doctors Responsible When Their Patients Overdose on Prescription Drugs?"

Other economic costs of illicit drug use include social welfare costs, workplace accidents, property damage, incarceration of otherwise productive individuals, goods and services lost to crime, work hours missed by victims of drug-related crime, and costs of law enforcement.

Government approaches to the drug problem have traditionally fallen into two broad categories: supply reduction and demand reduction. A newer approach to the drug problem is harm reduction, an approach used in alcohol treatment programs as well.

Supply Reduction Strategies

Strategies to reduce the supply of drugs are aimed at controlling the quantity of illicit substances that enter or are produced in the United States. An example is *interdiction*, the interception of drugs before they enter the country, as when customs officials use dogs to sniff out drugs at airports or when the Coast Guard boards ships to search for drugs as they enter U.S. waters.

The U.S. government also puts pressure on governments in other countries to suppress the production and exportation of drugs. Unfortunately, the plants that yield drugs are important and profitable cash crops for peasant farmers in many countries, and the drug smuggling business is controlled by criminal interests that are often beyond the control of the government. Efforts to reduce the drug supply at the international level have led to human rights abuses, an expansion of oppressive regimes, and increased corruption among police, government, and military personnel.

The government also attempts to prevent domestic production of drugs by raiding suspected underground drug labs or stamping out enterprises that grow marijuana on a large scale. Another domestic supply-side strategy is to obstruct the distribution of drugs, such as when a massive police presence is used in an area where drugs are sold.

Starting the Conversation

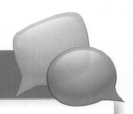

Should We Hold Doctors Responsible When Their Patients Overdose on Prescription Drugs?

Q: What has your experience been with prescription painkillers, if any?

In 2012, a physician in southern California was arrested and charged with murder in three fatal overdoses by patients taking drugs she prescribed. Prosecutors accused the doctor of recklessly prescribing narcotic painkillers and other addictive drugs to her patients—including OxyContin, Vicodin, Xanax, and Valium—"without a legitimate purpose." Previously, she had settled several wrongful death lawsuits with families of people who overdosed on the drugs she prescribed.

In November 2011, Dr. Conrad Murray was convicted of involuntary manslaughter in the death of pop star Michael Jackson. Murray had administered the powerful anesthetic propofol to the star to help him sleep. His actions were found to "be recklessly outside the bounds of accepted medical practice." Jackson was said to be taking numerous prescription drugs at the time of his death, including anti-anxiety medications and painkillers.

These criminal cases are unusual. Negative medical outcomes are usually not criminalized, and prescribing physicians have generally not been held responsible when someone dies as a result of their actions. Although several physicians have been prosecuted on drug-dealing charges, it's rare for a physician to be charged with criminal gross negligence, much less manslaughter or murder.

Deaths from prescription drug overdoses have soared in the last decade; since 2003, more overdose deaths have resulted from opioid analgesics (painkillers) than from heroin and cocaine combined. In many large cities, overdose deaths are more common than homicides. Overdoses often result from the combined effects of several drugs, often in conjunction with alcohol. Actor Heath Ledger, for example, died from a lethal combination of Oxy-Contin, Valium, Xanax, Ritalin, Vicodin, and sleep aids.

Numerous factors have contributed to this trend. More drugs have been developed, and pharmaceutical companies use aggressive sales campaigns to market them, including direct-to-consumer campaigns. Doctors prescribe these drugs in well-meaning efforts to relieve suffering, particularly among the growing number of older and overweight patients with chronic pain and musculoskeletal problems. The number of prescriptions doctors write has greatly increased over the past two decades. From 1991 to 2010, prescriptions for stimulants such as Ritalin and Adderall increased from 5 million to nearly 45 million, and prescriptions for opioid painkillers like OxyContin increased from 75.5 million to 209.5 million. This means that there are more drugs around, and they are easier to get.

In addition, attitudes toward prescription drugs are different from attitudes toward illicit drugs. Both physicians and the public seem to underestimate the dangers of prescription drugs, perhaps because they are not associated with street crime or violence. Many people assume that anything prescribed by a doctor is safe.

All of this has left some physicians unsure of how to respond to their patients in pain. They have effective medications at hand, but they also have concerns about patients' taking the drugs correctly, sharing their medications, protecting the medication from others, and becoming addicted. Their concerns extend to fear of losing their license or being charged with a crime.

A major component of a 2011 government plan to respond to the prescription drug abuse epidemic is physician education, focusing on raising awareness of the dangers of prescription drug use and the possibility of addiction, overdose, and death. These efforts would include training requirements for doctors. In the absence of such requirements, physicians continue to write prescriptions for narcotics and other addictive drugs for their patients, in most cases without being held responsible for negative outcomes.

Q: Do you think physicians are responsible when their patients become addicted to prescription painkillers or overdose on them? If so, are they also responsible for people who borrowed or stole the drugs from the patient?

Q: What are the disadvantages of holding physicians criminally responsible for the outcomes of their medical actions?

Q: What responsibility, if any, do you think pharmaceutical companies have in this situation?

Sources: "Doctor Charged in Fatal Prescription Overdose," by L. Girion, S. Glove, and H. Branson-Potts, March 1, 2012, *Los Angeles Times*, http://articles.latimes.com/2012/mar/01/local/la-me-drug-doctor-20120302; "Epidemic: Responding to America's Prescription Drug Abuse Crisis," The White House, 2011, www.whitehouse.gov/sites/default/files/ondcp/issues-content/prescription-drugs/rx_abuse_plan.pdf; "Topics in Brief: Prescription Drug Abuse," National Institute on Drug Abuse, 2011, www.drugabuse.gov/publications/topics-in-brief/prescription-drug-abuse.

Demand Reduction Strategies

Demand-side strategies include penalizing users through incarceration; preventing drug use, primarily through education; and treating individuals once they have become dependent on drugs.

Incarceration for Drug-Related Crimes Penalizing users means enforcing the laws against drug possession, arresting offenders, and putting people in prison. The assumptions behind this approach are that incarceration will reduce drug-related crime by getting users off the streets and that the threat of punishment will deter others from using drugs. Most states mandate harsh prison terms for the possession or sale of relatively small quantities of drugs, regardless of whether the person is a first-time or repeat offender.

As a result of such policies, U.S. prisons are crowded with people convicted of drug-related crimes; in fact, more than half of the people in U.S. prisons meet diagnostic standards for substance use disorders. The United States imprisons a larger percentage of its population than does any other nation. Elsewhere, low-level crimes like drug possession do not draw a prison sentence. Recently, however, some states are reducing penalties for possession of smaller amounts of certain drugs, such as marijuana, and for first-time offenses as a way to reduce incarceration rates and also steer people towards treatment.

Because prisoners are a captive audience, it would make sense to provide treatment while they are in jail, but only a small percentage of prisoners—between 7 and 17 percent—who need drug treatment receive it. Incarceration as a drug use reduction strategy does little to address the larger problem of drug use in our society.[22]

Prevention Strategies   A second demand-side strategy is prevention through education. Prevention strategies focus on reducing the demand for drugs by increasing an individual's ability to decline drug use when confronted with an opportunity to experiment. Programs involve primary, secondary, or tertiary prevention, depending on their targeted audience. *Primary, or universal, prevention programs* are designed to reach the entire population without regard to individual risk factors. Public service commercials on television asking us to imagine a world without cigarettes or billboards referring to crystal meth as "crystal mess" are examples of primary prevention strategies.

Secondary, or selective, strategies focus on those subgroups that are at greatest risk for use or abuse, with the aim of increasing protective factors and decreasing potential risk factors. An example is a class that teaches problem-solving skills to adolescents.

Tertiary, or indicated, strategies target at-risk individuals rather than groups, again focusing on protective factors such as academic, interpersonal, social, or job skills. An example is a program that tutors individual students in ways to manage emotions and maintain self-esteem without drugs.

A prevention strategy used in the workplace is drug testing, usually random urine screening. The goal of drug testing is not to catch drug users and fire them but to create an environment in which it is clear that drug use is not condoned. Companies also want to limit their liability by reducing the likelihood that an employee will make a mistake that causes someone harm. Federal law requires that people in jobs involving transportation, such as air traffic controllers, train engineers, and truck drivers, undergo regular testing to ensure public safety. U.S. military personnel also undergo regular drug testing. Although some see the practice as an infringement of privacy rights, so far it has withstood judicial challenges.

On college campuses, a number of steps can be taken to prevent drug use and to reduce harm to those students who do use (see the box, "Recognize Signs of a Drug Problem").

Action Skill-Builder

Recognize Signs of a Drug Problem

As a college student, you are in an environment where one in five people uses illicit drugs—mostly marijuana, but also cocaine, ecstasy, and LSD. A smaller number misuse prescription drugs, ranging from Adderall to Vicodin. Some people can use drugs recreationally without experiencing problems, but others cannot—they find themselves continuing to use a drug even though it's causing problems at school, at work, or in relationships. Because of the changes drugs cause in the brain, most people don't realize they are slipping into dependence, and what began as a choice becomes a need.

Most colleges focus on alcohol abuse and have fewer programs specifically aimed at helping students recognize early signs of drug dependence. If you have a friend, roommate, or classmate who is beginning to have a problem with drugs, you may notice some of these signs:

☐ A noticeable change in behavior, such as withdrawal or agitation.

☐ Mood swings, irritability, or angry outbursts.

☐ A change in sleep habits, needing either more or less.

☐ Nodding out during conversations or in class on a regular basis.

☐ Lack of interest in activities that used to be a source of enjoyment.

☐ Decline in academic performance.

☐ An increase in physical complaints or pain.

☐ Preoccupation with a drug or sense of urgency around its use; activities scheduled around drug use.

☐ Financial problems or unexplained need for money; an increase in requests to borrow money.

☐ Physical signs such as vomiting, constricted pupils, slurred speech.

If you notice these behaviors in a friend, here are a few things you can do:

☐ Speak up. Express your concerns; ask questions; give your friend a reality check. Keeping silent does nothing to help your friend acknowledge and address the problem.

☐ Be prepared for excuses and denial by listing specific examples of your friend's behavior that worry you.

☐ Know where help is available on campus or in the community so you can suggest resources.

☐ Don't enable your friend. Don't make excuses or help him or her avoid consequences. Continue to be supportive and look out for your friend's best interest.

☐ Take care of yourself. Make sure you have someone to talk to or someplace you can go for support.

Source: "Drug Abuse and Addiction," Helpguide.org, 2012, retrieved March 20, 2012, from www.helpguide.org/mental/drug_substance_abuse_addiction _signs_effects_treatment.htm.

A comprehensive approach, known as *environmental management*, can be implemented to modify an environment that often benignly accepts or overlooks drug use and experimentation during college. The most effective approaches seem to have a number of common factors:[2]

- Sending clear messages that drug use is not acceptable.

- Changing the climate of drug tolerance on campus, if it exists.

- Engaging parents.

- Identifying and intervening with at-risk students.

- Providing alternative activities.

- Involving students in the planning of prevention programs.

For those individuals who will experiment regardless of changes made on campus, harm reduction strategies are important. Implementing such strategies should not be seen as "giving permission" to students to use; rather, it reduces the likelihood that they will harm themselves or others. The following are some harm reduction strategies that have been implemented on college campuses:

- Providing containers in college buildings for the safe disposal of needles and syringes.

- Providing condoms so that students will not transmit infectious diseases if drug use leads to sexual activity.

- Making naloxone (Narcan) available in case of opioid overdose. Naloxone is an opiate antagonist that can counteract life-threatening depression of the respiratory system.

One of the best ways to understand and control your drug use is to first do a self-assessment to see the part drugs play in your life. Complete the self-assessment and questions in this chapter's Personal Health Portfolio to determine the impact drugs have on your life and whether you are in need of treatment by a professional.

Drug Treatment Programs The third type of demand-side strategy is helping people to stop using drugs after they

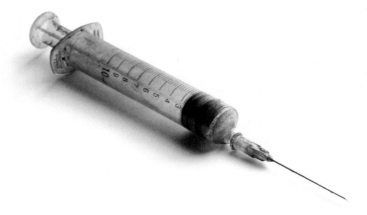

have started, that is, providing treatment. Evidence indicates that treatment is a more effective strategy for reducing drug use than locking up dealers or cutting off supplies at our borders.[23,24] As with alcohol, treatment is available in a variety of formats, ranging from hospital-based inpatient programs to self-help/mutual-help groups such as Narcotics Anonymous (NA).

Most experts agree that treatment is a long-term process, often marked by relapses and requiring multiple treatment episodes. The first step is acknowledging that there is a problem and getting into a program. No single treatment is appropriate for everyone; matching services to individual needs is important.

Treatment is more successful when the program lasts at least three months, includes individual counseling, and addresses all aspects of the client's life, including medical treatment, family therapy, living skills, and occupational skills. In counseling, clients work to increase motivation, build relapse prevention skills, improve problem-solving and interpersonal skills, and develop life-enhancing behaviors. Participating in self-help support programs during and following treatment often helps maintain abstinence.[25]

Harm Reduction Strategies

Harm reduction strategies are based on the idea that attempting to completely eliminate substance use is futile and that efforts should be focused on helping addicts reduce the harm associated with their substance use.[26,27] Advocates of the harm reduction approach assert that drug users are in need of treatment rather than punishment. Examples of harm reduction strategies are needle exchange programs, in which addicts are provided with sterile needles in exchange for their used ones, and drug substitute programs, in which individuals are maintained on addictive but less debilitating drugs, such as methadone for heroin addicts (see the box, "Needle Exchange Programs: Public Health Policy or Political Football?").

Other harm reduction strategies include controlled availability (certain drugs are available through a government monopoly), medicalization (drugs are available by prescription but only to individuals who are already addicted to them), and decriminalization (the penalty for possession of certain drugs is reduced or eliminated if the quantity held is below a certain limit).

Proponents of harm reduction strategies claim that they represent a more realistic approach to the drug problem and would allow resources to be directed away from punishment, which is ineffective, and toward treatment, which is effective. Opponents of harm reduction strategies argue that they are thinly disguised forms of drug legalization and that any softening of a zero tolerance position would result in an epidemic of drug use. Although effective harm reduction programs are in place in England and Canada, harm reduction is rejected as an official policy by the U.S. government.

Public Health Is Personal

Needle Exchange Programs: Public Health Policy or Political Football?

Needle exchange programs began informally in the 1970s and were widely adopted in the 1980s and 1990s by many U.S. states and by countries around the world in response to the HIV/AIDS epidemic. However, the U.S. Congress made sure no federal funds would be used to support these programs by passing a ban on such funding in 1998. After years of advocacy by public health and harm reduction activists, the ban was repealed by Congress in 2009, but it was reinstated by a differently configured Congress in 2011. Why is there so much political action around this public health issue?

Needle exchange (or syringe exchange) programs allow injection drug users to obtain clean hypodermic needles and related injection equipment at little or no cost; many programs require them to turn in used needles for the same number of new needles. Advocates of needle exchange programs assert that the programs reduce the spread of HIV and hepatitis C, remove used needles from the environment, and bring drug users into contact with health care providers who can guide them toward treatment if they are interested. Opponents of needle exchanges programs argue that this type of harm reduction approach only enables and encourages individuals to practice harmful behaviors by giving them "permission" to use; they assert that the programs attract drug sellers to neighborhoods and have a negative impact on living conditions and commerce.

Overall, the evidence indicates that needle exchange programs do reduce the sharing of needles and the spread of HIV and hepatitis C, although recent research suggests that they may not be as effective at reducing the spread of disease as previously thought. The programs have not been shown to increase drug use or cause harm. The consensus among public health officials is that needle exchange programs are effective in reducing needle sharing and disease transmission; the programs are supported by the CDC, the American Medical Association, the National Academy of Science, the American Public Health Association, the World Health Organization, and numerous other scientific bodies.

Despite the scientific support, there is intense resistance to implementing these programs, primarily for political reasons. Advisors have cautioned U.S. presidents that supporting the programs might "send the wrong message" and open them to charges of being "soft on drugs." Some members of Congress oppose needle exchange programs on moral and religious grounds. U.S. cities and states continue to run these programs as one part of their HIV/AIDS prevention strategies, but in Washington the debate continues: should social policy be based on scientific evidence, or should it be shaped by partisan politics?

connect
ACTIVITY

Sources: "Congress Votes to Restore Needle Exchange Funding Ban," by D. Smith, 2011, http://stopthedrugwar.org/chronicle/2011/dec/19/congress_votes_restore_needle_ex; "Expert Panel Strategizes to Repeal the Federal Ban on Funding for Syringe Exchange," by M. Mazzotta, 2012, http://sciencespeaksblog.org/2012/02/09/expert-panel-strategizes-to-repeal-the-federal-ban-on-funding-for-syringe-exchange.

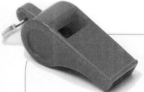

You Make the Call

Should Marijuana Be Legalized for Recreational Purposes?

Currently, 21 states and the District of Columbia have laws in place that legalize the use of marijuana for medical purposes, and many others are considering similar laws regarding medical marijuana. A somewhat different debate is also taking place—whether marijuana should be legalized for nonmedical use. This debate grew louder in 2010, when California became the first state to consider legalization of marijuana for adult recreational use. Since then, Colorado and Washington have legalized marijuana for recreational use. In national surveys 48 percent of Americans say they have tried marijuana, and 6.5 percent of high school seniors report daily use.

Proponents of legalization contend that marijuana is safer than alcohol and tobacco. An estimated 76,000 people die each year due to excessive alcohol consumption, and more than 400,000 die each year from the effects of smoking. Marijuana has not been the primary cause of any recorded deaths and was a secondary cause in only 279 deaths during an eight-and-a-half-year period. Proponents cite statistics connecting alcohol with violence and point out that marijuana does not make people belligerent. Alcohol is involved in two-thirds of domestic violence cases, and an estimated 40 percent of rape and sexual assault perpetrators are under the influence of alcohol at the time of the crime. Opponents respond that we should not legalize another substance that will cause harm, even if it is relatively less harmful than alcohol or tobacco. They point to the negative health consequences of smoking marijuana, which include heart and respiratory problems, as evidence that marijuana is not a benign drug.

Proponents also argue that the legalization of marijuana would result in financial benefits for the government. The federal government would gain revenue from income taxes on profits made by marijuana businesses. States would no longer have to use money and resources to enforce current marijuana laws and would gain revenue from taxes on the sale of marijuana. The California Legislative Analyst's Office estimates that the legalization of marijuana would result in $1.4 billion a year in additional tax revenue for the

Continued…

Concluded...

state. Some of these tax monies could even be used to bolster underfunded prevention and treatment programs, proponents say.

Opponents respond that the additional revenue would not result in a financial boon because states would have to spend more money on treatment programs, and individuals and society would have to bear the costs of marijuana-related health problems. Opponents argue that legalization would increase the number of young people using marijuana and likely lead to higher rates of use of more addictive drugs. The federal government currently classifies marijuana itself as a Schedule I drug, meaning that it has a high potential for abuse. More teens are in treatment for marijuana use than for any other drug, and increasing the availability of marijuana to adults would increase the opportunities for children and teens to obtain it for themselves, opponents say.

As the graph of a 2013 Gallup poll shows, the percentage of Americans who favor legalization is steadily increasing. Harmless fun or dangerous drug—what do you think?

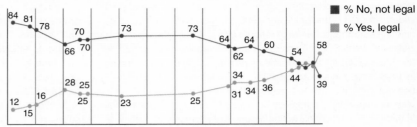

Americans' Views on Legalizing Marijuana, 1969–2013

■ % No, not legal
■ % Yes, legal

Pros

■ The number of states that have legalized medical marijuana and the most recent poll numbers show that public opinion is shifting favorably toward legalizing the drug.

■ Marijuana is a relatively safe drug when compared with legal drugs like alcohol and tobacco.

■ Legalizing marijuana will save money on law enforcement and generate tax revenue.

Cons

■ Marijuana is not a harmless drug. It can cause many health problems, including heart, respiratory, and short-term memory problems.

■ Legalization would make the drug more available to children and teens.

■ Taxing the sale of marijuana would not result in a net increase in federal and state revenues because health care costs from marijuana-related problems would outweigh any gains.

Sources: "Record-High 50% of Americans Favor Legalizing Marijuana Use," *Gallup Politics,* 2012, www.gallup.com/poll/150149/record-high-americans-favor-legalizing-marijuana.aspx; "Deaths from Marijuana v. 17 FDA-Approved Drugs," ProCon.org, 2009, http://medicalmarijuana.procon.org/view.resource.php?resourceID=000145; "Don't Legalize Marijuana," by S. Miller, 2010, *The Los Angeles Times,* http://articles.latimes.com/2010/jan/28/opinion/la-oe-miller28-2010jan28; "How Safe Is Recreational Marijuana?" by R. Khamsi, *Scientific American 308*(6), www.scientificamerican.com/article/how-safe-recreational-marijuana. Graph from "For the First Time, Americans Favor Legalizing Marijuana," by A. Swift, *Gallup Politics online,* October 22, 2013, www.gallup.com/poll/165539/first-time-americans-favor-legalizing-marijuana.aspx.

In Review

Why do people use drugs, and what are current patterns of drug use?
As with alcohol, people use drugs to feel better, often as a recreational activity; however, some people become addicted and lose control of their drug use. The most commonly used illicit drug is marijuana, but the nonmedical use of prescription-type drugs has increased dramatically in recent years.

What are the different categories of drugs, and what are the differences between drug misuse and abuse?
Drugs can be categorized as legal or illicit. Drugs developed for medical purposes are pharmaceutical drugs; some are available only by prescription, while others are available over the counter. Drug misuse is the use of prescription drugs for purposes other than those for which they were prescribed or the use of any drug or chemical for any purpose other than its intended one. Drug abuse is the use of a substance in an amount, situation, or manner that causes problems for the user or for others.

How do drugs affect the body?
As psychoactive substances, drugs affect the brain and the central nervous system (CNS). Effects vary depending on the route of administration, the chemical properties of the drug, the characteristics of the person, and the environment. Drug addiction causes changes in the brain, particularly the brain structures that make up the pleasure and reward circuit and those parts of the brain involved in rational thought and judgment.

What are the different categories of drugs?
Drugs are classified as CNS stimulants (e.g., cocaine, methamphetamine), CNS depressants (barbiturates, benzodiazepines), opioids (heroin, oxycodone), hallucinogens (LSD), inhalants (paint thinner, glue), and cannabinoids (marijuana).

What are the main approaches to the drug problem?
The main approaches are supply reduction strategies (e.g., interdiction), demand reduction strategies (incarceration, prevention through education, treatment), and harm reduction strategies (e.g., needle exchange programs). Because college administrations are often focused more on alcohol-related problems than on drug-related problems, students may have to be more proactive in identifying and helping friends who are developing a drug problem.

Sexual Health

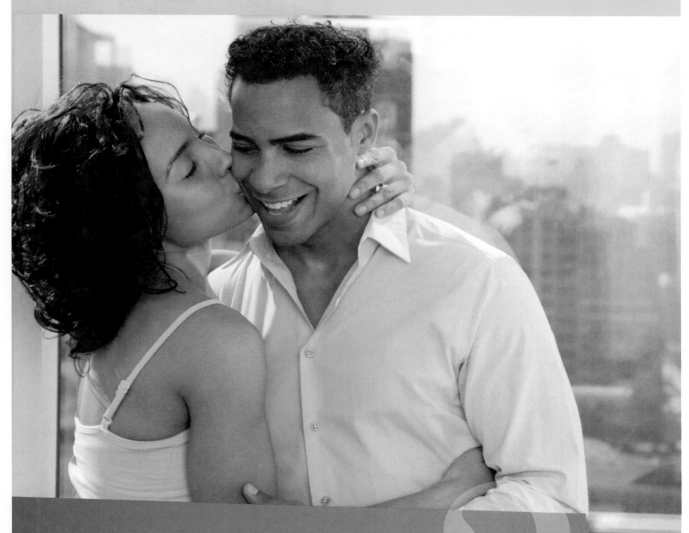

Ever Wonder...

- how the sex drive actually works?

- how to talk to a prospective partner about your sexual histories?

- how often most college students have sex, and how often they use condoms?

Sexuality is a vital aspect of physical and psychological wellness. In the context of intimate relationships, sexuality plays a role in some of life's most meaningful experiences. Sexual activity is a source of pleasure, excitement, and connection with other people, and it is even good for your health. Studies show that an active sex life reduces the risk of heart disease, decreases risk of depression, provides temporary relief from chronic pain, boosts the immune system, and lowers the risk of death.[1] But sexuality is a complex human behavior, and it can be associated with negative experiences, such as worries and anxieties, relationship discord, health issues, and societal problems.

Sexual health includes satisfying intimate relationships based on mutual respect and trust and the ability and resources to procreate if so desired. It involves acceptance of one's own sexual feelings and tolerance for those of others. It also includes knowledge about sexuality and access to the information needed to make responsible decisions. The Chapter 11 health portfolio addresses personal health decisions.

BIOLOGY, CULTURE, AND SEXUAL PLEASURE

Although sexual anatomy and physiology are similar in all human beings, sexual behavior and expression vary tremendously across societies, cultures, and eras. There are even differences in what is considered sexually pleasurable from one culture and time to another. Sexual pleasure has been defined as positively valued feelings induced by sexual stimuli.[2] Sensory signals arriving in the brain are not inherently pleasurable; rather, the brain interprets them as pleasurable. This interpretation and evaluation of stimuli by the brain as sexually pleasurable is influenced by everything the individual has learned about sex in his or her society and culture, including expectations, attitudes, and values.

In the United States, sexual attitudes are marked by an ongoing tension between the two poles of sexual restrictiveness and sexual freedom. The so-called sexual revolution of the 1960s gave way to a more conservative climate in the 1980s and 1990s. Prevailing attitudes toward sex and sexual pleasure in the early 21st century will be determined, in part, by college students and other young adults.

Sexual Anatomy and Functioning

Although sexuality serves many purposes in human experience, the biological purpose of sexuality is reproduction. In this section, we explore some of the biological aspects of sexuality.

Sexual Anatomy   The male and female sex organs arise from the same undifferentiated tissue during the prenatal period, becoming male or female under the influence of hormones (discussed later in this section). In this sense, the sexual organs of males and females are very similar, and their purpose and functions are complementary. The female sex organs

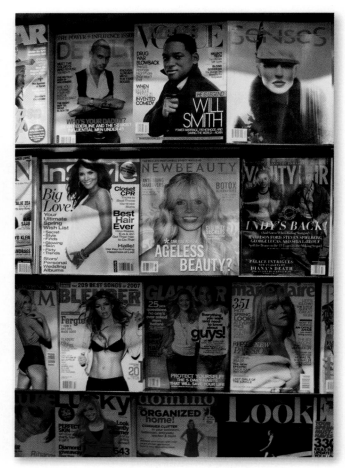

■ What we find sexually exciting, attractive, and acceptable is largely determined by the messages we get from our culture.

are responsible for the production of ova and, if pregnancy occurs, the development of the fetus. The male sex organs are responsible for producing sperm and delivering them into the female reproductive system to fertilize the ovum.

Female Sex Organs and Reproductive Anatomy   The external genitalia of the female are called the vulva and include the mons pubis, the labia majora and labia minora, the clitoris, and the vaginal and urethral openings (Figure 11.1). The mons pubis is a mound or layer of fatty tissue that pads and protects the pubic bone. The labia majora (major lips) and labia minora (minor lips) are folds of tissue that wrap around the entrance to the vagina. The labia minora form a protective hood, or prepuce, over the clitoris. The clitoris is a highly sensitive, cylindrical body about 3 centimeters in length that fills with blood during sexual excitement. Consisting of a glans, corpus, and crura, the clitoris is located at the top of the vulva between the lips of the labia minora.

The urethral opening, the passageway for urine from the urinary bladder, is located immediately below the clitoris. The hymen is a thin membranous fold, highly variable in appearance, which may partially cover the opening of the vagina.

External Organs (Vulva)

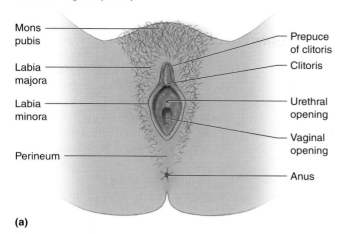

Mons pubis
Labia majora
Labia minora
Perineum
Prepuce of clitoris
Clitoris
Urethral opening
Vaginal opening
Anus

(a)

Internal Organs

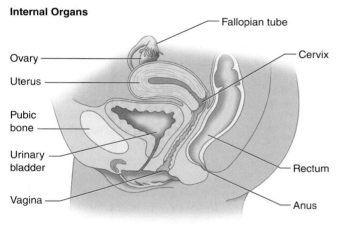

Ovary
Uterus
Pubic bone
Urinary bladder
Vagina
Fallopian tube
Cervix
Rectum
Anus

(b)

figure 11.1   Female sexual and reproductive anatomy.
(a) External structures; (b) internal structures.

The hymen has no known biological function and is frequently absent. The perineum is the area between the bottom of the vulva and the anus. It contains many nerve endings.

The internal sex organs of the female include the vagina, cervix, uterus, fallopian tubes, and ovaries. The vagina is a hollow, muscular tube extending from the external vaginal opening to the cervix. The walls of the vagina are soft and flexible and have several layers. The existence of an area called the G-spot on the lower front wall of the vagina is a subject of debate; if it is present, it may feel like an elevated bump. Located on either side of the vagina under the labia are the crura, extensions of the clitoris.

The cervix is the lower part of the uterus; it extends into the vagina and contains the opening to the uterus. The cervix produces a mucus that changes with different stages of the menstrual cycle. The uterus is the organ in which a fertilized egg develops into an embryo and then a fetus. Approximately the size of a pear, the uterus is made up of several layers of muscle and tissue. The endometrium is the layer that is shed during menstruation.

The ovaries are the female reproductive glands that store and release the ova (eggs) every month, usually one at a time—the process of ovulation. They also produce the female sex hormones estrogen and progesterone. The ovaries are located on either side of the uterus. Extending from the upper sides of the uterus are the fallopian tubes (or oviducts), the passageways through which ova move from the ovaries into the uterus. Their openings are lined with fimbria, appendages with beating cilia that sweep the surface of the ovaries during ovulation and guide the ovum down into the tubes.

The mammary glands, or breasts, are also part of female sexual and reproductive anatomy. They consist of 15 to 25 lobes that are padded by connective tissue and fat. Within the lobes are glands that produce milk when the woman is lactating following the birth of a baby. At the center of each breast is a nipple, surrounded by a ring of darker colored skin called the areola. The nipple becomes erect when stimulated by cold, touch, or sexual stimuli.

Male Sex Organs and Reproductive Anatomy   The external genitalia of the male include the penis and the scrotum, which contains the testes (Figure 11.2). The penis, when erect, is designed to deliver sperm into the female reproductive tract. The shaft of the penis is formed of three columns of spongelike erectile tissue that fill with blood during sexual excitement. The glans, or head of the penis, is an expansion of the corpus spongiosum (one of the three columns of erectile tissue in the penis shaft). The glans contains a higher concentration of nerve endings than the shaft and is highly sensitive.

The corona is a crownlike structure that protrudes slightly and forms a border between the glans and the shaft; it is also highly sensitive. The frenulum is a fold of skin extending from the corona to the foreskin. The foreskin, or prepuce, covers the glans, more or less completely. **Circumcision** involves removing this skin and leaving the head of the penis permanently exposed. The urethral opening, through which both urine and semen pass (at different times), is located at the tip of the penis in the glans. The urethra runs the length of the penis from the urinary bladder to the exterior of the body.

circumcision
Removal of the foreskin of the penis; a procedure often routinely performed on newborn male infants in the United States.

The scrotum, a thin sac composed of skin and muscle fibers, contains the testes. The scrotum is separated from the body to keep the testes at the lower temperature that is needed for sperm production. The area between the scrotum and the anus is the perineum; as in females, it contains many nerve endings.

The male internal reproductive organs include the testes, a series of ducts that transport sperm (the epididymis, vas deferens, ejaculatory ducts, and urethra), and a set of glands that produce semen and other fluids (the seminal vesicles, prostate gland, and Cowper's glands). The two testes, located

External Organs

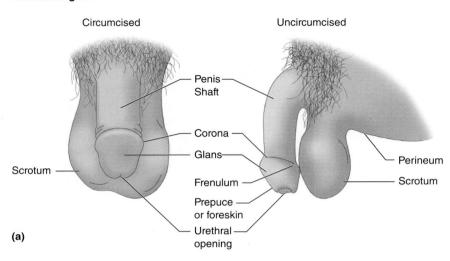

(a)

Internal Organs

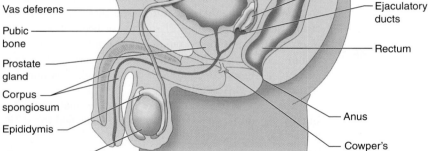

(b)

figure 11.2   **Male sexual and reproductive anatomy.**
(a) External structures; (b) internal structures.

in the scrotum, are the male reproductive glands; they produce both sperm and male sex hormones such as testosterone. Once sperm are produced in the testes, they enter the epididymis, a highly coiled duct lying on the surface of each testis. As they move along the length of the epididymis, immature sperm mature and develop the ability to swim.

When the male ejaculates, sperm are propelled from the epididymis into the vas deferens, another duct, which joins with ducts from the seminal vesicles to form the short ejaculatory ducts. The two seminal vesicles, located at the back of the bladder, produce about 60 percent of the volume of semen, the milky fluid that carries sperm

sex drive
Biological urge for sexual activity; also called sexual desire or libido.

vasocongestion
Inflow of blood to tissues in erogenous areas.

and contains nutrients to fuel them. The sperm and semen travel through the ejaculatory ducts to the prostate gland, a doughnut-shaped structure that encircles the urethra and contributes the remaining volume of semen. The semen is then ejaculated through the urethra. The two Cowper's glands, located below the prostate gland, produce a clear mucus that is secreted into the urethra just before ejaculation. The volume of semen in one ejaculation is about 2 to 5 milliliters, containing between 100 and 600 million sperm.

Sexual Response In order for reproduction to occur, ova and sperm have to be brought into close association with each other. The psychological and motivational mechanism for this is the human sexual response, which includes sex drive, sexual arousal, and orgasm.

Sex Drive **Sex drive**—sexual desire, or libido—is defined as a biological urge for sexual activity. The principal hormone responsible for the sex drive in both males and females is testosterone, produced by the testes in males and by the adrenal glands in both sexes. Testosterone stimulates increased release of the neurotransmitters dopamine and serotonin in the brain; they are thought to be involved in making external stimuli arousing. Dopamine and serotonin levels peak at orgasm and then decline.[3] Serotonin is thought to have an effect on feelings of sexual satisfaction and orgasm. The hormones epinephrine (adrenaline) and norepinephrine (nonadrenaline), released by the adrenal glands, are involved in arousal and increased heart rate, blood pressure, respiration, and other autonomic nervous system functions.

People usually seek to satisfy the sex drive through physical stimulation and release, either with a partner or through masturbation. Besides hormones, sex drive is also influenced by sexual imagery and sexual fantasies, which in turn are influenced by one's culture. Sex drive can be stimulated by sights, sounds, smells, tastes, and myriad other external stimuli, as well as by one's own thoughts and fantasies. The goal of arousal varies by culture. Western cultures typically focus on attaining orgasm. Some cultures encourage the suppression of the sex drive; other cultures emphasize spiritual and sensual outcomes as the goals of sexual activity.[3]

Sexual Arousal Sexual arousal on the physiological level involves vasocongestion and myotonia. **Vasocongestion** is the inflow of blood to tissues in erogenous areas. In men, the arterioles supplying blood to the erectile tissue of the penis are normally constricted. Sexual arousal causes nerves in the penis to release nitric oxide, which in turn activates an enzyme that relaxes the arterioles and allows the penis to fill with blood. Engorgement compresses the veins in the penis and prevents blood from flowing out. In women, a similar process causes engorgement of the clitoris, labia, vagina, and nipples; vaginal lubrication also increases. **Myotonia** is a voluntary or involuntary muscle tension occurring in response to sexual stimuli. Both vasocongestion and myotonia build up during sexual excitement and decrease afterward.[4]

The Human Sexual Response Model In the 1960s, sex researchers William Masters and Virginia Johnson conducted detailed studies of sexual activity and developed a four-phase model of the human sexual response (Figure 11.3) The four phases are excitement, plateau, orgasm, and resolution.[5,6]

The excitement stage begins with stimulation that initiates vasocongestion and myotonia. The first sign of excitement in men is penis erection. In women, signs include vaginal lubrication and, frequently, nipple and clitoral erection. Heart rate and respiratory rate generally increase in both men and women.

The plateau phase is a leveling-off period just before orgasm. Increased muscle tension continues during the plateau phase. The heart rate remains elevated and breathing is deep. The penis increases in size and length, and the upper two-thirds of the vagina widens and expands.

A more complex view of sexual response is the dual control model, which is based on brain function. Sexual excitement and sexual inhibition are viewed as separate systems. People with low propensity for sexual excitement or high sex inhibition are more likely to experience difficulty in sexual response to sexual stimuli. High-risk sexual activity, such as not practicing safe sex, is a more likely outcome for people with high sexual excitement and low sexual inhibition. Most people score in the middle for excitation and inhibition, but there is great variability from one person to the next. For example, men tend to score higher on the sexual excitement and lower on sexual inhibition than women, and gay men score higher on excitation and lower on inhibition than straight men.[3]

Orgasm **Orgasm** is a physiological reflex in which a massive discharge of nerve impulses occurs in the nerves serving the genitals, usually in response to tactile stimulation, causing rhythmic muscle contractions in the genital area and a sensation of intense pleasure. In men, contractions occur in the penis, ducts, glands, and muscles in the pelvic and anal regions; orgasm is accompanied by the ejaculation of semen. In women, contractions occur in the uterus, vagina, and pelvic and anal regions.

Resolution is the return to an unexcited, relaxed state. Men enter a **refractory period**, lasting from minutes to hours, during which vasoconstriction of the arterioles supplying the erectile tissue causes the penis to become flaccid (soft) again. During the refractory period, the man is not able to

have another orgasm. Most young men can have one to three orgasms in an hour, as can some older men.

In women, orgasm is not followed by a refractory period, so women can experience multiple orgasms during a single sexual experience. Multiple orgasms may be experienced as part of the general climactic wave or as a series of orgasms as much as five minutes apart.

An alternative model suggests that many women, especially those in long-term relationships, may not experience sexual desire (conscious sexual urges) moving to sexual arousal. Instead, sexual arousal more commonly precedes sexual desire. Sexual desire occurs only after a sufficient period of sexual arousal and is more of a responsive event than a spontaneous event.[5] The choice to initiate sexual arousal is often more dependent on intimacy needs (needs for emotional closeness, bonding, love, affection) than on a need for physical sexual arousal or release. Intimacy benefits and appreciation for the sexual well-being of the partner serve as the motivational factors to move from sexual neutrality to sexual arousal.[7] This model may also apply to some men in long-term relationships.

The Experience of Orgasm Although orgasm is physically experienced in the genitals, it is also a mental and emotional event. The subjective experience of orgasm can be influenced by an infinite variety of physical, emotional, psychological, interpersonal, and environmental factors.

Most people experience a feeling of deep warmth or pressure when orgasm is imminent or inevitable. Orgasm is usually felt as waves of intense pleasure accompanied by contractions in the penis, vagina, or uterus. The sensations may be localized to the genitals, or they may be generalized over the whole body.

About a third of women reach orgasm from the sensations produced in the vagina by the thrusting of the penis, but many women need direct stimulation of the clitoris to reach orgasm.[7,8] Most intercourse positions do not include such direct pressure or stimulation, so intercourse alone may not be completely satisfying for a woman. Even women who reach orgasm regularly only climax about 50 to 70 percent of the time. Active stimulation of the clitoris with fingers or a vibrator can help women reach orgasm. When a woman is unable to reach orgasm, it is usually due to inhibition or lack of needed stimulation (see Figure 11.4). Women are more likely to experience orgasm if the sexual encounter includes oral sex or anal sex. About 95 percent of men experience orgasm in sexual encounters that include vaginal intercourse.[8]

Some people pretend to have reached orgasm during sex when they haven't. One study found

myotonia
Voluntary or involuntary muscle tension occurring in response to sexual stimuli.

orgasm
Physiological reflex characterized by rhythmic muscle contractions in the genital area and a sensation of intense pleasure.

refractory period
Time following orgasm when a man cannot have another orgasm.

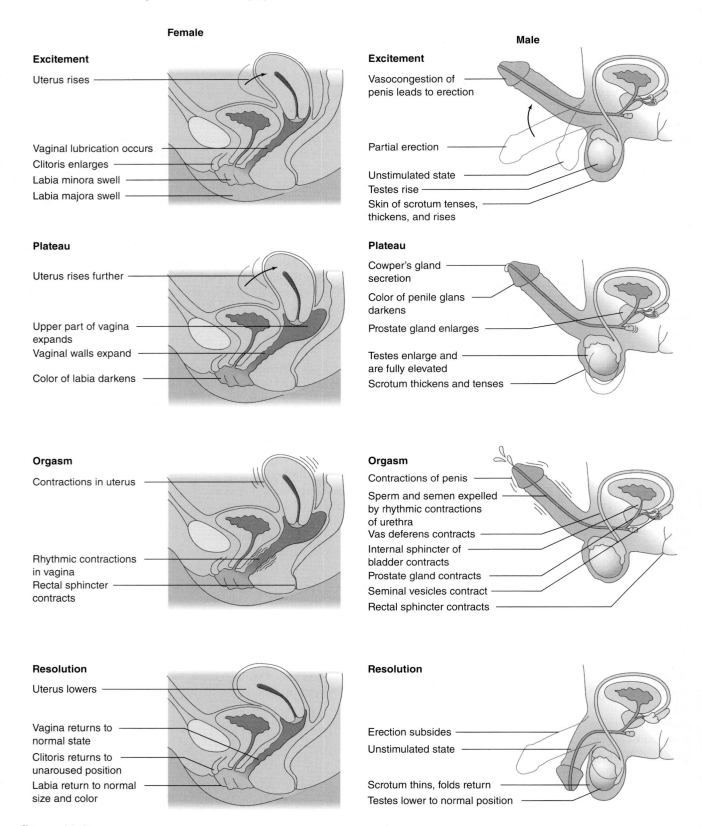

figure 11.3 **The human sexual response model.**

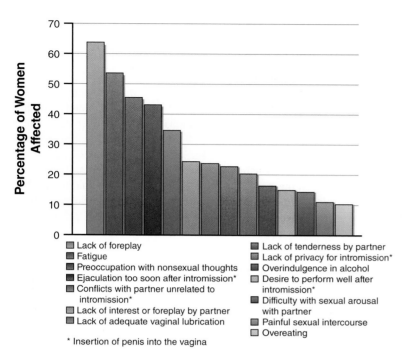

figure 11.4   **Factors inhibiting women's orgasm during intercourse.**

Adapted from Human sexuality: Diversity in contemporary America, by W. Yarber, B. Sayad, and B. Strong, 2012, New York: McGraw-Hill.

that about 60 percent of heterosexual college women and 71 percent of lesbian or bisexual women had faked an orgasm. In contrast, 17 percent of heterosexual men and 27 percent of gay or bisexual men had faked an orgasm.[9] The primary reason women fake orgasms is to protect the feelings of their sexual partner, but other reasons include the desire to expedite boring or painful intercourse and fear of their own sexual inadequacy. Faking an orgasm can undermine a relationship. A satisfying relationship includes having honest discussions about what helps both partners enjoy sex the most.

Sexual Development and Health Across the Lifespan The biology of sexual development is directed by hormones throughout the lifespan. Male sex hormones, called **androgens**, are secreted primarily by the testes, and female sex hormones, called **estrogens** and **progestins**, are secreted by the ovaries. Hormones play a role in the prenatal development of sex organs and again at puberty, when secondary sex characteristics appear and the reproductive system matures: the sex organs become larger, and pubic and underarm hair appears. In boys, the voice deepens, facial hair begins to grow, and the onset of **ejaculation** occurs. Boys begin to experience nocturnal emissions (orgasm and ejaculation during sleep), and the testes start to produce sperm. In girls, breasts develop, body fat increases, and **menarche**, the onset of menstruation, occurs.

Every month between the ages of about 12 and about 50, except during pregnancy, women experience monthly menstrual periods. During the first half of the cycle, the lining of the uterus thickens with blood vessels in preparation for the possibility of pregnancy, and an ovum matures in one of the ovaries. About halfway through the cycle, the ovum is released (ovulation) and is carried into the uterus. If sperm are present, the ovum may be fertilized and begin to develop into an embryo. If an ovum isn't fertilized, the uterine lining is shed, causing **menses**, and the cycle begins again.

Some girls and women experience uncomfortable physical symptoms during their periods, such as cramps and backache, and some experience physical and emotional symptoms before their periods, such as headache, irritability, and mood swings, referred to as premenstrual tension or premenstrual syndrome (PMS). If symptoms are severe and interfere with usual work, family, or social activities, the woman may be diagnosed with premenstrual dysphoric disorder (PMDD). The exact causes of PMS and PMDD are not known, but lifestyle changes—such as exercising, eating well, and avoiding alcohol—may help relieve symptoms. A physician may prescribe medications for more severe symptoms.

In middle age, hormonal changes cause a gradual reduction in ovarian functioning that culminates in menopause, the cessation of menstruation. During the time leading up to menopause, a period of three to seven years called perimenopause, many women experience symptoms caused by hormonal fluctuations, such as hot flashes, night sweats, irritability, and insomnia. A decrease in estrogen production can cause less visible symptoms as well, such as a reduction in bone density and changes in blood levels of cholesterol. These changes contribute to women's increased risk of osteoporosis and heart disease later in life. Uncomfortable symptoms of perimenopause and menopause can be improved in many cases by lifestyle changes like increased physical activity and stress management.[10]

Men do not experience a dramatic change in reproductive capacity in midlife as women do; the testes continue to produce sperm throughout life. Some researchers believe, however, that middle-aged men experience a period during which testosterone levels fluctuate and there may be changes in sexual functioning, irritability, mild to moderate mood swings, and other symptoms. For both men and women, however, biological changes in the sexual response phases have only a marginal effect on sexual interest and activity. The more sexually active a person is, the less effect these biological changes have.[11]

androgens
Male sex hormones, secreted primarily by the testes.

estrogens
Female sex hormones; secreted by the ovaries.

progestins
Female sex hormones; secreted by the ovaries.

ejaculation
Emission of semen during orgasm.

menarche
Onset of menstruation.

menses
Flow of menstrual blood; the menstrual period.

Sexuality and Disability Although individuals with disabilities may experience limitations in their sexuality or may have to develop new or alternative forms of sexual activity, most people with disabilities can have a rewarding sex life. For people with physical limitations, different forms of sexual expression may be possible. A person with spinal cord injury may not be able to have an orgasm, but he or she may be able to have intercourse, experience sensuous feelings in other parts of the body, or have a child. As in any relationship, the key is nurturing emotional as well as sexual intimacy. Information and education can help individuals with disabilities, as can counseling that focuses on building self-esteem and overcoming shame, guilt, fear, anger, and unrealistic expectations. Changes in sexual functioning and desire can also be caused by chronic disease, such as diabetes, arthritis, cancer, and cardiovascular disease, as well as by the medications used to treat them. For example, diabetes can cause nerve damage and circulatory problems that affect erectile functioning in men. Individuals and couples may have to make significant adjustments in their forms of sexual expression to accommodate such disabling conditions.[3,10,11] Information and education are also important for members of the general public, who too often fail to acknowledge the full humanity of individuals with disabilities, including their sexuality. The Development Disabilities Assistance and Bill of Rights Act of 2000 clearly states that sexual rights for people with disabilities should be the same as for people without disabilities, including the right to sexual expression, the right to have or not have children, and the right to privacy.

celibacy
Continuous abstention from sexual activities with others.

abstinence
Abstention from sexual intercourse, usually as a way to avoid conception or STDs.

foreplay
Touching that increases sexual arousal before sexual intercourse.

Varieties of Sexual Behavior and Expression

Rather than thinking in terms of "normalcy," social scientists think in terms of behavior that is typical and behavior that is less typical.

■ Pop star Lady Gaga, whose songs often feature provocative lyrics, surprised her fans in 2010 when she announced she was celibate, which she did in part to help promote HIV awareness among women. At a promotional event for MAC cosmetics' "Viva Glam" campaign to fight AIDS, she said, "Even Lady Gaga can be celibate. You don't have to have sex to be loved."

Typical and Common Forms of Sexual Expression Typical forms of sexual behavior and expression in U.S. society include celibacy, erotic touch, self-stimulation, oral-genital stimulation, and intercourse.

Celibacy Continuous abstention from sexual activities with others is called **celibacy**. People may be completely celibate (do not engage in masturbation) or partially celibate (engage in masturbation). Moral and religious beliefs lead some people to choose celibacy. Lack of a suitable sexual partner or sexual relationship may be another reason for celibacy.[8]

Some people use the term *abstinence* interchangeably with *celibacy,* but **abstinence** usually means abstention only from sexual intercourse. As such, abstinence is promoted as a way to avoid sexually transmitted diseases and unintended pregnancy.

Erotic Touch Touch is a sensual form of communication that can elicit feelings of tenderness and affection as well as sexual feelings. It is an important part of **foreplay**, touching that increases sexual arousal and precedes sexual intercourse. Some areas of the body are more sensitive to touch than others. Skin in the nonspecific erogenous zones of the body (the inner thighs, armpits, shoulders, feet, ears, and sides of the back and neck) contains more nerve endings than do many other areas; these areas are capable of being aroused by touch. Skin in the specific *erogenous zones* (penis, clitoris, vulva, perineum, lips, breasts, and buttocks) has an even higher density of nerve endings, and nerve endings are closer to the skin surface.[8] The landscape of erotic touch includes holding hands, kissing, stroking, caressing, squeezing, tickling, scratching, and massaging.

A popular view of pleasure-oriented touching is the "gears of connection" metaphor that identifies five touch dimensions: affection, sensuality, playfulness, erotic nonintercourse, and intercourse. First gear (affective touching) includes such interactions as holding hands, hugging, and kissing. Second gear (sensual) involves touching the body but not the genitals. Third gear (playful) includes playful touching nongenital and genital touching. Fourth gear (erotic) includes manual and oral genital touching, rubbing, and vibrator stimulation. And fifth gear (intercourse) is the final dimension of pleasure-oriented touching. The model emphasizes savoring each of the five touching dimensions rather than rushing through the first four gears to reach the final gear.[3]

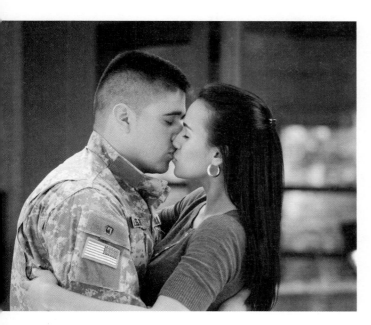

■ The lips are a highly sensitive part of the body, making kissing an intimate act.

Kissing Typically, kissing is a person's earliest interpersonal sexual experience. Kissing is the most accepted of all sexual activities because it represents a romantic expression of affection as well as sexual desire. The lips and mouth are erotic parts of the human body. Touching, tasting, and smelling with the lips and mouth activate our unconscious memories and associations. Scientists conjecture that the testosterone in a male's saliva can stimulate female sex hormones that make them more receptive to sex.[12]

In both emotional and practical terms, women and men tend to think about kissing differently. Women typically place more importance than men on kissing for beginning and sustaining a relationship. They are less likely than men to believe it is acceptable to kiss on the first date or that a woman should make the first move for a kiss. Women were more likely to say no to sex with someone whose kissing they don't like. In contrast, men may place more emphasis on kissing as a means to advance to oral sex or intercourse.[13] For some people, regardless of gender, kissing can make or break a relationship. One study found that 59 percent of men and 66 percent of women were attracted to someone until they discovered they did not like the way the person kissed.[1]

Self-Stimulation The two most common self-stimulation sexual activities, called **autoerotic behaviors**, are sexual fantasies and masturbation. Sexual fantasies are mental images, scenarios, and daydreams imagined to initiate sexual arousal. They range from simple images to complicated erotic stories.

The fact that the body can become aroused when a person thinks about sex highlights the fact that the brain is a major player in sexual functioning. Fantasies are effective and harmless ways of exploring sexual fulfillment.

Masturbation is self-stimulation of the genitals for sexual pleasure. It is usually done manually or with a vibrator or other sex toy. The stigma attached to masturbation is left over from a previous era, when it was considered sinful and dangerous to one's health, probably because its purpose was pleasure rather than procreation. Today, masturbation is better understood and more widely accepted as a natural and healthy sexual behavior. Masturbation is a part of sex therapy programs designed to help people overcome sexual problems, and mutual masturbation is promoted as a way to practice safer sex.[14]

Mutual masturbation and other ways people use their fingers and hands are less risky for STIs than sex involving the exchange of body fluids. There are still STI risks. The use of latex or nitrite gloves or finger cots reduce the transmission of bacteria and other pathogens that can be found on the skin or under the nails. Cutting nails or padding nails with cotton before putting on a glove can prevent making a hole in the glove. It is also a good idea to lubricate hands or gloves to prevent chafing or skin damage.[3,15]

Oral-Genital Stimulation **Cunnilingus** is the oral stimulation of the female genitals with the tongue and lips. **Fellatio** is the oral stimulation of the male genitals with the tongue, lips, and mouth. Oral stimulation can be part of foreplay, or it can be a sexual activity leading to orgasm. Some people find oral-genital stimulation very pleasurable; in fact, many women find that it is easier for them to reach orgasm through cunnilingus than through vaginal intercourse. Other people refrain from oral-genital stimulation because of religious or moral beliefs or simply because it makes them uncomfortable. Some women hesitate about cunnilingus because they are concerned about possible vaginal odors or their partner's enjoyment. A common concern with fellatio is whether the man should ejaculate into his partner's mouth. This is a matter of personal preference; the person receiving fellatio should respect the feelings of his partner.[14]

Oral sex is not an entirely safe form of sex because infections can be transmitted via the mouth. Unprotected oral sex can transmit HIV, herpes, HPV, gonorrhea, chlamydia, syphilis, and hepatitis B. These sexually transmitted infections (STIs) are discussed in-depth in Chapter 13. STIs can lead to very serious diseases; for example, HPV is a major risk factor for oral and throat cancers. Using some form of protection during oral sex is recommended. Condoms lubricated with nonoxynol-9 (N-9) are not safe either for vaginal or for oral sex.[16] Dental dams are effective forms of protection and, along with condoms, are discussed later in the chapter.

autoerotic behaviors
Self-stimulating sexual activities, primarily sexual fantasies and masturbation.

masturbation
Self-stimulation of the genitals for sexual pleasure.

cunnilingus
Oral stimulation of the female genitals with the tongue and lips.

fellatio
Oral stimulation of the male genitals with the tongue, lips, and mouth.

Anal Intercourse A small percentage of heterosexual couples and a larger percentage of gay male couples practice anal intercourse, the penetration of the rectum with the penis. About a third of people aged 15 to 44 have practiced anal intercourse, with higher rates among Whites than among Hispanics or Blacks. It is also more prevalent among people with more education.[3] The anal area has a high density of nerve endings and is sensitive to stimulation. Because the skin and tissue of the anus and rectum are delicate and can be easily torn, anal intercourse is one of the riskiest sexual behaviors for the transmission of infections, particularly HIV. Condom use is strongly recommended during anal intercourse. One study estimated the probability of HIV infection in a single unprotected act of receptive anal intercourse at 3.4 percent. The risk of contracting HIV through vaginal intercourse is much lower, less than 0.01 percent per act.[3]

Sexual Intercourse Sexual intercourse, also known as coitus, is by far the most common form of adult sexual expression. It is a source of sexual pleasure for most couples. In sexual intercourse, a man typically inserts his erect penis into a woman's vagina and thrusts with his hips and pelvis until he ejaculates. A woman who is aroused responds with matching hip and pelvic thrusts, but she may or may not reach orgasm solely from penetration and thrusting, as mentioned earlier.

Sexual intercourse can be performed in a variety of positions. The most common is the so-called missionary position, in which the man lies on top of the woman. In this position, the penis can penetrate deeply into the vagina. When the woman lies on top of the man, penetration may not be as deep, but the woman has more control, an important psychological factor for some women. When the woman sits or kneels on top of the man, penetration is deeper and the woman can increase clitoral stimulation by rocking back and forth.[8]

In the rear-entry position, the woman lies face down and the man lies on top of her, or both lie on their sides. Although penetration is not as deep in this position, there is more opportunity for clitoral stimulation by either the woman or the man. Side-by-side positions may be popular for sexual partners with significant weight differences, pregnant women, partners with chronic pain disorders like arthritis, and partners who do not enjoy deep thrusting.[8]

Atypical Sexual Behaviors and Paraphilias Some sexual practices are much less common statistically in our society than those already described. If they are practiced between consenting adults and no physical or psychological harm is done to anyone, they are simply considered atypical. Examples are sex games in which partners enact sexual fantasies, use sex toys (vibrators, dildos), or engage in phone sex (talk about sex, describe erotic scenarios). Another kind of sex game is bondage and discipline, in which restriction of movement (e.g., using handcuffs or ropes) or sensory deprivation (using blindfolds or masks) is employed for sexual enjoyment. Most sex games are safe and harmless, but partners need to openly discuss and agree beforehand on what they are comfortable doing.

Atypical sexual practices that do not meet the criteria described (being consensual and causing no harm) are called paraphilias; they are classified as mental disorders. Generally speaking, they involve victimization and are illegal. Some examples include exhibitionism (exposing one's genitals to strangers), voyeurism (observing others' sexual activity without their knowledge), telephone scatologia (making obscene phone calls), sexual sadism/masochism (inflicting psychological or physical suffering), and pedophilia (sexual attraction to and activity with children). Treatment of individuals with these disorders typically focuses first on reducing the danger to the patient and potential victims and then on strategies to suppress the behavior. Relapse prevention is essential because these behaviors are usually long-standing.[8]

SEXUAL DYSFUNCTIONS

At some point in their lives, many people experience some kind of **sexual dysfunction**—a disturbance in sexual drive, performance, or satisfaction. Up to 50 percent of couples report having experienced sexual dissatisfaction or dysfunction.[17] Sexual difficulties may occur at any point in the sexual response, although lack of sexual desire is cited as the most frequent problem in marriage and long-term relationships.[17] Most forms of sexual dysfunction are treatable.

Female Sexual Dysfunctions

Common sexual dysfunctions in women include pain during intercourse, sexual desire disorder, female sexual arousal disorder, and orgasmic dysfunction.

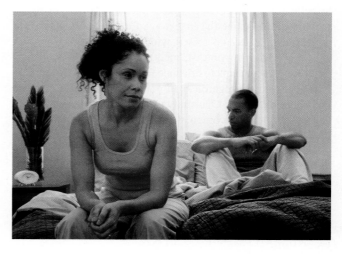

■ Sexuality has physical, psychological, emotional, and interpersonal dimensions. Although sexual problems can have medical or physical causes, they often occur because of relationship problems.

---

sexual dysfunction
Disturbance in sexual drive, performance, or satisfaction.

Pain During Intercourse Some women experience pain during intercourse as a result of **vaginismus**, intense involuntary contractions of the outer third of the muscles of the vagina that tighten the vaginal opening when penetration is attempted. The muscle spasm may range from mild (causing discomfort during intercourse) to severe (preventing intercourse altogether). Vaginismus may be caused by the physiological effects of a medical condition, such as a pelvic or vaginal infection; by psychological factors, such as fear of intercourse; or by lack of vaginal lubrication. A physician may recommend **Kegel exercises**, the alternating contraction and relaxation of pelvic floor muscles, to relieve vaginismus.[17]

Sexual Desire Disorder Sexual desire disorder is characterized by lack of sexual fantasies and desire for sexual activity. Because individuals have different normal levels of sexual desire, a problem is considered to exist only if a person is dissatisfied with her own or her partner's level of sexual desire. Low sexual desire can have physical causes, such as medications or hormonal changes, or it can be caused by psychological, emotional, and relationship problems.

Female Sexual Arousal Disorder This disorder is characterized by an inability to attain or maintain the lubrication–swelling response of sexual arousal to the completion of sexual activity. The symptoms do not occur because of insufficient or misplaced sexual stimulation. Like sexual desire disorder, this disorder is considered a problem only if the individual experiencing it considers it a problem.

Orgasmic Dysfunction Orgasmic dysfunction is defined as the persistent inability to have an orgasm following normal sexual arousal. Between 25 and 35 percent of women report having had difficulty with orgasm on one or more occasions, and 10 to 15 percent of women report that they have never had an orgasm.[18] Some women can achieve orgasm through masturbation or oral sex but not with penile penetration. Although orgasm is not necessary for conception or enjoyment of sex, difficulty achieving orgasm can become a frustrating experience.

Orgasmic dysfunction may be influenced by psychological and emotional factors, by lack of knowledge and experience, or by the person's beliefs and attitudes about sex.[3,19] Certain medications, including some antidepressants, also reduce the ability to reach orgasm. Therapy for orgasmic dysfunction focuses on encouraging women to experiment with their own bodies to discover what stimulates them to orgasm. They are then encouraged to transfer this learning to their sexual relationships.

Treatment of Female Sexual Dysfunctions Much of what is known about the neurophysiology of sexual arousal, desire, and orgasm has come from research on men and has been applied to women.[19] But women's sexuality is different from men's and much more complex than previously thought. Currently, there is a new interest in female sexuality on the part of scientists, sex therapists, and pharmaceutical companies, partly as a result of the success of Viagra in relieving men's sexual problems.[20]

One approach to treatment of sexual problems in women is testosterone replacement therapy. As noted earlier, testosterone is responsible for sex drive in both men and women. Sensibly prescribed, medically necessary testosterone can increase a woman's sex drive, but possible side effects include increased risk of heart disease and liver damage.[9]

Viagra has been tried in women to treat low sexual desire, but results have been disappointing. A few studies suggest that Viagra combined with low doses of testosterone replacement may have good results.[9] Despite setbacks, the drug market for treating female sexual dysfunction is likely to grow. In recent years, there has been an increase in personal lubricants targeted specifically for women (like Zestra), which may increase sexual arousal and orgasm by warming the clitoris.

Male Sexual Dysfunctions

Male sexual dysfunctions include pain during intercourse, sexual desire disorder, erectile dysfunction, and ejaculation dysfunction.

Pain During Intercourse Penile pain usually results from infections from sexually transmitted diseases. Herpes can cause painful lesions on the penis, and gonorrhea and chlamydia cause a penile discharge and pain with urination or ejaculation for most men. Peyronie's disease, an abnormal curvature of the penis, can also make intercourse painful. Infections of the prostate and epididymis also cause pain and should be treated.

Sexual Desire Disorder Sexual desire disorders are frequently caused by emotional problems, including relationship difficulties, depression, guilt over infidelity, worry, stress, and overwork. Reduced sexual desire also can have some physical causes, such as changes in testosterone level.

Erectile Dysfunction In men with **erectile dysfunction (ED)**, smooth-muscle cells constrict the local arteries and reduce blood flow into the penis to a trickle, preventing a buildup of blood. The penis remains flaccid if the smooth-muscle cells are contracted.

The causes of erectile dysfunction (formerly called impotence) can be psychological, physical or both. Less than 20 percent of ED cases have psychological causes.[8,21] Examples of such causes are anxiety about sexual performance and problems in the relationship with the partner.

---

vaginismus
Intense involuntary contractions of the outer third of the muscles of the vagina that prevent penetration or make it uncomfortable.

Kegel exercises
Alternating contraction and relaxation of pelvic floor muscles, performed to help relieve vaginismus, among other effects.

erectile dysfunction (ED)
Condition in which the penis does not become erect before sex or stay erect during sex.

Some of the physical causes of ED are low testosterone levels, medications (some antidepressants, blood pressure medications), drugs (alcohol, tobacco), injury, and nerve damage, such as from diabetes, injury, or prostate surgery.

Ejaculation Dysfunction Premature ejaculation, defined as ejaculation less than two minutes after the beginning of intercourse, is probably the most common type of ejaculation dysfunction.[21] (Men typically average two to seven minutes before ejaculation.) About one-third of sexually active men experience premature ejaculation; gay men have lower rates of premature ejaculation.[21] Like ED, premature ejaculation often results from anxiety about sexual performance or unreasonable expectations. For example, a man might be worried about maintaining an erection and rush to a climax.[21]

An effective technique for preventing premature ejaculation is to stop before orgasm, slow down, and then start again. The stop-start method trains the body to lengthen the duration of the sexual arousal state and can increase enjoyment.

Treatment of Male Sexual Dysfunction Treatment of sexual dysfunction in men often relies on testosterone. Men with a low testosterone level may benefit from testosterone replacement therapy. It is not prescribed for men with normal testosterone levels because it can increase blood pressure, affect blood cholesterol levels, and possibly increase risk for prostate cancer.[11]

Several drugs are now on the market for the treatment of ED. They work by increasing the concentration of the chemical that allows smooth-muscle cells in the erectile tissue to stay relaxed so that the spongy chambers of the penis can remain filled with blood. Viagra (Sildenafil) is taken an hour before sex and lasts about four hours. Use of Viagra is dangerous for men with preexisting health conditions such as heart disease, high blood pressure, and diabetes, and fatalities have been reported in connection with its use. Levitra (Vardenafil) and Cialis (Tadolifil) are chemically similar to Viagra but more potent and efficient. They work more quickly, last longer, and have fewer side effects.

A newly developed product is a condom containing a gel that helps men maintain a firmer erection while they are wearing it. The gel is a vasodilator absorbed through the skin to increase blood flow. This drug is not being marketed for erectile dysfunction; rather, it targets men who struggle to maintain an erection specifically while wearing a condom.

Drug approaches to sexual dysfunctions do not take into account the importance of relationships. They may offer a temporary confidence-builder, but they do not provide a long-term solution to issues that may lie behind sexual problems. Correcting unhealthy lifestyles, working on relationships, and cultivating a more realistic expectation of aging can improve mid- and late-life sexuality.

Misuse of ED Drugs by Young Men The misuse of Viagra and other ED drugs on college campuses has recently come to the attention of health experts. Viagra has been tagged the "thrill pill" on many campuses, where young men are taking it as a party drug at clubs, raves, and private parties. They mistakenly believe they will quickly and easily attain an erection that will allow them to have sex for hours. Erection drugs do not work unless nitric oxide is present in the penis, and nitric oxide is produced only in response to physical and mental stimulation. Any effect these drugs seem to have is more likely a placebo effect in healthy young men.

More important, the combination of ED drugs with alcohol or illicit drugs such as cocaine, amphetamines, or Ecstasy can be life-threatening. Even more dangerous is combining them with amyl nitrate ("poppers"). The combination of ED drugs with any stimulant drug dilates blood vessels, which can result in a sudden drop in blood pressure.[11,21]

PROTECTING YOUR SEXUAL HEALTH

Safer sex practices prevent the exchange of body fluids during sex. Two safer sex practices are using condoms and having sex that does not involve genital contact or penetration. A third practice is abstinence, considered the only way to completely guarantee protection against STDs. Another key to safeguarding your sexual health is communicating about sex.

Using Condoms

The **condom** (or *male condom*) is a thin sheath, usually made of latex, which fits over the erect penis during sexual intercourse. It provides a barrier against penile, vaginal, or anal discharges and genital lesions or sores. Although condoms do not provide complete protection against all STDs, they greatly reduce the risk of infection when used correctly (see the box, "Learn How to Use a Condom").

Protection against STIs is also offered by the **female condom**, a soft pouch of thin polyurethane that is inserted into the vagina before intercourse. The female condom has a soft flexible ring at both ends. The ring at the closed end is fitted against the cervix, and the ring at the open end remains outside the body. The female condom covers more of the genital area, so it may provide more protection against an STD lesion or sore than the male condom does. Spermicidal foam can be used with both male and female condoms to kill some bacteria, including HIV, herpes, gonorrhea, and chlamydia.

Most spermicides contain nonoxynol-9 (N-9). Oxtoxynol-9 (O-9) is also commonly used and has similar properties. High doses or frequent use of spermicides

safer sex
Sexual activities that do not include exchange of body fluids.

condom
Thin sheath, usually made of latex, that fits over the erect penis during sexual intercourse to prevent conception and protect against STDs.

female condom
Soft pouch of thin polyurethane that is inserted into the vagina before intercourse to prevent conception and protect against STDs.

Action Skill-Builder

Learn How to Use a Condom

It's possible to put on a male condom or insert a female condom in 10 seconds or less if you are prepared. Consider practicing so you can do it with ease in the heat of the moment (and possibly in the dark). Remember, to reduce risk of pregnancy and STD transmission, a condom must be in place prior to any contact between genital areas.

Male Condom

1. Open the condom package, being careful to not tear the condom.

2. Place the rolled condom over the head of the erect penis (or you can use a banana to practice). If you or your partner have foreskin, gently retract it prior to putting on the condom.

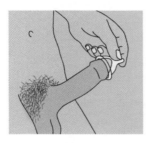

3. Pinch the reservoir tip to remove air and leave one-half inch of the condom as a space for semen.

4. Unroll the condom in a downward direction, smoothing out any air bubbles.

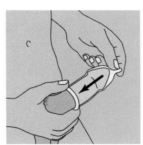

5. Once the condom is unrolled and secure at the base of the penis, you may apply a water-based lubricant, if desired, at any time. K-Y Jelly and Astroglide are two popular options.

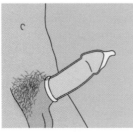

6. After ejaculation, hold the condom around the base of the penis until the penis has been completely withdrawn to avoid any leakage of semen.

7. Gently pull the condom off while still holding at the bottom edge to reduce the risk of spilling semen.

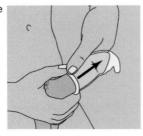

Female Condom

1. Open the condom package, being careful to not tear the condom.

2. If desired, apply a water-based lubricant at the closed end of the condom.

3. Find a position that is comfortable for you (squatting, on your back, sitting).

4. Pinch the smaller ring at the closed end of the condom and flex it gently to fit into the vaginal canal and push it as far up as you can. When the condom is in place, the smaller ring covers the cervix and the larger ring remains outside the vagina.

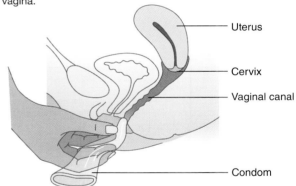

Uterus

Cervix

Vaginal canal

Condom

5. After ejaculation, remove the condom by squeezing and twisting the outer ring so that it stays closed and the semen is contained.

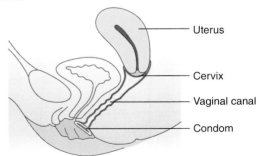

Uterus

Cervix

Vaginal canal

Condom

6. Pull the condom out of your vagina.

Disposing of a used condom.

Wrap it in toilet paper or tissue and discard it in a trash bin. Do not flush it down the toilet; this will clog the sewage system.

Consumer Clipboard

Purchasing Condoms

Condoms are an accessible, inexpensive, easy-to-carry, over-the-counter method of contraception, but the choices can be overwhelming. Here are some things to consider before you buy.

Check the expiration date.
If stored properly, condoms may last four to five years. To protect them from deterioration, store in a cool, dark place.

Choose a shape.
Most condoms have a reservoir tip, which helps contain semen. Beyond that, different shapes are designed to meet different personal preferences. For simple protection, a traditional condom with straight sides does the trick. Form-fitted models hug the tip of the penis so that they stay in place. Contours, flares, or bulbs around the head of the condom leave extra room and can feel more natural for the wearer, especially if he is uncircumcised. Ribs or studs along the shaft of the condom are generally intended to create pleasurable friction for women, but they can enhance both partners' pleasure.

Decide about spermicide.
Nonoxynol-9 is the most commonly used spermicide in condoms. As noted to the right, it may also increase the risk of HIV transmission and possibly the transmission of other STDs.

Consider the country of origin.
Condoms made in the United States require FDA approval. Those manufactured anywhere else should contain approval marks from the country in which they were made.

Think about thickness.
Condoms made of thinner material are less noticeable during sex and, if used correctly, are just as effective as standard thickness condoms. Anal intercourse puts extra strain on a condom; standard condoms are effective for preventing STDs during anal sex if used properly, but use thicker ones for extra peace of mind.

Find the right size.
Too small, and a condom is uncomfortable. Too big, and it slips off during sex. There are no standard condom sizes, and brands vary in length and width. Be prepared to try a few different brands and sizes to find the right fit. Manufacturers' websites may offer some specific guidelines to get you started.

Want lubrication, or not?
Either is safe, but a little extra moisture might be a lot more comfortable for you or your partner. Use of condoms lubricated with the spermicide nonoxynol-9 (N-9) is not recommended because of evidence that N-9 can irritate tissues and result in greater risk of HIV transmission.

Pick a material.
Latex is the most common material and the only one proven to reduce risk of sexually transmitted infections. Polyurethane condoms reduce risk of pregnancy for those with latex allergies, but their effectiveness in reducing the risk of STDs is still unproven. Natural membrane condoms only reduce risk of pregnancy and do not reduce risk of STDs.

---

can cause damage to the vaginal epithelium (layers of skin cells), and inflammation of the vagina and cervix. This damage makes a woman more vulnerable to STIs. They also make it easier for her to transmit STIs to her sexual partner. To avoid these problems, use non-lubricated condoms with a water-based or silicone-based lubricant, or use non-spermicide condoms.[16] For oral sex, do not use N-9 or O-9 condoms. They have a disgusting taste and will cause your tongue to go numb if kept in the mouth for a long time.

There are many types of novelty condoms on the market. They include glow-in-the-dark condoms, flavored condoms, studded condoms, warming condoms, edible condoms, colored condoms, quickstrip condoms, kiss of mint condoms, French Ticklers, tingling pleasure condoms, disc recording condoms, and going green condoms for the environmental savvy. It is important to read the label of novelty condoms to see if they are approved by the FDA for preventing STIs and pregnancy; condoms manufactured outside the United States should contain approval marks from the country in which they were made. Some flavored condoms contain lubricants with sugar that disrupt normal yeast levels in the

vagina, which increases the risk for infection.[16] Avoid oil-based food products as oral sex aids when using a latex condom because oil will cause the condom to quickly degrade (see the box, "Purchasing Condoms").

Many people believe it is only the male who does not want to use a condom. However, women may be reluctant to have their sexual partner use a condom because of (1) latex allergies, (2) problems with nonoxynol-9, or (3) not enough lubricant. If more lubricant would make sex more comfortable, use a nonlubricated condom and apply a water-based or silicone-based lubricant that does not contain nonoxynol-9. For allergic sensitivity prevention, try different brands of latex condoms and condoms made of nonlatex materials.

Latex is a kind of rubber typically made from plant protein. Allergies are typically to one particular type of plant protein. One alternative is polyurethane condoms, which are made from a type of latex-free plastic and can be used with oil-based lubricants. However, polyurethane condoms are more expensive than latex condoms, break more frequently during sex, and may more easily slip off. The effectiveness of these condoms for preventing STIs is still being studied.

Who's at Risk?

Sexual Activity and Condom Use Among College Students

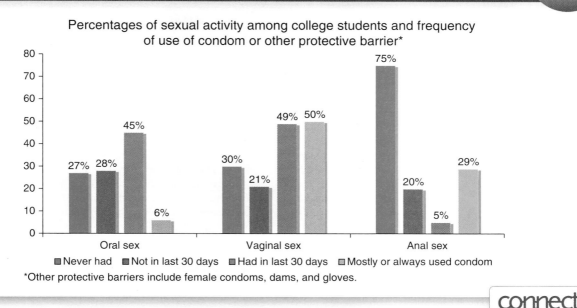

Percentages of sexual activity among college students and frequency of use of condom or other protective barrier*

Oral sex: Never had 27%, Not in last 30 days 28%, Had in last 30 days 45%, Mostly or always used condom 6%

Vaginal sex: Never had 30%, Not in last 30 days 21%, Had in last 30 days 49%, Mostly or always used condom 50%

Anal sex: Never had 75%, Not in last 30 days 20%, Had in last 30 days 5%, Mostly or always used condom 29%

■ Never had ■ Not in last 30 days ■ Had in last 30 days ■ Mostly or always used condom

*Other protective barriers include female condoms, dams, and gloves.

Source: "Spring 2013 Reference Group Executive Summary," American College Health Association, National College Health Assessment Survey, 2013, www.acha-ncha.org/docs/ACHA-NCHA-II_ReferenceGroup_ExecutiveSummary_Spring2013.pdf.

They are not likely to be as effective as latex condoms and should only be considered as a substitute for individuals with latex allergies. A third choice is polyisoprene condoms, called SKYN; these are made from synthetic rubber and have no plant proteins. They are as strong and safe as conventional latex condoms. They are more stretchy than polyurethane condoms and thus have lower breakage and slippage rates. The FDA has approved polyisoprene condoms for preventing pregnancy and STIs. Lambskin condoms are a fourth alternative, and people like the feel of them. These condoms are effective for preventing pregnancy but not STIs.[15]

Condoms and **dental dams** (a small latex square placed over the vulva) should be used during oral sex because bacteria and viruses can be transmitted in semen and vaginal fluids. Plastic wrap placed over the vulva, or a piece of latex cut from a latex glove, is an alternative to a dental dam. Protection is especially important if there are any cuts or sores in the mouth; even bleeding gums can increase the risk of getting an infection.

The American College Heath Association surveyed college students in 2012 and found that the use of condoms and other barrier devices varied by type of sexual contact[22] (see the box, "Sexual Activity and Condom Use Among College Students").

Communicating About Sex

Conversations about sexual topics are important to your health, your partner's health, and the success of your relationship. If you are about to begin a sexual relationship, take the time to tell your partner your sexual health history and find

out about his or hers. Here are some questions to guide your conversation:

- Are you having sex with anyone else? Are you willing to be monogamous with me?

- Have you ever had an STD? If so, how long ago, and what treatment did you get? Do you now have a clean bill of health?

- How many sexual partners have you had? As far as you know, did any of them ever have an STD?

- When was the last time you were tested for STDs? Would you be willing to get tested along with me?

- Are you willing to use condoms every time we have sex?

If you are not satisfied with the answers you get, take care of yourself by insisting on further conversations and behavioral changes before you begin a sexual relationship.

dental dams
Small latex squares placed over the vulva during oral sex.

SEX AND CULTURE: ISSUES FOR THE 21ST CENTURY

Many societal issues involving sex are as old as civilization itself, such as prostitution and sex trafficking (see the box, "Sex Trafficking"). We also face new issues, such as sexting and Internet pornography, as described in this section, due to contributions from technological advances and cultural shifts.

Public Health Is Personal

Sex Trafficking

Sex trafficking is, according to the Office of Refugee Resettlement, a "modern day form of slavery in which a commercial sex act is induced by force, fraud, or coercion, or in which the person induced into performing sexual acts is under the age of 18." Victims of sex trafficking include women and men, girls and boys, but the majority of victims are women and girls.

Victims are lured into the sex trafficking trade in many ways, including a job promise in a different country; bondage situations created by false marriage proposals; kidnapping; and family, husbands, or boyfriends selling victims into the sex trade. Victims are often subjected to debt-bondage, an illegal practice in which victims are forced to pledge their services to pay off transport costs and living expenses. Methods used to condition victims involve starvation, confinement, physical assault, sexual assault, threats to kill or hurt victim's family members, drug addiction, social isolation, psychological tactics, and threatening to shame victims by informing family and friends of their sex trade activities. Sex traffic victims face many physical health risks, including drug addiction, body trauma injuries, STIs, HIV, sterility, and infectious diseases. Psychological harm is also evident, such as PTSD, depression, acute anxiety, and insomnia. Victims may develop a form of traumatic bonding with their captors, the use of both fear and gratitude (being allowed to live) by the sex trafficker to maintain coercive control.

Sex trafficking is the third largest criminal empire in the world. It is an international business, with most victims coming from Southeast Asia, from Central and South America, and from parts of the old Soviet Union. The United States, however, is not immune from sex trafficking. The FBI estimates that almost 300,000 American youth are at risk for sex trafficking. Many of these victims come from homes in which they were physically abused, sexually abused, or abandoned. Victims range from age 9 to 19, and their average age is 12 to 14 years old. It is estimated that there are more than 100,000 American youth sex trafficked each year, and yet there are fewer than 5,000 trafficking convictions. Victims are forced into commercial sexual exploitation such as prostitution, pornography, sex operations, stripping, live-sex shows, mail-order brides, military prostitution, and sex tourism.

The Trafficking Victims Protection Act of 2000 was passed to make human trafficking in the United States a federal crime. This law focuses on prevention through public awareness, protection by issuing foreign national victims a temporary visa, and prosecution under new federal crime laws that enact severe penalties. The law also states that Americans are subject to prosecution in the United States if arrested for paying children for sex in foreign countries.

Social support services are being developed to confront sex trafficking. Education about sex trafficking is receiving attention through the I Stop Traffic Awareness Campaign. This campaign has produced documentary films and several public service announcements on human trafficking. The I Stop the Traffic website provides information about how people can become involved in helping to stop this pressing public health issue.

Sources: I Stop Traffic Awareness campaign, http://istoptraffic.com/; "Fact Sheet: Sex Trafficking," Office of Refugee Resettlement, www.acf.hhs.gov/programs/orr/resource/fact-sheet-sex-trafficking-english; *Human Sexuality: Diversity in Contemporary America* by W. L. Yarber and B. W. Sayad, 2013 New York: McGraw-Hill.

Hooking Up

A major trend on college campuses is the decline of traditional dating and the rise of the "hook-up" culture that is devoid of emotional intimacy and romantic relationships. *Hook-up culture* is defined as casual sexual contact between nondating partners without expectation of forming committed relationships.[23] In a hook-up culture, students rarely go on formal dates. Instead, they frequent parties or bars in large groups, consume alcohol and/or drugs, and hook up with casual friends or strangers. It is estimated that between 66 and 80 percent of college students hook up at some point during their college careers. A *serial hook-up* is hooking up with the same person multiple times over several months, even years. One study found that 28 percent of college students had 10 or more hook-ups.[23,24]

Sexual scripts for heterosexual couples who hook up have shifted toward placing less emphasis on vaginal sex and more emphasis on oral sex and anal sex. College-aged women are more likely to pleasure their male partner with oral sex than the college male is likely to do so for his female partner.[25–27] College women are less likely to orgasm than their male hook up partner. The deprioritization of women's sexual pleasure may be tied to women consenting to sexual encounters and behaviors that they do not desire.[24]

Men like hook-ups more than women do. One study found that 26 percent of women reported a positive reaction after hooking up, 49 percent had a negative reaction, and 25 percent were ambivalent. In contrast, 50 percent of men reported a positive reaction, 26 percent a negative reaction, and 23.6 percent an ambivalent reaction.[25–27] Black college students are less likely to participate in hook-ups than White students. As the statistics also show, many college women and men do not enjoy the hook-up experience and view hook-ups as fast, uncaring, perfunctory, and promoting nonpleasurable sex, drunken sex, and coercive sex.

Role-playing on the college party circuit has fueled the hook-up culture. Many party themes center on pornography and prostitution, starting with "Pimps and Hos"; variations have included "Politicians and Prostitutes," "Santa and His Reindeer Ho, Ho, Hos," "Superheroes and Supersluts," and "Horny Housewives and Randy

Life Stories

Madison: Hooking Up

Madison and Tomas were both sophomores and had been dating each other exclusively for a year. They met their freshman year and almost instantly bonded. Madison had had some sexual experiences before college, but Tomas was her first real boyfriend. Madison was shy and Tomas was outgoing—qualities that they both liked about each other. A lot of their friends hooked up with people at parties and had casual sex, but Madison and Tomas were happy with their exclusive relationship. Their friends thought they were a little boring and "old-fashioned" but also envied them for being satisfied with their relationship.

For spring semester of sophomore year, Tomas was planning to attend a study abroad program in Italy. A week before he was leaving, he told Madison that he wanted to be open to other relationships while they were apart. He said he cared about her but saw the trip as a chance to find out if they were "meant to be together." He wanted to have new experiences, including sexual experiences, if they came along, and he didn't want to feel as if he was cheating on her while he was away.

Madison was caught by surprise. She said okay, but only because she didn't know what else to say. She felt confused and rejected. After Tomas left, she figured she might as well use this time to explore new relationships herself—at least it would help get her mind off Tomas. She started partying more with her friends and tried to cast off her shy persona. She would have a few drinks (or more) and make herself dance and flirt. She was surprised to find

she got a lot of attention. It made her feel attractive and popular—and like she was getting back at Tomas. The first time a guy made it clear he wanted to hook up with her, she turned him down, but the next time she accepted. She found it exciting but also awkward, especially when the alcohol wore off. She enjoyed the sex but missed the intimacy she shared with Tomas—the talking, laughing, and sense of closeness and trust. She was also dismayed that the guy she hooked up with didn't call or e-mail her. She felt rejected all over again and dreaded running into him on campus.

Tomas sent her messages on Facebook with upbeat descriptions of all the fun things he was doing and said that he missed her. Neither of them brought up the topic of seeing other people or hooking up. Reading messages from Tomas, Madison realized how much she missed him and how much hooking up was not helping her with her feelings. In fact, it was making her feel worse. She decided to ask Tomas to clarify his feelings about her so she could make some decisions about her own actions. She also decided that hooking up was not for her, at least not right now.

- Do you think Madison's experience of hooking up is typical? What other experiences do you think people have with this practice?
- Do you think women suffer more than men after a hook-up? If so, why?
- Where does hooking up fit into your personal value system, if at all?

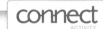

Handymen." Many college students refer to theme parties as "porn parties." Party scenarios generally call for women to show up in skimpy dress and wasted from alcohol. Alcohol has become the "X" factor for hook-ups; in Chapter 16, we will look at how alcohol in hook-ups increases the risk for sexual assaults. The consistent party sexual script places men in a role of power and women in a submissive role. Theme parties give participants an excuse not to feel responsible for the outcomes of their sexual behavior.[3] In addition to theme parties as a means of facilitating hook-up culture, student entrepreneurs have created hook-up websites where students can post anonymously as long as they have an ".edu" e-mail address. Students who frequent such sites often say they do not have time for relationship commitments. They think of college as a temporary place for fun and career preparation.

The downside of the hook-up culture has been significant increases in sexually transmitted diseases and emotional and mental health issues, including sexual regret, negative or ambivalent emotional reactions, psychological distress, depression, and anxiety (see the box, "Madison: Hooking Up"). Women tend to suffer from these consequences more than men do. Perhaps the most costly consequence of a hook-up culture is the failure to develop the qualities that are essential for healthy, long-term relationships—trust, respect, admiration, honesty, caring, and communication.[24,26]

Abstinence

Many college students who want to remain abstinent face social pressure to conform to a hook-up culture. The students who do not conform can be stigmatized, marginalized, or alienated. There is, however, a growing, vocal group of conservative college students who believe in abstinence until marriage. The Anscombe Society at Princeton University, for example, received extensive media attention for its call for a commitment to chastity by its members until marriage. Harvard's True Love Revolution is based on a similar platform. These associations are in direct opposition to the hook-up culture that permeates college campuses.[3,26]

The Love and Fidelity Network is dedicated to educating, training, and equipping college students with resources that uphold traditional marriage, family, and sexual values. It wants to ignite a movement on college campuses that values committed relationships and fidelity as opposed to the hook-up culture of casual sex. Some opponents of the abstinence movement claim it is centered on antigay bigotry. Even if these charges are true, they do not reflect the views a significant number of students who are not part of the abstinence movement but are displeased with the hook-up culture. Most colleges and universities have chosen to tiptoe around this debate.

The priority should be helping college students develop critical thinking skills that enable them to navigate sexuality and romantic relationships.[3,26]

Cybersex

Cybersex—virtual sexual encounters on the Internet—includes online porn (pictures, audio, video, text), real-time interactions (chat rooms, exchanging images and files), and multimedia software (X-rated movies, sexual games, online erotic media). Some argue that cybersex impairs real relationships and robs people of the ability to experience sexual pleasure through interpersonal communication and intimacy. Partners of people who participate in these activities say they feel as betrayed as they would by actual infidelity. Compulsive use of pornographic websites is now a significant factor in many divorces.[28] Other risks include arrest for trying to make a connection with a person under the age of 18, being attacked after agreeing to meet a stranger first encountered in a chat room, and public embarrassment.

Internet Pornography Although pornography has always existed, the Internet has expanded its audience and vastly increased its availability and consumption. According to one report, one in four Internet users looks at a pornography website in any given month, and 66 percent of men aged 18 to 34 visit a pornography site every month. Among college-age students, 87 percent of men and 31 percent of women reported using pornography sites in the last year.[3]

As shown by this statistic, some women have entered what has traditionally been a male domain, leading to the production of so-called femme porn. This genre of pornography usually has more of a story line, involves erotic fantasies, and includes emotional intimacy.[3] In contrast, the vast majority of Internet pornography has become increasingly explicit and violent.

Many people defend the right of adults to choose what they want to view on the Internet without restriction or censorship, and the courts have upheld their constitutional right to do so. On the other hand, there are concerns about possible harmful consequences of Internet pornography. Viewing pornography also seems to have negative effects on relationships. There is also debate about whether pornography promotes violence against women and sexual exploitation of children. Some social scientists have suggested that exposure to depictions of sexual violence and exploitation can increase criminal behavior, especially on the part of men with psychological problems or other vulnerabilities. Although a direct relationship has not been established between pornography and sexual violence, studies do show that viewing pornography affects viewers' attitudes, feelings, and behaviors as well as their sense of sexual norms.[29,30]

Sexting An emerging issue for teens is sexting—sending nude, sexually explicit messages (text, photo, or video) electronically, mostly by cell phone. The National Campaign to Prevent Teen and Unplanned Pregnancy estimates that 20 percent of 13- to 19-year-olds are sexting, and one in five people of all ages have sent sexually explicit messages on their smartphones. The Harris Interactive Poll found that people between the ages of 18 to 34 account for 57 percent of all people admitting to sexting. Only 3 percent of those people said they would be concerned about inappropriate photos or dirty messages being shared or getting into the wrong hands. This surprisingly low number ignores the risks of sexting.[3,31] Many young people are not aware of the potential serious legal consequences of sexting. Under federal and state laws, people who send nude or sexual images or video of minors may be subject to the possession, manufacturing, and distribution of child pornography. One 18-year-old male was sentenced to five years' probation and required to register as a sex offender for sending nude pictures of his 16-year-old girlfriend to dozens of her friends and family after an argument. Recently, some state governments have changed their child pornography laws so that underage teens who send nude pictures of themselves—and those who receive them—will not face serious legal consequences as convicted pedophiles and sex offenders.

About 80 percent of college students engage in sexting.[3,31] Although sexting between adults is legal, the images being distributed without their knowledge can cause embarrassment, humiliation, and harassment. Anthony Weiner's infamous sexting twitter destroyed his campaign for mayor of New York City. Jilted exes have been known to release explicit photos and videos in what is called "revenge porn," a phenomenon discussed next in the chapter.

College students who engage in sexting may think they are more tech savvy than older people like Anthony Weiner. But this belief gives them a sense of false security. They do not fully consider the real-life consequences if their phones are misplaced, stolen, or hacked. Nor do they consider that sexting to a trusted partner may expose them to a revenge porn website if the relationship turns sour. Images leave a digital footprint that can last for years, potentially damaging prospects for future relationships and careers.

Before hitting the send button, consider these five cautions: (1) do not assume anything you send or post is going to remain positive, (2) anything you send into cyberspace never truly goes away, (3) do not give into pressure to do something that makes you uncomfortable, (4) consider the recipient's reaction, and (5) nothing is truly anonymous.

Revenge Porn Revenge porn websites differ from other pornography sites because the culprit uploading the explicit photos is usually a jilted ex-lover/partner or an individual seeking to humiliate or expose the victim. The most common form of revenge porn is a "sext" from one former lover to another. These sites offer sexted images accompanied by a screen shot of the victim's Facebook profile, which typically includes address, place of employment, schools, family members, and other personal information. The consequences can be devastating for the victim.

California has introduced legislation to criminalize revenge porn. This bill would make electronically distributing

Starting the Conversation

Will Computers Reduce the Human Quality of Sexual Interactions?

Human–computer sexual interaction (HCSI) refers to the ways that humans use the computer for sexual interactions. Sex tech falls under HCSI and categories of sex tech include the following:

1. *Sexual communications.* Includes sexting, e-mail, video, and other technologies (e.g., sexting). Communication may be with a specific person or with the general public.

2. *Creating sexual opportunities.* Social network services are used to find sexual partners or to negotiate sexual interactions (e.g., hook-up websites).

3. *Real-life sexual activities.* Computer sex-play roles are used to change and enhance sexual pleasure in solo and partner sex play.

4. *Exploring sexual orientation.* Anonymity enables the users to develop alternate persons online to experience different sexual interactions (e.g., using avatars in virtual space).

5. *Sexual education.* Sex tech that is used for professional reasons has recently received more attention. Websites are being developed to offer sex education for youth and adults.

6. *Sexual entertainment.* Includes viewing pornographic videos, playing sex video games, and visiting virtual strip clubs on the Internet.

7. *Teledildonics.* Computer-mediated software and hardware facilitate remote sex between two or more people, as discussed in the chapter.

There is certainly educational value in sex tech. But the use of sex tech for sexual pleasure has generated a series of moral questions. Is sex tech a form of infidelity? How much sex tech is too much sex tech? Is sex tech addictive? The underlying question is whether sex tech is real sex—as is the view of some people. However, sex tech provides meaningful interactions that can be both healthy and unhealthy. For example, watching an online pornographic video may provide temporary amusement and escape. Whether watching online pornography is healthy depends on personal values and beliefs about sexuality. Perhaps the more disturbing question is whether the many forms of HCSI sex tech will make sex with humans less enjoyable or even obsolete. The rapid development of HCSI sex tech is posing some interesting questions. So, what do you think?

Q: Can computers enhance the quality of sexual interaction?

Q: Will enjoying HCSI sex tech lead to a loss of desire for "in person" sex with a partner?

Q: Is HCSI sex tech a healthy alternative for people who are unsatisfied with their real-life sexual interactions?

Sources: "The Truth about Sex Tech," by C. Silverberg, May 8, 2009, *About.com*, http://sexuality.about.com/od/sex_tech_faq/a/sex_tech_myths.htm; "What Are Examples of Sex Tech?" by C. Silverberg, May 8, 2009, *About.com*, http://sexuality.about.com/od/sex_tech_faq/f/sex_tech_examples.htm.

sexual pictures or videos of a former partner without the subject's consent a misdemeanor, punishable by a $1,000 fine and/or up to a month in jail. This bill was inspired by the death of a 15-year-old student who committed suicide after graphic photos of her being allegedly sexually assaulted by three teenage boys while passed out at a party were circulated in her high school.[32] Many other states are considering legislation that would make revenge porn websites illegal; see the discussion, "Should Revenge Porn Websites Be Illegal?" at the end of the chapter.[32]

Teledildonics Teledildonics is a type of human–computer sexual interaction (HCSI) in which computer software and hardware are used to facilitate remote sex between two or more people. Teledildonics has been described as using a sex toy controlled by someone who is not in the room. It is viewed as an extension of cybersex that involves tactile interaction between two people. Teledildonic theory was introduced in the 1980s as a practical application of virtual reality sex. For example, a person may one day be able to put on a tactile sensation suit and then use virtual reality goggles to simulate sex touch with another person. Today, one sex partner can email a series of move instructions that the other partner can download into a programmable

vibrator.[33] The question is whether HCSI sex toys expand the opportunities for people to sexually connect to others or to oneself, or if they dehumanize sexual interactions (see the box, "Will Computers Reduce the Human Quality of Sexual Interactions?").

Party and Play

The use of recreation drugs for sexual pleasure has long been a part of the American culture. These drugs have included amyl nitrite (poppers), cocaine, Ecstasy, marijuana, cantharides (Spanish Fly), and, recently, methamphetamine. Some scientists believe any sexual-pleasure effects of these drugs are largely placebo. Other scientists believe that changes in brain chemistry do have an effect on sexual pleasure. Long-term use of recreational drugs has been proven to cause low sexual desire, infertility, organ damage, heart damage, and many other health problems. Public health officials are particularly concerned about the use of crystal meth in "party-and-play" sex marathons, particularly among gay men. These parties are also called "slamming."[34]

Crystal meth increases the urgent need to have sex, provides the ability to have sex for hours and even days, and leads to an inability to ejaculate or reach orgasm. It lowers sexual inhibitions and may cause users to behave recklessly or become forgetful. Sex marathons often result in vaginal and anal tearing and trauma to sex organs that increase the risk for STIs and HIV. Crystal meth can also cause erectile dysfunction, called "crystal dick," which leads users to engage in more receptive anal sex and fisting (shoving fist into partner's anal cavity). A recent trend is to combine crystal meth with poppers, Ecstasy, and Viagra. Although party-and-play sexual marathons have been more visible in the gay community, the health dangers posed to heterosexual couples participating in sexual marathons have also become a concern.[34]

Compulsive Sexual Behaviors

Some users of pornography and cybersex are at risk for *sex addiction,* defined as compulsive, out-of-control sexual behavior that results in severe negative consequences. Sex addicts lose time every day to the isolating activities of fantasy and masturbation, and the Internet is a particularly seductive medium. Hours spent on the Web are hours not spent on real-life activities, including time spent developing intimate relationships with real partners.

There is some controversy over whether sex addiction is a real phenomenon, but some addiction experts believe that sex addicts, like other types of addicts, experience changes in brain chemistry that affect what is found motivating and rewarding. The current version of the American Psychiatric Association's *Diagnostic and Statistical Manual of Mental Disorders* (*DSM*) does not include sex addiction, but it does list it as requiring more research. Individuals with this disorder spend so much time in sexual activities that it interferes with their job and other important parts of their lives.

If you think you might be at risk for sex addiction, talk to a mental health professional at your campus counseling center. Sex addiction can cause serious physical, emotional, spiritual, family, financial, and legal problems, but treatment is available. You can also learn more about sex addiction at the Sexual Recovery Institute (www.sexualrecovery.com).

A related phenomenon is the compulsive avoidance of sex, dubbed "sexual anorexia" and described as the flip side of sex addiction. Named for its parallels with the eating disorder anorexia nervosa, sexual anorexia involves an intense fear of sexual contact or intimacy, preoccupation with sexual matters, rigid and judgmental attitudes toward sex, and shame and self-hatred over sex.[35] Those at risk for this disorder include people who have experienced past sexual abuse, sexual assault, or other sexual trauma; people who were raised in sexually repressive families; and people who are fearful of underlying homosexual tendencies. People who watch pornography compulsively may also be at risk for sexual anorexia because they are no longer able to respond sexually to a real partner. Sexual anorexia is not just a low sex drive; it is a physical, mental, and emotional condition that can benefit from professional help.[36]

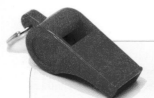

You Make the Call

Should Revenge Porn Websites Be Illegal?

In the days of the Wild West, a personal affront often resulted in a shoot-out. Today, cyberspace has given a new form to revenge called revenge porn. After a nasty break-up, ex-boyfriends, ex-girlfriends, ex-husbands, and ex-lovers post explicit pictures/videos that are accompanied by identification details, such as where the person lives, works, and Facebook pages. Revenge porn has become so popular that there are now websites dedicated to it, such as UGotPosted and IsAnyoneUp. The creator of IsAnyoneUp claimed he received more than 10,000 revenge porn image submissions in a three-month period. Devoted followers of the site even created a Twitter page featuring uploaded pictures of the site's "hash tag" tattooed on their bodies.

Most people are disturbed by the paucity of civil and criminal privacy laws that protect people from being a victim of revenge porn, and some states are now considering bills that would make revenge porn operators criminally liable. The Fourth Amendment gives American citizens the right to be secure in their persons, houses, papers, and effects. But this amendment does not protect people who "give" naked pictures by hitting Send on their

Continued…

Concluded...

computer or consent to a picture or video being taken. This property belongs to the recipient. Although children are protected by the Child Protection and Obscenity Enforcement Act, adults can do little unless the photo or video was taken without their knowledge and not in a public setting, constituting a violation of privacy.

Section 230 of the Communications Decency Act has a safe-harbor provision that protects site operators and editors from being liable for third-party content if they had no involvement in creating the content. This is the technical reason revenge porn websites are legal.

Victims may not be able to sue revenge porn website operators, but laws may be available to pursue the person who uploaded the photo or video. Pictures of underage people, stalking, computer harassment, and copyright infringement are legally actionable. The safe-harbor provision might be bypassed under federal and state stalking and cyberstalking laws. An example of a violation would be a site that developed a mapping app containing the person's home and work addresses. A final legal course of action might be the Publicity Rights Intellectual Property Violation Act. Websites that use advertising for revenue could be classified as a commercial operation, and the victim could argue that his or her "likeness" is being used for profit without permission. It is important to note that many states are wrestling with how to apply this legislation. Revenge porn sites could claim the fair use doctrine as a defense.

Civil and criminal legal recourse against revenge porn sites appears unlikely at this time. However, the IsAnyoneUp creator recently lost a $250,000 civil lawsuit to a revenge porn victim. This case was significant as it demonstrated the judicial system is willing to exhaust legal possibilities to prosecute revenge porn. There is also likely to be a class action civil law suit that may spell the end to revenge porn websites.

But not everyone agrees with making revenge web porn illegal. Critics see this action as having a chilling impact on first amendment rights.

What do you think?

Pros

- Revenge porn is not freedom of expression. It is a willing violation of privacy to inflict emotional harm on the victim.
- Once a picture or video is posted on the Internet, it is impossible to completely scrub it from computer access.
- Victims are at risk for offline stalking and physical attack. They do not feel safe leaving their homes.
- Victims have lost jobs and admissions to colleges and universities because of revenge porn postings.

Cons

- The safe harbor provision clearly protects the First Amendment rights of website operators. Free speech should be criminalized only in the narrowest sense.
- People who record pictures or videos of themselves in a compromising position that are later leaked to the public do not deserve sympathy. They caused the embarrassment and humiliation by their own actions.
- Civil remedies are a better course of action than criminal remedies. There are a number of civil right statutes for protection against revenge porn.
- The real party at fault is the ex who sent the picture or video to the revenge porn website. The ex should be held criminally responsible and not the revenge porn website.

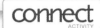

Sources: "Revenge Porn Websites: A Legal Look," http://kellywarnerlaw.com/revenge-porn-websites-a-legal-look/; "Revenge Porn: California Legislators Go After Troubling New Trend," by A. Sankinaaron, June 5, 2013, *Huffington Post,* www.huffingtonpost.com/2013/06/05/revenge-porn-california_n_3391638.html; "Victims Push Laws to End Online Revenge Posts," September 24, 2103, *New York Times,* www.nytimes.com/2013/09/24/us/victims-push-laws-to-end-online-revenge-posts.html.

In Review

What is sexual health in terms of human biology and culture, and what are common varieties of sexual behavior?
Sexual health includes satisfying intimate relationships based on mutual respect and trust, the ability and resources to procreate if so desired, acceptance of one's sexual feelings and tolerance for those of others, and knowledge about sexuality and access to the information needed to make responsible decisions. Sexual behavior, expression, and pleasure vary across cultures and eras. Common forms of sexual expression include celibacy, abstinence, erotic touch, kissing, self-stimulation, oral-genital stimulation, anal intercourse, and sexual intercourse. Less common forms are atypical sexual practices, such as sex toys and sex games, which are consensual and cause no harm and paraphilias, which are not consensual and are classified as mental disorders and crimes.

What are sexual dysfunctions in males and in females?
Sexual dysfunctions can have physical, psychological, emotional, or relationship causes. Some are deemed problems only if the person or the partner considers it a problem. Female sexual dysfunctions include pain during intercourse, sexual desire disorder, female sexual arousal disorder, and orgasmic dysfunction. Male sexual dysfunctions include pain during intercourse, sexual desire disorder, erectile dysfunction, and ejaculation dysfunction. Testosterone and other drugs are common therapies for both females and males.

What are the best ways to protect your sexual health?
Using condoms, practicing abstinence, avoiding alcohol in sexual situations, and practicing good communication skills are the best ways to protect your sexual health.

What are important sex-related issues in the 21st century?
Hooking up and abstinence are two common issues on college campuses. New issues in the last few decades relate to cybersex, including Internet pornography, sexting, revenge porn, and teledildonics. The use of methamphetamines in party-and-play sexual marathons has recently become a concern. Compulsive sexual behaviors, notably sex addiction and sexual anorexia, are conditions that can benefit from professional help.

12 Reproductive Choices

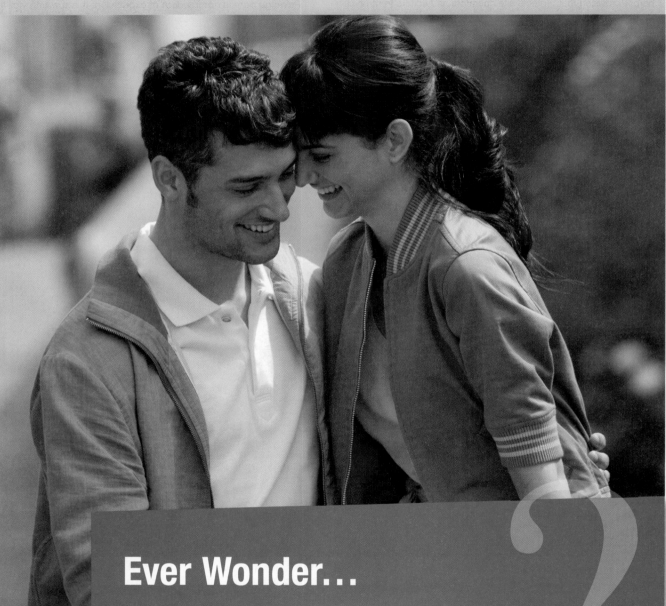

Ever Wonder...

- what the best form of contraception is?
- how to have the "contraception talk" with your partner?
- how much it costs to raise a child?

Who's at Risk?

Unintentional Pregnancy

What factors might play a role in differences in rates of unintentional pregnancy? Consider the ecological model of health and wellness presented in Chapter 1 (Figure 1.3).

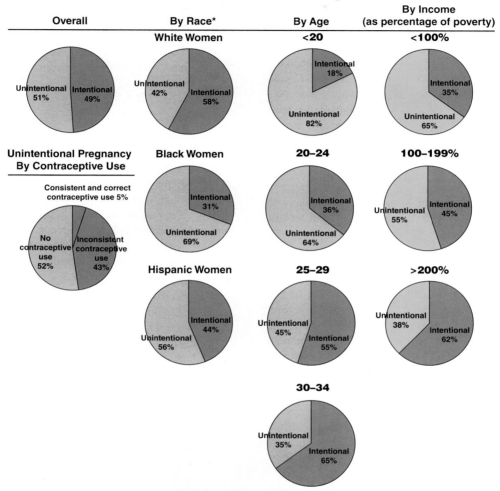

Intentional and Unintentional Pregnancies

* Rate for American Indian/Alaska Natives not reported in Finer & Zolna study; however, rate for urban AI/ANs is significantly higher than for non-Hispanic whites.

Sources: "Shifts in Intended and Unintended Pregnancies in the United States, 2001-2008" by Finer, L. B. and M. R. Zolna, 2014. *American Journal of Public Health,* Feb 104 Suppl 1: S43-8; *Unintended Pregnancy in the United States,* Fact Sheet, Guttmacher Institute, December 2013, www.guttmacher.org/pubs/FB-Unintended-Pregnancy-US.html; *Reproductive Health of Urban American Indian and Alaska Native Women: Examining Unintended Pregnancy, Contraception, Sexual History and Behavior, and Non-voluntary Sexual Intercourse,* Urban Health Institute, Seattle Indian Health Board, February 2012, www.uihi.org/wp-content/uploads/2010/09/nsfg-report_final_2010-09-22.pdf.

Are you ready to be a parent? If your answer is no, and you are in a heterosexual relationship, many safe and effective methods of contraception are available that you and your partner can use to avoid an unintended pregnancy. If your answer is yes, a wealth of knowledge is available that you can use to increase the likelihood that your pregnancy is a positive experience and that your baby is healthy. If you want to have children sometime in the future, planning for it now—by using contraception and choosing healthy lifestyle behaviors—can give you peace of mind and the knowledge that you are doing everything you can to protect the health of your future family. This chapter builds on the topics discussed in Chapters 3 and 11—relationships and sexual health—to discuss reproductive choices and issues in creating a family.

CHOOSING A CONTRACEPTIVE METHOD

Choosing and using a contraceptive method that is right for you is important for one very significant reason: it lowers your risk of unintended pregnancy. About half of all pregnancies in the United States are unintended, and many are unwanted, either because the couple does not want a child at this time or because they don't want a child at all. Unintended pregnancies occur among women of all ages and ethnic groups, but rates are highest among low-income, minority (Black, American Indian, Alaska Native, and Hispanic) women in the 18- to 24-year-old age group. See the box, "Unintentional Pregnancy," to compare the rates among different groups. Unintended pregnancies nearly always cause stress and life disruption and are associated with poorer health outcomes. Compared with women having planned pregnancies, women with unintended pregnancies are less likely to receive adequate **prenatal care**, are more likely to drink alcohol and smoke, and are more likely to have babies with **low birth weight** (less than 5.5 pounds).[1]

Advances in reproductive technology have led to the development of many acceptable and reliable contraceptive methods. In this section we take a look at several of these methods. Complete the activities in this chapter's Personal Health Portfolio to determine which contraceptive method may best suit your needs.

prenatal care
Regular medical care during pregnancy, designed to promote the health of the mother and the fetus.

low birth weight
Birth weight of less than 5.5 pounds, often as a result of preterm delivery.

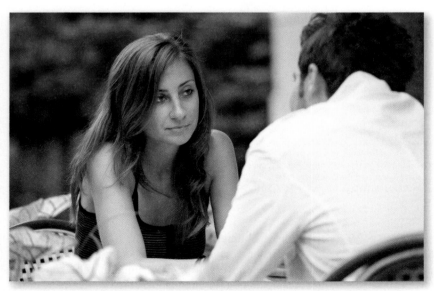

■ Having a talk about contraception may be uncomfortable at first, but you and your partner will both be glad you had it. Think about what you want to say ahead of time and use good communication skills.

Communicating About Contraception

If you are in a sexual relationship, you and your partner should decide together how to best protect each other from sexually transmitted infections (STIs) and unintended pregnancy. If you have casual sex or hook up with people you do not know well, it may be more of a challenge to have this discussion. If this is the case for you, you may want to consider abstinence from intercourse until you are in a relationship where the conversation is possible.

How do you have the conversation? See the box, "Discussing Contraception," for some steps you can take.

Which Contraceptive Method Is Right for You?

Given all the options available for contraception and the number of variables that have to be taken into account in choosing a method—effectiveness, cost, convenience, permanence, safety, protection against STIs, and consistency with personal values—deciding which method is the best one for you can be difficult. Making the right choice is important, because half of unintended pregnancies occur in a month when the woman has been using contraception.[1,2] Here are some questions to consider:

■ *Is your main concern preventing pregnancy? Or do you also need to worry about sexually transmitted infections?* If you are concerned about STIs, you need to use condoms. However, if you are in a mutually faithful, monogamous relationship and neither you nor your partner has an STI, then a barrier method may not be necessary. You may want to consider birth control pills, an injectable contraceptive, or an intrauterine device (IUD).

■ *Do you sometimes have sex under the influence of alcohol or drugs? Do you hook up with partners and not always know their sexual history?* In these situations, you are at risk for both STIs and pregnancy. The best option is dual contraception—a barrier method plus a hormonal method or IUD. Condoms are the best way to reduce risk for STIs. A hormonal contraceptive or IUD is important because its efficacy does not rely on your decision-making abilities at the time of intercourse.

■ *Are you planning to have children with this partner at some time in the future?* The male and female condoms, the diaphragm, the cervical cap, and the contraceptive sponge are all safe, nonpermanent methods. The slightly lower efficacy of a method used only at the time of intercourse may be acceptable if you and your partner are in agreement you want children together, even though not just yet.

Action Skill-Builder

Discussing Contraception

In a recent study on hooking up, half of college students reported being carried away in the moment. Looking back on it, they did not understand how they became so sexually involved. Lack of planning is associated with a higher risk of unprotected sex, but being prepared to talk about it can save you future regrets and worries. An open conversation about birth control is a sign of respect for yourself and your partner.

Before you have the conversation:

☐ *Consider which method you think is best for you and your type of relationship.* It will be easier to discuss if you feel educated and confident about what you want to use.

☐ *Prepare yourself for the conversation.* Consider how you will start the conversation, and think about your partner's potential responses. If you are comfortable doing so, role-play the discussion with a friend.

☐ *Don't make assumptions about whether your partner is on birth control or ready to use a condom.* Plan to ask specifically about that. Contraception is not just a woman's responsibility. Ninety percent of college women feel contraceptive responsibility should be shared, and yet only half report it actually is shared.

When you have the conversation:

☐ *Talk about the relationship.* Do you both have the same expectations about your relationship status—are you going to be monogamous, or does either of you plan to be sexually involved with other people?

☐ *Discuss what you would want to do if your birth control fails.* Can you agree on a contingency plan in the event of a pregnancy?

☐ *Have this conversation prior to the initiation of any sexual contact!* This requires being honest with yourself as well as your partner(s) about what you expect from the relationship.

☐ *Be prepared to take more time before starting a sexual relationship.* You and your partner may not agree on a method to use, or you may have very different beliefs regarding what you would do if you or your partner became pregnant.

The unintended consequences of unprotected sex affect both men and women, and thus the responsibility should be shared.

Sources: "Hooking Up and Sexual Risk Taking Among College Students: A Health Belief Model Perspective," by T. M. Downing-Matiga and B. Geisinger, 2009, *Qualitative Health Research, 19* (9), pp. 1196–1209; "Perceptions of Contraceptive Responsibility Among Female College Students: An Exploratory Study," by L. R. Brunner Huber and J. L. Ersek, 2011, *Annals of Epidemiology, 21* (3), pp. 197–203.

■ *Do you already have children and know that you do not want any more?* Surgical sterilization is a highly effective method with no hassles after the initial procedure.

■ *How much can you afford to pay for contraception?* There are several factors to consider here. For example, how often do you need contraception? If you have sex daily, the cost of buying condoms for every time can quickly add up, whereas the one-time cost of an IUD or sterilization may be less. If you have sex once a month or less, the opposite may be true. If you need to use two forms of contraception—one to prevent STIs and one to decrease your chances of pregnancy—again, the costs can add up. Don't forget to take into account the financial and emotional cost if you or your partner gets pregnant with the form of contraception you select. It might be the cost of having an abortion, or it might be the cost of raising a child.

■ *Are you worried about the safety and health consequences of contraception?* These are important concerns, but people are often surprised to learn all the contraceptive options available today are relatively safe. To put the risks in perspective, consider that the risk of being killed in a car crash in a given year is 1 in 5,900; the risk of dying from a pregnancy carried past 20 weeks is 1 in 10,000; and the risk of dying from the use of birth control pills for a nonsmoking woman aged 15 to 44 years is 1 in 66,700.[3]

■ *Is your choice influenced by your religious, spiritual, or ethical beliefs?* Some people are not comfortable with any method that interferes with natural processes. Abstinence, periodic abstinence, or a fertility awareness-based method may be the right choice for them.

Abstinence

The only guaranteed method of preventing pregnancy and STIs is *abstinence* (see the box, "Choosing a Contraceptive for Family Planning"). As noted in Chapter 11, abstinence is usually defined as abstention from sexual intercourse; that is, there is no penile penetration of the vagina. In heterosexual couples who have vaginal intercourse and use no contraceptive method, 85 percent of the women will become pregnant in one year.[3]

Abstinence requires that both partners feel empowered and free from sexual coercion. It requires control and commitment—that is, the ability or the determination not to change one's mind in the heat of the moment, especially in situations where one or both partners are intoxicated.

Hormonal Contraceptive Methods

Hormonal methods come in a variety of forms—pills, injections, patches, vaginal rings, and implants—and work by preventing ovulation. They also alter cervical mucus, making it harder for sperm to reach ova, and they affect the uterine lining so that a fertilized egg is less likely to be implanted. They are prescribed or administered by a health

Consumer Clipboard

Choosing a Contraceptive for Family Planning

When it comes to reducing the risk of STIs, condoms are king. But if your main concern is avoiding pregnancy, you have a myriad of methods of contraception to choose from. All have benefits and drawbacks, and some are more effective than others. In making the choice, it is important to consider all of the factors—effectiveness, the medical and practical pros and cons of each method, and the cost.

Most effective ↑ ... ↓ **Least effective**

Failure Rate by Average Users*	Method of Birth Control	Factors to Consider	Cost**
0.05%	Implant (Nexplanon)	Lasts 3 years. Minor procedure required to place and remove the device. Reversible. No provider maintenance necessary until removal. Contains no estrogen.	$$
0.15	Sterilization (male)	No further action needed after procedure, but difficult to reverse. No significant long-term side effects.	$$$
0.2	IUD—progesterone (Mirena, Skyla)	Effective for 3–5 years. Always in place. Woman may experience decreased menstrual flow. Possible complications rare. Provider must place the device, but no provider maintenance necessary until removal. Reversible	$$$
0.5	Sterilization (female)	No further action needed after procedure, but difficult to reverse. No significant long-term side effects. Requires surgery/anesthesia. Risk of ectopic pregnancy if failure.	$$$
0.8	IUD—copper (ParaGard)	Effective for 10 years. Always in place. Reversible. Woman may experience pain/heavy menstrual flow. Possible complications rare. Provider must place the device, but no provider maintenance necessary until removal.	$$$
6	Injection (Depo-Provera)	Only required action is a provider visit every 3 months. Side effects include weight gain and decreased bone density over time. Contains no estrogen.	$$
9	Oral contraceptives (birth control pills)	Easy to use. Requires a prescription and must be taken daily. Safe for most women, but in rare cases serious health problems occur. Noncontraceptive benefits include improvement in acne, reduction in menstrual cramps, blood loss, and reduction in risk for ovarian and endometrial cancers.	$$
9	Transdermal patch (Ortho Evra patch)	Easy to use. Requires a prescription and must be maintained on a weekly basis. Safe for most women, but in rare cases serious health problems occur. Greater risk of blood clots than with pill or other hormonal methods. Noncontraceptive benefits include improvement in acne, reduction in menstrual cramps, blood loss, and reduction in risk for ovarian and endometrial cancers.	$$
9	Vaginal contraceptive ring (NuvaRing)	Easy to use. Requires a prescription and must be maintained on a monthly basis. Safe for most women, but in rare cases serious health problems occur. Noncontraceptive benefits include improvement in acne, reduction in menstrual cramps, blood loss, and reduction in risk for ovarian and endometrial cancers.	$$
12	Diaphragm	Same as cervical cap.	$$
12	Sponge (Today) w/o prior pregnancy	Available over the counter. Immediately effective upon insertion, and must be used with every act of intercourse. May cause allergic reaction but is rarely associated with toxic shock syndrome.	$
14	Cervical cap (FemCap) w/o prior pregnancy	Requires provider appointment/prescription. May reduce risk of some STIs. May be inserted prior to onset of sexual activity and must be used with every act of intercourse. May cause allergic reaction but is rarely associated with toxic shock syndrome.	$$
18	Male condom	Accessible, easily carried, and available over the counter. Best method for reducing risk of STI transmission. Requires placement on penis prior to insertion of penis.	$
21	Female condom	Easily carried, available over the counter. Can be inserted before intercourse, though some women find insertion difficult. Not as readily available as the male condom and more expensive.	$$
22	Withdrawal***	Available to all. An exercise in self-control. Interrupts sexual expression.	None
24	Fertility awareness–based methods	Requires both partners to learn about the fertility cycle. No drugs or devices to buy, and no side effects. Variations in cycle may make methods difficult for some women.	None
28	Spermicides	Available over the counter. May increase effectiveness of barrier methods if used as secondary contraceptive method. Must be inserted with every act of intercourse. May cause irritation or allergic reaction. May increase transmission of HIV.	$
85	No method†	No protection against pregnancy or STIs.	***

*Actual use takes into account user variability, whereas "perfect use" would be effectiveness if a user did not miss any pills or occasionally not use a condom; actual use and "perfect use" are similar for methods that require little action on part of user but can vary greatly when action is required at time of intercourse. **See discussion in text regarding cost; this is initial upfront cost but varies by sexual activity and time using method; longer-acting methods become less expensive when averaged over time used. ***Many do not consider withdrawal a form of contraception. See text discussion. †"No method" has no initial cost but carries with it a high risk of pregnancy and associated costs.

Sources: Adapted from "Contraceptive Failure in the United States," by J. Trussell, 2011, *Contraception, 83* (5), pp. 397–404; "Contraceptive Procedures," by A. Beasley and A. Schutt-Aine, 2013, *Obstetrics and Gynecology Clinics, 40* (4), pp. 697–729.

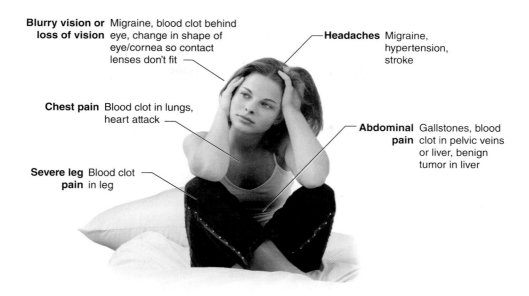

Blurry vision or loss of vision Migraine, blood clot behind eye, change in shape of eye/cornea so contact lenses don't fit

Headaches Migraine, hypertension, stroke

Chest pain Blood clot in lungs, heart attack

Abdominal pain Gallstones, blood clot in pelvic veins or liver, benign tumor in liver

Severe leg pain Blood clot in leg

figure 12.1   Serious side effects of hormonal contraceptives.
Serious side effects are very rare, but if you are taking hormonal contraceptives, you need to be aware of the warning signs.

provider. The advantages of hormonal methods include their effectiveness, their ease of use, their limited side effects, and the fact that they do not permanently affect fertility. They do not require any action at the time of intercourse. In addition, they offer some general health benefits. They reduce menstrual cramping and blood loss, premenstrual symptoms, ovarian cysts, endometriosis, and the risk of endometrial and ovarian cancer. They can also improve acne.

A major disadvantage associated with hormonal contraceptives is that they offer no protection against STIs. In some women, they can also cause some minor side effects, including symptoms of early pregnancy (nausea, bloating, weight gain, and breast tenderness), mood changes, lowered libido, and headaches. Serious side effects are rare and more common in women who are older, who smoke, or who have a family history of early heart disease, stroke, or clotting disorders (Figure 12.1). Hormonal contraceptives require a visit to a health care provider to determine which method is best for you and to ensure you do not have a contraindication for use.

■ The development of "the pill" and its approval by the FDA in 1960 ushered in an era of more relaxed sexual attitudes and behaviors— the so-called sexual revolution. Today, birth control pills remain the most popular form of contraception among unmarried women.

Birth control pills (oral contraceptives) are the most popular reversible form of contraception. They usually contain a combination of estrogen and progesterone. A pack of birth control pills typically contains a month's worth of pills. Some formulations contain only progesterone; they are slightly less effective but can be used by women who can't take estrogen (e.g., because they are breastfeeding or have a family history of blood clots).

When birth control pills were initially introduced, they were designed to mimic a woman's typical menstrual cycle with seven days of placebo pills at the end of each month. The lack of hormones in these pills causes the uterine lining to shed. As the use of hormonal contraceptives has become more accepted, so too has the idea that it may be nice to *not* menstruate each month. Sixty percent of women report they would be interested in skipping their monthly period. In response, hormonal contraceptives have begun to include options that skip the placebo period and extend the hormonal pill cycles so that women only menstruate four times a year—or not at all. If a woman who is not taking hormonal contraceptives skips a period, it can signify a hormone imbalance that may be due to weight gain or loss, stress, some other health conditions, too much exercise, or pregnancy. However, when it is due to the use of hormonal contraceptives, it does not appear to cause an increased risk to health, only

Starting the Conversation

What About an IUD?

Q: If a woman is sexually active and is not currently planning a pregnancy, should she use a long-acting contraceptive?

If you want to reduce your risk of injury from a car crash, driving (or riding) in a car with engineered safety features, such as air bags, auto-lock brakes, and automated seatbelts will make you safer than relying on speed control and defensive driving alone. If employers want to reduce the risk of hearing loss in their workers, engineered features that reduce risk of loud exposure in work sites are more effective than individual hearing protection. Health and safety technology is generally more effective if it does not depend on individual behavior but instead works automatically and consistently.

So why when it comes to reproductive health would women not use the technology that is most effective at preventing pregnancy? Intrauterine devices and hormonal implants are the most effective form of reversible contraception currently available on the market and yet are used by only 5 percent of U.S. women desiring contraception—lagging far behind use in other countries.

Intrauterine devices have been available since the mid-1950s. However, due to design flaws associated with the Dalkon Shield (the IUD available from the 1950s to the 1970s), IUDs became associated with pelvic inflammatory disease and a risk of permanent infertility. If you mention intrauterine devices to your mother, she is likely to immediately tell you about this history! However, with redesign, the three IUDs now available on the market are well tolerated, and risks of serious side effects are very rare. The ParaGard copper IUD has been FDA-approved for use in the United States since 1984. Once inserted, it remains in place for 10 years. The Mirena IUD was approved for use in the United States in 2000. It contains the hormone progesterone, which is slowly released and, once inserted, the IUD remains in place for 5 years. The Skyla IUD was approved for use in the United States in

2013. It also contains progesterone, which is slowly released; the Skyla IUD remains in place for 3 years. All are approved for use in sexually active women from age 16 until menopause.

In contrast to the pill, patch, vaginal ring, condoms, or other barrier methods, IUDs do not have a difference between "perfect use" and "actual use." This is because once they are placed, they require no further action on the part of the user for 3 to 10 years. And, when the time comes for a planned pregnancy, they are easily removable with rapid return to fertility. Younger women (under age 21) may particularly benefit from an IUD—they are twice as likely to get pregnant on the pill, patch, or ring as older women. Think about how variable your daily routine can be—different classes, job schedule, bedtime, and wakeup time. When you try to take a pill at the same time each day, it can be very difficult to remember. And yet, when you miss a pill or two a month (as is reported by 25 percent of young women), you risk pregnancy.

It is important to remember, however, that IUDs do not protect against sexually transmitted infections. Women who have new sexual partners will still need to use condoms to reduce disease transmission.

Intrauterine devices do need to be placed by a health provider. Thus, limited knowledge about their availability and initial upfront cost has played a role in reduced use in the United States. With expansion of coverage for contraception as part of the Affordable Care Act, the cost of placement should no longer be a barrier for most women.

Long-acting reversible contraceptives appear to be the technological wave of the future for contraception. With almost no contraindications and improved access with insurance changes, women may want to consider this effective option.

Q: How have technological advances reduced your risk for undesired health outcomes?

Q: How reliable are you at using contraceptives? Does the idea of not thinking about it at all after an initial visit sound appealing?

Sources: "Effectiveness of Long-Acting Reversible Contraception," by B. Winner, J. F. Peipert, Q. Zhao, et al., 2012, New England Journal of Medicine, 366 (21), 1998–2007; "Disparities in Contraceptive Access and Provision," by F. Casey and V. Gomez-Lobo, 2013, Seminal Reproductive Medicine 31, pp. 347–359; "Contraceptive Procedures," by A. Beasly and A. Schutt-Aine, 2013, Obstetrics and Gynecology Clinics, 40 (4), pp. 697–729.

a slightly higher risk of more irregular spotting or bleeding for the first six months of use.[4]

Some newer ways of delivering hormones are becoming popular, especially among college women who find it difficult to take a daily pill due to irregular sleep, a hectic daily schedule, or daily stress. The *transdermal patch* works by slowly releasing estrogen and progesterone into the bloodstream through the skin. A woman places a new patch on her skin every week for three weeks; during the fourth week, she does not use a patch and has a light period. Potential side effects are similar to those of the pill, except that the patch results in higher levels of estrogen in the blood (about 60 percent higher than with a typical birth control pill) and may be associated with an increased risk of blood clots compared to pills.[5]

The *vaginal contraceptive ring* is a soft, flexible plastic ring that is placed in the vagina and slowly releases estrogen and progesterone. It is left in place for 21 days and then removed. After 7 days, a new ring is inserted. Women and their partners report that they rarely feel the ring during intercourse. The advantage of the ring is the monthly application; side effects are similar to those of birth control pills.

The only *injectable contraceptive* currently available in the United States is Depo-Provera. A progesterone-only injection, it is administered as a shot in a health care provider's office every three months. It is highly effective and requires little action on the part of a woman except regular visits to her provider. Depo-Provera can cause menstrual changes with irregular bleeding early on and amenorrhea (no periods) in 50 percent of women after one year. Most women consider this an advantage. Disadvantages specific to Depo-Provera include weight gain (about 5.4 pounds on average in the first year) and decreased bone density with prolonged use (longer than two years).

A *contraceptive implant* is a small, flexible plastic rod that contains progesterone. It is inserted under the skin on the inner side of the upper arm and slowly releases hormones. The only implant currently available in the United States is Nexplanon. Once inserted, it can be left in place for three years, thus eliminating user error. It may be less effective for women with a body mass greater than 30 percent of ideal, but in general is the most effective form of reversible contraception.

At this time there are no hormonal contraceptive methods available for men. Differences between men's and women's reproductive physiology, the lack of research success, the reluctance of pharmaceutical companies to invest in more research, and the lengthy process of securing FDA approval for new drugs all pose seemingly insurmountable obstacles. A primary problem for researchers is that suppressing the production of 10,000 sperm per second is more challenging than suppressing the production of one egg per month. Although a majority of men believe that contraception is the responsibility of both partners, the technology of male contraception has lagged far behind that of female contraception.

The IUD

Long-acting reversible contraception, provided by an **intrauterine device (IUD)** or a contraceptive implant, is being increasingly recommended for college-age women (see the box, "What About an IUD?"). After insertion, these methods work extremely well for years without the woman having to do anything else. Fertility quickly returns upon removal.[6] Two types of IUD are available in the United States, the copper IUD (ParaGard) and the progesterone IUD (Mirena or Skyla). Both are small, T-shaped devices that a health care provider inserts through the cervix into the uterus. A correctly placed IUD is shown in Figure 12.2.

The IUD is believed to work by altering the uterine and cervical fluids to reduce the chance that sperm will move up into the fallopian tubes, where they can fertilize an ovum. In addition, some women using the progesterone-containing IUD do not ovulate.

IUDs are highly effective and require little maintenance after they are in place. Because it is possible for an IUD to shift its position in or to be expelled from the uterus, women are taught to check that the device is still properly located each month. They may experience a change in menstrual patterns with IUDs. The copper IUD may cause slightly heavier periods and cramping; the progesterone IUD may cause irregular spotting initially and then the cessation of periods at one year for 20 percent of women. Neither

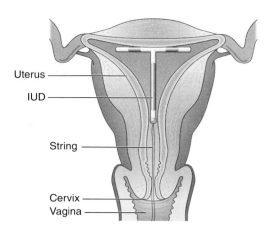

figure 12.2 **T-shaped IUD correctly positioned in the uterus.**

appears to increase the risk of pelvic inflammatory disease unless a woman is infected with gonorrhea or chlamydia at the time of insertion. Both kinds of IUD can be used in women who have not previously been pregnant.

Barrier Methods

Contraceptive methods known as **barrier methods** physically separate the sperm from the female reproductive tract. These methods include the male condom, the female condom, the diaphragm, the cervical cap, and the contraceptive sponge. To increase their effectiveness, the diaphragm and cervical cap should be used with **spermicide**, chemical agents that kill sperm. Spermicide usually comes in a foam or jelly and can be purchased at a grocery store or drugstore. The sponge already has spermicide in it.

The chance of becoming pregnant while using a barrier method is low if the method is used consistently and correctly—that is, the barrier is used 100 percent of the time and spermicide is correctly applied. Unfortunately, this is often not the case.

Condoms—Male and Female The only form of contraception proven to decrease the risk of contracting an STI are condoms. Neither provides 100 percent protection from STIs, but they do reduce risk. The *male condom* is a thin sheath, usually made of latex, that is rolled down over the erect penis before any contact occurs between the penis and the partner's genitals. The *female condom* is a pouch of thin polyurethane that is inserted into the vagina before intercourse. Newer male, female, and anal silicone condoms are under development.[7] For more information on condoms, including how to use them, see Chapter 11.

intrauterine device (IUD)
Small T-shaped device that when inserted in the uterus prevents conception.

barrier methods
Contraceptive methods based on physically separating sperm from the female reproductive tract.

spermicide
Chemical agent that kills sperm.

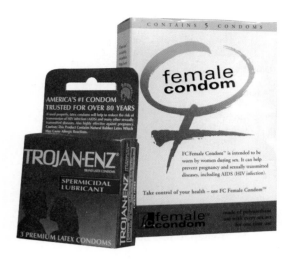

■ The advantages of condoms are that they are portable, available over the counter, and inexpensive. Condoms provide some protection against STIs, including HIV.

Female Barrier Methods The vaginal **diaphragm** is a circular rubber dome that is inserted in the vagina before intercourse; correct placement is shown in Figure 12.3. It fits between the pubic bone and the back of the vagina and covers the cervix. Spermicidal jelly or foam is placed in the dome, or cup, of the diaphragm before it is inserted; thus, the spermicide covers the cervix, where it provides the best protection. Nonoxynol-9 is the most common spermicide available in the United States. Spermicide can cause irritation for some people and, due to the irritation, may increase risk of HIV transmission. Spermicide must be reapplied into the vagina if a second act of sex occurs. The diaphragm is removed 6 to 12 hours after sex. Diaphragm use has been associated with an increased risk for urinary tract infections.

diaphragm
Circular rubber dome that is inserted in the vagina before intercourse to prevent conception.

cervical cap
Small, cuplike rubber device that covers only the cervix and is inserted in the vagina before intercourse to prevent conception.

A woman has to be fitted with the correctly sized diaphragm by a health care provider, who will show her how to insert and remove it. A new "one-size" diaphragm has been developed and approved for sale in Europe.

■ The FemCap cervical cap (left) and the diaphragm (right) work by creating a physical barrier at the cervical opening, preventing sperm from entering the uterus. Both are used with spermicidal cream or jelly.

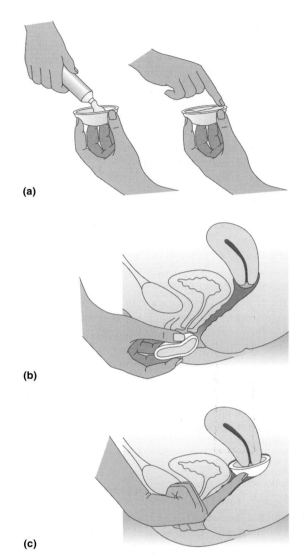

(a)

(b)

(c)

figure 12.3   Use of the diaphragm.
(a) With clean hands, place about 1 tablespoon of spermicide (jelly or cream) in the diaphragm, spreading it around inside the diaphragm and on its rim. (b) Using the thumb and forefinger, compress the diaphragm. Insert it into the vagina, guiding it toward the back wall and up into the vagina as far as possible. (c) With the index finger, check the position of the diaphragm to make sure that the cervix is covered completely and the front of the rim is behind the pubic bone.

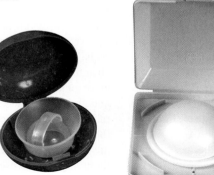

An application has been submitted to the Food and Drug Administration for its sale in the United States. Initial trials show that the single-size silicone diaphragm is as effective as traditional diaphragms and has the advantage of not requiring a visit to a health care provider.[8]

The **cervical cap** is a small, cuplike device that covers the cervix and prevents sperm from entering the uterus. As with a diaphragm, the cervical cap requires a fitting by a health care provider; it is replaced annually. Currently the FemCap is the only available model in the United States. It is made of nonallergenic silicone and comes in three sizes. A small amount of spermicide is placed in a groove on the vaginal side of the cap prior to insertion. It should be left in place for 6 to 48 hours after intercourse.[3]

The **contraceptive sponge** is a small, polyurethane foam device that is presaturated with 1 gram of the spermicide nonoxynol-9. The sponge is moistened with water and inserted into the vagina. It fits snugly over the cervix, becomes effective immediately, and remains effective for 24 hours. It should be left in place for at least six hours after intercourse and should then be removed. The sponge is available over the counter without prescription; one size fits all. The sponge should not be used during menstruation or if the user or her partner is allergic to sulfa medicines or polyurethane. It may be less effective in women who have had a pregnancy.

Toxic shock syndrome (TSS) is a very rare, potentially life-threatening bacterial infection that has been associated with the use of contraceptive sponges and diaphragms. In the 1980s, there was a sudden increase in the number of cases of TSS, most affecting young women who were using superabsorbent tampons. The infection is caused by an overgrowth in the vagina of the bacterium *Staphylococcus aureus* (or more rarely with *Streptococcal* infection). The risk is very low, but to reduce risk further, women should change tampons frequently (at least every four to eight hours) and should not leave female barrier methods of contraception in place beyond the recommended time. Symptoms of TSS include sudden high fever, vomiting or diarrhea, muscle aches, headache, seizures, and a rash that looks like a sunburn and eventually leads to peeling of the skin on the hands and feet.

Fertility Awareness–Based Methods

Women can usually become pregnant in a window of time around ovulation (release of an ovum). **Fertility awareness–based methods** of contraception rely on the identification of the fertile days in the menstrual cycle and abstaining from sex (or using a barrier contraceptive) during the fertile time. The Standard Days Method of fertility awareness relies on the fact that ovulation usually occurs 14 days *before* the menstrual period begins (Figure 12.4). For a woman with a 28-day cycle, ovulation usually occurs on day 14. However, for a woman with a shorter or longer cycle, the time difference is in the first part of the cycle (from menstruation to ovulation), not in the second part of the cycle (from ovulation to menstruation). For example, if a woman has a 21-day cycle, ovulation will usually occur on day 7. If a woman has a 32-day cycle, ovulation will usually occur on day 18.

The ovum is most likely to become fertilized within 24 hours after release from the ovary if it is to happen at all;

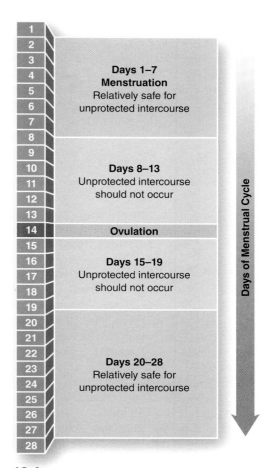

figure 12.4   **Fertility awareness–based methods.**
These methods use the menstrual cycle to determine when fertilization is likely to occur and when unprotected sexual intercourse should be avoided. If a woman does not have a 28-day cycle, the variability in her cycle will be in the part of the cycle from menstruation to ovulation.

however, the ovum can remain viable for four days. Sperm can survive up to seven days in cervical mucus. Thus any sperm deposited in the vagina after day 8 of the menstrual cycle could still be around on day 14, when the woman ovulates (in a 28-day cycle). To avoid pregnancy, the couple would need to avoid intercourse or use another method of contraception between day 8 and day 19.

The Standard Days Method requires that the woman have a regular cycle (same number of days every month) because abstinence or barrier methods must be used for seven days before ovulation. Cycle beads (as well as a Cycle Beads app) have been developed as a tool to help women track their cycles and fertile times.

contraceptive sponge
Small polyurethane foam device presaturated with spermicide that is inserted in the vagina before intercourse to prevent pregnancy.

toxic shock syndrome (TSS)
A rare, life-threatening bacterial infection in the vagina associated with the use of tampons and female barrier contraceptive methods.

fertility awareness–based methods
Contraceptive method based on abstinence during the window of time around ovulation when a woman is most likely to conceive.

Another method of fertility awareness is called the Two Day Method. This method takes advantage of the fact that ovulation is accompanied by certain signs that a woman can learn to recognize. One sign is that cervical mucus becomes thinner and stretchier, resembling egg white, and increases in quantity before ovulation, so the vagina feels wetter. Another sign is that because of hormone activity, basal body temperature rises by about half a degree when ovulation occurs and remains higher until the end of the cycle. A woman can take her temperature each morning with a basal temperature thermometer to see when this increase occurs. In the Two Day Method, a woman checks for vaginal secretions twice a day. If she notices secretions for two days in a row, she is in her fertile period and should abstain from sex or use a barrier contraceptive method.[9] Couples also use these signs to pinpoint the time of ovulation when they are trying to conceive.

Fertility awareness–based methods may be the only acceptable options for some people due to personal or religious reasons. However, there is debate over their effectiveness as a method of contraception. Some studies list the failure rate at 3 to 5 percent with perfect use and 25 percent with actual use; other studies conclude that the failure rate is unclear and recommend that couples be informed about the lack of evidence regarding effectiveness and be counseled about other options if they are willing to consider them.[3]

Withdrawal

Withdrawal, or *coitus interruptus,* is the removal of the penis from the vagina prior to ejaculation. As a method of contraception, it is controversial. It is not included on the list of recommended contraceptives issued by the American College of Obstetrics and Gynecology or the Planned Parenthood Federation of America. However, while it is significantly less effective than hormonal methods, some studies show levels of effectiveness similar to those of barrier

withdrawal
A contraceptive method in which the man removes his penis from the vagina before ejaculating.

emergency contraception (EC)
A contraceptive method used after unprotected sex to prevent pregnancy.

methods (approximately 18 to 27 percent of women will become pregnant in a year of using only withdrawal as a contraceptive).[3,10,11]

Withdrawal is highly dependent on the characteristics of the users. Success is dependent on a man's ability to determine when he is about to ejaculate and to have the self-control to withdraw with impending orgasm. However, sperm can be present in pre-ejaculate, so this method can fail even if a man withdraws prior to ejaculation. Both partners need to be committed to interruption of intercourse at the time of the man's orgasm. Failure rates appear to be higher in unmarried couples. While not generally recommended, withdrawal may be better than no method at all.[10]

Emergency Contraception

Also referred to as the *morning-after pill, post-sex contraception,* or *backup birth control,* **emergency contraception (EC)** can prevent pregnancy after unprotected vaginal intercourse. It is most effective if taken within 48 to 72 hours and must be taken within five days of unprotected intercourse. EC reduces the chance of pregnancy by preventing ovulation and fertilization. It may reduce the likelihood of implantation, but this is not proven. EC will not cause the termination of an existing pregnancy and thus is not an *abortogenic* (abortion-causing) agent.

Emergency contraception may be used when another method fails, such as when a condom breaks or a diaphragm or cervical cap slips out of position. It is also useful in cases of forced sex, including rape and incest. Plan B One-Step is an emergency contraceptive now available over the counter for women aged 17 or older. It consists of one pill, containing progesterone only. Other progesterone-only formulations or estrogen-progesterone combinations are available by prescription.

Emergency contraception is an important tool in preventing unintended pregnancy. It has been shown to be extremely safe in almost all women. Its over-the-counter status has increased accessibility, but many college women still remain uninformed about how to access it and when to use it if they have an unprotected sexual encounter. Colleges have tried to increase student education about its safety and availability. Women using emergency contraception should be advised to start effective contraception after use.[12,13]

Emergency contraception pills are less effective in women who are overweight or obese (BMI > 25). In these women, the copper IUD would be the emergency contraceptive

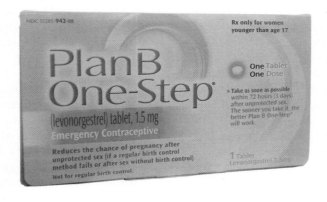

■ Emergency contraception can be taken to prevent pregnancy after unprotected sex or used as a backup when another form of contraception fails, as when a condom breaks.

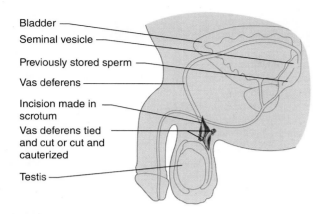

figure 12.5   **Vasectomy.**
With only local anesthesia needed, this surgical procedure offers permanent sterilization.

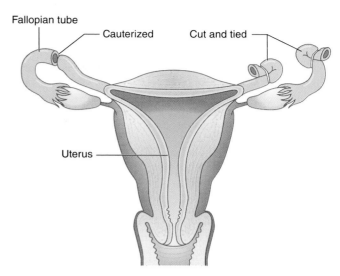

figure 12.6   **Tubal ligation.**
This surgical procedure is often performed via laparoscopy, which involves creating two small incisions, one for the scope device and the other for the surgical instruments. It usually requires only local anesthesia.

of choice. It may be inserted within five days of unprotected sex and has the advantage of providing ongoing contraception.[14]

Sterilization

Sterilization is a surgical procedure that is considered a permanent form of contraception. Worldwide, it is the most commonly used form of contraception and is especially popular among couples who do not want to have any more children. Despite counseling prior to sterilization, surgical reversal is sometimes requested due to changing circumstances. The likelihood of pregnancy after a surgical reversal varies widely, with success rates from 10 to 70 percent, and cannot be guaranteed.[15,16] Besides condoms, sterilization is currently the only form of contraception available to men.

The male sterilization procedure is **vasectomy**. In this procedure, a health care professional makes a small incision or puncture in the scrotum, then ties off and severs the vas deferens, the duct that carries sperm from the testes to the seminal vesicle, where sperm would mix with semen (Figure 12.5). Vasectomy is usually a relatively quick procedure performed with a local anesthetic.

The most common female sterilization procedure is **tubal ligation**. In this procedure, a physician makes an incision in the abdomen, then severs and ties or seals the fallopian tubes, the ducts through which ova pass from the ovaries to the uterus (Figure 12.6). The procedure can be done via a surgical method called *laparoscopy*. A laparoscope, a tube that the surgeon can look through with a tiny light on the end, is inserted through a small incision, and the surgical instruments are inserted through another small incision. Recovery usually takes somewhat longer than recovery from a vasectomy. Tubal ligation is also associated with more risk of complications than vasectomy.

Tubal ligation does not alter a woman's menstrual cycle or hormone levels. The ovaries continue to function, but ova are prevented from traveling through the fallopian tubes to the uterus and thus cannot be fertilized. Another option for permanent sterilization in women, called Essure, involves the placement of a micro-rod in each of the fallopian tubes. Tissue begins to develop around the micro-rods, and after three months this tissue barrier prevents sperm from reaching the egg.

Although in rare cases pregnancy does occur after a vasectomy or tubal ligation, sterilization procedures should be considered permanent.

UNINTENDED PREGNANCY

If you or your partner becomes pregnant unexpectedly, you have to make a monumental decision in a very short period of time. The options are to (1) carry the pregnancy to term and raise the child, (2) carry the pregnancy to term and place the child in an adoptive family, or (3) terminate the pregnancy. Read about how one couple handled this complicated decision in the box, "Jack and Michelle: Unexpected Pregnancy."

sterilization
Surgical procedure that permanently prevents any future pregnancies.

vasectomy
Male sterilization procedure, involving tying off and severing the vas deferens to prevent sperm from reaching the semen.

tubal ligation
Female sterilization procedure involving severing and tying off or sealing the fallopian tubes to prevent ova from reaching the uterus.

Life Stories

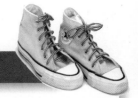

Jack and Michelle: Unexpected Pregnancy

Jack was a senior in college and was looking forward to graduation. He had applied to medical school and was confident he would get in, but he did not yet know where he would be going. He wanted to move to a new part of the country and meet new people, but a call from his ex-girlfriend Michelle cast a sudden shadow over his plans for the future.

Michelle told him that she was pregnant. They had seen each other for a few months but had broken up about three weeks earlier. He couldn't believe that it could be true, yet he knew she wouldn't lie to him. When they started dating, she was taking birth control pills, but they had agreed to use condoms as an extra precaution. However, a couple of times, after they had been out late at parties and drinking, they had had sex without a condom. He hadn't thought much about it, as he considered the condoms a backup method. He didn't realize she had stopped taking the pill.

Now Jack felt really confused. He was glad Michelle had called him, and when they met to talk about options, it was pretty clear to him that she did not want to consider an abortion. She had talked to her sister and parents, and they were ready to support and help her if she needed it. They were encouraging her to move home, but home was in a different state several hundred miles away. Jack did not feel ready to be a parent, but he did want to take responsibility. He was very close with his father and could imagine being close with his own child. He knew that if Michelle had the child, he would want to be involved. Still, this affected his plan to go to medical school, and it all felt really complicated.

Neither of them wanted to get back together—they both knew that their relationship would not last and that a child would not solve that. But when Michelle talked about going home, Jack got scared that he might never see the child. He wondered about his rights as a father.

- Do you have ongoing discussions about contraception with partners, or do you make assumptions about what a partner is using?

- Do you have discussions with your partner about what you would do in the event of an unintended pregnancy? If not, why not?

- Do you know what your legal rights and responsibilities are in your state as a woman or a man involved in an unintended pregnancy?

Signs of Pregnancy

ectopic pregnancy
A pregnancy in which a fertilized egg implants or attaches outside of the uterus, usually in a fallopian tube.

Some signs of pregnancy are common early on, even before a missed period, as a result of hormonal changes. They can include breast tenderness and swelling, fatigue, nausea and vomiting, light-headedness, and mood swings. Some women have light vaginal bleeding or spotting 10 to 14 days after conception—about the time of a normal period but shorter in duration. If you experience any of these symptoms after unprotected sex or a missed period, you may want to take a pregnancy test.

A rare complication in early pregnancy is **ectopic pregnancy**, when the fertilized egg implants or attaches outside of the uterus, usually in the fallopian tube. Signs of this potentially life-threatening condition are severe lower abdominal pain or cramping on one or both sides; vaginal spotting or bleeding with abdominal pain; or light-headedness, dizziness, or fainting (a possible sign of internal bleeding). If you experience any of these signs, contact your physician or go to the emergency room immediately.

Deciding to Become a Parent

Are you ready to become a parent? Here are some questions to consider:

- What are your long-term educational, career, and life plans? How would having a child at this time fit in with those plans?

- What is the status of your relationship with your partner? Is he or she someone you want to commit to and share parenthood with? If you are the mother, the greater part of the pregnancy experience will fall on you, but parenting will involve making decisions with your partner about childrearing. Do you have similar goals for a child? Can you communicate well with each other?

- Do you feel emotionally mature enough to take on the responsibility of raising a child? Parenthood requires patience, sacrifice, and the ability to put aside your own needs to meet the needs of another person.

- What are your financial resources at this point? Having a child is expensive. Factoring in inflation, a child born in 2012 will cost between $216,910 and $501,250 to raise through age 18.[17]

- If you are the father, do you plan to be financially, emotionally or physically involved? While you will probably be legally required to remain financially involved, children who have their father's involvement physically and emotionally are less likely to live in poverty, use drugs, be victims of child abuse, or engage in criminal behavior, and they have fewer emotional, psychological, and health problems.[18]

- How large is your social support system? Do you have family members and friends who will help you? Does your community have resources and support services?

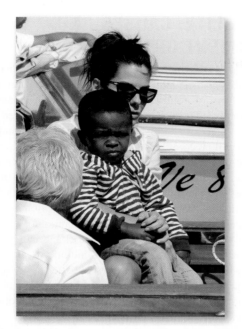

■ Adoption offers the possibility of parenting to people who are not able to conceive a child or who choose not to. Actress Sandra Bullock adopted her son in 2010.

Social support has been found to be one of the most important factors in helping couples make a successful adjustment to parenthood.

■ What is your health status and age? Do you smoke, drink, or use recreational drugs? Do you have an STI or other medical condition that needs to be treated? Are you under 18 or over 35? Babies born to teenagers and women over 35 have a higher incidence of health problems.

Adoption

Adoption can be a positive solution for an unintended pregnancy if you and your partner are not able or willing to become parents at this time in your lives. All forms of adoption require that both biological parents relinquish their parental rights.

In an *open adoption,* the biological parents help to choose the adoptive parents and can maintain a relationship with them and the child. The degree of involvement can range from the exchange of information through a third party to a close and continuous relationship among all parties throughout the child's life. This choice can make it easier for parents to give up a baby, and it allows the child to know his or her biological parents, siblings, and relatives. Many adoption agencies offer this option.

In a *closed adoption,* the more traditional form of adoption, the biological parents do not help choose the adoptive parents, and the adoption records are sealed. This type of adoption provides more privacy and confidentiality than

open adoption does. In some states, the child may access the sealed records at the age of 18, and many states are in the process of passing legislation that would open previously sealed records, even for adoptions that occurred decades ago. One of the reasons for the proposed change is the realization that knowledge about one's biological parents can be important for both psychological and health reasons.

International adoptions have become increasingly common, with children being adopted from countries around the world. A major legislative change now allows children in international adoptions to automatically be granted U.S. citizenship at the time of their adoption.

Elective Abortion

Terminating the pregnancy through **elective abortion** is the third option for a woman with an unintended pregnancy. (This type of abortion is called *elective* to distinguish it from **spontaneous abortion**, or miscarriage.) Since 1973, elective abortion has been legal in the United States. In the case of *Roe v. Wade,* the U.S. Supreme Court ruled that the decision to terminate a pregnancy must be left up to the woman, with some restrictions applying as the pregnancy advances through three *trimesters* (divisions of the pregnancy into parts, each about three months long).

Since the passage of *Roe v. Wade,* many attempts have been made at state and national levels to limit access to legal abortion. The debate over abortion between pro-life and pro-choice activists is one of the most highly charged political issues of our time. The vast majority of abortions—92 percent—are performed during the first 12 weeks of pregnancy.[19,20]

International studies show that women around the world seek abortion regardless of the legality of the procedure. However, the lowest rates of abortion occur in countries where abortion is legal (western Europe), and the highest rates of abortion occur in countries where abortion is illegal (Latin America). When abortion is illegal, it is more likely to be unsafe and to be associated with a higher rate of maternal death.[21]

Unintended pregnancy raises complex emotions. Fifty-nine percent of women having an abortion have one or more children already; they report that the concern for or responsibility to others and cost are the major factors in why they choose abortion.[19,22] This may help explain why the majority of women who have an abortion report a feeling of relief after the abortion. Multiple studies have confirmed that pregnancy termination does not increase risk of mental health concerns.[19]

Women who are pregnant and considering abortion should seek health care counseling as soon as possible to discuss all their options, the risks associated with the

elective abortion
Voluntary termination of a pregnancy.

spontaneous abortion
Involuntary termination of a pregnancy, or miscarriage.

procedure, and the technique to be used. The most common technique currently in use is surgical abortion, but the use of medical abortion is increasing.

Surgical Abortion   In **surgical abortion**, the embryo or fetus and other contents of the uterus are removed through a surgical procedure. (Between two and eight weeks of gestation, the term *embryo* is used; after the eighth week, the term *fetus* is used.) The most common method of surgical abortion performed between the sixth and twelfth weeks is vacuum aspiration; it is used for about 72.4 percent of all abortions performed in the United States. A physician performs this procedure in a clinical setting, such as a medical office or hospital. The cervix is numbed with a local anesthetic and opened with an instrument called a dilator. After the cervix has been opened, a catheter, a tubelike instrument, is inserted into the uterus. The catheter is attached to a suction machine, and the contents of the uterus are removed.[22]

surgical abortion
Surgical removal of the contents of the uterus to terminate a pregnancy.

medical abortion
Use of a pharmaceutical agent to terminate a pregnancy.

infertility
Inability to become pregnant after not using any form of contraception during sexual intercourse for 12 months.

congenital abnormalities
Birth defects.

The procedure takes about 10 minutes and requires a few hours' recovery before the woman can return home. A follow-up appointment is needed about two weeks after the procedure to ensure that the body is healing and, if appropriate, to start a more effective form of contraception. When performed in a legal and safe setting, elective abortion does not increase the risk of infertility or of complications in future pregnancies. For later-stage pregnancies, usually when the mother's life is at risk, a procedure called dilatation and extraction or induction of labor is sometimes used.[22]

Medical Abortion   An alternative to surgical abortion is **medical abortion**, in which a pharmaceutical agent is used to induce an abortion. Medical abortions can be performed very early in pregnancy (less than seven weeks of gestation) or in late pregnancy (after 15 weeks). Between these gestational ages, the surgical techniques are recommended.

The drug mifepristone (RU-486) is used during the first seven weeks of gestation (or nine weeks of pregnancy, dated from the first day of the last menstrual period). It is taken in a pill and followed two or three days later by another drug, misoprostol, which induces contractions. Most women have cramping and bleeding and abort the pregnancy within two weeks, although in some cases abortion may occur in a few hours or days. The success rate is nearly 90 percent, and serious complications are rare. For women seeking early pregnancy termination, the rates of medical abortion are increasing. After 15 weeks of gestation, different medications are used to induce labor. If abortion does not occur with medication, a surgical abortion is recommended.[20,22]

INFERTILITY: CAUSES AND TREATMENT OPTIONS

Approximately 10 percent of couples receive specialist care for **infertility**,[23] the inability to become pregnant after not using any form of contraception during sexual intercourse for 12 months. The longer childbearing is delayed, the higher the chances that conception will be difficult and that pregnancy will be complicated.

In about one-third of cases, infertility stems from male factors, such as low sperm count or lack of sperm motility. In another one-third of cases, infertility results from blockage in the woman's fallopian tubes, often scarring that has occurred as a result of pelvic inflammatory disease or another complication of an STI. Blockage can also be caused by an unsterile abortion or by endometriosis, a condition in which uterine tissue grows outside the uterus. In the remaining one-third of cases, the problem is lack of ovulation, abnormalities in the cervical mucus or in anatomy, or unknown causes.

Treatment options for infertility are increasingly being used by couples experiencing difficulty conceiving and by single and lesbian women. Treatments include surgery to open blocked fallopian tubes or correct anatomical problems, fertility (hormonal) drugs to promote ovulation and regulate hormones, and more advanced reproductive techniques. Intrauterine (artificial) insemination is a process whereby sperm are collected and placed directly into a woman's uterus by syringe. This procedure can be helpful if a man has a low sperm count or low sperm mobility. Donor sperm can be used if a man has a genetic abnormality or if the patient is a single woman or a lesbian.

In vitro fertilization is a technique by which hormones are used to stimulate egg production in the ovaries, multiple eggs are collected through a surgical procedure, the eggs are fertilized in the clinic, and the fertilized eggs are transferred to the woman's uterus. Other fertilization techniques include gamete intrafallopian transfer and zygote intrafallopian transfer. Both techniques involve induction of multiple eggs with hormones, surgical collection, and manual reintroduction into the fallopian tubes.

PREGNANCY AND PRENATAL CARE

Research is now indicating that adverse events and conditions during pregnancy can not only cause **congenital abnormalities** (birth defects) but also influence development throughout life, affecting cognitive development in childhood and health risks, including mental health risks, in adulthood. The best approach to ensuring good health is to give every child the best possible start in life.

Pregnancy Planning

When is the best time to have a child? Although this is a highly personal decision influenced by many factors—educational and career plans, relationship status, health issues, and others—evidence indicates that the least health risk occurs when women have pregnancies between the ages of 18 and 35. Before age 18, a woman's body is still growing and developing. The additional demands of pregnancy and nursing can impair her health, and the baby is more likely to be born early and have a low birth weight.

After age 35, a woman is more likely to have difficulty getting pregnant, because fertility declines as a woman gets older. Women over 35 are also more likely to have medical problems during pregnancy, including miscarriage, and to have a baby who is born prematurely, has low birth weight, or has a genetic abnormality like Down syndrome.

Male fertility also declines with age. After age 35, men are twice as likely to be infertile as men in their early 20s. Men over age 40 have an increased risk of fathering a child with autism, schizophrenia, or Down syndrome.[24]

Prepregnancy Counseling

Couples who practice family planning can take advantage of **prepregnancy counseling**, which typically includes an evaluation of current health status, health behaviors, and family health history. A woman who smokes, uses drugs, or drinks alcohol will be encouraged to quit *before* trying to become pregnant, as will her partner. Existing health conditions will be treated and medications adjusted to the safest options for pregnancy. This can be especially important if a woman is taking medications for high blood pressure, seizure disorder, or some psychiatric disorders. If obesity is an issue, a woman may be counseled about a weight management program. If a couple appear to be at increased risk for a genetic disease on the basis of their ethnic background or family history, they may be referred at this point for genetic counseling and testing.

Nutrition and Exercise

Because so many women become pregnant unintentionally, every sexually active woman who might become pregnant should be aware of the importance of healthy lifestyle factors. A balanced, nutritious diet before and during pregnancy helps ensure that mother and child get required nutrients. A baby needs calcium for its growing bones, and this is linked to the mother's calcium intake. Getting folic acid in food or in a folate supplement is also recommended to reduce the risk of neural tube defects (problems in the development of the brain and spinal cord). Women should increase their folic acid intake

■ Prenatal care includes regular, moderate physical activity.

one month *before* getting pregnant so that they have a high level of folic acid in their bodies at the time of conception. It is recommended that all women of childbearing age who may become pregnant consume at least 400 micrograms of folic acid a day, usually in the form of a supplement.[25]

Foodborne infections can have more serious effects in pregnant women than in the general population. Pregnant women are advised to avoid unpasteurized foods, soft cheese (for instance, Brie, Camembert, and feta), and raw or smoked seafood. Pregnant women, women who might become pregnant, nursing mothers, and young children are advised to monitor their fish and shellfish intake because of contamination with mercury.[25] For guidelines on safe fish consumption, see Chapter 5, "Fats—A Necessary Nutrient."

Weight gain goals during pregnancy vary based on prepregnancy weight. A woman in the healthy weight range needs to increase calorie intake by only 300 calories a day to achieve a goal weight gain of 25 to 35 pounds. An underweight woman should gain 28 to 40 pounds, and an overweight woman, 11 to 20 pounds. Regular exercise during pregnancy is recommended to help maintain muscle strength, circulation, and general well-being. Women can usually maintain their prepregnancy level of activity. In the second and third trimesters, women should be cautious about exercise that might cause injury or trauma (such as contact sports or downhill skiing) and favor safer forms of exercise like walking and swimming.[26]

Maternal Immunizations

Women should be up-to-date on routine vaccinations *before* pregnancy. Especially important are vaccination for rubella (German measles) and hepatitis B. Rubella can cause spontaneous abortion or serious birth defects, including deafness and blindness. Hepatitis B is a highly infectious disease that causes liver damage and can be transmitted from mother to child during pregnancy and delivery (called **vertical transmission**). Pregnant women are also at high risk of complications from influenza and should get a flu shot during the flu season. Pregnant

prepregnancy counseling Counseling before conception that may include an evaluation of current health behaviors and health status, recommendations for improving health, and treatment of any existing conditions that might increase risk.

vertical transmission Transmission of an infection or disease from mother to child during pregnancy and delivery.

women should receive a booster of Tdap (tetanus, diphtheria, and acellular pertussis vaccination) prior to delivery. All people who will have close contact with the infant should also be sure they are up to date on their Tdap vaccination. The Tdap vaccination protects the infant from a number of infections, including *Bordetella pertussis,* the bacterium that causes whooping cough, which can cause serious illness or death in infants.[27]

Medications and Drugs

The uterus is a highly protected place, but most substances that the mother ingests or that otherwise enter her bloodstream eventually reach the fetus. These include prescription medications as well as other drugs and toxic substances. Some substances, called **teratogens**, can cause physical damage or defects in the fetus, especially if they are present during the first trimester, when rapid development of body organs is occurring.

Tobacco and alcohol are the most commonly used drugs during pregnancy. Tobacco use is associated with increased risk of spontaneous abortion, low birth weight, early separation of the placenta from the uterine wall, and infant death. Babies living in homes where adults smoke have a higher incidence of respiratory infections and **sudden infant death syndrome (SIDS)**.

Consuming 3 or more ounces of alcohol daily (about six drinks) during pregnancy is associated with **fetal alcohol syndrome (FAS)**. This condition is characterized by abnormal facial appearance, slow growth, mental retardation, and social, emotional, and behavior problems. A safe level of alcohol consumption during pregnancy has not been established, and binge drinking, even occasionally, may carry significant risk.

Illicit drugs have a variety of effects on a fetus, depending on the chemical action of the drug. Cocaine causes blood vessels to constrict in the placenta and fetus, increasing the risk of early separation of the placenta from the uterine wall, low birth weight, and possible birth defects. Heroin, OxyContin, and other narcotics can cause retarded growth or fetal death as well as behavior problems in a child exposed to it in the womb. A baby whose mother used narcotics during pregnancy is born addicted and experiences withdrawal symptoms, which can include seizures, irritability, vomiting, and diarrhea. Illicit drugs are also dangerous because they are often contaminated with harmful substances, such as glass, poisons, and other drugs.[28]

teratogens
Substances that can cause physical damage or defects in the fetus, especially if they are present during the first trimester, when rapid development of body organs is occurring.

sudden infant death syndrome (SIDS)
Unexpected death of a healthy baby during sleep.

fetal alcohol syndrome (FAS)
Combination of birth defects caused by prenatal exposure to alcohol, characterized by abnormal facial appearance, slow growth, mental retardation, and social, emotional, and behavior problems.

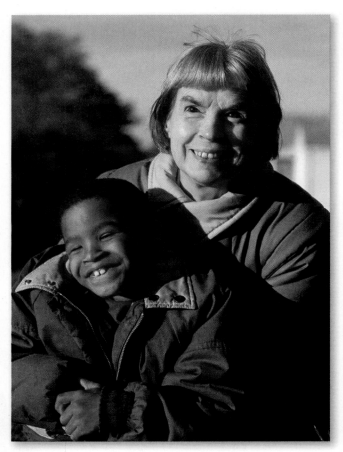

■ Alcohol consumption during pregnancy can cause permanent damage to the fetus, with physical, learning, and behavioral effects. Here, a blind parent holds her adopted son, whose brain is damaged from fetal alcohol syndrome. Some of the facial characteristics associated with FAS include a short nose, low nasal bridge, and thin upper lip.

Prenatal Care and Delivery Choices

Every pregnant woman should visit her health care provider regularly for *prenatal care.* After the first visit, the health care provider uses the subsequent visits to monitor the fetus for normal growth and development and the woman for complications of pregnancy.

Pregnant women have a number of options for health care providers, ranging from midwives to perinatologists, and for delivery: giving birth at home, in a birthing center, or in a hospital. A woman's choice depends on her personal preferences, medical and health history, and the likelihood of complications during pregnancy.

Midwives usually take patients who are at low risk for medical or pregnancy complications. If complications develop during prenatal care or delivery, a midwife will refer the case to a family physician or an obstetrician. Midwives tend to view pregnancy and birth as a family event. They are usually trained in support techniques (such as breathing and relaxation techniques) so the woman can have a delivery without anesthetic medications, and they usually stay with the woman throughout labor.

Some family physicians provide pregnancy-related care. They may deliver babies in birthing centers or hospitals, but they rarely perform home births. Like midwives, many family physicians view pregnancy and birth as a family event, and some use the same kind of support techniques.

Obstetricians are trained to handle all kinds of pregnancies, from low risk to high risk. Perinatologists are obstetricians with additional training in the management of high-risk pregnancy. These specialists consult with and accept referrals from obstetricians. They are usually found at major medical centers. Most women see a perinatologist only if serious complications arise in the pregnancy.

Complications of Pregnancy Although it is shocking to hear that a woman has died in childbirth in the 21st century, such deaths do occur. The U.S. rates of maternal death are higher than the rates in 16 peer countries (Australia, Austria, Canada, Denmark, Finland, France, Germany, Italy, Japan, Netherlands, Norway, Portugal, Spain, Sweden, Switzerland, and the United Kingdom). Mortality is highest in ethnic and racial minority groups, highlighting the role of socioeconomic factors, such as lack of prenatal care, lack of access to health information, dietary differences and potentially underlying stress.[29] But even Americans in the highest socioeconomic levels experience poorer health than equivalent groups in other developed countries.

Different health risks are more common at different stages of pregnancy. Early complications of pregnancy include the diagnosis of an STI, usually treated with antibiotics or antiviral medications, and miscarriage. Approximately 15 to 50 percent of all pregnancies end in miscarriage, most during the first trimester.

Pregnancy predisposes some women to develop diabetes, called *gestational diabetes*. Most women are screened between 24 and 28 weeks, because the condition occurs midway through pregnancy. Women with gestational diabetes are advised to exercise, control their diet, and monitor glucose levels, but some women need to start taking insulin.

Toward the end of pregnancy, the risk for several complications increases. An especially dangerous condition is **preeclampsia**, characterized by high blood pressure, fluid retention, possible kidney and liver damage, and potential fetal death. Signs include facial swelling, headaches, blurred vision, nausea, and vomiting. If not treated, the condition can progress to **eclampsia**, a potentially life-threatening disease marked by seizures and coma.

Preterm or early labor is another complication of pregnancy. If a woman experiences contractions, cramping, pelvic pressure, or vaginal bleeding before 37 weeks, she should be evaluated to prevent preterm labor.[26]

Complications of Pregnancy for the Child Approximately 1.2 percent of all pregnancies end in infant death. Half of these deaths occur before the fetus is born, and 80 percent occur before the 28th week of pregnancy (**stillbirth**). After birth, the leading causes of infant death are preterm birth, low birth weight, and SIDS.

Rates of both low birth weight and infant mortality are significantly higher for African Americans in the United States than for members of other groups. Reducing such disparities through improved access to health information and prenatal care is a national health goal.[26,28]

Fetal Development

Within 30 minutes of fertilization in the fallopian tube, the single-celled fertilized ovum, called a *zygote,* starts to divide. By the end of five days, the cluster of cells has made its way down the tube into the uterus. By the end of a week, it attaches to the uterus and starts to send small rootlike attachments into the uterine wall to draw nourishment. By the end of the second week, it is fully embedded in the lining of the uterus.

The period from week 2 to week 8, called the embryonic period, is a time of rapid growth and differentiation. By four weeks, the cluster of cells has divided into cells of different types, forming an embryo, a **placenta**, and an **amniotic sac**. By eight weeks, all body systems and organs are present in rudimentary form, and some, including the heart, brain, liver, and sex organs, have started to function.

The period from the end of the eighth week after conception to birth is called the fetal period. By 16 weeks, the sex of the fetus can be readily determined, and the mother can feel fetal movements. By 24 weeks, the fetus makes sucking movements with its mouth.

By week 26, the eyes are open, and by week 30, a layer of fat is forming under the skin. At 36 weeks, the fetus has an excellent chance of survival. A baby is considered to be full term at 38 weeks of gestation, 40 weeks after the mother's last menstrual period. Full-term babies usually weigh about 7½ pounds and are about 20 inches long. An overview of fetal development is shown in Figure 12.7.

Diagnosing Problems in a Fetus

About 5 percent of babies born in the United States have a birth defect. Several tests have been developed to detect abnormalities in a fetus before birth. In the first trimester, all women are offered screening for Down syndrome, the most

preeclampsia
Dangerous condition that can occur during pregnancy, characterized by high blood pressure, fluid retention, possible kidney and liver damage, and potential fetal death.

eclampsia
Potentially life-threatening disease that can develop during pregnancy, marked by seizures and coma.

stillbirth
Infant death before or at the time of expected birth.

placenta
Structure that develops in the uterus during pregnancy and links the circulatory system of the fetus with that of the mother.

amniotic sac
Membrane that surrounds the fetus in the uterus and contains amniotic fluid.

Time	Changes/milestones
8 weeks (end of embryonic period)	*By week 8, pregnancy is detectable by physical examination.* Head is nearly as large as body. First brain waves can be detected. Limbs are present. Ossification (bone growth) begins. Cardiovascular system is fully functional. All body systems are present in at least basic form. Crown-to-rump length: 30 mm (1.2 inches) Weight: 2 grams (0.06 ounce)
9–12 weeks (3rd month)	*By week 10, fetus responds to stimulation.* Head is still large, but body is lengthening. Brain is enlarging. Spinal cord shows definition. Facial features begin to appear. Internal organs are developing. Blood cells are first formed in bone marrow. Skin is apparent. Limbs are well molded. Sex can be recognized from genitals. Crown-to-rump length: 90 mm
13–16 weeks (4th month)	*By week 14, skeleton is visible on X-ray.* Cerebellum becomes prominent. Sensory organs are defined. Blinking of eyes and sucking motions of lips occur. Face has human appearance. Head and body come into greater balance. Most bones are distinct. Crown-to-rump length: 140 mm
17–20 weeks (5th month)	*By week 17, mother can feel movement of fetus.* Fatty secretions (vernix caseosa) cover body. Lanugo (silky hair) covers skin. Fetal position is assumed. Limbs are reaching final proportions. Mother feels "quickening" (movement of fetus). Crown-to-rump length: 190 mm
21–30 weeks (6th and 7th months)	*By weeks 25–27, survival outside the womb is possible.* Substantial weight gain occurs. Myelination (formation of sheath around nerve fibers) of spinal cord begins. Eyes are open. Bones of distal limbs ossify. Skin is wrinkled and red. Fingernails and toenails are present. Tooth enamel is forming. Body is lean and well proportioned. Blood cells are formed in bone marrow only. In males, testes reach scrotum at 7th month. Crown-to-rump length: 280 mm
30–40 weeks (8th and 9th months)	*Between weeks 32 and 34, survival outside the womb is probable.* Skin is whitish pink. Fat is present in subcutaneous tissue. Crown-to-rump length: 360–400 mm Weight: 2.7–4.1 kg (6–10 pounds)

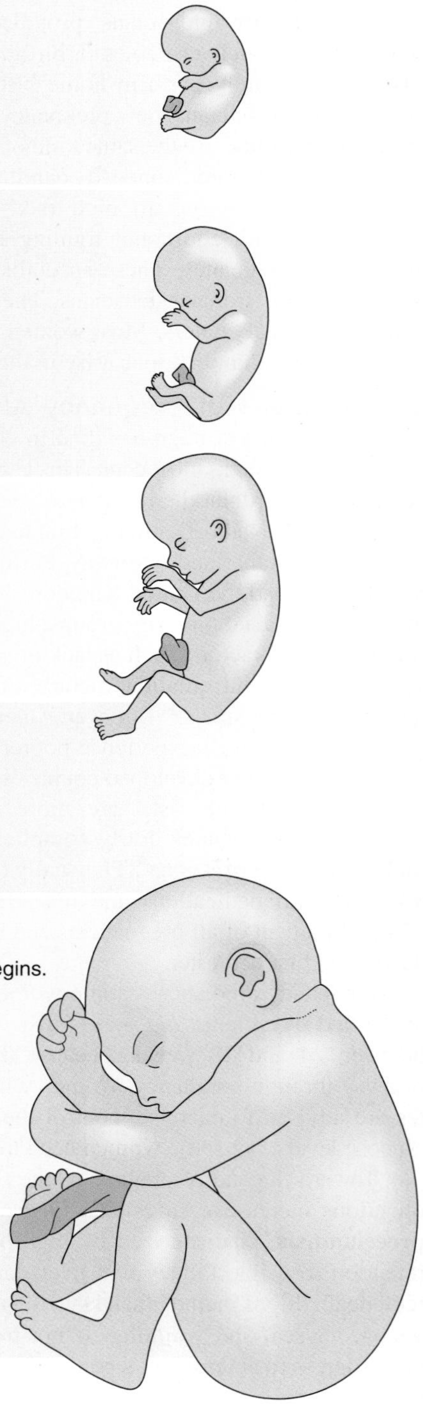

figure 12.7   Fetal development.

Sources: Data from *Human Anatomy and Physiology*, 6th ed., by E. N. Marieb, 2004, San Francisco: Benjamin-Cummings; *Understanding Children and Adolescents*, 4th ed., by J. A. Schickedanz et al., 2001, Boston: Allyn & Bacon.

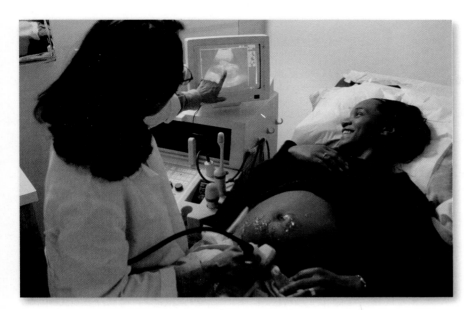

■ Ultrasound is a commonly used prenatal screening tool that can reveal the sex of the fetus, along with other information. Sonograms give expectant parents their first view of their child.

common chromosomal abnormality, with a maternal blood test and **ultrasound**, high-frequency sound waves that produce a visual image of the fetus in the womb. Ultrasound is commonly used to determine the size and gestational age of the fetus, its location in the uterus, and any major anatomical abnormalities. It can also reveal the sex of the fetus.

If the screening blood test and ultrasound raise concerns for possible chromosome abnormalities, either **chorionic villus sampling (CVS)** or **amniocentesis** can be performed to confirm results. In both tests, a needle is passed through the abdomen of the pregnant woman into the uterus. In CVS, a sample is taken from the chorionic villus, part of the placenta (fetal support system) in the uterus. In amniocentesis, a sample of amniotic fluid, the fluid that fills the pouch enclosing the fetus in the uterus, is taken. In both cases, fetal cells from the samples are subjected to chromosomal analysis. CVS can be performed between weeks 10 and 12, and amniocentesis can be performed between weeks 14 and 18.

CHILDBIRTH

By the ninth month, the pregnant woman is usually uncomfortably large and eager to have the baby, despite any apprehension she may harbor about the process of giving birth.

Labor and Delivery

Labor begins when hormonal changes in both the fetus and the mother cause strong uterine contractions to begin. The pattern of labor and delivery can be different for every woman, but often it begins with irregular uterine contractions.

When labor begins in earnest, the contractions will become regularly spaced and begin to get stronger and more painful. The contractions cause the cervix to gradually pull back and open (dilate), and they put pressure on the fetus, forcing it down into the mother's pelvis. This first stage of labor can last from a few to many hours.

When the cervix is completely open, the second stage of labor begins. The baby slowly moves into the birth canal, which stretches open to allow passage. The soft bones of the baby's head move together and overlap as it squeezes through the pelvis. When the top of the head appears at the opening of the birth canal, the baby is said to be *crowning*. After the head emerges, the rest of the body usually slips out easily.

The third stage of labor is the delivery of the placenta, which usually takes another 10 to 30 minutes. An overview of the process of labor and delivery is shown in Figure 12.8.

Many techniques have been developed to help women with the discomfort of the labor and delivery process. Childbirth preparation classes help women and their partners learn breathing and relaxation techniques to use during contractions. Several medication options are available in hospitals to further help with the discomfort.

Occasionally, the birthing process does not go smoothly. Sometimes, the infant is too big to pass through the mother's pelvis or is in the wrong position, either sideways, buttocks first, or face first. Occasionally, the placenta covers the cervix so the baby cannot move into the birth canal. And sometimes the infant just does not tolerate the stress of the process well.

In these situations, the health care provider usually recommends **cesarean section (C-section)**, the surgical delivery of the infant through the abdominal wall. Although many women are not enthusiastic about this option, it has saved many infants' and mothers' lives.

ultrasound
Technique for producing a visual image of the fetus using high-frequency sound waves.

chorionic villus sampling (CVS)
Technique for testing fetal cells for chromosomal abnormalities by removing cells from the chorionic villus, part of the placenta in the uterus.

amniocentesis
Technique for testing fetal cells for chromosomal abnormalities by removing a sample of amniotic fluid from the amniotic sac.

labor
Physiological process by which the mother's body expels the baby during birth.

cesarean section (C-section)
Surgical delivery of the infant through the abdominal wall.

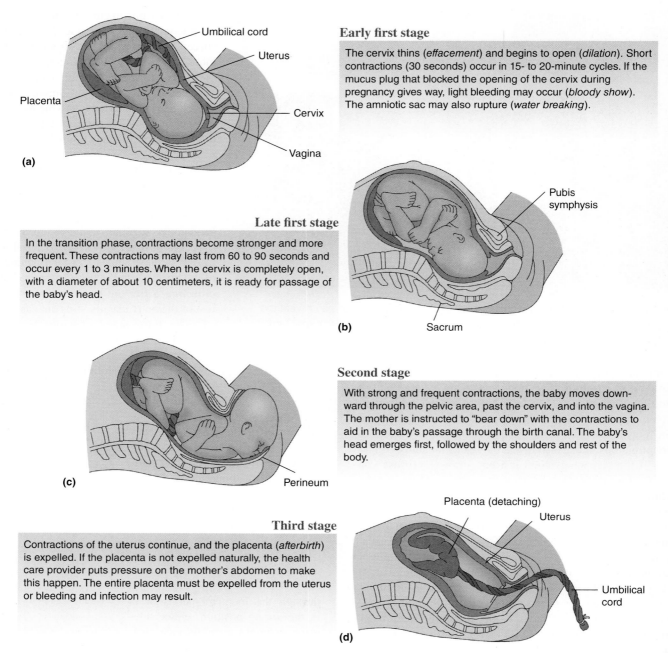

Early first stage

The cervix thins (*effacement*) and begins to open (*dilation*). Short contractions (30 seconds) occur in 15- to 20-minute cycles. If the mucus plug that blocked the opening of the cervix during pregnancy gives way, light bleeding may occur (*bloody show*). The amniotic sac may also rupture (*water breaking*).

Late first stage

In the transition phase, contractions become stronger and more frequent. These contractions may last from 60 to 90 seconds and occur every 1 to 3 minutes. When the cervix is completely open, with a diameter of about 10 centimeters, it is ready for passage of the baby's head.

Second stage

With strong and frequent contractions, the baby moves downward through the pelvic area, past the cervix, and into the vagina. The mother is instructed to "bear down" with the contractions to aid in the baby's passage through the birth canal. The baby's head emerges first, followed by the shoulders and rest of the body.

Third stage

Contractions of the uterus continue, and the placenta (*afterbirth*) is expelled. If the placenta is not expelled naturally, the health care provider puts pressure on the mother's abdomen to make this happen. The entire placenta must be expelled from the uterus or bleeding and infection may result.

figure 12.8   Labor and delivery.
(a) In the first stage of labor, the cervix thins and dilates, ending with (b) the transition phase. (c) Delivery of the baby occurs in the second stage. (d) In the third stage, the placenta is expelled.

Newborn Screening

Babies are evaluated at birth to determine whether they require any medical attention or will need developmental support later. The Apgar scale is used as a quick measure of the baby's physical condition: a score of 0 to 2 is given for heart rate, respiratory effort, muscle tone, reflex irritability, and color. The scores are added for a total score of 0 to 10. The baby's neurological condition may also be assessed, and various screening tests may be given, such as tests for hearing and for phenylketonuria, a genetic disorder that requires a special diet. Most babies are pronounced healthy and taken home within 24 to 48 hours of birth.

The Postpartum Period

The first few months of parenthood, known as the postpartum period, are a time of profound adjustment, as parents

Public Health Is Personal

The Importance of Early Childhood Education

As an infant, you are born into a family and environment that either provides you with tremendous opportunity or potential disadvantage. Research is increasingly showing that fetal and early childhood experiences are critical for lifelong health. Development of the brain is most intense from birth to three years of age. Early experiences can actually alter which genes are turned on or off and thus shape a child's developing brain structure.

Children exposed to positive early environments activate their brains learning and memory circuits and experience epigenetic changes that have the potential for lifelong positive health outcomes. For example, the number of words a child has by age 3 directly correlates with their ability to read by grade 3, which directly correlates with their likelihood of graduating from high school. Positive early childhood environments are directly linked to improved educational outcomes, increased earning potential, and reduced crime rates.

In contrast, children born into stressful environments—such as the experience of poverty, racism, or family or neighborhood violence—are more likely to have negative health outcomes. The brain changes in these situations may influence the stress response activation level of a child and impact lifelong responses to adversity. Poverty is a particularly relevant early childhood stressor given the fact that the United States has more children living in poverty than any of our peer developed countries. High stress and lack of academic preparedness in early childhood reduce the foundation children have when they enter kindergarten and increase the likelihood of poor school performance. This in turn increases the likelihood of criminal behavior, lack of preparedness for work or college, and ongoing cycles of poverty.

Young children need stimulating learning opportunities and positive relationships with adults. High-quality early care and education programs can provide these for children, yet such programs are limited. The "Strong Start for America's Children Act," introduced in Congress in November 2013, is a bipartisan proposal to support expansion of early childhood education from birth to age 5. This federal–state partnership will support the 39 states and District of Columbia that already provide state-funded pre-kindergarten programs and expand coverage to all states. The act has wide support from a broad cross-section of the country, including the military (because young adults will be better prepared to serve), law enforcement (because it may reduce crime), and business leaders (because workers will be better qualified). After all, who can argue with providing infants with quality, safe, and stimulating environments?

connect
ACTIVITY

Sources: *Early Experiences Can Alter Gene Expression and Affect Long-Term Development: Working Paper No.10*, National Scientific Council on the Developing Child, 2010, www.developing child.net; Lawmakers Introduce Bipartisan Legislation to Improve Early Education for America's Children, 2013 http://democrats.edworkforce.house.gov/press-release/lawmakers-introduce-bipartisan-legislation-improve-early-education-america%E2%80%99s-children; *U.S. Health in International Perspective: Shorter Lives, Poorer Health*, by S. H. Woolf and L. Aron, 2013, Washington, DC: National Academies Press.

learn how to care for their newborn (or **neonate**) and the newborn takes his or her place in the family. Early childhood development is critical to long-term health opportunities (see the box, "The Importance of Early Childhood Education"). A few issues that deserve attention are growth and nutrition, illness and vaccinations, and attachment.

Growth and Nutrition Babies have very high calorie requirements. One reason is their rapid rate of growth—they triple their birth weight by their first birthday—and another reason is the great relative mass of the infant's organs, especially the brain and liver, compared with muscle. Organs have much higher metabolic and energy requirements than muscle does.

Most medical organizations agree that breastfeeding is the best way to feed babies. Breast milk is perfectly suited to babies' nutritional needs and digestion; it also contains antibodies that reduce the risk of infections, allergies, asthma, and SIDS. For mothers, breastfeeding enhances bonding with the baby, contributes to weight loss after pregnancy, and may decrease the risk of ovarian cancer and breast cancer after menopause.

Breastfeeding can be more convenient and less expensive than bottle-feeding. New mothers who have difficulty with breastfeeding can get advice and support from a lactation consultant, their health care provider, or support groups like LaLeche League. When a woman is breastfeeding, she may not get her menstrual period for up to six months after giving birth; however, ovulation can still occur, so breastfeeding is not a reliable form of birth control.

neonate
Newborn.

Because of illness, breast infection, or other reasons, about 10 percent of women are unable to breastfeed, and they bottle-feed their infants instead. Bottle-feeding provides adequate nutrition and enables parents to know how much food the baby is consuming.

Illness and Vaccinations Childbirth and the neonatal period are times of increased risk of infection for an infant. Starting at 2 months, children receive vaccinations against several childhood diseases that, in the past, caused serious illness and death. They include diphtheria, pertussis (whooping cough), tetanus, measles, rubella (German measles), mumps, and polio, among others. The vaccinations are inexpensive and safe, especially when compared with the physical, emotional, and social costs of childhood diseases. Most states require that children be vaccinated before they are allowed to start public school.

Adjustment and Attachment Although babies are tiny, they quickly become the center of attention in the household. They spend their time in recurring states of crying, alertness, drowsiness, and sleep. Parents spend much of their time feeding their newborn (at first, every two hours or so), changing diapers, and trying to soothe the crying infant. The strong emotional bond between parents and infant known as **attachment** develops during this period, and the infant begins to have feelings of trust and confidence as a result of a comforting, satisfying relationship with parental figures. This sense of trust is crucial for future interpersonal relationships and social and emotional development. Thus a healthy infancy lays the foundation for a healthy life.

attachment
Deep emotional bond that develops between an infant and its primary caregivers.

About 13 percent of women experience depression in the first year after giving birth, referred to as *postpartum depression.* Rapid hormone changes after delivery, broken sleep patterns, self-doubt about one's ability to provide for an infant, a sense of loss of control, and changes in one's support system can all contribute to feelings of sadness, restlessness, loss of interest, guilt, difficulty focusing, and withdrawal. Postpartum depression can have significant effects on a woman's relationships with her partner and baby. Effective treatments exist for depression, and women and their partners should be aware of the signs and symptoms of the condition.

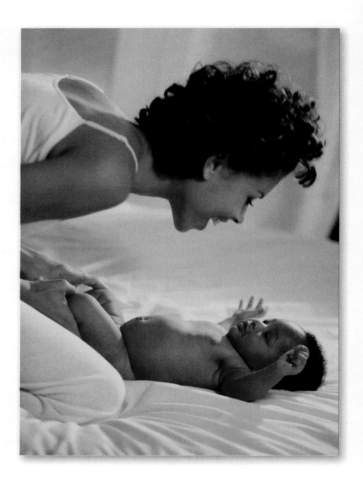

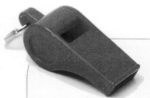

You Make the Call

Should the U.S. Provide Paid Family Leave After the Birth of a Child?

What do the United States, Swaziland, Liberia, and Papua New Guinea have in common? They are the only four countries in the world to not offer some form of paid parental leave. The United States is the only industrialized country in the world to not have paid parental leave. In 1993, the Family Medical Leave Act was signed into law and allowed U.S. workers to take up to three months of paid or unpaid leave when seriously ill or to care for a baby or a sick relative. The assumption at that time was that employers would make the choice to provide paid family leave but, in reality, only 9 percent of U.S. companies provide any paid leave for childbirth (or adoption of an infant). The employees who have access to paid leave tend to be higher-income earners while those who have no paid leave are employees with lower incomes and are the least likely to be able to afford to take time off work. In 2013, Senator Kirsten Gillibrand and Representative Rosa DeLauro introduced the Family and Medical Insurance Leave Act (also referred to as the FAMILY Act), which proposes an insurance plan to provide paid family and sick leave to all employees.

What do other countries offer? It ranges from 12 weeks of paid leave in Pakistan, South Africa, and Mexico to 44 weeks of paid leave in the United Kingdom, Italy, and Norway. Our closest neighbor to the north, Canada, offers the highest level: 50 weeks of paid family leave.

Advocates give a number of reasons for paid leave. From a business perspective, paid leave makes sense financially because it acknowledges the reality that workers will have children and sick family members. Planning for paid leaves will help workers make smoother transitions to the new role of parent (or caregiver for a sick family member), and they will be more prepared to return to work smoothly. They will feel more valued as a worker and in turn have more loyalty and work harder. This will reduce employee turnover and the resulting loss in production.

There are also health arguments for paid time off. Women who feel a financial strain because they have no paid time off from work are more likely to return to work within 12 weeks of delivery.

Continued...

Concluded...

However, women who return to work 13 weeks or later after the birth of a child are more likely to breastfeed and bond more closely with their infant. Breastfeeding improves the newborn's immunity and helps the mother lose pregnancy-related weight. Paid leave decreases financial stress and supports parent–infant relationships that promote positive early childhood development.

Another argument is that paid leave is a justice issue for women. Women are 47 percent of the work force, and 40 percent of households with children under the age of 18 are headed by a mother who is the primary breadwinner, so women need paid leave to care for newborn or sick children. Women should not have to choose between providing financially for their family and taking time to be with a new child or sick family member.

Opponents argue that time off work will be disruptive to the workforce and place undue financial burden on employers. Employee leave reduces production levels, and hiring temporary workers to replace workers on leave increases expenses. In addition, some argue that requiring companies to pay for maternity leave would discriminate against women of childbearing age—making it more difficult for women to find work.

What do you think? Is it time for a change?

Pros

- It makes business sense to plan for and support employees taking time off for their family.
- Paid leave benefits parent–child bonding and children's health.
- It is unjust to ask parents to choose between financial stability and caring for a newborn or sick family member.

Cons

- This is a burden placed on employers that will reduce the ability of companies to compete on a global scale.
- Providing paid time off will encourage employees to take longer leaves, which will be more disruptive to the workforce.
- Worksites will discriminate more against women if they are required to contribute to family leave.

Sources: "3 Reasons Why Card-Carrying Capitalists Should Support Paid Family Leave," May 23, 2012, *Forbes,* www.forbes.com/sites/work-in-progress/2012/05/23/3-reasons-why-card-carrying-capitalists-should-support-paid-family-leave/3/; "Why America Needs Sen. Gillibrand and Rep. DeLauro's Family Act," December 13, 2013, Insurancenewsnet, http://insurancenews -net.com/oarticle/2013/12/13/why-america-needs-sen-gillibrand-and-rep-delauros-family-act-a-436448.html#.UrCedv6A19M; "The Family and Medical Leave Act at 20: Still Necessary, Still Not Enough," February 5, 2013, *The Atlantic,* www.theatlantic.com/sexes/archive/2013/02/ the-family-and-medical-leave-act-at-20-still-necessary-still-not-enough/272605/.

In Review

What are the commonly available contraceptive methods?
The most reliable method is abstinence. The next most reliable method of reversible contraception is long-acting contraception with an IUD or implant. Other methods include hormonal methods (birth control pills, the transdermal patch, the contraceptive ring, the injectable contraceptive, and the contraceptive implant), barrier methods (male and female condoms, the diaphragm, the cervical cap, and the contraceptive sponge), fertility awareness–based methods, emergency contraception, and male and female sterilization. Methods vary in their effectiveness, cost, convenience, permanence, safety, protection against STIs, and consistency with personal values.

What are the options in the event of unintended pregnancy?
The three options are having and keeping the baby, placing the baby for adoption, and having an abortion. The vast majority of elective abortions, nearly 90 percent, are performed during the first 12 weeks of pregnancy. Abortions can be performed surgically or medically (with drugs).

What are the options when a couple cannot conceive?
Treatments are increasingly available for infertility and include surgery, fertility drugs, intrauterine fertilization, in vitro fertilization, and other advanced technologies.

What are the basics of prenatal care?
Prepregnancy care can include genetic counseling and vaccinations against common infectious diseases, especially rubella and hepatitis B. Once a woman is pregnant, prenatal care includes good nutrition and exercise, avoidance of substances that could harm the fetus, and regularly scheduled health care visits. Problems in the fetus can be diagnosed prenatally by advanced technologies.

What happens during prenatal development?
The fertilized egg (zygote) implants in the uterine wall and begins a period of rapid growth and differentiation. During the first trimester, all the body systems form and start functioning (e.g., the heart starts beating), the limbs are molded, and the sex of the fetus can be recognized. During the second trimester, the fetus continues to develop, and the proportion of the body to head becomes more balanced. The third trimester is a period of rapid weight gain. At birth, the typical baby weighs about 7½ pounds and is about 20 inches long.

What happens during labor and delivery?
During the first stage of labor, strong uterine contractions cause the cervix to shorten and open and push the baby down into the mother's pelvis. During the second stage of labor, the baby moves into the birth canal and emerges from the mother's body, usually head first. During the third stage of labor, the placenta is delivered.

What concerns arise during the postpartum period?
Breastfeeding is considered the best way to feed a baby, but bottle-feeding is an acceptable alternative. Newborns are especially vulnerable to infections; they start receiving routine vaccinations at about 2 months. The newborn period is one of profound adjustment for all family members.

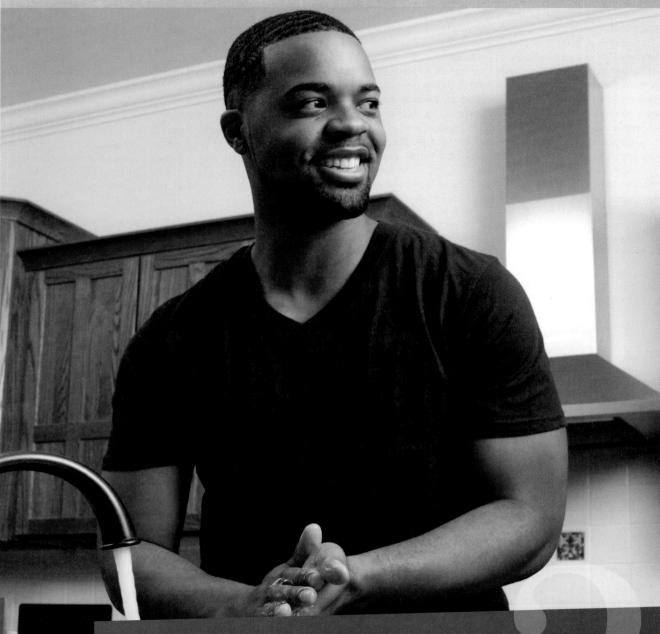

13 Infectious Diseases

Ever Wonder...

- if you are up to date on your vaccines?
- how antimicrobial resistance might affect you?
- which STIs can be cured and which can't?

Prior to 1900, infectious diseases were the leading cause of death in the United States, with 30 percent of all deaths occurring among young children. Public health measures, including vaccinations, and antibiotics are responsible for the reduction in the death rate from infectious diseases in the United States to about 2 percent by the end of the 20th century. Perhaps the greatest reductions in infectious diseases have come from improved sanitation and hygiene practices, especially clean water supplies. In recent years, however, death rates from infectious diseases have started to creep up again, as a result of newer diseases such as AIDS, the reemergence of existing diseases once thought vanquished, and new challenges such as drug resistance. This chapter provides an overview of infectious diseases, including sexually transmitted infections (STIs), and offers guidelines for protecting yourself from infections.

THE PROCESS OF INFECTION

Microorganisms, the tiniest living organisms on earth, do what all living organisms do: eat, reproduce, and die. An **infection** occurs when part of a microorganism's life cycle involves you. An infection is considered an illness or disease if it interferes with your usual lifestyle or shortens your life.

The process of infection often follows a typical course, with the length of each stage depending on the pathogen (Figure 13.1). Infections can also result in different outcomes. Some infections cause a sudden illness with a high risk of death, such as infection with the Ebola virus. Some stimulate your body's immune response, causing the death of the microorganism, as occurs with the common cold virus. Still others may persist without signs of illness for years and yet be passed on to other people, as is the case with the human immunodeficiency virus (HIV). Finally, some infections are dormant or walled off by the immune system, as in the case of tuberculosis, and held at bay in a latent phase for as long as the immune system is healthy.

Latent infections may activate at a later point. Other infections are incompletely cleared by the body and continue at a low level indefinitely.

The Chain of Infection

The **chain of infection** is the process by which an infectious agent, or **pathogen**, passes from one organism to another. Pathogens often live in large communities, called *reservoirs,* in soil or water or within organisms. Many pathogens cannot survive in the environment and require a living *host.* To cause infection, pathogens must have a *portal of exit* from the reservoir or host and a *portal of entry* into a new host (Figure 13.2).

A pathogen can exit a host in respiratory secretions (coughing, sneezing); via feces, genital secretions, blood or blood products, or skin; or through an insect or animal bite. The pathogen enters the new host in similar ways: through skin-to-skin contact, genital-to-genital contact, inhalation of respiratory droplets, exposure to blood products, or insect or animal bites. If the transfer from host to host or from reservoir to host is carried out by an insect or animal, that organism is called a **vector**.

Altering or breaking the chain of infection at any point can increase or decrease the risk of infection. For example, urban development that encroaches on deer populations increases the chance of humans contracting tick-borne disease; raising chickens close to the house can increase risk of novel influenza viruses; and contracting genital herpes affects the portal of exit or the portal of entry for HIV, increasing the risk of HIV transmission.

infection
Disease or condition caused by a microorganism.

chain of infection
Process by which an infectious agent passes from one organism to another.

pathogen
Infectious agent capable of causing disease.

vector
Animal or insect that transmits a pathogen from a reservoir or an infected host to a new host.

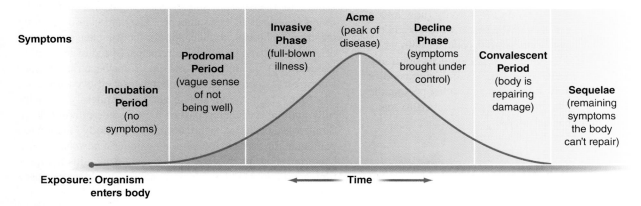

Symptoms

Incubation Period (no symptoms)

Prodromal Period (vague sense of not being well)

Invasive Phase (full-blown illness)

Acme (peak of disease)

Decline Phase (symptoms brought under control)

Convalescent Period (body is repairing damage)

Sequelae (remaining symptoms the body can't repair)

Exposure: Organism enters body

Time

figure 13.1   Stages of infection.
At the peak of the disease, either the immune system gains control, medical treatment occurs, or death ensues.

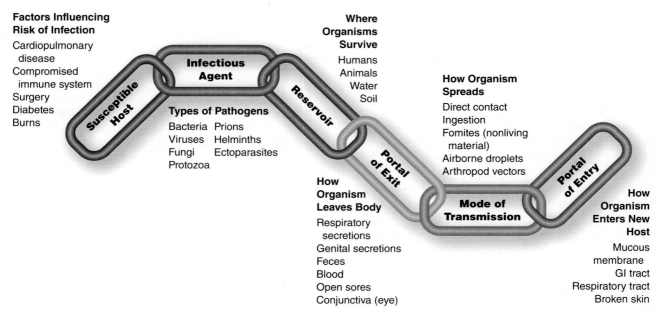

figure 13.2   The chain of infection.
Breaking the chain at any point decreases the risk of infection.

virulence
Speed and intensity with which a pathogen is likely to cause an infection.

epidemic
Widespread outbreak of a disease that affects many people.

normal flora
Bacteria that live in or on a host at a particular location without causing harm and sometimes benefiting the host.

Meanwhile, chlorinating drinking water reduces the number of pathogens and the size of reservoirs for waterborne infections; using condoms disrupts both the portal of exit and the portal of entry for infectious agents that may be present in semen or vaginal secretions; and controlling mosquito populations eradicates vectors and disrupts a pathogen's mode of transmission.

The extent or spread of an infection depends on several factors, including the **virulence** (speed and intensity) of the pathogen, the mode of transmission (how an infection spreads from person to person), the ease of transmission, the duration of infectivity (how long a person with infection can spread it to other people), and the number of people an infected person has contact with while he or she is infectious. If an infected person does not transmit the infection to anyone else, that person's disease dies out. If the person transmits it to at least one other person, the infection continues. If the infection is transmitted to many people, an **epidemic** may occur.

Pathogens

Millions of different pathogens cause human infections, but they fall into several broad categories (Figure 13.3).

Viruses Viruses are some of the smallest pathogens. They are also among the most numerous; it is estimated that there are more different types of viruses than all other living organisms combined.

Viruses consist of a genome (a genetic package of either DNA or RNA), a capsid (protein coat), and in some cases an outer covering or envelope. They are unable to reproduce on their own; they can replicate only inside another organism's cells. Viruses do not survive long outside of humans or other hosts. A virus infects a host cell by binding to its receptors and injecting its genetic material into the cell. Once inside, the virus can have a number of different effects. It can make many copies of itself, burst the cell, and release the copies to infect more cells. It can persist within the cell, slowly continuing to cause damage or becoming inactive and reactivating at a later time. Some viruses integrate themselves into a cell's DNA and alter the growth pattern of the cells. This process can lead to the development of a tumor or cancer.[1]

Bacteria Bacteria are single-celled organisms that can be found in almost all environments. They are classified based on shape (spherical, rodlike, spiral), the presence or absence of a cell wall, and growth requirements. Speed of replication varies from 20 minutes to two weeks. Some bacteria can enter a dormant or spore state in which they can survive for years.

Many bacteria inhabit a person harmlessly or helpfully and are considered part of the person's **normal flora**. Sometimes, bacteria that are normal in one body location are pathogens in another location, as when *Escherichia coli,* a bacterium that inhabits the large intestine and aids in digestion, enters the bladder, where it causes a bladder or urinary tract infection.

Prions Prions, the least understood infectious agents, are known to be responsible for the neurodegenerative disease

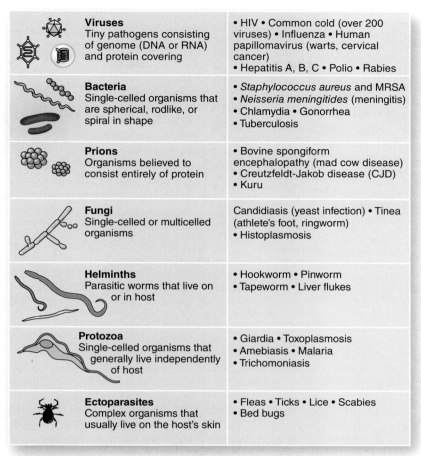

Viruses Tiny pathogens consisting of genome (DNA or RNA) and protein covering	• HIV • Common cold (over 200 viruses) • Influenza • Human papillomavirus (warts, cervical cancer) • Hepatitis A, B, C • Polio • Rabies
Bacteria Single-celled organisms that are spherical, rodlike, or spiral in shape	• *Staphylococcus aureus* and MRSA • *Neisseria meningitides* (meningitis) • Chlamydia • Gonorrhea • Tuberculosis
Prions Organisms believed to consist entirely of protein	• Bovine spongiform encephalopathy (mad cow disease) • Creutzfeldt-Jakob disease (CJD) • Kuru
Fungi Single-celled or multicelled organisms	Candidiasis (yeast infection) • Tinea (athlete's foot, ringworm) • Histoplasmosis
Helminths Parasitic worms that live on or in host	• Hookworm • Pinworm • Tapeworm • Liver flukes
Protozoa Single-celled organisms that generally live independently of host	• Giardia • Toxoplasmosis • Amebiasis • Malaria • Trichomoniasis
Ectoparasites Complex organisms that usually live on the host's skin	• Fleas • Ticks • Lice • Scabies • Bed bugs

figure 13.3 **Main types of pathogens.**

bovine spongiform encephalopathy (BSE), or mad cow disease. The term *prion* was coined as a shortened form of *proteinaceous infectious particle.* Prions are believed to be made entirely of protein. They are found in brain tissue and appear to alter the function or shape of other proteins when they infect a cell, initiating a degeneration of brain function. Prions appear to spread by the ingestion of infected brain or nerve tissue.[1]

Fungi A fungus is a single-celled or multicelled organism. Several kinds of fungi, including yeasts and molds, cause infection in human beings. Fungi reproduce by budding or by making spores; many fungal infections result from exposure to spores in the environment, such as in the soil or on tile floors. Fungal infections rarely spread from person to person.

Dermatophytes are a group of fungi that commonly infect the skin, hair, or nails. They are sometimes called "ringworm" or "tinea" infections. There are many different species that can infect humans, and they are usually described by the location they infect rather than the specific species, such as athlete's foot, nail fungus, or jock itch. Another type of fungus, the yeast *Candida,* may be part of a person's normal flora but can overgrow and cause an infection in the vagina (vaginal candidiasis), the mouth (thrush), or throughout the body (systemic candidiasis). All of the fungi can become serious infections in a person with a compromised immune system (e.g., someone with HIV infection or AIDS, someone undergoing chemotherapy for cancer, or someone taking immunosuppressant drugs following an organ transplant).[1]

Helminths Helminths, protozoa, and ectoparasites are broadly grouped in the category *parasites*—organisms that live on or in a host and get food at the expense of the host. Helminths, or parasitic worms, include roundworms, flukes, and tapeworms. They are large compared with other infectious agents, ranging in length from 0.4 inch to greater than 30 feet. People usually become infected with parasites by accidentally ingesting worm eggs in food or water or by having the skin invaded by worm larvae. Worldwide, especially in developing countries, parasitic worms cause a huge disease burden. For example, hookworm, which attaches to the human intestine and causes blood loss, can lead to anemia and malnutrition, particularly in children.[1, 2]

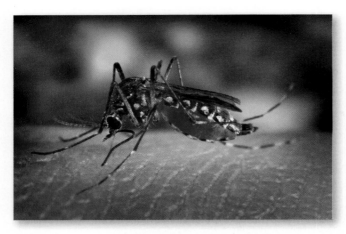

■ Skin is an excellent physical barrier, but the female mosquito is able to penetrate it with her proboscis. Mosquitoes serve as vectors for several diseases caused by bloodborne pathogens, including encephalitis, West Nile virus, and malaria.

immune system
Complex set of cells, chemicals, and processes that protects the body against pathogens when they succeed in entering the body.

innate immune system
Part of the immune system designed to rapidly dispose of pathogens in a nonspecific manner.

acquired immune system
Part of the immune system that recognizes specific targets.

acute inflammatory response
Series of cellular changes that bring blood to the site of an injury or infection.

Protozoa Protozoa are single-celled organisms; most can live independently of host organisms. Protozoal infections are a leading cause of disease and death in Africa, Asia, and Central and South America. They may be transmitted by contaminated water, feces, or food, as is the case in giardia, toxoplasmosis, and amebiasis; by air, as is the case in *Pneumocystis carinii* pneumonia; by sexual contact, as is the case in trichomoniasis; or by a vector, such as the mosquito in the case of malaria.[1,2]

Ectoparasites Ectoparasites are complex organisms that usually live on or in the skin, where they feed on the host's tissue or blood. They cause local irritation and are frequently vectors for serious infectious diseases. Examples are fleas, ticks, lice, mosquitoes, bed bugs, and scabies.[1,2]

THE BODY'S DEFENSES

A single square inch of skin on your arm is home to thousands of bacteria. A sneeze projects hundreds of thousands of viral particles into the air. Bacteria can double in number every 20 minutes, and a virus can replicate thousands of times within a single human cell. Although you are substantially larger than microorganisms, you feel the power of their numbers each time you catch a cold. Considering these facts, our ability to overcome invasion and survive infectious diseases is remarkable.

External Barriers

The skin is the first line of defense against infection. Most organisms cannot get through skin unless it is damaged, such as by a cut, burn, or infection, or if passage is aided by an insect bite or needle stick. Most portals of entry into the body, such as the mouth, lungs, nasal passages, and vagina, are lined with mucous membranes. Although these linings are delicate, mucus traps many organisms and prevents them from entering the body. Nasal passages and ear canals have hair that helps trap particles. The lungs are protected by the cough reflex and by cilia, tiny hairlike structures that rhythmically push foreign particles up and out. Damage to these physical barriers increases risk of infection.

If pathogens get past these barriers, they often encounter chemical defenses. Saliva contains special proteins that break down bacteria, and stomach acids make it difficult for most organisms to survive. The small intestine contains bile and enzymes that break down pathogens. The vagina normally has a slightly acidic environment, which favors the growth of normal flora and discourages the growth of other bacteria. The body protects pores and hair follicles in the skin by excreting fatty acids and lysozyme, an enzyme that breaks down bacteria and reduces the likelihood of infection. The physical and chemical barriers to infection are illustrated in Figure 13.4.

The Immune System

The **immune system** is a complex set of cells, chemicals, and processes that protects the body against pathogens when they succeed in entering the body. It has two subdivisions: the **innate immune system**, a rapid response designed to catch and dispose of foreign particles or pathogens in a nonspecific manner, and the **acquired immune system**, a highly specialized response that recognizes specific targets.

The Innate Immune System The body's initial reaction to tissue damage, whether it is due to trauma or infection, is an **acute inflammatory response**, a series of changes that increase the flow of blood to the site. A complicated series of molecular and cellular events occurs when the innate immune system is activated. Signs of the inflammatory response are redness, warmth, pain, and swelling.

The cells of the innate immune system are neutrophils, macrophages, and natural killer cells. Neutrophils and macrophages are white blood cells that travel in the bloodstream to areas of infection or tissue damage. These phagocytes ("cell eaters") digest damaged cells, foreign particles, and bacteria. Natural killer cells are white blood cells that recognize and destroy virus-infected cells or cells that have become cancerous.

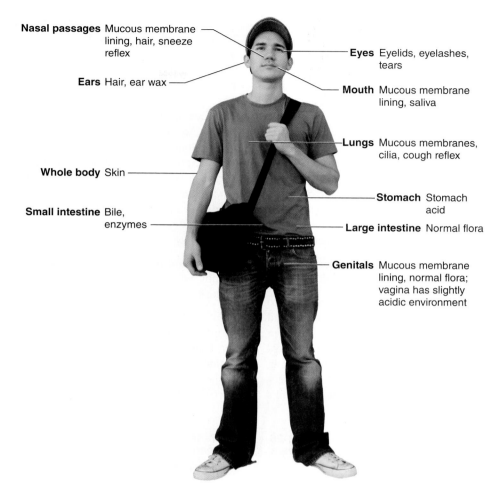

Nasal passages Mucous membrane lining, hair, sneeze reflex

Ears Hair, ear wax

Whole body Skin

Small intestine Bile, enzymes

Eyes Eyelids, eyelashes, tears

Mouth Mucous membrane lining, saliva

Lungs Mucous membranes, cilia, cough reflex

Stomach Stomach acid

Large intestine Normal flora

Genitals Mucous membrane lining, normal flora; vagina has slightly acidic environment

figure 13.4 **Physical and chemical barriers to infection.**

The Acquired Immune System Your acquired (or adaptive) immunity develops as you are exposed to potential infections and vaccinations. Each time the cells of the acquired immune system are exposed to a pathogen, they form a kind of memory of it and can mount a response the next time they encounter it.

The important white blood cells of the acquired immune system are **lymphocytes**, which circulate in the bloodstream and lymphatic system. If the lymphocytes encounter an **antigen** (a marker on the surface of a substance that is foreign to the body), they rapidly duplicate and "turn on" their specific function. The two main types of lymphocytes are *T cells* and *B cells*.

T cells monitor events that may be occurring inside cells. If a cell is infected, alterations to molecules on its surface indicate it is now "nonself." *Helper T cells* "read" this message and trigger the production of killer T cells and B cells; helper T cells also enhance the activity of the cells of the innate immune system and of B cells once they are activated. *Killer T cells* attack and kill foreign cells and body cells that have been infected by a virus or have become cancerous. *Suppressor T cells* slow down and halt the immune response when the threat has been handled.

B cells monitor the blood and tissue fluids. When they encounter a specific antigen, they mature to become cells that produce **antibodies**—proteins that circulate in the blood and bind to specific antigens, triggering events that destroy them.

Immunity Once you have survived infection by a pathogen, you often acquire **immunity** to future infection by the same pathogen. The reason is that some B and T cells become *memory cells* when exposed to an infectious agent; if they encounter the same antigen in the future, they can respond rapidly, destroying the invader before it can cause illness. Immunization is based on

lymphocytes
White blood cells that circulate in the bloodstream and lymphatic system.

antigen
Marker on the surface of a substance foreign to the body that identifies the substance to immune cells as "nonself."

antibodies
Proteins that bind to specific antigens and trigger events that destroy them.

immunity
Reduced susceptibility to a disease based on the ability of the immune system to remember, recognize, and mount a rapid defense against a pathogen it has previously encountered.

vaccines
Preparations of weakened or killed microorganisms or parts of microorganisms that are administered to confer immunity to various diseases.

this principle: The immune system is exposed to enough of an infectious agent to trigger an immune response. On subsequent exposures, the immune system mounts a rapid response, preventing disease.

The concept of immunization was first introduced in 1796 by English physician Edward Jenner. Jenner realized that people who had been infected with cowpox (a disease that causes mild illness in humans) seldom became ill or died when exposed to smallpox (a related but often fatal disease). Jenner's observation led to the development of **vaccines**, preparations of weakened or killed microorganisms or parts of microorganisms that are administered to confer immunity to various diseases. Since 1900, vaccines have been developed for many infectious diseases, and significant reductions in death rates from these diseases have occurred (Figure 13.5).[3,4]

Vaccination serves two functions. The first is to protect an individual by stimulating an immune response. The second is to protect society. Widespread vaccination shrinks the reservoir of infectious agents, protecting the community through "herd" immunity. In other words, if someone with a disease enters a community where most people are vaccinated against the disease, it cannot spread because few people are susceptible. The widespread use of the smallpox vaccine, for example, led to the elimination of naturally occurring smallpox worldwide. All future generations benefit from the earlier smallpox vaccination campaigns and no longer require vaccination themselves. Deaths from vaccine-preventable diseases are at an all-time low, but high vaccination levels are necessary to maintain this effect.[4] If vaccination levels drop, these diseases will spread more easily because there will be more susceptible people.

Risk Factors for Infection

Your risk for infections depends on numerous factors, some within your control and others beyond your individual control.

Controllable Risk Factors You can reduce your risk of infection by adopting behaviors that support and improve the health of your immune system. One such behavior is eating a balanced diet; poor nutrition is associated with a higher risk of infectious disease. Other behaviors that support a healthy immune system are exercising, getting enough

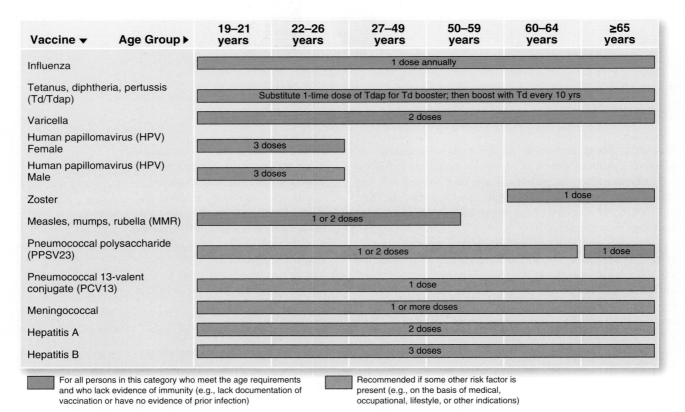

Vaccine ▼ Age Group ▶	19–21 years	22–26 years	27–49 years	50–59 years	60–64 years	≥65 years
Influenza	1 dose annually					
Tetanus, diphtheria, pertussis (Td/Tdap)	Substitute 1-time dose of Tdap for Td booster; then boost with Td every 10 yrs					
Varicella	2 doses					
Human papillomavirus (HPV) Female	3 doses					
Human papillomavirus (HPV) Male	3 doses					
Zoster					1 dose	
Measles, mumps, rubella (MMR)	1 or 2 doses					
Pneumococcal polysaccharide (PPSV23)	1 or 2 doses					1 dose
Pneumococcal 13-valent conjugate (PCV13)	1 dose					
Meningococcal	1 or more doses					
Hepatitis A	2 doses					
Hepatitis B	3 doses					

▨	For all persons in this category who meet the age requirements and who lack evidence of immunity (e.g., lack documentation of vaccination or have no evidence of prior infection)	▨	Recommended if some other risk factor is present (e.g., on the basis of medical, occupational, lifestyle, or other indications)

figure 13.5   Recommended adult immunizations.
Additional information about specific recommendations and vaccines can be found at www.cdc.gov/vaccines.
Source: "Recommended Adult Immunization Schedule—United States, 2013," Centers for Disease Control and Prevention, 2013, *Mortality and Morbidity Weekly Report, 62* (1).

Action Skill-Builder

How to Keep Your Hands Clean

Your hands go everywhere. They touch the public bathroom doorknob; they rummage through your backpack as it sits on the classroom floor; they grasp the sweaty handles of the elliptical at the gym; they touch the screen of your smartphone to answer a call; and they convey your worn five-dollar-bill to the cashier at the cafeteria. Then they grip your sandwich or the spoon you use to eat your lunch. Because our hands are there no matter how dirty the job, it's no surprise that hand-washing is one of the first lessons we learned as children. It is an easy and effective way to protect yourself and others from germs. Here are some steps to help you brush up on this time-honored tradition:

☐ Use warm water and enough soap to produce a bubbly lather. Any type of soap will do. Soaps containing antibiotics are not necessary and not recommended.

☐ Scrub the backs and fronts of your hands with the lather, from your fingertips all the way up to your wrists. Don't forget to scrub between your fingers and under your nails.

☐ Wash for a minimum of 20 seconds to ensure that even the toughest microorganisms get scrubbed off your skin.

☐ Rinse the soap from your hands with warm water, starting with the wrists. Point your fingers down so the dirty soap and water go directly into the sink rather than dribbling up your forearms.

☐ Dry your hands with a clean towel or allow them to air dry.

☐ Do not touch the faucet, the area around the sink, or the bathroom door; doing so will recontaminate your hands. You can use the paper towel to turn off the faucet and open the door.

If your hands are not visibly soiled, or if no soap and water is available, use a hand sanitizer that contains at least 60 percent alcohol. Apply enough sanitizer to cover all surfaces of your hands. Rub hands together until all the moisture is absorbed.

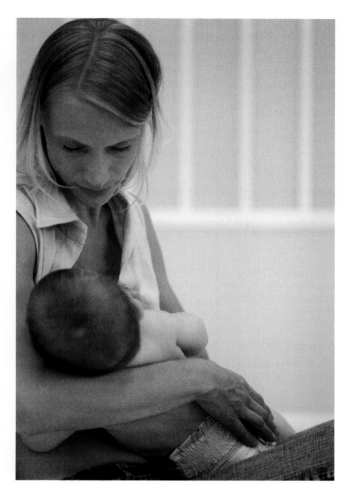

■ Antibodies for some diseases are passed from mothers to babies in breast milk. Breastfeeding has been shown to reduce the incidence of infections, allergies, and diarrhea in infants and even to promote good health later in the child's life.

sleep, and managing stress. Vaccination, when available, can boost your immune system and facilitate a quicker response to pathogens. Good hygiene practices like hand washing reduce the risk of many infections (see the box, "How to Keep Your Hands Clean"), and protecting your skin from damage keeps many pathogens out of your body. Avoiding tobacco and environmental tobacco smoke improves your defenses against respiratory illness.

Uncontrollable Risk Factors Age plays a role in vulnerability to infection, with higher risks at both ends of the lifespan. Newborns and young children are at increased risk because they have not been exposed to many infections;

pregnancy and breastfeeding confer **passive immunity**—a mother's antibodies can pass to the fetus or child to provide temporary immune protection. Older people are at increased risk due to the gradual decline in the immune system that can occur with aging. Other factors that increase vulnerability include undergoing surgery, having a chronic disease such as diabetes or lung disease, and being bedbound.

Genetic predisposition may play a role in susceptibility to infectious disease. It is unclear why certain people develop an overwhelming, life-threatening illness when exposed to a pathogen while others develop only a mild fever. Certain sociocultural factors are associated with higher risk for infectious disease; in many situations, these are not controllable risk factors. Overcrowded living environments (including residence halls, fraternities, and sororities)

passive immunity
Temporary immunity provided by antibodies from an external source—such as passed from mother to child in breast milk.

increase the risk for any infectious disease that is spread from person to person, such as influenza, meningitis, and tuberculosis. Poverty is associated with increased risk for many illnesses, probably owing to poor nutrition, stress, and lack of access to health care, among other factors.

Disruption of Immunity

Because the immune system is so complex, it occasionally malfunctions. Two such disruptions are autoimmune diseases and allergies.

anaphylactic shock
Hypersensitive reaction in which an antigen causes an immediate and severe reaction that can include itching, rash, swelling, shock, and respiratory distress.

Autoimmune Diseases Sometimes, a part of the body is similar enough to an antigen on a foreign agent that the immune system mistakenly identifies it as "nonself." For example, in autoimmune thyroid disease, the immune system makes antibodies against cells in the thyroid, which stimulates overproduction of thyroid hormone. Other times, the immune control system fails to turn off an immune response once an infection is over. In both cases, a process of self-destruction can ensue, causing damage to body cells and tissues. Autoimmune diseases vary in their effects, depending on which part of the body is seen as foreign. Autoimmune diseases include hyperthyroidism, rheumatoid arthritis, psoriasis, multiple sclerosis, scleroderma, and lupus erythematosus. Genetics is known to play a role in some autoimmune diseases.[1] For unknown reasons, most autoimmune diseases are more common in women than in men.

Allergies Allergic reactions occur when the immune system identifies a harmless foreign substance as an infectious agent and mounts a full-blown immune response. Allergic responses to substances like pollen or animal dander, for example, include a runny nose, watery eyes, nasal congestion, and an itchy throat. In extreme cases, the body goes into **anaphylactic shock**, a life-threatening systemic allergic response requiring immediate medical attention.

Asthma, a condition characterized by wheezing and shortness of breath, is caused by inflammation of the bronchial tubes and spasm of

the muscles around the airways in response to an allergen or other trigger. Because viruses can trigger an asthma attack, it's especially important for people with asthma to get flu shots annually. Asthma is covered in greater detail in Chapter 14.

Immunity and Stress As described in Chapter 2, stress can weaken the immune system. College students report high levels of stress as they juggle competing demands, and they frequently have more colds and other infections than they did in high school. Short-term stress, such as a single exam, can actually enhance the immune system's functioning by activating the body's responses. However, stress that lasts for more than a few days or for months, such as a difficult housing situation, a heavy course load, financial concerns, disruption of sleep, or final exams, suppresses the immune system's functioning and can increase risk for infections in the short term and chronic conditions in the long term.[5, 6]

CHANGING PATTERNS IN INFECTIOUS DISEASE

In 1969, the surgeon general of the United States declared before Congress that it was time to close the book on infectious diseases. Dramatic declines in the death rate from infectious diseases during the 20th century (Figure 13.6) inspired this bold statement. Within a little more than 10 years, however, the first cases of what would soon be identified as human immunodeficiency virus (HIV) infection were causing perplexity and alarm in hospitals in several U.S. cities. Since then, the appearance of other new infections, changes in patterns of infection, and the development of antibiotic resistance in many strains of bacteria have demonstrated that infectious diseases remain an important health concern.

Food-Related Pathogen Transmission

Have you or your friends become locavores? *Locavores* are people who attempt to eat only foods that have been grown, processed, and produced locally, generally within 100 miles of their home.[7] This movement has developed in response to the fact that most of the foods we eat travel a thousand miles or more before reaching our table. Foods are grown in one part of the country (or in a foreign country), shipped to a central processing plant, packaged, and then distributed to locations from coast to coast. This widespread distribution of food lowers some costs and makes

■ The incidence of asthma has increased dramatically in recent years, particularly among ethnic minorities, low-income populations, and children living in inner cities.

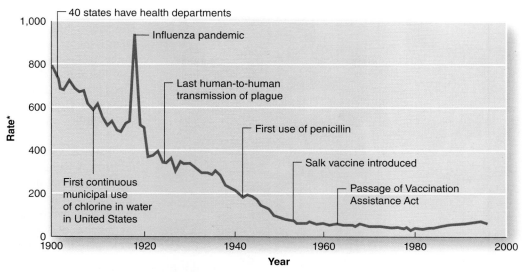

figure 13.6 **Death rate from infectious diseases, United States, 20th century.**
Sources: Adapted from "Achievements in Public Health, 1990–1999: Control of Infectious Disease" (MMWR serial online), 1999, *Morbidity and Mortality Weekly Report, 48* (29), p. 621, www.edc.gov/mmwr; "Trends in Infectious Disease Mortality in the United States During the 20th Century," by G. L. Armstrong, L. A. Conn, and R. W. Pinner, 1999, *Journal of the American Medical Association, 281,* pp. 61–66; "Water Chlorination Principles and Practices: AWWA Manual M20," American Water Works Association, 1973, Denver, CO: AWWA.

production more convenient, but it may decrease nutrient value, increase environmental impact, and increase the risk that contaminated food will cause infectious disease in large numbers of people.

More than 250 organisms are associated with food-related illnesses. They include viruses, bacteria, prions, and parasites. A national network of public health officials monitors reported cases of foodborne illness in the United States and investigates unusual increases in cases involving particular strains of pathogens. For example, in October 2013, an outbreak of salmonella poisoning with 416 cases in 23 states and Puerto Rico was traced to chicken from a factory in California.[8] For guidelines on food safety, see the tips provided in Chapter 5.

Behavior-Related Pathogen Transmission

Disease transmission has also been affected by changes in behavior, including travel, climate change, sexual behavior, and illicit drug use.

Travel and Infectious Diseases Before the advent of modern transportation systems—for example, when it took weeks to cross the ocean on a ship—a passenger who became sick en route could be quarantined (separated from others to prevent transmission of disease). Nowadays, you can travel immense distances in hours, potentially carrying incubating pathogens with you. University students and staff are particularly vulnerable to disease transmission because higher education is an international endeavor, with

academics traveling to distant parts of the world in pursuit of their interests.

The severe acute respiratory syndrome (SARS) outbreak in 2003 is an excellent example of how travel affects the spread of disease and how public health agencies detect and contain disease outbreaks. In March 2003, the World Health Organization activated a Global Outbreak Alert (a system for monitoring outbreaks) concerning an atypical pneumonia that was believed to have originated in southern China at the end of 2002. By February 2003, it had spread to Hong Kong, Vietnam, Singapore, Germany, and Canada. By the time the disease was contained in July 2003, there had been 8,098 probable cases and 774 deaths in 26 countries.

SARS is caused by a previously unknown coronavirus (the same species of virus that causes the common cold) and is spread directly from person to person by coughing, sneezing, and skin contact. Air travel was identified as a key reason for its rapid spread. With no vaccine or treatment available, isolation and quarantine of potentially infected people was the key to stopping the spread of infection.

During the outbreak, airlines and travelers were alerted to the early symptoms, which can progress fairly rapidly to a severe form of pneumonia. Travelers boarding planes that were departing from cities with SARS cases were screened for symptoms and prevented from traveling if symptomatic. If a traveler became ill in flight, health officials boarded the plane upon arrival to examine and possibly quarantine the individual. Travelers were advised to avoid cities with SARS cases, and many locales suffered financially until the advisory ended. Countries around the world remain on alert for a recurrence.

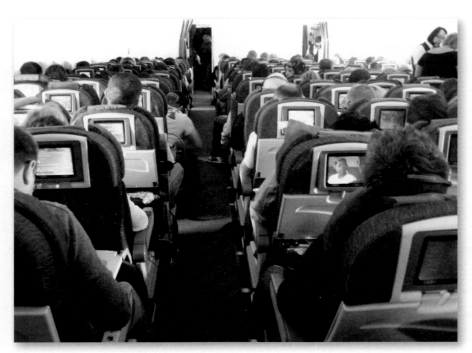

■ By allowing people to travel immense distances in short time periods, air travel facilitates the global spread of infectious disease.

International surveillance and preparedness have significantly improved as a result of this experience.[9] The World Health Organization's Global Alert and Response Network is an international collaboration of institutions and organizations that pool data and resources in order to rapidly identify, confirm, and respond to infectious diseases of international importance. The network's coordinated approach is critical, given the potential for rapid international transmission (see the box, "Are the Issues Raised by Medical Thrillers Realistic?"). The U.S. Center for Disease Control Travel Health website is also an important resource that posts up-to-date travel alerts, recommendations, and warnings.[10]

Climate Change and Infectious Diseases The geographic distribution of diseases is dependent on the environment. With climate change increasing average temperatures and precipitation and bringing more extreme weather events, patterns of infectious disease are likely to change. This is especially true for water- and vector-borne diseases. Increased rainfall and flooding will potentially exacerbate bacterial or parasitic diseases due to runoff from farms or changes in water temperature that make it easier for some pathogens to survive. Severe storms, such as Hurricane Katrina and Hurricane Sandy, are likely to increase and lead to more immediate infectious disease concerns with the breakdown of community infrastructure and sewage treatment. Changes in precipitation and an increase in average temperatures will affect diseases transmitted by ticks and mosquitos, such as Lyme disease, malaria, and West Nile virus, because the number of vectors will increase and the geographic area in which they can survive will increase.[11, 12]

Sexual Behavior and Infectious Diseases Sexual behavior also affects the transmission of disease. Three factors make a difference in how likely it is that a person will be exposed to a sexually transmitted disease (STI): partner variables, personal susceptibility variables, and sex act variables.

Partner variables that increase the risk of being exposed to an STI include the total number of sex partners a person has, how frequently he or she acquires new sex partners, and the number of sexual partners in the same period of time. Certain types of partners are associated with an increased risk of infection; the highest risks are associated with commercial sex workers (people who are paid to have sex) and unknown partners (e.g., a person someone hooks up with at a party or a bar).[13]

Variables associated with increased susceptibility to infection include gender, age at first intercourse, and general health. Women are at greater risk than men due to anatomy (the larger mucosal surface of the vagina and the cervix in comparison to the penis). Young women are at particular risk because the cervix is more susceptible to infection in the first few years after the start of menstruation. Overall health is important because it affects the strength of the immune response and the integrity of the mucosal surfaces. For instance, people who have one sexually transmitted infection may be more likely to contract a second infection, as discussed later in this chapter.

Different types of sexual acts also affect disease transmission. Nonpenetrative sex (fondling, mutual masturbation) has the lowest risk, followed in increasing order of risk by oral sex, penile-vaginal intercourse, and penile-anal intercourse. Other factors can also increase or decrease the risk of transmission. The risk of exposure increases with the number of sexual acts. The amount of lubrication, either natural from foreplay or applied, affects risk because abrasions to the mucosa make it easier for the STI to be transmitted. Forced sex or violent sex increases the risk of abrasions and of STI transmission.

The most effective way to avoid contracting STIs is to abstain from intimate sexual activities until you are ready to be in a mutually monogamous, long-term relationship with an uninfected partner. If you do not abstain between long-term relationships with uninfected partners, limit the number of partners and be sure to use condoms. Correct and consistent condom use can reduce transmission of some—but not all—STIs. And finally, get tested if you are at risk for sexually transmitted infections—most STIs have no symptoms.

Starting the Conversation

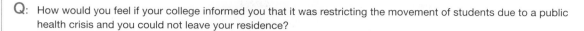

Are the Issues Raised by Medical Thrillers Realistic?

Q: How would you feel if your college informed you that it was restricting the movement of students due to a public health crisis and you could not leave your residence?

In the movie *Contagion,* a woman goes on a business trip to China, where she is infected with a recently mutated and highly contagious virus. She returns to the United States and unknowingly infects others along the way. She dies within days, as do people who came in contact with her in Hong Kong and then traveled to cities around the world. As panic takes hold, the National Guard is called out to restrict travel across state lines, transportation shuts down, and state and national public health departments impose quarantines on cities and towns, allowing no one to enter or leave.

Director Steven Soderbergh received assistance and cooperation from several prominent public health officials and from the CDC in making the movie, which realistically portrays many of the issues that may arise in the event of a pandemic (an epidemic that spreads around the world). One such issue is the possible suspension of certain individual rights that are normally guaranteed by international law, including freedom of association, freedom of assembly, and freedom of movement. In the face of a highly contagious, rapidly spreading, lethal infection for which there is no vaccine and no cure, social distancing and quarantine may be the only measures that can slow the spread of disease.

Another issue is the possible suspension of the rights to privacy and confidential health care. In the movie, the infected woman stops over in Chicago to see an ex-lover, who also becomes infected and dies. In the course of investigating a cluster of cases in Chicago, public health officials question her husband about whom she might have known there, and he becomes aware of her infidelity. Her right to privacy is superseded by the need to share information in the interest of the community.

In real life, notifications may be sent out concerning a category of infectious diseases called "mandatory reportable diseases." These infections are tracked by health departments, and health care providers are required to report them to state and local health departments and sometimes to the CDC. Health care providers also try to locate and notify people who may have been exposed to the infection, even if the patient with the infection is reluctant to notify them. Mandatory reportable diseases include many sexually transmitted diseases, so recent sexual partners of the patient may receive notification from the health department. Although the patient would not be identified by name, it might not be difficult for those receiving notification to figure out his or her identity.

In situations like these, the rights of individuals are protected as much as possible, but the interests of the community often override individual concerns. In this regard, *Contagion* got it just right.

Q: How do you think you would handle isolation if you were suddenly quarantined? Would you be prepared to stay in one place for an extended period of time?

Q: Is it fair, in your opinion, for a health department to notify others without your consent if you may have exposed them to an infectious disease?

Sources: "New Movie Puts Public Health, Infectious Diseases in Spotlight: Behind the Scenes of 'Contagion,'" by K. Krisberg, September 2011, *The Nation's Health, 41,* pp. 1, 10; "Reportable Diseases," by National Institute of Health, www.nlm.nih.gov/medlineplus/ency/article/001929.htm.

Illicit Drug Use: The Case of Hepatitis C When users of illicit drugs share needles and syringes, some blood from the first user is injected into the bloodstream of the next user, creating an effective means of transmitting blood-borne infections. Several viral infections, specifically HIV, hepatitis B, and hepatitis C, are easily transmitted through shared needles. We discuss HIV and hepatitis B later in the chapter; here, we consider hepatitis C.

All hepatitis viruses cause inflammation of the liver, with symptoms such as fatigue, weakness, loss of appetite, and jaundice (a yellow discoloring of the skin and eyes). The hepatitis C virus was discovered in 1989. Before 1990, approximately 10 percent of blood transfusion recipients developed hepatitis, nearly always from hepatitis C. After blood banks started screening for hepatitis C, transfusion-related infection dropped.

Hepatitis C is not a highly infectious virus and requires introduction directly into the bloodstream for transmission. Risk factors include intravenous drug use or sharing of other drug paraphernalia that may have infected blood on it; receipt of blood or blood products prior to 1990; sex with a person infected with hepatitis C (although sexual transmission is rare); or sharing personal items, such as a razor or toothbrush, with a person who has hepatitis C. It also can be transmitted through contaminated tattoo or body piercing equipment.

The incubation period for hepatitis C infection is about four to six weeks, but only about 20 percent of infected people will develop symptoms. The virus causes a chronic, low-level infection in 75 to 85 percent of people, and after about 20 years, one in five infected people will develop liver failure, scarring of the liver (cirrhosis), or liver cancer. Hepatitis C is the leading cause of liver failure requiring liver transplantation. A two-drug regimen can be used to treat hepatitis C infection, but not all patients respond, so decisions are made on an individual basis.[14]

Individuals reduce their risk for hepatitis C by not using injection drugs and by maintaining mutually monogamous sexual relationships with noninfected partners. Those who

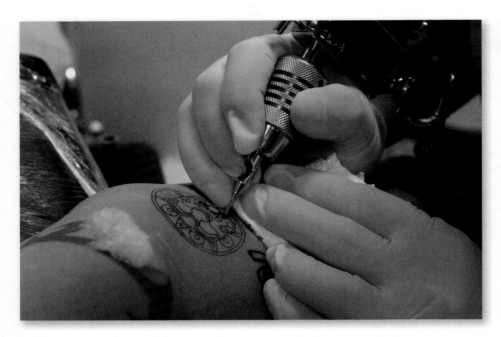

■ Anything that causes a break in the skin carries the potential for infection. Tattooists who don't follow infection control measures like wearing gloves, changing gloves between clients, and disinfecting their equipment can place their clients at risk for diseases like MRSA and hepatitis C.

antibiotic
Drug that works by killing or preventing the growth of bacteria.

antibiotic resistance
Lessened sensitivity to the effects of an antibiotic.

do use drugs should reduce risk by not sharing needles or syringes or, at the very least, cleaning them with bleach after every use. People with hepatitis C can reduce the risk of disease progression by avoiding alcohol, limiting the use of medications that affect the liver (such as acetaminophen), and getting vaccinated for hepatitis A and B. Community programs have helped reduce risk by linking drug users with treatment programs and by encouraging safe injection programs for addicts until they are able to receive treatment. Community programs can also raise awareness about this asymptomatic disease and encourage testing of persons at risk.

Antibiotic Resistance

When penicillin, the first **antibiotic**, was discovered in 1928, it was declared a miracle drug. It was widely used during World War II and saved the lives of many wounded soldiers. By the 1950s, however, the bacterium *Staphylococcus aureus* was already showing signs of resistance to penicillin. A new antibiotic, methicillin, was introduced in 1960 and proved effective, but resistance began developing by 1961. Methicillin-resistant *Staphylococcus aureus* (MRSA) is becoming common on college campuses and will be discussed in detail in the section "Infectious Diseases on Campus." Since the discovery of penicillin, hundreds of new antibiotics have been developed.[15]

The 21st century may mark the beginning of a postantibiotic era as **antibiotic resistance** grows (as well as antiviral and antifungal resistance). Sharp increases in antibiotic resistance have been noted, whether infections are acquired in hospitals, nursing homes, or the community. Some bacteria are becoming resistant to all known antibiotics.[15,16] Two factors are believed to account for bacterial resistance: the frequency with which resistant genes arise naturally among bacteria through mutation and the overuse of antibiotics.

Resistant genes arise naturally because bacteria reproduce quickly, and mutations in their DNA occur frequently. The appearance of resistant genes in bacteria through mutation is amplified when a population of bacteria is exposed to an antibiotic. The most sensitive bacteria die quickly, while those with some resistance survive. Once the nonresistant bacteria are out of the way, the resistant bacteria have more space and food, and they quickly produce more resistant bacteria. They can also share resistant genes with other bacteria. Inappropriate use of antibiotics in health care, home care, and food production increase risk for resistance. Measures to cut down on inappropriate use are critical (see the box, "Reducing Antibiotic Resistance").

Vaccination Controversies

Many of you and your health care providers have never seen a case of measles, mumps, polio, diphtheria, or rubella. Vaccine-preventable childhood diseases that devastated previous generations are at an all-time low. In addition, new vaccines are being developed constantly as a way to combat disease and as a method to hopefully reduce the risk of antibiotic resistance. However, as diseases become less common, some people have begun to question the necessity and safety of the vaccines.

In response, public health officials have been quick to point out that although cases of these diseases may be infrequent, high rates of vaccination (greater than 90 percent of people in a community) are necessary to keep the diseases at bay. Other than smallpox (which was eradicated by worldwide vaccination efforts), the viruses and bacteria that cause them still exist. As rates of vaccination drop, the likelihood of a disease recurrence increases. For example, if you or a classmate travel to a part of the world where a vaccine-preventable childhood disease still occurs, you could bring

Public Health Is Personal

Reducing Antibiotic Resistance

As an individual, you play an active role in reducing antimicrobial resistance to antibiotics. When you are sick, discuss with your health care provider whether the cause is viral or bacterial to determine if antibiotics are really necessary. Don't pressure your doctor to prescribe antibacterial antibiotics when the cause is a virus (as in the case of colds and flu) because antibacterial antibiotics kill only bacteria, not viruses. If you do have a bacterial infection and antibacterial antibiotics are necessary, be sure to complete the full course of treatment and don't miss doses. If you miss doses or stop early, it enables the growth of bacteria that have the ability to survive more easily in the presence of antibacterial antibiotics. In addition, avoid the use of antibiotics in home products, such as soaps and cleaning agents, for the same reason that low levels of antibiotics enable the survival of bacteria with resistance.

However, even if every person used antibacterial antibiotics only when necessary, antibiotic resistance would still occur because an estimated 70 percent of antibiotics produced in the United States are used on livestock. Some of it is to treat animals for actual diseases; however, a significant amount is used in low doses mixed into animal feed or drinking water to promote growth and weight gain in cattle, poultry, hogs, and other food animals. Long-term use of low doses of antibiotics is much more likely to promote bacterial resistance than short courses of high-dose treatments. Antibiotic-resistant bacteria in food animals can cause human disease or pass resistant genes on to other bacteria, which in turn cause human disease. Consequently, individual action alone cannot solve the problem of antibiotic resistance. Public health actions are necessary to ensure that antibiotics will be available and successful in treating human (and animal) disease when it occurs.

In 1969, the first evidence that low levels of antibiotics used in feed production promote antibacterial resistance was published in Europe. In 1977, the U.S. Food and Drug Administration (FDA) proposed the withdrawal of penicillin and tetracycline (two classes of antibiotics important to treating animal and human illnesses) from feed. This proposal was withdrawn, however, due to lack of data proving harm to human health (although there was no evidence proving it was safe). Since then, scientists around the world have studied the relationship and now have strong evidence to support the following findings:

1. The use of antibiotics in food-producing animals allows antibiotic-resistant bacteria to thrive while antibiotic-susceptible bacteria are suppressed or die.

2. Resistant bacteria can be transmitted from food-producing animals to humans through the food supply.

3. Resistant bacteria can cause infections in humans.

4. Infections caused by resistant bacteria can result in adverse health consequences for humans.

In December 2013, the FDA put forth a guidance document designed to protect "medically important antimicrobial drugs"—a term generally used to mean antibiotics that are necessary for the treatment of human diseases. The guideline recommends that certain antibiotics no longer be available over the counter for the animal production industry and that they no longer be used in feed and water at low levels for production. This directive will phase in veterinary oversight to ensure prudent and responsible use of antibiotics in the feed animal industry. Although not binding by law, the FDA is counting on the animal pharmaceutical companies to voluntarily comply. With the overwhelming evidence supporting the elimination of unnecessary use of antibiotics, it is in all of our interests that the animal feed industries also comply.

Sources: "Antibiotic Resistance Threats in the United States 2013," Centers for Disease Control and Prevention, 2013, www.cdc.gov/drugresistance/threat-report-2013/pdf/ar-threats-2013-508.pdf#page=32; "Guidance for Industry: The Judicious Use of Medically Important Antimicrobial Drugs in Food Producing Animals," U.S. Food and Drug Administration, 2013, www.fda.gov/downloads/AnimalVeterinary/GuidanceComplianceEnforcement/GuidanceforIndustry/UCM216936.pdf.

---

the pathogen back to your local community and the disease could spread quickly if local vaccination rates are low.

In recent years, there has been increasing opposition to vaccinations by some people who believe risks associated with vaccines are too great. The controversy was exacerbated in 1998 when Dr. Andrew Wakefield, a British medical researcher, published a study supposedly confirming a link between the measles, mumps, and rubella (MMR) vaccine and autism. After 10 years, no other researchers had been able to reproduce his findings, and, in 2010, his work was declared fraudulent. Wakefield was found guilty of ethical, medical, and scientific misconduct and banned from practicing medicine in the United Kingdom. However, the damage was done: because of the alarm he raised, vaccination rates dropped steeply, and cases of measles and other diseases increased.[17]

Although some minor, temporary side effects may occur after vaccination—such as a local reaction, fever, discomfort, irritability, and, more rarely, allergic reactions—serious reactions to currently recommended vaccinations are very rare. The risk of the vaccine must be weighed against the risk of the disease. For example, the risk of developing encephalitis (brain inflammation) after a dose of the MMR vaccine is less than 1 in 1 million, whereas the risk of developing encephalitis from measles is 1 in 1,000 and the risk of death from measles is 2 in 1,000.[18]

As new vaccines are developed and introduced, they are constantly monitored in efforts to improve vaccine safety. The CDC and the FDA jointly run the Vaccine Adverse Event Reporting System, which collects and analyzes information on possible adverse events that occur after vaccinations.

INFECTIOUS DISEASES WORLDWIDE AND ON CAMPUS

Of the hundreds of thousands of infectious diseases that occur throughout the world, a handful, relatively speaking, are responsible for most cases of illness and death. However, most of the infectious diseases common on college campuses are more easily prevented and treated.

Global Infectious Diseases

From an infectious disease perspective, the world has become a small community. Diseases do not respect borders or boundaries. New diseases and pathogens arise, such as H1N1 flu, and other diseases reemerge as public health concerns, such as tuberculosis. New ways of monitoring the spread of infectious diseases also emerge with global tracking systems. In this section, we consider the four leading causes of infectious disease mortality around the world: pneumonia, diarrhea, tuberculosis, and malaria.

latent infection Infection that is not currently active but could reactivate at a later time.

Pneumonia Pneumonia—infection of the lungs or lower respiratory tract—is the leading cause of death in children and the third most common cause of death (behind heart disease and stroke) for all ages, worldwide.[19,20] Young children and older adults are at greatest risk for pneumonia; besides age, factors that increase risk include exposure to environmental pollutants and use of tobacco, alcohol, or drugs, all of which reduce the lungs' ability to clear infection. Close living situations, such as college dormitories or military barracks, can also increase risk.

Pneumonia can be viral or bacterial (it can also be caused by other organisms). The pathogens are usually inhaled in infected air droplets transmitted from an infected person who is coughing or sneezing nearby. Symptoms of pneumonia include fever, cough, chest pain, shortness of breath, and chills. Viral pneumonia tends to come on more gradually and is often milder than bacterial pneumonia, but both types can be serious and deadly.

Vaccines are available to reduce the risk of contracting pneumonia, and some antiviral and antibacterial medications can shorten the course of the illness. Prevention strategies include avoiding tobacco smoke and crowded living conditions, practicing good hygiene, and following vaccination recommendations. Antibiotic resistance is a growing problem in treating pneumonia. Up to 40 percent of the *Streptococcus* bacterium that causes pneumonia is resistant to penicillin, and approximately 96 percent of influenza A, one of the viruses that causes pneumonia, is resistant to two of the four antiviral drugs used for treatment—both of these causes are vaccine preventable (see the box, "Preventing Influenza with Annual Vaccinations").[16]

Diarrhea Worldwide, diarrhea is the second leading cause of death among children under age 5, killing an estimated 700,000 children per year.[19] Severe diarrhea leads to dehydration and electrolyte imbalances, and repeated episodes lead to malnutrition and growth delay. Multiple organisms cause diarrhea, including viruses and bacteria; rotavirus is responsible for 27 percent of diarrhea deaths worldwide. In the developed world, sanitation and clean water have substantially reduced the risk and severity of diarrhea illness. Prevention depends on effective sanitation systems and access to clean water and food. In addition, a vaccine against rotavirus has been recommended for all infants starting at age 2 months.[21]

Tuberculosis Worldwide, *Mycobacterium tuberculosis* (TB) is the most common infectious disease, with approximately 30 percent of the world population infected, although rates have been decreasing since 2002. The disease is caused by a mycobacterium, a subset of bacteria, and is spread primarily through aerosolized droplets coughed out of the lungs of an infected person and breathed in by another person. Once the mycobacterium is inhaled, a healthy immune system creates a wall around it and prevents it from growing or spreading. In this **latent infection**, the bacterium is in the body but not causing any signs of disease or infection.

About 5 to 10 percent of infected people develop the active disease at some point in their lives, meaning that the bacterium is no longer controlled and can replicate, spread, and be transmitted to other people. Symptoms of active tuberculosis include cough, fatigue, weight loss, night sweats, fever, and coughing up blood. The active disease is more likely to develop if the immune system is impaired, as in HIV infection.

Tuberculosis has reemerged as a major health problem because of the rapid spread of HIV. Anyone with a new case of active tuberculosis should be screened for possible co-infection with HIV. Changes in population patterns have also influenced the spread of TB. Poverty and crowded living situations enhance the spread of disease. In the United States, the people at highest risk for tuberculosis are recent immigrants (particularly from Asia, Africa, Mexico, and South and Central America), homeless people, prison populations, and people infected with HIV.

Active tuberculosis is treated with a combination of four anti-tuberculosis drugs taken for six months (making it a difficult treatment to complete, although 85 percent of cases are successfully treated). Multi-drug-resistant TB (MDR-TB) has become a major public health concern in recent years with 3.7 percent of new cases and 20 percent of previously treated cases being resistant. An even more resistant strain, called extensively drug-resistant tuberculosis (XDR-TB), has recently developed in 41 countries, and reports of cases of completely resistant tuberculosis are emerging. In these cases, treatment options are very limited.[22,23]

International public health efforts are essential for the control of TB. Screening of people at risk for tuberculosis, access to appropriate medications, and tracking systems to ensure successful completion of treatment are essential.

Consumer Clipboard

Preventing Influenza with Annual Flu Vaccinations

Ever wonder why every October you start to see advertisements promoting this year's flu vaccine? None of the other vaccinations require annual updates. So why does influenza? Influenza is an RNA virus and has several different strains. The major types of influenza that infect humans are called A and B. Influenza A has several different subtypes based on two types of proteins on the outer surface of the virus—a hemagglutinin (H) protein and a neuraminidase (N) protein such that human influenza A will be identified as Influenza A, subtype H1N1 or subtype H3N2. During the annual flu season, several types of influenza (A or B), and subtypes H1N1 or H2N2, will circulate and cause illness. Influenza has an amazing propensity to genetically change. There are frequent minor changes of the viral genome—called *genetic drift.* These changes are small and occur frequently in both influenza A and B. If you get the flu one year (or a flu shot), you develop immunity to that particular subtype. However, the genetic drift may make next year's virus different enough that your immune system doesn't quite recognize it. Because the changes are small, genetic drift does not usually lead to pandemics with major mortality because, often, there is a little crossover with immunity to prior viral strains.

Infrequently, abrupt major changes in the influenza A viral genome occur and are called *genetic shift.* These major changes create a new H or N subtype and the virus becomes so different that most people have no immunity to the new strain. These major genetic shifts were responsible for major influenza pandemics that have altered the history of mankind. In 1918, Spanish influenza swept across the globe and led to the death of 20 to 40 million people (cited as the most devastating epidemic in world history). This virus was an influenza A H1N1 subtype. Again in 1947 and 1978, pandemics occurred with the similar H1N1 subtype. In 1957, an H2N2 pandemic swept the globe and, in 1968, an H3N2 subtype.

How can influenza A make such major changes? Influenza A can infect birds, pigs, horses, humans, whales, and bats. Each species has its primary influenza subtypes. Wild bird populations are the major reservoir for influenza A, and all subtypes have been identified in wild birds. Pigs can be infected with their own subtypes (called swine influenza strains) and human or avian (bird) influenza strains. If a pig is infected with two subtypes of influenza at the same time, major genetic recombination can occur, creating totally novel viral subtypes. If the new virus spreads to humans—and if it can spread from human to human and cause disease—a new major pandemic may occur.

Each year, scientists look at patterns of influenza circulation and spread at 130 influenza centers in 101 countries and try to predict which strains will be the major players for the upcoming year. The World Health Organization identifies the major players, and each country then identifies which they will include in their vaccine. The U.S. Food and Drug Administration will identify three or four subtypes—typically two influenza A subtypes and one or two influenza B subtypes—for use in U.S. flu vaccinations. Because it takes about six months to produce sufficient vaccine, these decisions are often made in January of the preceding year. In a good year, the predictions will be accurate and the vaccine will work well. In "mismatched" years, the subtypes included in the vaccine do not match well with circulating viral subtypes and the vaccine is less effective.

Influenza can be a serious illness and lead to hospitalization and even death. In the past 30 years, annual U.S. flu-associated deaths have ranged from 3,000 to 49,000. The flu vaccine is now recommended for all people age 6 months and older. Your options are extensive for which vaccine to choose and include a standard trivalent shot (two influenza A subtypes and one influenza B subtype), a high-dose trivalent shot (for people age 65 and older), a trivalent shot that is egg-free for people who have an egg allergy, a quadrivalent shot (two influenza A and two influenza B subtypes), or a quadrivalent nasal spray. The vaccine shots are all inactivated vaccines and cannot cause actual influenza disease; they can sometimes cause soreness at the injection site, low-grade fever, and muscle aches as the immune system is boosted to develop immunity. The nasal spray is a weakened live virus that cannot cause influenza but can cause short-lived symptoms of a mild runny nose, muscle aches, and low-grade fever.

Source: "Seasonal Influenza," Centers for Disease Control, (n.d.), www.cdc.gov/flu/index.htm.

People with latent infection are treated to reduce the risk that they will develop active tuberculosis. Researchers are trying to develop simpler treatments, and new vaccines are being studied that will reduce the risk of infection and progression to active disease.

Malaria Malaria is a mosquito-borne disease caused by four species of the Plasmodium parasite. Approximately 207 million people were infected in 2012, with 627,000 deaths, mostly among young children. Currently, about 80 percent of malaria cases and 90 percent of malaria deaths occur in Africa, predominantly sub-Saharan Africa.[24]

Malaria symptoms, which include high fever, chills, sweats, headache, nausea, vomiting, and body aches, develop 7 to 30 days after a bite from an infected Anopheles mosquito. Symptoms are often cyclic, recurring every few days. Severe malaria can lead to confusion, seizures, coma, heart failure, kidney failure, and death.

Prevention strategies include eliminating mosquito breeding grounds (e.g., standing water), applying insecticides, using screens and mosquito netting, and staying inside during peak mosquito hours (dawn and dusk). People who travel to malaria-endemic areas should use mosquito repellent and take chemoprophylaxis—a medication taken before, during, and for a period of time after travel. Malaria used to be endemic in parts of the southeastern United States, but the CDC, working with local health agencies, undertook a program that targeted mosquito breeding grounds and

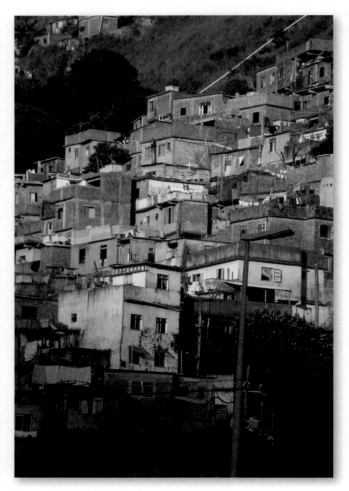

■ Crowded living conditions, poor sanitation, and poverty create perfect conditions for the transmission of infectious diseases, including tuberculosis. These hillside structures in Rio de Janeiro are home to thousands of impoverished people squatting on public land.

included other anti-mosquito measures. Efforts to eradicate malaria worldwide are under way, with researchers attempting to develop a vaccine, new treatments, and new preventive measures. These efforts are especially important with the development of resistance to antimalarial medications and the concerns that climate change may alter where the mosquito that transmits malaria is found.[12,24]

Infectious Diseases on Campus

Infectious diseases also cause illness on college campuses (Table 13.1). College students consistently list colds, flu, and sore throat among the top 10 impediments to academic performance.[25] Assess your risk for infectious disease by completing the immunizations table and answering the questions in this chapter's Personal Health Portfolio.

Pertussis (Whooping Cough) *Whooping cough* is the common name for an infection of the respiratory tract caused by the pertussis bacterium. It is highly contagious, transmitted by inhaling respiratory droplets from an infected person's cough or sneeze. Initial infection may seem similar to a common cold, with nasal congestion, runny nose, mild fever, and a dry cough, but after one to two weeks, the coughing occurs in spells lasting a few minutes and ending in a "whooping" sound as the person gasps for air. The cough can persist for months. Pertussis is treated with antibiotics if diagnosed early.

Most infants and young children are vaccinated against pertussis, but immunity begins to wear off after 5 to 10 years, leaving adolescents and young adults susceptible to infection. Studies on college campuses show that among students with a prolonged cough, approximately 30 percent may have pertussis. It is now recommended that all adolescents and adults receive a booster Tdap vaccination (tetanus, diphtheria, and acellular pertussis) to enhance their immunity against this infection.[26]

Reported cases of pertussis have increased 20-fold in the past 30 years. Because of the high risk of pertussis to newborns, pregnant women should receive a booster during pregnancy regardless of when they last had a booster, as should anyone who spends time around newborns.[27]

***Staphylococcus Aureus* Skin Infections** *Staphylococcus aureus* (often called "staph"), a common bacterium carried on the skin or in the noses of healthy people, is one of the most common causes of skin infection. Some strains of staph are becoming increasingly resistant to antibiotics. Initially seen in hospitals, methicillin-resistant *Staphylococcus aureus* (MRSA) is becoming common in community settings. MRSA is transmitted from person to person by skin-to-skin contact, through the sharing of personal items,

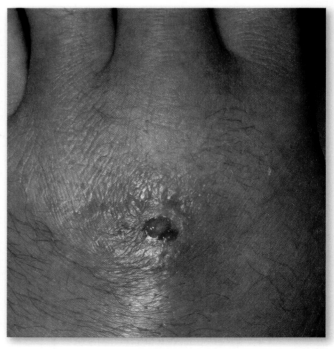

■ A skin infection caused by MRSA is easy to get and hard to treat.

TABLE 13.1 Infectious Diseases on Campus

Illness	Cause (Pathogen)	Incubation	Symptoms	Home Treatment	When to Seek Medical Care	Prevention
Common cold	More than 200 different viruses, including rhinovirus, adenovirus, coronavirus	1–4 days	Runny nose (mucus often clear initially, then thicker, darker), nasal congestion, mild cough, sore throat, low-grade fever (<101° F), sneezing.	Usually ends on its own; fluids, rest, OTC decongestants, antihistamines, cough suppressants, antipyretics, analgesics; avoid alcohol and tobacco.	Inability to swallow, worsening symptoms after 3rd day, difficulty breathing, stiff neck.	Wash hands thoroughly and frequently, avoid sharing personal items, eat a balanced diet, exercise, get adequate sleep.
Influenza ("the flu")	Influenza A or B virus	1–5 days	Sudden-onset fever (usually >101° F), headache, tiredness (can be extreme), body aches, cough, sore throat, runny or stuffy nose.	Usually ends on its own; same home treatments as for common cold; in addition, antiviral medications can be used by prescription.	Immediately if at risk for complications, e.g., pregnant women, people with chronic lung or heart disease, asthma. Otherwise, if difficulty breathing, severe headache or stiff neck, confusion, fever for more than 3 days, new pain in one area (ear, chest, sinuses).	Annual flu shot in October or November, frequent hand washing; avoid close contact with sick people.
Strep throat	*Streptococcus* bacteria	2–5 days	Sudden-onset sore throat and fever (often >101° F); mild headache, stomachache, nausea; red and white pus on tonsils, sore lymph nodes in neck; absence of cough, stuffy nose, other cold symptoms.	Salt water gargles, analgesics, antipyretics, throat lozenges.	If symptoms are consistent with strep, visit health care provider, who can prescribe antibiotics to reduce duration of symptoms and reduce risk of complications.	Same as common cold.
Acute sinus infection	Virus: cold virus most common cause. Bacteria: *Streptococcus, Haemophilus* influenza; less common cause, often as complication of cold or allergies.	Varies	Pain or pressure in the face, stuffy or runny nose, upper teeth pain, fever; may have headache, bad breath, yellow or green nasal discharge.	Same as for common cold: decongestants or antihistamines; nasal irrigation; most sinus infections resolve on their own with opening and drainage of the sinuses.	Fever >101° F after 3 days; no improvement in facial pain or pressure after 2 days of home treatment with decongestant; cold symptoms continue beyond 10 days or worsen after 7 days.	Same as common cold. Early treatment of nasal congestion with decongestant or antihistamine.
Mononucleosis ("mono")	Epstein-Barr virus (EBV)	4–6 weeks	High fever (>101° F), severe sore throat, swollen glands, weakness and fatigue; loss of appetite; nausea, and vomiting can occur.	Usually resolves on its own; rest, fluids; avoid contact sports until symptoms resolve due to risk of spleen rupture.	Fever >101° F after 3 days, unable to maintain fluids; low energy, body aches, swollen glands for more than 7–10 days. Severe pain in belly can indicate spleen rupture, is a medical emergency.	Do not kiss or share utensils or foods with someone who has mono; EBV is spread from saliva.

(continued)

TABLE 13.1 Infectious Diseases on Campus *(continued)*

Illness	Cause (Pathogen)	Incubation	Symptoms	Home Treatment	When to Seek Medical Care	Prevention
Bronchitis or cough	Virus: same as common cold. Bacteria: rare. Other lung irritants: tobacco smoke.	Varies	Initial dry, hacking cough; in a few days, may produce mucus; maybe low fever and fatigue; often develops 3–4 days after start of a cold; may last 2–3 weeks.	Rest, fluids, cough drops, and avoidance of lung irritants such as tobacco; over-the-counter cold medications may help.	Shortness of breath; history of asthma or chronic lung disease; signs of pneumonia: high fever, shaking chills, shortness of breath; also, if symptoms last more than 4 weeks.	Avoid tobacco smoke; get annual flu shot; wash hands thoroughly and frequently.
Meningitis and encephalitis	Virus: usually not as serious as bacterial; some forms can be spread by mosquitos Bacteria: rare, must be treated immediately to avoid brain damage and death.	Varies	Stiff and painful neck, fever, headache, vomiting, difficulty staying awake, confusion, seizures.	Home treatment is not appropriate until a health care provider determines if cause is virus or bacteria. If viral cause, home treatment to relieve fever and pain symptoms is appropriate.	Immediately if signs of meningitis are present.	Immunization against some pathogens, including measles, mumps, rubella; chicken pox; *Neisseria meningitides* (meningococcal vaccine). Special immunizations for certain areas of the world; insect repellent. Bacterial: Antibiotics after coming in close contact with infected person.
Cellulitis	Bacteria: Most common are *Streptococcus* and *Staphylococcus aureus*	Varies	Infected area will be warm, red, swollen, and painful. If infection spreads, may have fever, chills, swollen glands.	Warm compresses; keep area clean and dry; topical antibiotics if only small area of skin involved.	Usually treated with antibiotics; any symptoms should be evaluated by a health care provider.	Healthy skin protects against infection; keep cuts, burns, insect bites clean and dry; treat chronic skin conditions (e.g., eczema, ulcers, psoriasis); avoid skin-to-skin contact with infected people; avoid IV drug use, piercing, and tattoos.

and through contact with contaminated surfaces. Outbreaks of infection have been reported among athletes and people in shared living situations (such as on college campuses).

Usually staph infections are mild, taking the form of a pimple or small boil (sometimes mistaken for a spider bite). Sometimes these infections can spread, creating a large abscess (pocket of infection), which can require incision, drainage, and treatment with antibiotics. Less often, staph can cause infection of the blood, lungs, or muscle. These cases usually require hospitalization and intravenous antibiotic treatment.

Good hygiene practices can reduce the risk of staph infection. Keep your hands clean by washing frequently with soap and water, or use an alcohol-based hand sanitizer. Shower after exercising, and avoid sharing personal items such as towels, razors, clothing, and uniforms. Keep cuts and scrapes clean and covered until healed. If you have been diagnosed with a staph infection, avoid skin-to-skin contact (including contact sports) until the area has healed.[28]

Urinary Tract Infections Urinary tract infections (UTIs) are the most common bacterial infection in women, and half of all women will have one in their lifetime. They occur in men too, but less frequently. The vast majority of UTIs are caused by the bacterium *E. coli,* although they can be caused by other bacteria. Symptoms include pain or burning with urination, pain in the lower abdomen, urgency and frequency of urination, and, if the kidneys become involved, pain in the back and fever. Recent sexual activity and history of UTI are risk factors for infection. If a woman is at risk for STIs or has vaginal symptoms, such as discharge or irritation, she should be tested to rule out STIs. Treatment includes fluids and antibiotics, although *E. coli* is becoming increasingly resistant to commonly used antibiotics.[29]

SEXUALLY TRANSMITTED INFECTIONS

Sexually transmitted infections (STIs) are infections that are spread from one person to another predominantly through sexual contact. Most health experts prefer the term *sexually transmitted infection (STI)*, because often there are no symptoms, and by definition, a disease is an infection that causes symptoms. However, the CDC continues to use the term *sexually transmitted disease.*

The primary pathogens responsible for STIs are viruses and bacteria. We begin this section with HIV infection, one of the most serious threats to public health worldwide, and then we discuss the other STIs by type of pathogen. See Table 13.2 on pages 306–307 for information relating to the incubation period, symptoms, complications, screening and diagnosis, and treatment of each STI discussed.

HIV/AIDS

Acquired immunodeficiency syndrome (AIDS) is caused by the human immunodeficiency virus (HIV). Since the first case was diagnosed in 1981, more than 20 million people have died from HIV/AIDS. The pandemic is considered the most serious infectious disease challenge in public health today. At the end of 2012, an estimated 35.3 million people worldwide were infected, two-thirds of them in sub-Saharan Africa (Figure 13.7). In 2012, 2.3 million new infections and 1.6 million deaths occurred. The overall number of new infections has declined globally, but new infections have increased in the Middle East, Northern Africa, Eastern Europe, and Central Asia.[30]

In sub-Saharan Africa, the epidemic is in the general population, with women representing 61 percent of the

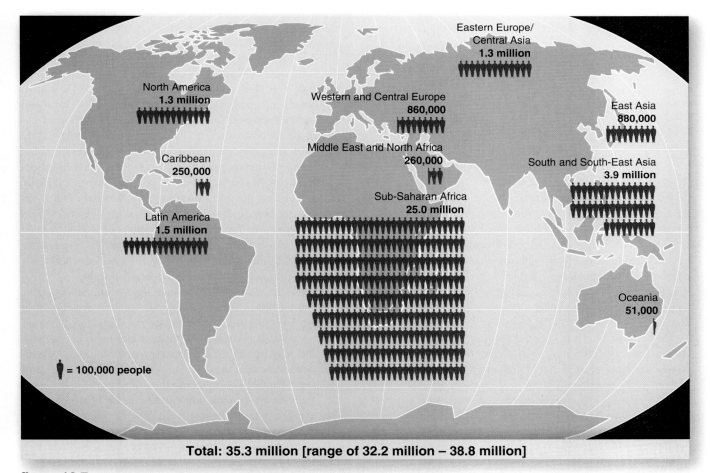

Total: 35.3 million [range of 32.2 million – 38.8 million]

figure 13.7   **Adults and children estimated to be living with HIV in 2012**
Source: HIV/AIDS Data and Statistics, World Health Organization, HIV Department, March 2014, p. 5, www.who.int/hiv/data/en/.

Who's at Risk?

Disproportionate Risk for HIV Infections

Certain groups are at disproportionate risk for HIV infections. The following graph shows the subpopulations that reported the most new HIV cases in 2010 in the United States.

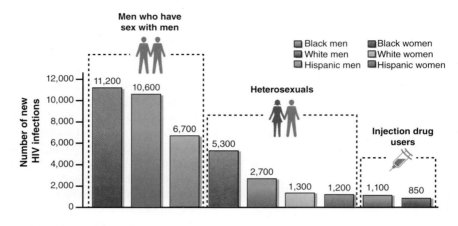

Source: "HIV/AIDS in the United States," Centers for Disease Control and Prevention, 2012, www.cdc.gov/nchhstp/newsroom/docs/2012/HIV-Infections-2007-2010.pdf.

---

opportunistic infections
Infections that occur when the immune system is weakened. These infections do not usually occur in a person with a healthy immune system.

people living with HIV, and transmission is predominantly via heterosexual contact. In other parts of the world, HIV remains concentrated in populations of increased risk, such as men who have sex with men, injection drug users, and sex workers and their sexual partners.[30]

An estimated 1.3 million people are living with HIV in North America. Rates of diagnosis of new infection in the United States have declined; however, certain populations are at increased risk. In the United States, men who have sex with men account for 63 percent of all new HIV infections, and high-risk heterosexual sex accounts for 25 percent. About 8 percent of newly diagnosed HIV infections involve intravenous drug use. Racial and ethnic minority populations continue to be affected disproportionately, with new infections among young black men who have sex with men continuing to increase (see the box, "Disproportionate Risk for HIV Infections").[31,32]

HIV most likely originated from a similar virus, the simian immunodeficiency virus found in chimpanzees in Africa. It is believed to have jumped from animal host to human host approximately 50 to 75 years ago. The virus may have entered a human being from the bite of an infected chimpanzee or during the slaughtering of a chimpanzee. Once in a human host, the simian immunodeficiency virus evolved through mutation into human immunodeficiency virus.[33] There are two main strains of the virus: HIV-1 is the predominant strain in North America and most of the rest of the world; HIV-2 is found primarily in Africa.

Course of the Disease HIV targets the cells of the immune system, especially macrophages and CD4 cells (a subcategory of helper T cells). Once inside these host cells, the virus uses the cell's DNA to replicate itself and disable the host cell. During the initial infection with HIV, known as *primary infection,* the virus replicates rapidly. Within 4 to 11 days of exposure, several million viral copies may circulate in the bloodstream. The immune system mounts a rapid response in an attempt to control and remove the virus, but HIV is able to mutate quickly and avoid complete eradication.

Between 40 and 90 percent of people infected with HIV experience an acute infection phase approximately four to six weeks after exposure, with symptoms such as fever, weight loss, fatigue, sore throat, swollen lymph nodes, night sweats, muscle aches, rash, and diarrhea. The symptoms may last for a few weeks and are easily mistaken for those of other infections, such as influenza, mononucleosis, or herpes.

After the early phase, the immune system and the virus come to a balance with the establishment of a *viral load set point,* a level of virus that continues to circulate in the blood and body fluids. During this phase, a person is asymptomatic and may remain so for 2 to 20 years. The virus continues to replicate, and the immune system continues to control it without completely removing it.

Eventually, the immune system is weakened significantly and can no longer function fully, signaling the onset of AIDS. Symptoms of AIDS include rapid weight loss, cough, night sweats, diarrhea, rashes or skin blemishes, and memory loss. These symptoms are due to **opportunistic infections**—infections that occur when the immune system is no longer able to fight them off. Common opportunistic infections include *Pneumocystis carinii* pneumonia, Kaposi's sarcoma (a rare cancer), and tuberculosis.

A note of caution: The symptoms associated with acute HIV infection and AIDS are also associated with many other illnesses. A person experiencing such symptoms should not automatically assume they are signs of HIV infection or AIDS. However, if the person is at risk, he or she should get tested for HIV infection.

Methods of Transmission HIV cannot survive long outside of a human host, and thus transmission requires intimate contact. The virus can be found in varying concentrations in an infected person's blood, saliva, semen, genital secretions, and breast milk. It usually enters a new host either at a mucosal surface or by direct inoculation into the blood. HIV is not transmitted through casual contact, such as shaking hands, hugging, or a casual kiss, nor is it spread by day-to-day contact in the workplace, school, or home. Although HIV has been found in saliva and tears, it is present in very low quantities. It has not been found in sweat.

Risk of HIV transmission is influenced by factors associated with the host (the already infected person), the recipient (the currently uninfected person), and the type of interaction that occurs between the host and recipient (behaviors). An important host factor is the level of virus circulating in the blood. High levels of circulating virus, such as during the initial infection stage, increase the risk of transmission. In addition, some people may have a higher viral load set point during the equilibrium period. Antiviral treatment (see the section "Management of HIV/AIDS") lowers the level of circulating virus and may reduce the risk of transmission.

Sexual Conduct The primary exposure risk for 88 percent of cases of HIV infection in the United States is sexual contact.[32] HIV can enter the body through the mucosa or lining of the vagina, penis, rectum, or mouth. If the mucosa is cut, torn, or irritated (as can happen with intercourse or if there is another STI, especially genital herpes), the risk increases. The sexual behaviors associated with transmission are receptive anal sex, insertive anal sex, penile-vaginal sex, and oral sex.

Although discussing HIV status with a potential sexual partner may be awkward, its importance cannot be overemphasized. As noted, the time of highest circulating virus is shortly after initial infection; the person may not have any symptoms and may not know he or she is infected. In fact, 25 percent of HIV-positive people in the United States do not know they are infected. Unless you have a conversation about whether your potential partner has been tested for HIV, what risky behaviors he or she has engaged in, and what other sexual partners he or she has been involved with, you do not know what your risk is in starting a sexual relationship.[32]

Injection Drug Use The second most common method of HIV transmission is injection drug use, reported by 18 percent of people with AIDS in the United States. Another 3 percent report both injection drug use and being a man who has sex with other men as combined risk factors. Individuals can reduce their risk of HIV infection by avoiding injection drug use. People who are already using drugs can reduce their risk by using sterile needles and not sharing needles with others. Communities can play a role in decreasing the spread of HIV by implementing needle exchange programs and ensuring adequate access to drug treatment programs.

Contact With Infected Blood or Body Fluids HIV can be transmitted by direct contact with the blood or body fluids of an infected person. The risk of transmission depends on how much virus is in the body fluid, how much fluid gets onto the other person, and where the fluid contacts the other person. A small amount of infected blood on the intact skin of another person carries essentially no risk. A larger amount of blood on cut or broken skin or mucosal membranes has a greater risk. The accidental injection of infected blood through a needle stick has an even greater risk.

These types of exposure are most likely to occur in health care settings, and to reduce the risk of transmission of HIV, hepatitis B and C, and other bloodborne infections, these places take a **universal precautions** approach. Universal precautions include the use of gloves, gown, mask, and other protective wear (such as eyewear or face shields) by anyone who is likely to be exposed to the blood or body fluids of an infected person. These precautions should be taken with every patient.[34]

Perinatal Transmission Perinatal, or vertical, transmission—the transmission of HIV from an infected mother to her child—can occur during pregnancy, during delivery (when the fetus is exposed to the mother's blood in the birth canal), or after delivery (if the baby is exposed to the mother's breast milk). The risk of transmission from mother to child can be reduced through the use of antiretroviral medications during pregnancy and around the time of delivery. Infected mothers also reduce the risk to their babies by electing not to breastfeed.

In the United States, women are routinely offered HIV testing as part of prenatal care. Women who test positive are offered preventive therapy with antiretroviral medications to reduce their child's risk. In untreated pregnant women with HIV, approximately 30 percent of infants are infected; in treated women, less than 2 percent are infected.

HIV Testing The earlier HIV infection is recognized, the sooner treatment can begin, the longer the person is likely to remain symptom free, and the fewer people he or she is likely to expose to the virus. The only way to confirm HIV infection is by laboratory testing.

universal precautions A set of precautions designed to prevent transmission of bloodborne infections. Blood and certain body fluids of all patients are considered potentially infectious for HIV and hepatitis B and C. Protective barriers, such as gloves, aprons, and protective eyewear, are used in health settings.

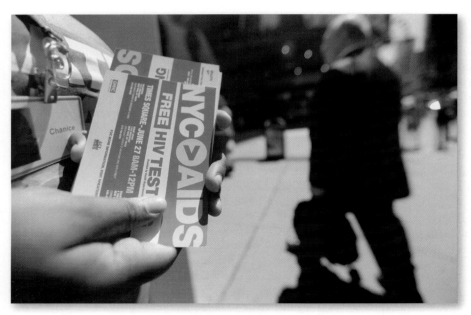

■ The CDC recommends that people aged 13 to 64 get tested for HIV at least once during routine medical care.

To increase the number of HIV cases that are diagnosed early, the CDC recommends that everyone between the ages of 13 and 64 be tested for HIV infection at least once during routine medical care. Testing is strongly recommended for anyone who has engaged in any of the following behaviors or has had a partner who has done so:

■ Injected drugs, including steroids.

■ Had unprotected vaginal, anal, or oral sex with men who have had sex with men.

■ Had multiple partners or anonymous partners or has exchanged sex for drugs or money.

■ Been diagnosed with an STI.

Anyone who continues to engage in these risk behaviors should be tested at least annually. Men who have sex with men should consider testing every three to six months if they have multiple partners or anonymous partners. All pregnant women should be screened for HIV. June 27 is National HIV Testing Day in recognition of the importance of testing.[35,36]

Most HIV tests are designed to detect antibodies to HIV circulating in the bloodstream. After an HIV exposure, it can take two to eight weeks for a sufficient quantity of antibodies to be produced for an HIV test to detect them. This time is referred to as a "window period"—a time when an HIV test may result in a false negative.

Some tests include a screen for HIV antigen (part of the virus) in addition to the antibody. In this case, HIV infection can be detected much earlier. It is important to know which test you are getting because if it is the one that looks only for antibodies and you are within the first three months after a potential exposure, you will need to repeat the test three months later.

HIV screening has never been easier because multiple new tests now can be done. Tests can use oral swabs or urine instead of blood, and some can deliver results in about 20 minutes. An over-the-counter home test called the Home Access HIV-1 Test System has been licensed and approved by the FDA. In the privacy of your home, you collect a small amount of blood from a finger prick, place the blood on a card, mail the card to a registered laboratory, and telephone for results using an identification number. Consumers are warned to use only FDA-approved test kits, because others may not be as accurate. If the result of an oral, urine, or home test is positive, you will be referred to a health clinic for a confirmatory test. If you are HIV negative, share your results with your partners and encourage them to be tested if they do not know their status.[37]

Management of HIV/AIDS The development of new medications and improved understanding of the HIV disease process have prolonged survival for some people infected with HIV. Educating people in low- and middle-income countries and getting them medication has been a major challenge, but international efforts have shown tremendous progress in recent years.[30]

Antiretroviral Agents The most important medications in HIV treatment are antiviral drugs—or, more accurately, antiretroviral drugs because HIV is a type of virus called a retrovirus. Antiretroviral medications do not cure the infection, but they slow the rate at which the virus replicates and destroys the immune system, thus prolonging life, improving the quality of life for people who are HIV-positive, and reducing risk of transmission.

Drug Cocktails If a single antiretroviral medication is used, resistant strains develop fairly quickly. To combat resistance, scientists have developed complicated drug combinations, called **drug cocktails**, that usually include a medication from two to four of the drug categories. A viral strain is less likely to develop several mutations allowing it to evade the combination of drugs than to develop one or a few mutations allowing it to evade a single drug. However, the complexity, cost, and risk of side effects for the person taking the drugs are all increased.

drug cocktails
Complicated drug combinations used to overcome drug resistance in different strains of HIV.

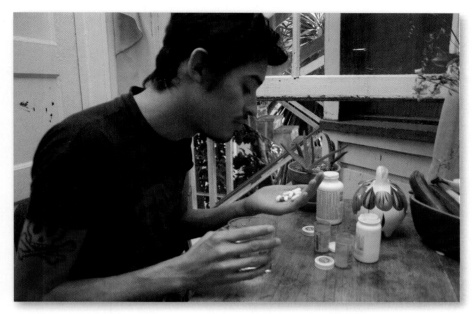

■ People with HIV manage the disease with antiretroviral medications. Multiple drugs are used since the virus can quickly become resistant to individual drugs.

New Prevention Strategies Since the identification of the virus, researchers have been attempting to develop safe and effective measures to reduce risk of infection. An HIV vaccine would be ideal but is challenging. The immune system does not seem to be able to clear HIV and produce immunity; instead, in most people the virus produces life-long infection. Furthermore, the virus is a moving target; it mutates frequently and develops new strains rapidly. That said, multiple vaccine trials are under way.[38]

Preexposure prophylaxis is now recommended for people who are HIV negative but in high-risk situations, including those who have sex with a partner with HIV infection, a recent diagnosis of a bacterial STI, or a high number of sexual partners, and among commercial sex workers and intravenous drug users who share needles. Preexposure prophylaxis is the daily use of a two-drug combination antiretroviral medication (the same one that is used in HIV treatment).[39] In addition, adult male circumcision is recognized as an intervention to reduce risk of HIV infection from penile-vaginal sex, possibly due to the fact that removing the foreskin results in a toughening of the skin covering the penis. The benefits are not seen in men who have sex with men, most likely due to the fact that the risk of contracting HIV is greatest during receptive anal sex.[40]

Bacterial STIs

Bacterial STIs are generally curable infections if identified early. Undiagnosed, they can cause serious consequences, including pelvic inflammatory disease, reduced fertility, ectopic pregnancy, and increased risk for HIV transmission.[39]

Chlamydia The most commonly reported bacterial STI is chlamydia. Rates of infection are increasing in the United States, with an estimated 1.4 million cases diagnosed annually. Young women are at greatest risk for chlamydia, with rates three times that of young men. Eight percent of women aged 15 to 24 visiting family planning clinics are infected. Although all racial and ethnic groups are affected, Black women have rates seven times higher than those of White women.[39]

All sexually active women under age 26 should be screened annually for chlamydia, as should women who are at increased risk because they have a new sexual partner or multiple sexual partners or are infected with another STI. Identification and treatment of infection reduces the risk of complications such as pelvic inflammatory disease and infertility.

There is debate about the cost effectiveness of screening all sexually active men under age 26. Men have less long-term aftereffects from chlamydia infection and thus routine screening efforts are targeted at women. Men should be tested if they have symptoms or have a new sexual partner or if their sexual partner has been diagnosed with chlamydia. Men who have sex with men should be tested annually for rectal, penile, or throat infection (depending on their sexual practice). Rates of chlamydia infection are increasing among men, and men can be infected yet have no symptoms.

Gonorrhea The second most commonly reported bacterial STI is gonorrhea. As with chlamydia, the highest rates occur in young women. In addition, rates in Blacks are 17 times higher those in Whites. Rates of gonorrheal infection decreased to a low in 2010 but have been rising, with an estimated 320,000 cases diagnosed in 2011.[41]

Regular screening is recommended for women at high risk of infection—those who are under 25 and have had two or more sex partners in the past year, who exchange sex for money or drugs, or who have a history of repeated episodes of gonorrhea.

It is less clear if asymptomatic men should be screened because most men eventually develop symptoms. However, young men with new partners and men who have sex with men should consider annual testing (or more frequent testing if they have multiple partners or anonymous partners).[42]

Gonorrhea is treated with antibiotics, but drug resistance is a significant problem. Cephalosporins are the only class of antibiotics now available to treat gonorrhea infection, and there have been reports of strains resistant to all

TABLE 13.2 Common Sexually Transmitted Infections

Infection	Incubation	Signs and Symptoms	Complications	Screening and Diagnosis*	Treatment	Prevention
Bacterial						
Chlamydia (*Chlamydia trachomatis*)	1–3 weeks	No symptoms for 75% of women and 50% of men. **If symptoms:** watery discharge, burning with urination.	Women: pelvic inflammatory disease (PID), chronic pelvic pain, infertility, ectopic pregnancy. Men: epididymitis (red, swollen testicles) and, rarely, sterility. **If untreated in pregnant women:** premature birth; eye and lung infections in newborns.	Urine or sample collected from penis, cervix, rectum, or throat (site based on sexual practice). Women <26: annually. MSM: annually (or more often). Men <26 consider annually if new partners.	Antibiotics. Sex partners need testing and treatment prior to resuming sexual intercourse.	Condoms.
Gonorrhea (*Neisseria gonorrhoeae*)	2–5 days	No symptoms in most women and some men. **If symptoms:** Men: pain or burning with urination; discharge from penis; itching inside penis. Women: pain or burning with urination; vaginal discharge, bleeding between periods; pain during sex. Rectal infection: discharge, soreness, bleeding, or pain. Throat infection: sore throat.	Pelvic inflammatory disease (PID), chronic pelvic pain, infertility, and ectopic pregnancy in women. Epididymitis (red, swollen testicles) and infertility in men; can spread to blood and joints. **If untreated in pregnant women:** risk of newborn eye, joint, and blood infection.	Urine or sample collected from cervix, penis, rectum, or throat (site based on sexual practice). Annually in women <26. Annually (or more frequently) in MSM; consider annually in men <26 if new partners.	Antibiotics, sex partners need testing and treatment prior to resuming sexual intercourse.	Condoms.
Syphilis (*Treponema pallidum*)	**Primary stage:** 10–90 days **Secondary stage:** 3–6 weeks after primary stage **Late stage:** years after initial untreated infection	No symptoms for most people. **If symptoms: Primary stage:** single round, firm, and painless sore (chancre) at exposure site; sore resolves without treatment in 3–6 weeks. **Secondary stage:** skin rash with non-itchy, rough, reddish brown spots on palms and soles; may have fever, swollen lymph nodes, headache, fatigue; resolves without treatment.	**Late stage:** without treatment, infection remains in body and 15% of people will develop deterioration of the brain, arteries, bones, heart, and other organs; death possible. **If untreated in pregnant women:** risk of fetal death or infant developmental delay, seizures, or other complications.	Blood test for antibodies to syphilis. MSM: annually (or more often). Heterosexuals and WSW: test if positive for another STI.	Antibiotics will cure if diagnosed within the first year of infection.	Avoidance of high-risk behaviors; condoms.
Viral						
HIV (human immunodeficiency virus)	4–6 weeks	No symptoms for 10–60% of people. **If symptoms:** fever, fatigue, sore throat, lymph node swelling, muscle aches; may include weight loss, rash, night sweats, and diarrhea; often mistaken for other illnesses.	Acquired immunodeficiency syndrome (AIDS) 2–20 years after initial infection if untreated; symptoms include opportunistic infections, weight loss, rashes, and skin changes. **Pregnant women:** can be transmitted to fetus; reduced risk with treatment of mother.	Blood, saliva, or urine test. Annually if intravenous drug user, new sexual partners, or diagnosed with another STI. MSM with multiple or anonymous partners: consider every 3 to 6 months. All pregnant women.	No cure; management with antiretroviral medications that reduce rate of viral replication and slow rate of immune system decline.	Condoms; post-exposure prophylaxis (taking an antiretroviral medication as soon as possible after high-risk sexual encounter or assault can reduce risk of infection).

TABLE 13.2 Common Sexually Transmitted Infections *(continued)*

Infection	Incubation	Signs and Symptoms	Complications	Screening and Diagnosis*	Treatment	Prevention
Bacterial						
HPV (human papilloma-virus; more than 40 strains)	Weeks to months	No symptoms for most people. **If symptoms:** Genital warts: small bumps or clusters of bumps in genital area. Cervical cancer: irregular bleeding.	In 90% of cases, immune system clears infection within 2 years; cancers of cervix, vulva, vagina, anus, and penis. **Pregnant women:** very rarely, newborn can develop throat infection during vaginal birth.	Genital warts: visual identification. Cervical cancer: routine Pap testing starting at age 21 for all women.	Warts: topical medications or cryotherapy (freezing). Cervical cancer: see Chapter 15.	Vaccination for women and men; Pap test for women reduces risk of cervical cancer; condoms reduce risk, but virus can infect areas of genitalia not covered by male and female condoms.
Genital herpes (herpes simplex virus type 1 or type 2)	2–7 days	No symptoms for most people. **If symptoms:** one or more blisters on or around the mouth, genitals, or rectum, which break open, leaving a painful sore that resolves after 2–4 weeks (for first infection); may have associated fever and lymph node swelling.	Recurrent outbreaks, usually less severe than initial one and decrease in severity with time. **Pregnant women:** potential life-threatening infection in newborn if infection during pregnancy or outbreak at time of vaginal birth.	Culture of ulcer or blood test. Routine screening controversial if no symptoms.	No cure; antiviral medications can shorten and prevent outbreaks.	Antiviral medications reduces risk of transmission, which can occur even when lesions are not present. Condoms reduce risk, but virus can infect areas of genitalia not covered by male and female condoms.
Hepatitis B	6 weeks–6 months	No symptoms for 30% of people. **If symptoms:** fever, loss of appetite, nausea, vomiting, abdominal pain, dark urine, yellow color of skin or eyes.	Chronic hepatitis B: increased risk of liver failure due to scarring of liver and liver cancer. **Pregnant women:** can transmit infection to newborn.	Blood tests can look for virus and evidence of immune response.	No treatment for acute infection; several medications for chronic infection but are not suitable for all people.	Vaccination recommended routinely for most people, and can be effective if given within 24 hours after exposure. Condoms.
Protozoan						
Trichomonia-sis (*Trichomonas vaginalis*)	5–28 days	No symptoms in most men. **If symptoms:** Men: slight burning of penis or mild discharge. Women: frothy, yellow-green vaginal discharge with strong odor; vaginal soreness or itching.	**If untreated in pregnant women:** increased risk of premature delivery.	Identification under a microscope. Test if symptoms.	Antibiotics; treatment of both partners prior to resuming sexual activity.	Condoms.

*Heterosexual women and women who have sex with women (WSW) follow the same recommendations for screening guidelines; men who have sex with men (MSM) should consider increased frequency of screening at three- to six-month intervals if multiple or anonymous partners.

Sources: "Sexually Transmitted Disease Surveillance, 2010," Centers for Disease Control and Prevention, 2010, Atlanta: U.S. Department of Health and Human Services; "Sexually Transmitted Diseases Treatment Guidelines 2010," Centers for Disease Control and Prevention (n.d.), retrieved from www.cdc.gov/STI/treatment/default.htm.

antibiotics. Given this rising problem, gonorrhea infections should be treated with two antibiotics instead of one to reduce risk of further resistance.[42]

Pelvic Inflammatory Disease Pelvic inflammatory disease (PID) is an infection of the uterus, fallopian tubes, and/or ovaries. The infection occurs when bacteria from the vagina or cervix spread upward into the uterus and fallopian tubes. The bacteria involved are usually from STIs, such as chlamydia or gonorrhea, but they can be bacteria that are normally found in the vagina.

Symptoms of PID include fever, abdominal pain, pelvic pain, and vaginal bleeding or discharge. If PID is suspected, a combination of antibiotics is prescribed to cover gonorrhea, chlamydia, and vaginal bacteria. If symptoms are severe, hospitalization may be required. About 18 percent of women with PID develop chronic abdominal or pelvic pain that lasts more than six months.

PID can cause severe consequences and can be life threatening if untreated. Most of the long-term problems arise from scarring in the fallopian tubes, which increases the risk of ectopic pregnancy and infertility.[41,42]

Syphilis Rates of syphilis decreased throughout the 20th century but increased from 2001 to 2009. In 2010, overall rates decreased again and have since leveled off. Seventy-two percent of current syphilis cases are diagnosed in men who have sex with men. Racial disparity in syphilis has decreased but remains pronounced especially in younger age groups, with 15- to 19-year-old Black men having rates 16 times the rate for White men of the same age. For 15- to 19-year-old women, Black women have 30 times the rates of White women.[41] Syphilis progresses through several stages. If left untreated, it can lead to serious complications, including death.

Screening is recommended for all pregnant women at their initial prenatal care visit and for anyone at increased risk for syphilis infection. This includes men who have sex with men, commercial sex workers, and anyone who tests positive for another STI, exchanges sex for drugs, or has sex with partners who have syphilis.[42]

Bacterial Vaginosis Bacterial vaginosis (BV) is an alteration of the normal vaginal flora; *Lactobacillis,* the usually predominant bacteria, is replaced with different bacteria, causing a vaginal discharge and unpleasant odor. It is not clear why women develop bacterial vaginosis. Although it is not considered an STI, women who have never had sex rarely experience the condition. In addition, women who have sex with women have increased rates of BV. Treatment of male partners does not alter the rate of recurrence for women.

Screening for BV is recommended only if a woman has symptoms and treatment of partners is not indicated. BV is diagnosed by an evaluation of the vaginal flora under a microscope. Treatment is recommended not just because the symptoms are unpleasant but also because BV has been

associated with increased risk of PID, complications in pregnancy, and transmission of HIV. The condition is treated with the antibiotic metronidazole, which can be taken orally or vaginally.[42]

Viral STIs

Viral STIs cannot be cured, making prevention even more important than in cases of bacterial STIs. Vaccination is an option for some of the viral STIs, and symptoms can be treated.

Human Papillomavirus Human papillomavirus (HPV) is the most common STI in the United States. There are more than 40 types of HPV. Some types are associated with genital warts, others with cancers of the cervix, vulva, penis, anus, mouth, throat, and other areas. Strains associated with cancer are called high-risk strains; of these, two strains (HPV-16, HPV-18) are associated with 70 percent of cervical cancer cases. Strains associated with genital warts are called low-risk strains; of these, two strains (HPV-6, HPV-11) are most commonly associated with 90 percent of genital warts.

HPV is transmitted by skin-to-skin contact, usually through penetrative vaginal or anal sex, but it can be transmitted with oral sex and from woman to woman. Weeks to months after exposure to low-risk strains of HPV, both men and women can develop genital warts—flat or raised, small or large, pinkish lesions—on the penis, scrotum, vagina, anus, or skin around the genital area. They can be treated with topical medications, but this treatment is primarily for cosmetic reasons and may not alter the risk of transmission because the virus is most likely present in areas where warts are not visible.

Men are not routinely screened for high-risk HPV infection. Most women with HPV are diagnosed through screening with the Papanicolaou smear (Pap test), which can detect cervical cancer or precancerous lesions. After infection with HPV, the cells of the cervix undergo specific changes that can be identified under a microscope. If mild abnormalities in the cervical cells are noted, HPV testing can be performed to determine if a high-risk (cancer-causing) strain of HPV is present.

Estimates of U.S. women infected with HPV are 35 percent of women aged 14 to 19; 29 percent, aged 20 to 29; 13 percent, aged 30 to 39; 11 percent, aged 40 to 49; and 6.3 percent, aged 50 to 65.[41] Among women with HPV infection, the majority will clear the infection within two years. A small percentage of women will go on to have persistent infection and increased risk for cervical cancer. Risk appears to be higher in women who smoke and who have impaired immune systems, such as is caused by HIV infection. Given the high rates of spontaneous clearance and the very low rates of cervical cancer in young women, the recommended age for starting Pap screening has been raised from 18 to 21, regardless of the age of onset of sexual activity; then every three years until age 30 if normal and every five years from age 30 to 65 if Pap is normal and HPV testing is negative.[43]

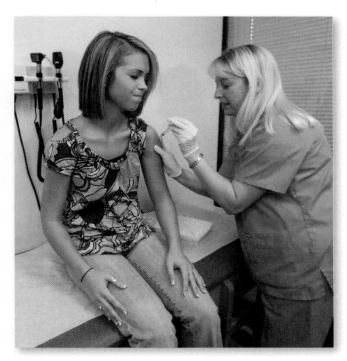

■ The vaccine Gardasil, approved for females and males 9 to 26 years of age, protects against strains of HPV that cause 70 percent of cervical cancer cases and 90 percent of genital warts cases.

Men and women who have receptive anal intercourse are at high risk for anal HPV infection and anal cancer. A test called an anal Pap can be used to collect a sample of cells from the rectum to be evaluated for precancerous changes. Currently, anal Pap or anal HPV testing is not recommended as a routine screening for men, but some organizations are beginning to recommend it for men who have sex with men.[44,45]

Consistent and correct use of condoms may reduce the risk of transmission of HPV but may not provide full protection because HPV can infect skin not covered by the condom. Two vaccines are available to reduce risk of HPV infection and are optimally effective when given prior to the onset of sexual activity. Gardasil protects against HPV strains 6, 11, 16, and 18; it is approved for females 9 to 26 years of age and males 9 through 26 years of age. Cervarix is the second vaccine and protects against two strains of HPV (16 and 18). It is currently approved only for females 10 through 25 years of age.[46,47]

Genital Herpes Genital herpes is caused by the herpes simplex virus (HSV), which has two strains, HSV-1 and HSV-2. Both strains can infect the mouth, genitals, or skin. HSV-1, however, is often associated with lesions in and around the mouth (cold sores). This type of herpes is frequently acquired in childhood from nonsexual transmission. An estimated 16 percent of U.S. adults have genital HSV-2 infection, and many do not know that they are infected.[41,48]

Because there is no cure for HSV infection, prevention is particularly important (see the box, "Nate: Dealing With a Herpes Diagnosis"). Condoms partially protect people against infection with HSV, but they are not 100 percent effective. Condoms must be used at all times when there is genital-to-genital contact and not just when a lesion is present because the virus can be spread even without evidence of a sore. Several different vaccines for HSV are currently under study. Antiviral medications are available that shorten the course of outbreaks and reduce their frequency. These medications may also reduce the risk of transmission to sexual partners.[42]

Hepatitis Hepatitis (inflammation of the liver) can be caused by several viruses, but the most common ones are hepatitis A, B, and C. Hepatitis C was discussed earlier in the context of injection drug use, the most common route of acquiring the infection. Hepatitis A and B are both easily transmitted through sexual acts. Hepatitis A is transmitted through fecal-oral contact and can be spread through contact with contaminated food or water. The people at greatest risk for sexual transmission of hepatitis A are those who have oral-anal contact or penile-anal intercourse.

A safe and effective vaccine is available for hepatitis A and is now routinely recommended as part of the childhood vaccine series. Vaccination is recommended for adults who did not receive the vaccine in childhood and who are in a high-risk group, such as men who have sex with men, illicit drug users, people with chronic liver disease, and the general population in regions that have high rates of hepatitis A or before travel to such areas.[42]

Most hepatitis B infections in the United States are sexually transmitted, although the infection can also be spread by exposure to infected blood. Worldwide, hepatitis B is a major cause of liver disease, liver failure, and liver cancer; unlike hepatitis A, it can cause chronic liver disease. The chance of developing chronic disease varies by age at the time of infection, with risk decreasing with age of exposure. Chronic infection carries an increased risk of liver failure and liver cancer.

A safe and effective vaccine for hepatitis B is available, and universal vaccination of all children is recommended. Adolescents and adults who were not vaccinated in childhood and are sexually active should be vaccinated; some colleges encourage hepatitis B vaccinations for all entering students. Vaccinations are currently required for all health care workers, and all pregnant women are screened for the virus.[42]

Other STIs

Several other nonbacterial, nonviral infections are transmitted sexually or involve the genital area. Most are treatable infections.

Nate: Dealing With a Herpes Diagnosis

Nate, a second-year student at a community college, had just come home from the student health center after being diagnosed with genital herpes. A week ago he had noticed a sore on his penis and had gone to the doctor to get it checked out, even though he felt embarrassed. The doctor did a culture and gave him the results today. He also gave him a prescription for acyclovir, an antiviral medication that would help reduce the number of future outbreaks, though Nate would carry the virus with him forever.

Nate was still in shock at the results. He couldn't believe he had an STI. He found himself wondering how he got it—he had been with his current girlfriend, Stacy, for more than a year. The doctor had explained that he may have contracted herpes from a previous partner and just not had any symptoms yet. The doctor told him he needed to discuss his diagnosis with his girlfriend. That thought filled Nate with dread and embarrassment. He felt confused as he did not know if he had this virus from previous relationships or if he had contracted it from Stacy. What if Stacy had cheated on him and had given him the infection?

To make matters worse, Stacy had just left for a quarter-long internship in a city three hours away. They had been arguing a lot before she left, and they hadn't talked much since then.

He worried about how she was going to react. Would she suspect him of cheating and possibly break up with him? His mind raced forward—if they broke up and he started dating again, he would eventually have to tell other women that he had herpes. He couldn't *not* tell them and have sex with them—he would never do something like that—but what if they didn't want to date him or have sex with him after he told them?

Nate brought his thoughts back to the present situation. He felt stuck and alone. He missed Stacy—she was the one he told everything. Even though they had been fighting, he didn't want to break up. He knew he needed to talk with her to work through their problems and tell her about his diagnosis. He sent her a text asking if they could talk later that day and spent the rest of the afternoon planning what to say.

- How do you think you would feel if you were diagnosed with an STI? How hard would it be to tell your current and/or former partners? How about your future partners?

- What are a person's ethical obligations under these circumstances? Are they different in different situations (e.g., a hook-up) or with different people?

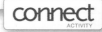

Trichomoniasis Trichomoniasis is caused by a protozoan and is transmitted from person to person by sexual activity. Sexual partners of the infected person need to be contacted and treated to prevent the further spread and recurrence of the infection.[42]

Candidiasis Candidiasis is usually caused by the yeast *Candida albicans*. Symptoms of yeast infection include vaginal discharge, itching, soreness, and burning with urination. Yeast infections are not usually acquired through sexual intercourse, but they can be mistaken for an STI because the symptoms are similar. *C. albicans* can be a normal part of the vaginal flora and may overgrow in response to changes in the vaginal environment, such as those caused by antibiotics or diabetes.

Candidiasis is treated by antifungal medications available over the counter that can be taken orally as a pill or applied to the vagina as a tablet suppository or as a cream. If a woman is unsure of the diagnosis, has recurrences, or is at risk for STIs, she should have the diagnosis confirmed by a health care provider before she treats herself. Treatment of partners is not generally needed.[42]

Pubic Lice and Scabies Pubic lice and scabies are ectoparasites that can be sexually transmitted. Pubic lice (or "crabs") infect the skin in the pubic region and cause intense itching. Scabies can infect the skin on any part of the body and, again, cause intense itching. In adults, both pubic lice and scabies are most often sexually transmitted, but in children, scabies is usually acquired through nonsexual contact.

Both infections are treated with a medicated cream or shampoo containing permethrin. Bedding and clothing must be decontaminated to prevent reinfection.

PREVENTION OF INFECTIOUS DISEASES

There are many steps that you as an individual can take to protect yourself from infectious diseases. Each of these measures will in turn reduce the risk of spread and the rates of disease in your community.

- *Support your immune system by eating a balanced diet, getting enough exercise and sleep, managing stress, not smoking, and adopting other practices that are part of a healthy lifestyle.*

- *Cover your cough.* If you need to cough or sneeze, cover your mouth with a tissue or cough/sneeze into your upper arm (not your hand!). Put used tissues into a wastebasket.

- *Avoid touching your face or mouth.* Every time you touch doorknobs, counters, and other objects, you are potentially picking up germs on your hands. Avoid transmitting these to your nose or mouth by not touching your face unless you have just washed your hands.

- *Get an annual flu shot and booster vaccines as recommended.* Follow government recommendations for vaccinations for both adults and children.

- *Minimize your use of antibiotics.*

- *If you have been exposed to an infectious disease, minimize the chances that you will pass it on to someone else.* For example, if you have a cold or the flu, follow good hygiene practices such as washing your hands frequently, stay home from work, and avoid crowded public places. If you have been exposed to an STI, take appropriate action—get tested and complete treatment if needed. Do not resume sexual activity until your partner is treated, and consider safer sex practices.

- *Practice the ABCDs of STI prevention:* **A**bstain from sex until you are ready for a long-term committed relationship, and abstain between relationships; **B**e faithful, and maintain a mutually monogamous relationship with an uninfected partner; use **C**ondoms; promote **D**etection of any STIs by being tested and following recommended screening guidelines. If you have been exposed to an STI or have symptoms, see your physician for testing and treatment, and tell any sexual partners that they have been exposed so that they can be treated too. If you are in high risk relationships, consider preexposure prophylaxis for HIV.

- *If you are planning a trip to a new part of the country or a new country, learn what infectious diseases are common there and how you can decrease your risk of infection.*

- *Reduce the likelihood that new diseases will take hold in your community, with such actions as getting rid of any standing water in your yard where mosquitoes could breed.*

Infectious diseases will always be part of human existence. By being vigilant, we can reduce their negative impact on our lives.

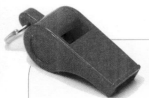

You Make the Call

Should Colleges Tighten Vaccination Requirements?

In October 2011, an outbreak of mumps occurred on the campus of the University of California, Berkeley, with an estimated 40 students having confirmed cases. Although mumps is usually mild, it occasionally has serious complications, and it is extremely contagious. The student health center encouraged students to come in for a booster shot of measles-mumps-rubella (MMR) vaccine regardless of immunization status. UC Berkeley recommends (but does not require) that students receive two doses of MMR prior to enrollment.

In 2013, Princeton University had eight confirmed student cases of serogroup B meningococcal disease and, unrelated, the University of California, Santa Barbara, had four confirmed student cases. On both campuses, the serogroup B strain was not covered by the standard U.S. meningococcal vaccine recommended for adolescents and college students, so the FDA allowed temporary voluntary use of a serogroup B vaccine used in Europe, Canada, and Australia.

These cases exemplify the ethical dilemma frequently faced by society, in which individual freedom is pitted against the collective welfare of the community, or the "common good." College campuses are uniquely vulnerable to these dilemmas. Colleges and universities are small communities of people living in close contact with each other, whether in residence halls, off-campus housing, classrooms, or shared eating facilities. In addition, students, faculty, and staff frequently travel around the world for recreation, academic research, and family opportunities. As such, they have an increased likelihood of exposure to infectious disease. Returning students, faculty, and staff can bring infections back to campus, where they may spread rapidly.

In the mumps case, UC Berkeley merely recommended students receive a second MMR vaccine. In the meningococcal meningitis cases, both campuses offered a vaccine approved for use in other countries. Some health experts have proposed stricter requirements in such situations, including the following:

- *Immunizations for a range of diseases could be required prior to entry onto campus.* Currently, most colleges require one or two doses of MMR and recommend but do not require immunization for such diseases as meningococcal infection, varicella (chickenpox), pertussis (whooping cough), influenza, and other childhood and adult infectious diseases. To increase "herd immunity" and reduce the risk of outbreaks, colleges could require immunization for all these diseases.

- *Travel to high-risk areas by students, faculty, and staff could be restricted.* Currently, the CDC and the World Health Organization offer travel warnings, precautions, and news of outbreaks in the states and around the world; occasionally, they recommend that travelers avoid certain areas or countries if an outbreak risk is high. Colleges could similarly limit or restrict travel.

- *Travelers returning from certain parts of the world could be prevented from entering campus for a certain period of time.* The CDC recommends that travelers returning from countries with outbreaks of new and emerging diseases monitor themselves for symptoms for 10 days prior to returning home or stay at home for 10 days after re`turning. Colleges could enforce this restriction on campus.

Continued…

Concluded...

■ *Individuals with infectious diseases could be quarantined.* This course of action has been proposed in the event of a pandemic flu outbreak. Colleges could house students, faculty, or staff in separate facilities for the duration of their illness so that the disease could be contained.

Each of these proposals has its advantages and its drawbacks. Some people think colleges and universities should tighten their restrictions to protect the community and promote the common good. Others see such restrictions as violations of personal freedom, if not civil rights. What do you think?

Pros

■ Required vaccination reduces the risk of disease for the entire college community. When vaccination levels are high overall, even the few who aren't or can't be vaccinated are protected by herd immunity because widespread vaccination shrinks the reservoir of infectious agents.

■ College campuses are unique, tightly linked communities with a high risk of contagion should an infectious agent be introduced.

■ Colleges have a responsibility to protect students and other community members from unnecessary risk. Requiring vaccination and taking other restrictive measures helps ensure health and safety for everyone.

Cons

■ Individuals should have freedom of choice about health risks and what they do with their bodies. They should not have to take personal risks, such as those associated with vaccination, for the good of the community.

■ Travel advisories by the CDC and the World Health Organization are usually issued as recommendations. Colleges do not have the right to enforce a different standard.

■ Isolation and quarantine are difficult to enforce, and the threat of such treatment may discourage people from seeking appropriate medical care. Thus, these measures could actually increase the risk of infectious disease outbreaks.

connect
ACTIVITY

Sources: "Recommendations for Institutional Prematriculation Immunization," American College Health Association, 2013, from www.acha.org/topics/vaccine.cfm; "A Resource Guide for Parents," U.C. Berkeley, http://calparents.berkeley.edu/guide/advising/todo.html. "Serogroup B Meningococcal Vaccine and Outbreaks" Center for Disease Control and Prevention, 2013, www.cdc.gov/meningococcal/outbreaks/vaccine-serogroupB.html.

In Review

What causes infection, and how does the body protect itself from infectious diseases?
Several different types of pathogens cause infection and illness in humans, categorized as viruses, bacteria, prions, fungi, helminths, protozoa, and ectoparasites. Infection occurs when one of these microorganisms gains entry to the body and reproduces, sometimes causing symptoms of illness. The body has external barriers to keep pathogens out and a complex immune system to destroy them when they get in.

How are infectious diseases changing?
Technological advances—for example, blood banks, organ transplants, and centralized food distribution—have created new opportunities for widespread disease transmission, as have global travel, changes in sexual behavior, injection drug use, and tattooing and piercing. Overuse of antibiotics has led to the appearance of resistant strains of many bacteria.

What are the most common infectious diseases?
Currently the top four infectious diseases worldwide are pneumonia, diarrhea, tuberculosis, and malaria. On college campuses in the United States, the top four are pertussis (whooping cough), mumps, *Staphylococcus aureus* skin infections, and urinary tract infections.

What are the most serious and most common sexually transmitted diseases?
HIV/AIDS is the most serious STI because it is fatal, although it is now possible, with medications, to live with HIV infection as a chronic condition for many years. The virus attacks and eventually overwhelms the immune system, leaving the body vulnerable to opportunistic infections like tuberculosis. The bacterial STIs—which include chlamydia, gonorrhea, pelvic inflammatory disease, syphilis, and bacterial vaginosis—can be treated with antibiotics. The viral STIs—which include human papillomavirus, genital herpes, and hepatitis A and B—can be controlled but not cured. Other STIs include trichomoniasis, candidiasis, and pubic lice and scabies.

How can infectious diseases be prevented?
The best defense is being in good health, so a healthy lifestyle is important. Getting all recommended vaccinations also helps, as do avoiding exposure, practicing safer sex, and minimizing unnecessary use of antibiotics.

Cardiovascular Disease, Diabetes, and Chronic Lung Diseases

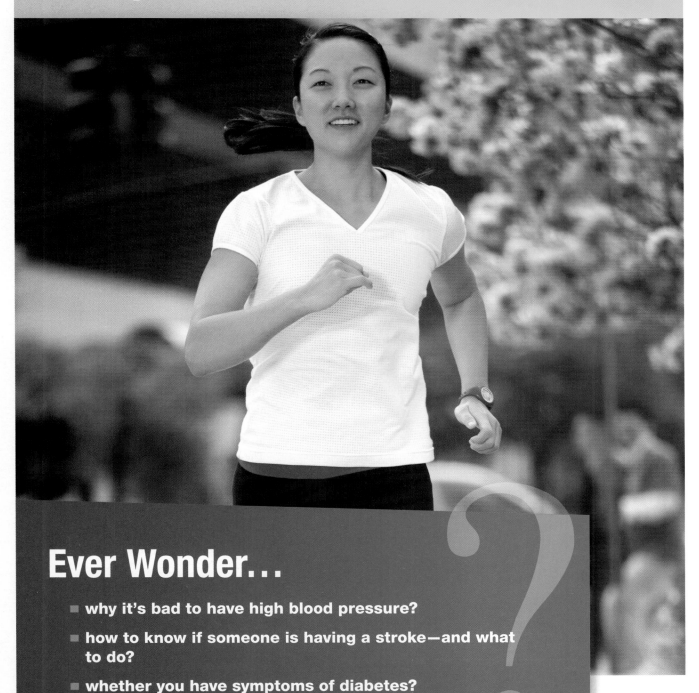

Ever Wonder...

- why it's bad to have high blood pressure?

- how to know if someone is having a stroke—and what to do?

- whether you have symptoms of diabetes?

N ot long ago, people believed that heart attacks and strokes were like bolts out of the blue, happening without warning. Today, we know that heart attacks, strokes, and other chronic diseases are the result of processes that begin much earlier, often in childhood. As public health measures have reduced mortality from infectious diseases and life spans have increased, chronic diseases—including cardiovascular disease (CVD), diabetes, chronic lung diseases, and cancer—have emerged as the leading cause of death in the United States and the rest of the developed world. This chapter presents an overview of CVD, diabetes, and chronic lung diseases, along with guidelines for living a healthy lifestyle that reduces the risk for these diseases.[1,2] Cancer is covered in Chapter 15.

CARDIOVASCULAR DISEASE (CVD)

The leading cause of death for men and women in the United States, **cardiovascular disease (CVD)** accounts for one in every three deaths. An estimated 82.6 million Americans live with cardiovascular disease, and more than half are under the age of 60. Fortunately,

cardiovascular disease (CVD)
Any disease involving the heart and/or blood vessels.

cardiovascular system
The heart and blood vessels that circulate blood throughout the body.

pulmonary circulation
Pumping of oxygen-poor blood to the lungs and oxygen-rich blood back to the heart by the right side of the heart.

systemic circulation
Pumping of oxygen-rich blood to the body and oxygen-poor blood back to the heart by the left side of the heart.

vena cava
Largest veins in the body; they carry oxygen-poor blood from the body back to the heart.

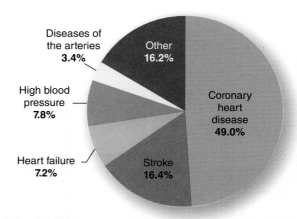

figure 14.2   **Percentage of deaths from types of CVD, United States, 2013.**
Source: "Heart Disease and Stroke Statistics—2013 Update," Chart 13-5, American Heart Association, 2013, Dallas: AHA.

the death rate from CVD for men has been decreasing for more than 30 years and more recently for women (Figure 14.1). The drop in the death rate is believed to be the result of lifestyle changes, improved recognition and treatment of risk factors, and improved treatment.[3] *Cardiovascular disease* is a general term that includes heart attack, stroke, peripheral artery disease, congestive heart failure, and other conditions (Figure 14.2).

The Cardiovascular System

The **cardiovascular system** consists of a network of blood vessels (arteries, veins, and capillaries) and a pump (the heart) that circulate blood throughout the body. The heart is a fist-sized muscle with four chambers—the right and left atria and the right and left ventricles—separated by valves.

The right side of the heart is involved in **pulmonary circulation**—pumping oxygen-poor (deoxygenated) blood to the lungs and oxygen-rich blood back to the heart. The left side of the heart is involved in **systemic circulation**—pumping oxygen-rich blood to the rest of the body and returning oxygen-poor blood to the heart (Figure 14.3).

In pulmonary circulation, oxygen-poor blood returning from the body to the heart enters the right atrium via large veins called the inferior and superior **vena cava**. After the right atrium fills, it contracts and moves the blood into the right ventricle. The right ventricle fills and contracts, moving the blood into the lungs via the right and left pulmonary arteries. The pulmonary artery branches into a network of smaller arteries and arterioles that eventually become the pulmonary capillaries. Capillaries are the smallest blood vessels; some capillary walls are only one cell thick, readily allowing the

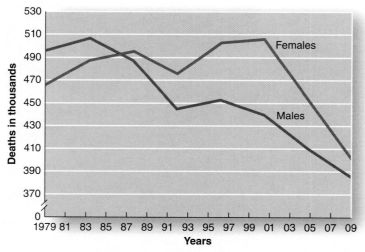

figure 14.1   **Cardiovascular disease mortality trends for males and females, United States, 1979–2009.**
Source: Centers for Disease Control and Prevention/National Center for Health Statistics, www.cdc.gov/nchs; "Heart Disease and Stroke Statistics—2013 Update," Chart 13-17, American Heart Association, 2013, Dallas: AHA.

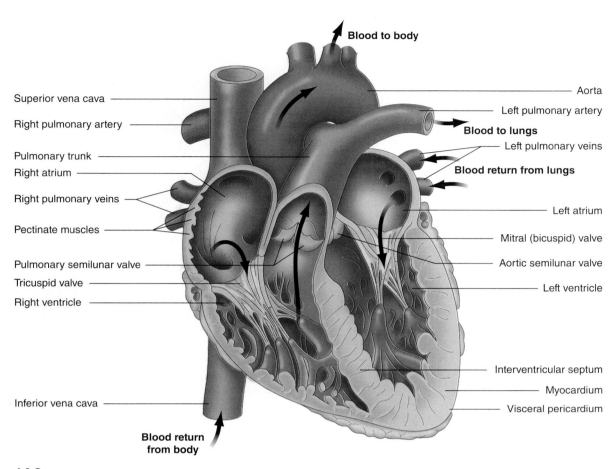

Blood to body

Superior vena cava

Right pulmonary artery

Pulmonary trunk

Right atrium

Right pulmonary veins

Pectinate muscles

Pulmonary semilunar valve

Tricuspid valve

Right ventricle

Inferior vena cava

Blood return from body

Aorta

Left pulmonary artery

Blood to lungs

Left pulmonary veins

Blood return from lungs

Left atrium

Mitral (bicuspid) valve

Aortic semilunar valve

Left ventricle

Interventricular septum

Myocardium

Visceral pericardium

figure 14.3   **The heart, showing interior chambers, valves, and major arteries and veins.**

exchange of gases and molecules. In the interweaving network of capillaries, the red blood cells in the blood pick up oxygen and discard carbon dioxide, a waste product from the cells. The capillaries then unite and form venules, and venules join to become pulmonary veins. The pulmonary veins return oxygen-rich blood from the lungs to the left atrium of the heart.

In systemic circulation, the left atrium fills and contracts to move oxygen-rich blood into the left ventricle. The left ventricle fills, contracts, and moves oxygen-rich blood into the body via the **aorta**, the largest artery in the body. The aorta branches into smaller and smaller arteries, and eventually, oxygen-rich, nutrient-rich blood enters the capillaries located throughout the body. At these sites, red blood cells release oxygen and nutrients to the tissues and pick up carbon dioxide to be carried back to the lungs. The capillaries unite to form veins and eventually connect to the inferior and superior vena cava, which returns the oxygen-poor blood to the heart. The cycle then repeats.

Like other muscles of the body, the heart needs oxygen and nutrients provided by blood; the blood being pumped through the heart does not provide nourishment for the heart muscle itself. Two medium-sized arteries, called **coronary arteries**, supply blood to the heart muscle (see Figure 14.4). The main vessels are the right coronary artery and the left coronary artery, each distributing blood to different parts of the heart. Blood flow is important, because when a vessel is narrowed, the muscle that it supplies does not get enough blood.

The four chambers of the heart contract to pump blood in a coordinated fashion. The contraction occurs in response to an electrical signal that starts in a group of cells called the **sinus node** or **sinoatrial (SA) node** in the right atrium. The signal spreads through a defined course leading first to contraction of the right and left atria, then to contraction of the right and left ventricles. The contraction and relaxation of the ventricles are what we feel and hear as the heartbeat. The contraction phase is called *systole* and the relaxation phase is called *diastole*.

aorta
Largest artery in the body; it leaves the heart and branches into smaller arteries, arterioles, and capillaries carrying oxygen-rich blood to body tissues.

coronary arteries
Medium-sized arteries that supply blood to the heart muscle.

sinus node or sinoatrial (SA) node
Group of cells in the right atrium where the electrical signal is generated that establishes the heartbeat.

Atherosclerosis

atherosclerosis
Thickening or hardening of the arteries due to the buildup of lipid (fat) deposits.

fatty streak
Accumulation of lipoproteins within the walls of an artery.

lipoprotein
Package of proteins, phospholipids (fat molecules with phosphate groups chemically attached), and cholesterol that transports lipids in the blood.

cholesterol
Type of fat that is essential in small amounts for certain body functions.

plaque
Accumulation of debris in an artery wall, consisting of lipoproteins, white blood cells, collagen, and other substances.

aneurysm
Weak or stretched spot in an artery wall that can tear or rupture, causing sudden death.

coronary heart disease (CHD)
Atherosclerosis of the coronary arteries.

Atherosclerosis is a thickening or hardening of the arteries due to the buildup of fats, cholesterol, cellular waste products, calcium, and other substances in artery walls. It is a progressive disease that takes years to develop and starts at a young age. Autopsies of people aged 15 to 35 who died from unrelated trauma have revealed that some young people already have the beginnings of significant atherosclerosis, which shows that it is never too early to think about heart health.[4]

Healthy arteries are strong and flexible. Arteries can harden and become stiff in response to too much pressure, a process generally referred to as *arteriosclerosis*. Atherosclerosis is a common form of arteriosclerosis, and the terms are often used interchangeably. Atherosclerosis starts with damage to the inner lining (e.g., by tobacco smoke, high blood pressure, or infection), creating a *lesion* where a **fatty streak** can form. Fatty streaks consist of an accumulation of **lipoproteins**, which are a combination of proteins, phospholipids (fat molecules with phosphate groups chemically attached), and **cholesterol** (a waxy, fatlike substance that is essential in small amounts for certain body functions). Lipoproteins can be thought of as packages that carry cholesterol and fats through the bloodstream.

When lipoproteins accumulate within the wall of an artery, they can undergo chemical changes that trigger an inflammatory response, attracting white blood cells. Once at the site, white blood cells take up the altered lipoproteins. Some white blood cells leave the site, cleaning lipids from the artery wall, but if blood lipoprotein levels are high, more lipoproteins continue to accumulate. Many of the white blood cells die within the lesion, depositing lipid-rich material—a fatty streak.

The process may stop at this point, leaving a dynamic lesion that can still undergo repair or can develop further in the artery wall. Together with the white blood cells, smooth muscle cells release collagen and other proteins to form a **plaque**, an accumulation of debris that undergoes continuing damage, bleeding, and calcification. Plaques cause the

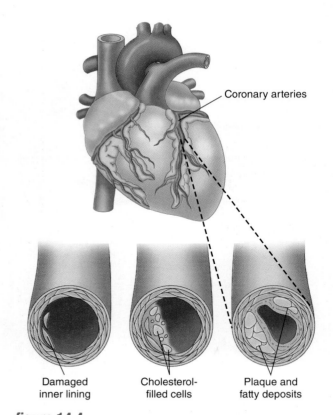

Coronary arteries

Damaged inner lining

Cholesterol-filled cells

Plaque and fatty deposits

figure 14.4 **The process of atherosclerosis.**
The process begins with damage to the lining of an artery and progresses to narrowing or blockage of the artery by fatty deposits and plaques.

artery wall to enlarge and bulge into the *lumen,* the channel through which the blood flows, slowing blood flow and reducing the amount of blood that can reach the tissue supplied by the artery (Figure 14.4). Plaques can also break off and completely block the artery, preventing any blood from flowing through.

Heart attacks, strokes, and peripheral vascular disease are all consequences of the narrowing of arteries caused by atherosclerosis. A diagnosis of one of these diseases suggests risk for the others. Atherosclerosis may also weaken an artery wall, causing a stretching of the artery known as an **aneurysm**. Aneurysms can rupture, tear, and bleed, causing sudden death.

Coronary Heart Disease (CHD) and Heart Attack

When atherosclerosis occurs in a coronary artery, the result is **coronary heart disease (CHD)** and, often, a heart attack. Coronary heart disease (also called coronary artery disease [CAD]) is the leading form of CVD, accounting for 1 in 6 U.S. deaths. An estimated 16.3 million Americans are living with CHD. Those who survive a heart attack are often left with damaged hearts and significantly altered lives.[3]

Consumer Clipboard

Aspirin Therapy for Heart Disease and Heart Attack

Nearly 36 percent of American adults—more than 50 million people—take aspirin regularly to reduce their risk of CVD. Because of its ability to inhibit blood clotting, aspirin is often recommended for anyone who has a history of heart attack, unstable angina, ischemic stroke, or transient ischemic attack. A regular regimen of aspirin is usually between 80 and 160 mg per day; a baby aspirin (81 mg) is often recommended for daily aspirin therapy. Someone experiencing the symptoms of a heart attack may be advised to chew a 325-mg aspirin tablet slowly. However, the decision to take aspirin should be made in collaboration with a physician because aspirin therapy has both benefits and risks.

Benefits

- Inhibits the formation of blood clots, which can clog or block arteries.
- Reduces the risk of heart attack.
- Reduces the risk of stroke.
- Reduces the damage to the heart during a heart attack.
- Decreases the pain and inflammation associated with CVD, such as angina or pain in the legs.
- Reduces the risk of death from all causes, particularly among older adults, people with heart disease, and people who are physically unfit.

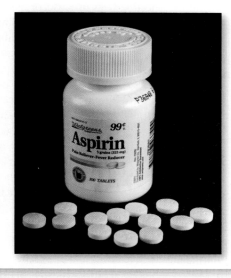

Risks

- Increases the risk of internal bleeding and stomach ulcers.
- Increases the risk of bleeding into the brain during a hemorrhagic stroke.
- Should not be taken by pregnant women.
- Should not be taken by anyone with an allergy to aspirin.
- Should not be taken by people about to undergo surgery.
- Should not be taken by children or youth under age 18 who are recovering from a viral infection like the flu or chickenpox.

Source: "Heart Disease and Aspirin Therapy," 2012, WebMD, www.webmd.com/heart-disease/aspirin-therapy.

When a coronary artery becomes narrowed or blocked, the heart muscle does not get enough oxygen-rich blood, a condition called **ischemia**. If the artery is completely blocked, the person has a heart attack, or **myocardial infarction (MI)**. The blockage may be caused by an atherosclerotic plaque that has broken loose or a blood clot (a *thrombus*) that has formed in a narrowed or damaged artery. The latter condition is called a **coronary thrombosis** and may cause sudden death. During a heart attack, the area of muscle supplied by the blocked coronary artery is completely deprived of oxygen. If blood flow is not quickly restored, that part of the heart muscle will die (see the box, "Aspirin Therapy for Heart Disease and Heart Attack").

The severity of a heart attack is determined by the location and duration of the blockage. If the blockage occurs close to the aorta, where the coronary arteries are just starting to branch, a large area of heart muscle is deprived of oxygen. If the blockage is farther out in a smaller coronary artery, the area of muscle supplied is smaller. The duration of the blockage is usually determined by the time between onset of symptoms and initiation of medical or surgical treatment to reopen the artery. Duration is directly dependent on how quickly a person recognizes the symptoms of a myocardial infarction and gets help.

A heart attack may occur when extra work is demanded of the heart, such as during exercise or emotional stress, but it can also occur during light activity or even rest. A classic symptom of a heart attack is chest pain, often described as a sensation of pressure, fullness, or squeezing in the midportion of the chest. However, symptoms vary, and 37 percent of women and 27 percent of men typically do not have chest pain or discomfort during a heart attack. Men and women can both have a range of symptoms, including pain radiating to the jaw, back, shoulders, or arms. However, women may be less likely to have classic symptoms of a heart attack. They may also be less aware that heart disease is a major health concern and thus less likely to seek help for their symptoms. Although awareness has increased over the past decade, only 54 percent of women are aware that heart disease is the leading cause of death for women. African American, Asian American, and Hispanic women were even less likely to know that heart disease is the leading cause of death, and their awareness of heart attack signs is low.[3–7]

ischemia
Insufficient supply of oxygen and nutrients to tissue, caused by narrowed or blocked arteries.

myocardial infarction (MI)
Lack of blood to the heart muscle with resulting death of heart tissue; often called a heart attack.

coronary thrombosis
Blockage of a coronary artery by a blood clot that may cause sudden death.

When coronary arteries are narrowed but not completely blocked, the person may experience **angina**—pain, pressure, heaviness, or tightness in the center of the chest that may radiate to the neck, arms, or shoulders. Half of all heart attacks are preceded by angina. The difference between a heart attack and angina is that the pain of angina resolves, whereas the pain of a heart attack continues. Angina can be controlled with medical treatment.

Many physical conditions can cause pain in the chest, including irritated esophagus, arthritis of the neck or ribs, gas in the colon, stomach ulcers, and gallbladder disease. Chest pain can also be caused by weight lifting or other heavy lifting or vigorous activity. If you are used to chest pain from any of these causes, you may be inclined to ignore angina or chest pain from a heart attack. Don't let complaisance or confusion delay your efforts to seek help if you experience the signs of a heart attack.

Arrhythmias The pumping of the heart is usually a well-coordinated event, controlled by an electrical signal emanating from the sinus node in the right atrium, as described earlier. The sinus node establishes a rate of 60 to 100 beats per minute for a normal adult heart. The rate increases in response to increased demand on the heart, such as during exercise, and slows in response to reduced demand, such as during relaxation or sleep. If the signal is disrupted, it can cause an **arrhythmia**, or disorganized beating of the heart. The disorganized beating is usually not as effective at pumping blood.

An arrhythmia is any type of irregular heartbeat. It may be an occasional skipped beat, a rapid or slow rate, or an irregular pattern. Not all arrhythmias are serious or cause for concern. In fact, most people have occasional irregular heartbeats every day; some people do not even notice them. However, arrhythmia may cause noticeable symptoms, including palpitations, a sensation of fluttering in the chest, chest pain, light-headedness, shortness of breath, and fatigue.

Arrhythmias occur for a variety of reasons, including damage to the sinus node, chemical imbalances, or the use of caffeine, alcohol, tobacco, cocaine, or medications.

Sudden Cardiac Death **Ventricular fibrillation** is a particular type of arrhythmia in which the ventricles contract rapidly and erratically, causing the heart to quiver or "tremor" rather than beat. Blood cannot be pumped by the heart when the ventricles fibrillate. The result is **sudden cardiac death**—an abrupt loss of heart function. An estimated 0.3 to 1 in 100,000 high school athletes and 5,900 infants and children die each year from sudden cardiac death. Vigorous exercise can be a trigger for lethal arrhythmia when an underlying heart abnormality is present. Under age 35, sudden cardiac death is usually due to congenital cardiac abnormalities (birth defects). Over age 35, the cause is usually coronary artery disease.[3]

Ventricular fibrillation can be reversed with an electrical shock from a defibrillator, which can restart the heart's normal rhythm. Automated external defibrillators (AEDs) are often installed in public places like gyms and airports. AEDs are designed for use by the general public, ideally by people who have received training at a CPR, first-aid, or first-responder class. Every minute counts, however; the chances of survival are reduced by 7 to 10 percent for every minute following cardiac arrest. About 310,000 Americans die each year from sudden cardiac death in emergency rooms or prior to reaching the hospital. Only 32 percent of these people receive bystander CPR (see the box, "What to Do During a Heart Attack or Stroke Emergency").

Stroke

When blood flow to the brain or part of the brain is blocked, the result is a **stroke, or cerebrovascular accident (CVA)**. Stroke is the fourth-leading cause of death in the United States, after heart disease, cancer, and chronic lung disease, and is a leading cause of severe, long-term disability.

angina
Intermittent pain, pressure, heaviness, or tightness in the center of the chest caused by a narrowed coronary artery.

arrhythmia
Irregular or disorganized heartbeat.

ventricular fibrillation
Type of arrhythmia in which the ventricles contract rapidly and erratically, causing the heart to quiver or "tremor" rather than beat.

sudden cardiac death
Abrupt loss of heart function caused by an irregular or ineffective heartbeat.

stroke, or cerebrovascular accident (CVA)
Lack of blood flow to the brain with resulting death of brain tissue.

■ Automated external defibrillators can be used by the general public and thus decrease the time that it takes to provide defibrillation to someone in cardiac arrest. A variety of models are shown here.

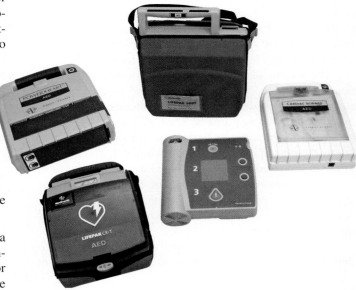

Action Skill-Builder

What to Do During a Heart Attack or Stroke Emergency

Would you know what to do if a friend, colleague, family member, or stranger had a heart attack or stroke? Recognizing the signs of a heart attack or stroke and responding and getting treatment quickly are critical to survival. Here are steps you can take to be prepared:

1. *Recognize the signs.* People are often embarrassed or in denial when they have a heart attack or stroke. If you know the signs, you can recognize the situation and let the person know how serious it is.

   a. *Heart attack:* chest discomfort that lasts more than a few minutes or that comes and goes, often in the center of the chest (can feel like pressure, squeezing, fullness, or pain); discomfort in other areas of the upper body (can include pain in one or both arms, the back, neck, jaw or stomach); shortness of breath; nausea; cold sweat; light-headedness, weakness, or faintness.

   b. *Stroke:* sudden numbness or weakness in the face, arm, or leg, especially on one side of the body; sudden confusion, trouble speaking or understanding; sudden trouble seeing in one or both eyes; sudden trouble walking, dizziness, loss of balance or coordination; sudden, severe headache with no known cause.

2. *Don't delay—call 9-1-1.* New treatments can break up the clots that cause heart attacks and strokes, but they must be started as soon as possible (within hours). Paramedics can begin treatments on the way to the hospital and are equipped to administer external defibrillation if needed.

3. *Take a cardiopulmonary resuscitation (CPR) class.* Most colleges, community centers, and fire stations offer CPR classes on a regular basis. Staying current on guidelines for activation of the emergency medical system, assessment, resuscitation, and use of an automated external defibrillator will help you stay calm and be ready. Training in the new "hands-only" CPR is now available.

Sources: American Heart Association, www.americanheart. org; "Symptom Presentation in Women with Acute Coronary Syndromes: Myth vs. Reality," by J.G. Canto, R.J. Goldberg, M.M. Hand, et al., 2007, *Archives of Internal Medicine, 167* (22), pp. 2405–2413.

Ischemic strokes account for 87 percent of all strokes and occur when an artery in the brain becomes blocked, in the same way that a heart attack occurs when a coronary artery is blocked, and prevents the brain from receiving blood flow (Figure 14.5). The blockage can be due to a **thrombus** (a blood clot that develops in a narrowed artery) or an **embolism** (a clot that develops elsewhere, often in the heart, travels to the brain, and lodges in an artery).[3]

Hemorrhagic strokes make up 13 percent of strokes and occur when a brain artery ruptures, bleeds into the surrounding area, and compresses brain tissue. Hemorrhagic strokes may be due to a head injury or a ruptured aneurysm. There are two types of hemorrhagic stroke. *Intracerebral hemorrhagic* strokes account for 10 percent and occur when the ruptured artery is within brain tissue. *Subarachnoid hemorrhagic* strokes account for 3 percent and occur when the ruptured artery is on the brain's surface and blood accumulates between the brain and the skull.[3]

As with the heart, different arteries supply different areas of the brain. The symptoms of a stroke depend on the area of the brain involved. However, these symptoms usually include the sudden onset of neurological problems, such as headaches, numbness, weakness, or speech problems.

A small percentage of people have **transient ischemic attacks (TIAs)** before having a stroke. Sometimes called "ministrokes," TIAs are periods of restricted blood supply that produce the same symptoms as a stroke, but in this case the symptoms resolve within 24 hours with little or no tissue death. A TIA should be viewed as a warning sign of stroke. After a TIA, 9 to 17 percent of people will have a stroke within the next 90 days. Early recognition and rapid treatment are as important for TIA and stroke as they are for heart disease. Treatment can improve survival and reduce complications but must be given quickly.[3]

ischemic strokes
Strokes caused by blockage in a blood vessel in the brain.

thrombus
Blood clot that forms in a narrowed or damaged artery.

embolism
Blood clot that travels from elsewhere in the body.

hemorrhagic strokes
Strokes caused by rupture of a blood vessel in the brain, with bleeding into brain tissue.

transient ischemic attacks (TIA)
Periods of ischemia that temporarily produce the same symptoms as a stroke.

■ Bret Michaels, Poison lead singer, reality TV star, and father to two girls, suffered a subarachnoid hemorrhagic stroke in April 2010. Michaels, who has Type-1 diabetes, said that the stroke felt like he had been shot in the back of the head.

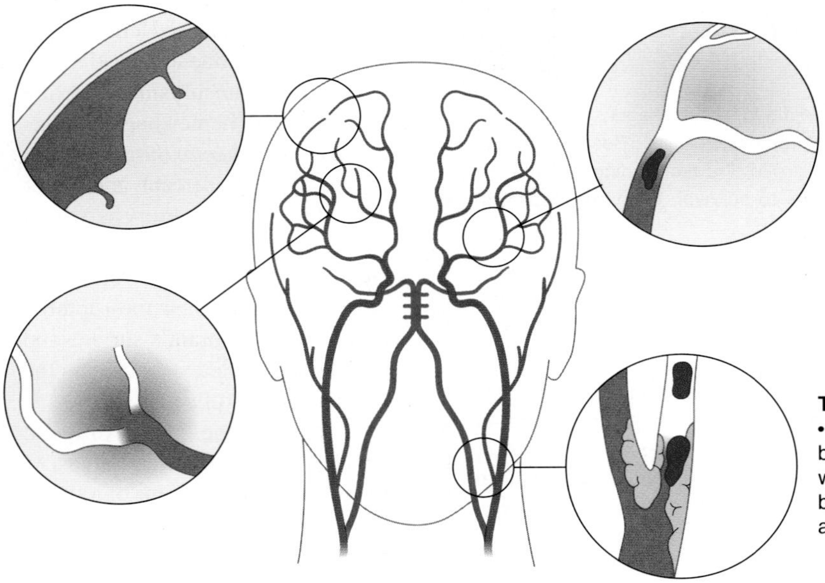

Hemorrhagic stroke
• Caused by ruptured blood vessels followed by blood leaking into tissue; more serious than ischemic stroke

Ischemic stroke
• Caused by blockage in brain blood vessels; potentially treatable with clot-busting drugs

Subarachnoid hemorrhage
• A bleed into the space between the brain and the skull

Embolic stroke
• Caused by *emboli*, blood clots that travel from elsewhere in the body to the brain blood vessels

Intracerebral hemorrhage
• A bleed from a blood vessel inside the brain

Thrombotic stroke
• Caused by *thrombi*, blood clots that form where an artery has been narrowed by atherosclerosis

figure 14.5   Types of stroke.
Source: Reprinted with permission from the *Harvard Health Letter,* April 2000. Copyright © Harvard University. For more information visit www.health.harvard.edu. Harvard Health Publications does not endorse any products or medical procedures.

Congestive Heart Failure

When the heart is not pumping the blood as well as it should, a condition known as **congestive heart failure** occurs. It can develop after a heart attack or as a result of hypertension (high blood pressure), heart valve abnormality, or disease of the heart muscle. When the heart cannot keep up its regular pumping force or rate, blood backs up into the lungs, and fluid from the backed-up blood in the pulmonary veins leaks into the lungs. A person with congestive heart failure experiences difficulty breathing, shortness of breath, and coughing, especially when lying down. Blood returning to the heart from the body also gets backed up, causing swelling of the lower legs. When blood fails to reach the brain efficiently, fatigue and confusion can result.

congestive heart failure
Condition in which the heart is not pumping the blood as well as it should, allowing blood and fluids to back up in the lungs.

mitral valve prolapse
Heart valve disorder in which the mitral valve, which separates the left ventricle from the left atrium, does not close fully, allowing blood to leak backward into the atrium.

Other Cardiovascular Diseases

Other conditions can affect the structure of the heart and blood vessels and their ability to function. Some of these conditions are congenital (present from birth), and others result from progressive diseases.

Heart Valve Disorders Four valves in the heart keep blood flowing in the correct direction through the heart (see Figure 14.3). A normally functioning valve opens easily to allow blood to flow forward and closes tightly to prevent blood from flowing backward. Sometimes a valve does not open well, preventing the smooth flow of blood, and sometimes a valve does not close tightly, allowing blood to leak backward.

These problems can be caused by congenital abnormalities, rheumatic heart disease (scarring of a heart valve that can follow untreated infection with streptococcus bacteria, usually strep throat), or an aging-related degeneration process. When valves are not functioning normally, the flow of blood is altered and the risks of blood clots and infection increase. Often, the person experiences no symptoms; if symptoms do occur, they can include shortness of breath, dizziness, fatigue, and chest pain.

The most common heart valve defect is **mitral valve prolapse** (the mitral valve separates the left atrium from the left ventricle). In this condition, the mitral valve billows backward and the edges do not fully close when the left ventricle contracts to move blood into the aorta, allowing blood to leak backward into the atrium (Figure 14.6). Mitral valve prolapse is common, affecting 5 to 10 percent of the population. People with certain types of mitral valve prolapse should take antibiotics before dental surgery and other procedures to reduce the risk of infection from bacteria introduced into the bloodstream.

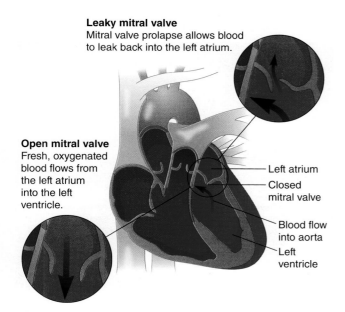

Leaky mitral valve
Mitral valve prolapse allows blood to leak back into the left atrium.

Open mitral valve
Fresh, oxygenated blood flows from the left atrium into the left ventricle.

Left atrium
Closed mitral valve
Blood flow into aorta
Left ventricle

figure 14.6 **Mitral valve prolapse.**

Congenital Heart Disease A variety of structural defects that are present at birth can involve the heart valves, major arteries and veins in or near the heart, or the heart muscle. An abnormality can cause the blood to slow down, flow in the wrong direction, or not move from one chamber to the next. Undetected cardiac abnormalities are the leading cause of death in competitive athletes. More than 35 types of heart defects have been described, and about 8 out of every 1,000 babies are born with a heart problem.[3,8]

Peripheral Vascular Disease The result of atherosclerosis in the arteries of the arms or legs (more commonly, the legs), **peripheral vascular disease (PVD)** causes pain, aches, or cramping in the muscles supplied by a narrowed blood vessel. Although it is usually not fatal, PVD causes a significant amount of disability, limiting the activity level of many older people because of pain with walking. If circulation is severely limited by the ischemia, the affected leg or arm may have to be amputated.

Cardiomyopathy **Cardiomyopathy**—disease of the heart muscle—accounts for 1 percent of heart disease deaths in the United States, with the highest rates occurring among men and Blacks. The most common form of cardiomyopathy is **dilated cardiomyopathy**, an enlargement of the heart in response to weakening of the muscle. The cause is often unknown, although a virus is suspected in some cases. Other factors that can weaken the heart muscle are toxins (alcohol, tobacco, heavy metals, and some medications), drugs, pregnancy, hypertension, and coronary artery disease.

Another form is **hypertrophic cardiomyopathy**, an abnormal thickening of one part of the heart, frequently the left ventricle. The thickened wall makes the heart abnormally

stiff, so the heart doesn't fill well. Although most people with hypertrophic cardiomyopathy have no symptoms, warning signs can include dizziness or passing out with exercise. The condition can cause heart failure, arrhythmia, and sudden death. In fact, 36 percent of cases of sudden death in young competitive athletes are due to hypertrophic cardiomyopathy. The cause of the condition is unknown in about 50 percent of cases, but in the rest, there is a genetic link. A family history of sudden death prior to age 50 is a risk factor.[3]

PROMOTING CARDIOVASCULAR HEALTH

Cardiovascular disease is a multifactorial disease (see Chapter 1), meaning that it is caused by a combination of genetic, environmental, and lifestyle factors interacting over time. Some risk factors are controllable, such as maintaining a healthy BMI, while others are not, such as being male or getting older. In 2011, the American Heart Association (AHA) developed the concept of "ideal cardiovascular health" and has mounted a campaign to improve the cardiovascular health of Americans by 20 percent and reduce the number of deaths from CVD by 20 percent by the year 2020. Ideal cardiovascular health is measured by seven health behaviors and risk factors: smoking status, healthy BMI, healthy diet, participation in physical activity, and healthy levels of blood pressure, blood glucose, and total cholesterol.[3] Unfortunately, only about 4 percent of the American public currently meet six of the seven target goals in the AHA definition of ideal cardiovascular health.

Major Controllable Factors in Cardiovascular Health

Controllable factors are ones that can be altered through individual behavior or community intervention. Given that cardiovascular disease develops gradually, we are never too young to start paying attention to these factors. Avoiding the development of CVD is preferable to treating it once it is evident.[1]

Avoid Tobacco Tobacco use is the leading risk factor for all forms of CVD. Cigarette smokers develop coronary artery disease at two to four times the rate of nonsmokers and have twice the risk of sudden cardiac death as nonsmokers.

peripheral vascular disease (PVD) Atherosclerosis in the blood vessels of the arms or legs.

cardiomyopathy Disease of the heart muscle.

dilated cardiomyopathy Enlargement of the heart in response to weakening of the muscle.

hypertrophic cardiomyopathy Abnormal thickening of one part of the heart, frequently the left ventricle.

Cigar and pipe smoking also increase the risk of coronary artery disease and perhaps the risk of stroke, although not as great an increase in risk as is associated with cigarettes.

Tobacco smoke increases risk in a variety of ways. Components of tobacco smoke damage the inner lining of blood vessels, speeding up the development of atherosclerosis. Toxins in tobacco smoke can stimulate the formation of blood clots in the coronary arteries and trigger spasms that close off the vessels. Smoking raises blood levels of LDL cholesterol ("bad" cholesterol) and decreases blood levels of HDL cholesterol ("good" cholesterol). Exposure to environmental tobacco smoke (secondhand smoke) is also a risk factor for CVD; risk appears to be proportional to the amount of daily exposure.

The risk for CVD decreases within a few years of quitting smoking.[9] Because nicotine is so addictive, the best prevention is never to start smoking. If you do smoke, quitting now can significantly reduce your risk of developing CVD.

Maintain Healthy Blood Pressure Levels **Blood pressure** is the pressure exerted by blood against the walls of arteries, and high blood pressure, or **hypertension**, occurs when the pressure is great enough to damage artery walls. Untreated high blood pressure can weaken the arteries, promote atherosclerosis, and force the heart to work harder, weakening it as well. Hypertension increases the risk for heart attack, stroke, congestive heart failure, and kidney disease; the higher the blood pressure, the greater the risk.

Blood pressure is determined by two forces—the pressure produced by the heart as it pumps the blood and the resistance of the arteries as they contain blood flow. When arteries are hardened by atherosclerosis, they are more resistant. Blood pressure is measured in millimeters of mercury (abbreviated as Hg) and stated in two numbers, such as 120/80 mmHg. The upper number represents **systolic pressure**, the pressure produced when the heart contracts; the lower number represents **diastolic pressure**, the pressure in the arteries when the heart is relaxed, between contractions. There is no definite line dividing normal blood pressure from high blood pressure, but categories have been established as guidelines on the basis of increased risk for CVD. The ideal is for the blood pressure to remain less than 120/80 mm/Hg. See Table 14.1.

Prehypertension is a category of blood pressure measurement higher than recommended but not meeting criteria

blood pressure
Force exerted by the blood against artery walls.

hypertension
Blood pressure that is forceful enough to damage artery walls.

systolic pressure
Pressure in the arteries when the heart contracts, represented by the upper number in a blood pressure measurement.

diastolic pressure
Pressure in the arteries when the heart relaxes between contractions, represented by the lower number in a blood pressure measurement.

Table 14.1 Blood Pressure Guidelines

Category	Systolic (mmHg)	Diastolic (mmHg)
Normal	Less than 120 *and*	Less than 80
Prehypertension	120–139 *or*	80–89

Hypertension
  Stage 1
  Stage 2
	140–159 *or*
	160 and above *or*
		90–99
		100 and above

Source: "The Seventh Report of the Joint National Committee on Prevention, Detection, Evaluation and Treatment of High Blood Pressure" (NIH Publication No. 03-5233), 2003, Bethesda, MD: National Heart, Lung, and Blood Institute, National Institutes of Health.

for hypertension; the category has been identified to target people at high risk of developing hypertension. An estimated 29.7 percent of the U.S. population aged 20 and older have prehypertension. Blood pressure in this range should prompt aggressive lifestyle change and increased monitoring to reduce future risk.

Hypertension is often referred to as the "silent killer" because it usually causes no symptoms. More than 78 million people in the United States (nearly one in three adults) and more than 1 billion people worldwide are estimated to have high blood pressure; rates are similar for men and women. Although people are becoming more aware of this condition, 18 percent of people with high blood pressure do not know they have it.[3,10]

In approximately 95 percent of cases, no single cause of hypertension can be identified. In Western societies, aging seems to be a factor, but this is not the case in other cultures. Genetics plays a role in some cases. Other factors that contribute to elevated blood pressure include high salt consumption, use of alcohol, low potassium levels, physical inactivity, and obesity. Less frequently, medical conditions can cause hypertension. Women can develop hypertension during pregnancy or while taking oral contraceptive pills. Among children and adolescents, rates of hypertension are increasing. The trend appears to be following the rising rates of obesity within these age groups.[3]

There are significant differences in the prevalence of high blood pressure in different racial and ethnic populations. In Blacks, hypertension not only is more common but also appears to follow a different course than it does in other groups. It develops earlier, is more severe, and is associated with more complications, such as heart attacks, stroke, and kidney failure. Blacks are on average more sensitive than Whites to the dietary effects of salt on blood pressure. This difference may contribute to the higher rate of stroke among Blacks. To date, there has not been a clear genetic explanation for the ethnic differences. Socioeconomic and behavioral factors may be involved as well, as discussed later in the chapter.[3,11]

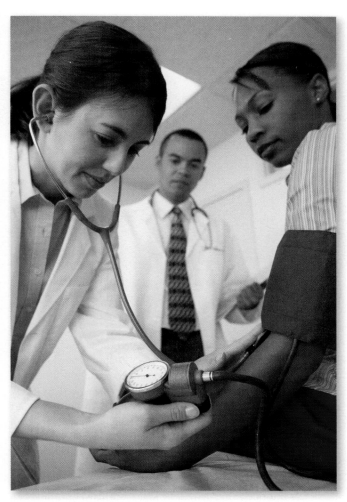

■ African Americans have higher rates of hypertension than the rest of the population, probably due to a combination of genetic, sociocultural, and behavioral factors. Regular screening can help keep blood pressure under control.

Regular screening for hypertension is recommended for individuals over age 15.[3] For anyone in the prehypertension or hypertension category, lifestyle changes are recommended, including weight reduction, dietary changes, low salt intake, physical activity, and moderate alcohol intake.[10] The DASH diet to reduce elevated blood pressure was developed from research by the National Heart, Lung, and Blood Institute and five medical research centers. The 2010 *Dietary Guidelines for Americans* recommends a limit of 1,500 mg of sodium per day for individuals with hypertension and those with a likelihood of developing it, including middle-aged and older adults and African Americans. If lifestyle changes alone do not reduce blood pressure, medications are recommended.

Maintain Healthy Cholesterol Levels The amount of cholesterol in your body is affected by what you eat and by how fast your body makes and gets rid of cholesterol. Because it is fatlike, cholesterol cannot circulate in the blood in a free-floating state; instead, it is combined with proteins and other molecules in packages called *lipoproteins*. Lipoproteins are categorized into five main classes according to density, with each class playing a different role in the body. The categories that have received the most study are total cholesterol and the LDL and HDL subcategories.

Levels of total cholesterol and LDL cholesterol are directly related to frequency of coronary heart disease; that is, as cholesterol levels rise, so does the incidence of heart disease (Table 14.2). Nearly half of the adult U.S. population have total cholesterol greater than 200 mg/dL, and 14 percent have more than 240 mg/dL. Among youth aged 12 to 17 years, one in five has at least one abnormal cholesterol level; the rate is nearly one in two for obese youth.[3]

Low-density lipoproteins (LDLs)—"bad" cholesterol—are clearly associated with atherosclerosis. The higher the level of LDLs, the higher the risk of atherosclerosis. In 2013, the American Heart Association and the American College of Cardiology published new guidelines for the treatment of high LDL cholesterol. This major shift is based on increased evidence showing that cholesterol-lowering statin medications significantly reduce risk of cardiovascular disease. The new guidelines identify four groups who benefit from statin treatment

low-density lipoproteins (LDLs) "Bad" cholesterol; lipoproteins that accumulate in plaque and contribute to atherosclerosis.

Table 14.2 Cholesterol Guidelines

Total cholesterol (mg/dL)	
Less than 200	Desirable
200–239	Borderline high
240 or greater	High
LDL cholesterol (mg/dl)	
Less than 100*	Near or above optimal
100–129	Optimal
130–159	Borderline high
160–189	High
190 or greater	Very high
HDL cholesterol (mg/dl)	
Less than 40	Low (undesirable)
60 or greater	High (desirable)
Triglycerides (mg/dl)	
Less than 150	Normal
150–199	Borderline high
200–499	High
500 or greater	Very high

*Achieving a goal of less than 70 is an option if there is a high risk for heart disease.

Source: "Executive Summary of the Third Report of the National Cholesterol Education Program Expert Panel on Detection, Evaluation, and Treatment of High Blood Cholesterol in Adults," 2001, *Journal of the American Medical Association, 285* (19), pp. 2486–2497.

instead of focusing on numbers. If you answer yes to any of the following, according to the new guidelines you would benefit from statin therapy.[3,12]

- Do you have a history of cardiovascular disease?

- Is your LDL cholesterol >190 mg/dl?

- Do you have diabetes AND are you over age 40 AND is your LDL cholesterol >70?

- Is your 10-year risk of heart attack greater than 7.5 percent?*

The National Cholesterol Education Program recommends that all adults over age 20 have their cholesterol checked at least once every five years. If your LDL cholesterol level, in combination with other risk factors, puts you at risk for CVD, your physician will work with you to develop a plan to reduce your cardiovascular risk. Exercising, maintaining a healthy weight, and dietary changes, including reducing total and saturated fat intake and increasing dietary fiber, are first-line actions. However, if these measures do not sufficiently lower your LDL level, cholesterol-lowering statin medications may be necessary.

High-density lipoproteins (HDLs)—"good" cholesterol—consist mainly of protein and are the smallest of the lipoprotein particles. HDLs help clear cholesterol from cells and atherosclerotic deposits and transport it back to the liver for recycling. High HDL levels provide protection from CVD.

HDL levels are determined mainly by genetics, but they are influenced by exercise, alcohol, and estrogen. They are higher among Blacks and among women, especially before menopause, and they change little with age. The protective effect of HDL is significant: a 1 percent decrease in HDL level is associated with a 3 to 4 percent increase in heart disease.[13]

high-density lipoproteins (HDLs) "Good" cholesterol; lipoproteins that help clear cholesterol from cells and atherosclerotic deposits and transport it back to the liver for recycling.

Be Physically Active Regular physical activity reduces the risk of CVD and many cardiovascular risk factors, including high blood pressure, diabetes, and obesity. Physical activity conditions the heart, reduces high blood pressure, improves HDL cholesterol levels, helps maintain a healthy weight, and helps control diabetes. Even low-intensity activities, such as walking, gardening, or climbing stairs, can be helpful. As discussed in Chapter 6, many adults in the United States are not active at levels that can promote health. In addition, exercise is very important for children, because it is associated with lower blood pressure and better weight control and because active children tend to become active adults.

*The 10-year risk is based on a combination of risk factors and can be calculated at http://cvdrisk.nhlbi.nih.gov/calculator.asp.

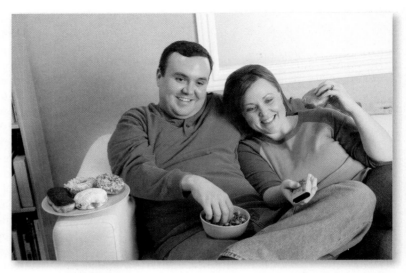

- Physical inactivity and obesity are two of the major controllable risk factors for cardiovascular disease.

Maintain a Healthy BMI Overweight and obesity are associated with increased risk for CVD and greater seriousness of the disease, so it's important to maintain a healthy body weight and body composition, as measured by body mass index (BMI). Excess weight puts a strain on the heart and contributes to other risk factors, such as hypertension, high LDL levels, and diabetes. The association among all these risk factors is found across ethnic groups, including Mexican Americans, non-Hispanic Blacks, and non-Hispanic Whites.

As discussed in Chapter 7, body fat distribution plays a role in CVD risk. Waist-to-hip ratio may play a greater role than BMI. People with central fat distribution—those who are apple-shaped, as suggested by an abdominal circumference of greater than 40 inches for men and greater than 35 inches for women—have a higher risk for diabetes, high blood pressure, and CVD.

Overweight people can improve their cardiovascular risk profile if they lose 10 to 15 percent of their total weight and maintain the loss. Diet and exercise are recommended ways to reduce overweight and obesity.[3]

Maintain Healthy Blood Glucose Levels Elevated levels of glucose circulating in the bloodstream, a symptom of diabetes (which is discussed later in this chapter), cause changes throughout the body, including damage to artery walls, changes in some blood components, and damage to peripheral nerves and organs. People with diabetes are two to four times more likely than people without diabetes to develop cardiovascular disease. Their arteries are particularly susceptible to atherosclerosis, and it occurs at an earlier age and is more extensive. The incidence of Type-2 diabetes has doubled in the past 30 years and is expected to double again by 2050.

Eat a Heart-Healthy Diet A diet that supports cardiovascular health, such as the DASH diet, emphasizes fruits,

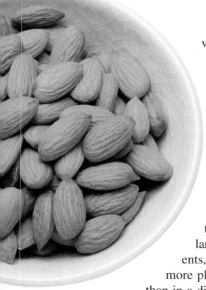

vegetables, whole grains, low-fat dairy products, fish, and lean meat and poultry. Balancing calories in with calories out is important, as is avoiding or limiting saturated fat, trans fat, dietary cholesterol, and added sugars.

Micronutrients (vitamins, minerals, and other substances in food) appear to play a role in cardiovascular health. Many micronutrients, especially antioxidants, are more plentiful in a plant-based diet than in a diet based on foods from animal sources. Foods high in important antioxidants are brightly colored fruits and vegetables and nuts and seeds (see Chapter 5). Experts recommend that micronutrients be consumed in foods rather than in supplements.

Specific foods have been shown to alter cholesterol levels. Soy products and legumes, such as lentils and chickpeas, have both been shown to decrease LDL levels. Garlic appears to have a similar effect on total cholesterol, although fresh garlic (one to two cloves per day) is recommended over synthetic garlic capsules. Foods rich in fiber also help reduce cholesterol levels; they include fruits, vegetables, oats, and barley.

Contributing Factors in Cardiovascular Health

In addition to the major controllable factors in cardiovascular health, other factors have been identified that contribute, or may contribute, to heart health.

Triglyceride Levels **Triglycerides** are another form in which fat exists in the body. They are derived from fats eaten or produced by the body from other energy sources, such as excess carbohydrates. High blood levels of triglycerides are a risk factor for CVD, although they are not linked to CVD as strongly as are high cholesterol levels. A triglyceride level of less than 150 is desirable (see Table 14.2). Triglyceride levels are reported as part of lipid (cholesterol) screening results.

triglycerides
Blood fats similar to cholesterol.

High triglyceride levels are associated with excess body fat, diets high in saturated fat and cholesterol, alcohol use, and some medical conditions, such as poorly controlled diabetes. The main treatment for high triglycerides is lifestyle modification, but medications can also be used.

Limited Alcohol Intake The relationship between alcohol and CVD is complicated because different levels of alcohol consumption have different effects. Heavy drinking,

defined as more than two drinks per day for men and one drink per day for women, can damage the heart, increasing the risk of cardiomyopathy, some arrhythmias, and neurological complications. Light to moderate alcohol intake, defined as fewer than two drinks per day for men and one drink per day for women, appears to have a protective effect against heart disease and stroke, increasing HDL levels.

The benefit associated with light to moderate alcohol use is seen regardless of the beverage, which suggests that the protective factor is alcohol itself, rather than another substance, such as the tannins in red wine. The disadvantages of alcohol consumption are that it may contribute to weight gain, higher blood pressure, and elevated triglycerides, as well as alcoholism in vulnerable individuals. The possible cardiovascular benefits have to be weighed against the disadvantages and potential harm associated with drinking.[3]

Psychosocial Factors As described in Chapter 2, traits and behavior patterns associated with the so-called Type A personality—specifically, anger and hostility—have been shown to contribute to CVD risk. These feelings cause the release of stress hormones. When anger, hostility, and stress in general are persistent and pervasive, the continuous circulation of stress hormones in the blood increases blood pressure and heart rate and triggers the release of cholesterol and triglycerides into the blood. All these changes may promote the development of atherosclerosis and, for those with atherosclerosis, increase vulnerability to heart attack or stroke.[14]

Depression has a bidirectional relationship with CVD; that is, depression increases risk of CVD, and CVD increases risk of depression. People who are depressed have a more difficult time choosing healthy lifestyle options, making lifestyle changes, initiating access to health care, and adhering to medication regimens. Early diagnosis and treatment of depression may help reduce risk of CVD in vulnerable individuals.[3,15]

If you frequently feel overwhelmed by stress, anger, or depression, try incorporating stress management and relaxation techniques into your daily life. Meditating can lower blood pressure and blood cholesterol levels; biofeedback may help reduce blood pressure; hypnosis may help control hypertension and other chronic health problems. You can also just try simplifying your schedule and slowing down.

Low socioeconomic status and low levels of educational attainment are associated with an increased risk for heart attack, stroke, congestive heart failure, hypertension, and other chronic diseases. Income inequality in a country—the gap between the rich and the poor—is directly related to national rates of death from CVD, coronary artery disease, and stroke. Numerous factors may help explain the link between poverty and poor health. For example, poverty limits people's ability to obtain the basic requisites for health, such as food and shelter, as well as their ability to participate in society, which creates psychological stress. Poverty also limits access to health-related information, health care,

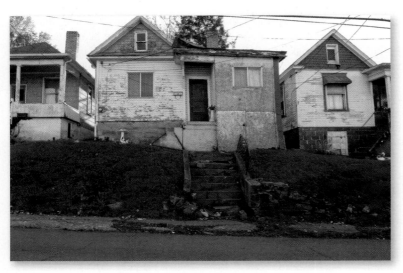

■ Low socioeconomic status is associated with greater risk for cardiovascular disease. Contributing factors may be the stress of poverty and discrimination and lack of access to health information and health care services.

medications, behavior change options, and physical activity. In addition, racism, prejudice, and discrimination can act as psychosocial stressors and lead to increased risk of CVD.[3,14–18]

People who lack social support or live in social isolation are at increased risk for many health conditions, including CVD. Strong social networks have been shown to decrease the risk of CVD, and social support, altruism, faith, and optimism are all associated with a reduced risk of CVD. In other words, people can improve their health by expanding their connections to family, friends, community, or church. It appears that the strength of people's relationships and their basic attitudes toward life play important roles in maintaining health and protecting against disease.[19]

Noncontrollable Factors in Cardiovascular Health

Some factors in heart health are not within the control of the individual, such as age, gender, and geographic influences (see the box, "Place Matters: Geographical Location and Noncommunicable Disease"). For individuals with noncontrollable risk factors, it's especially important that they choose behaviors that promote ideal cardiovascular health.

Age Age is probably the most important noncontrollable risk factor. There is a significant rise in deaths due to heart disease and stroke after age 65. Age alone does not cause CVD, however; there is great variation in CVD among older people of the same age.[3]

Gender Although heart disease has often been thought of as a man's disease, CVD is the leading cause of death for both men and women. There are some differences between the sexes, however. A 40-year-old man without evidence of heart disease has a one-in-two chance of developing CVD

in his lifetime, whereas a 40-year-old woman has a one-in-three chance. Women tend to develop heart disease about 10 years later than men, perhaps because of the protective effect of estrogen before menopause. After age 50 (the average age of menopause), the difference in risk between men and women starts to decrease.

The death rates for CVD are higher in women, both Black women and White women, than in men; this is true of heart attack, stroke, hypertension, and congestive heart failure. Three reasons have been identified. First, women tend to be older and frailer when they develop heart disease, so they are less likely to survive. Second, women are more likely to have either no symptoms before a heart attack or symptoms, such as stomach complaints, that make the diagnosis of heart disease more difficult. The third reason women's CVD death rates are higher is that treatment is more likely to be delayed. Because treatment is more effective the sooner it is started, this delay means that more damage occurs. One study showed that women delay seeking treatment as much as 3.5 hours longer than men. In addition, health care providers may not provide immediate treatment because they do not recognize the symptoms or are less likely to think about heart disease in women.[3]

Genetics and Family History Individuals who have a relative with a history of CVD have a higher risk of CVD themselves. High rates of CVD in a family may be related to genetics or lifestyle patterns or both. A large part of the family risk is due to other risk factors, such as hypertension, elevated lipids, and diabetes. As mentioned previously, a history in the family of sudden cardiac death at a young age may signify a genetic risk for cardiomyopathy or another congenital cardiac disease.[15,20]

Ethnicity and Race Minority and low-income populations in the United States carry a disproportionate burden of CVD. Blacks have a higher risk of CVD and stroke than do Whites, as well as higher rates of hypertension, obesity, and diabetes. Mexican Americans, American Indians, and Native Hawaiians also have a higher risk of CVD than do Whites, along with higher rates of obesity and diabetes.

Recent improvements in cardiovascular health have not been shared evenly by all racial or ethnic groups. Although the death rate from heart attack has declined across all groups, it has declined less among minority groups and women. Several pathways may lead to these health disparities, including differences in such risk factors as hypertension, genetics, stress, and psychosocial factors.[16,18,21]

Postmenopausal Status The hormone estrogen has long been thought to protect premenopausal women from CVD. When levels of estrogen fall during menopause, levels of HDL also decline, and body fat distribution shifts to a more central distribution pattern, similar to the male pattern.

Who's at Risk?

Place Matters: Geographical Location and Noncommunicable Disease

The United States ranks second to last among 17 peer countries when it comes to deaths from noncommunicable disease. When we look within the United States, we also see significant differences in deaths from heart disease by area of the country. Why do you think geographical location makes a difference in risk for heart disease? Consider the socioeconomic framework presented in

Chapter 1. How might health care, health behaviors, neighborhood environments, education, income, and public policies play a role?

Heart Disease Death Rates, 2002–2007, Adults Age 35+, by County

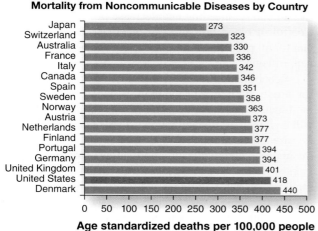

Mortality from Noncommunicable Diseases by Country

Country	Age standardized deaths per 100,000 people
Japan	273
Switzerland	323
Australia	330
France	336
Italy	342
Canada	346
Spain	351
Sweden	358
Norway	363
Austria	373
Netherlands	377
Finland	377
Portugal	394
Germany	394
United Kingdom	401
United States	418
Denmark	440

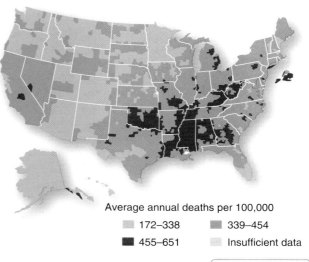

Average annual deaths per 100,000
- 172–338
- 339–454
- 455–651
- Insufficient data

Sources: Health in International Perspective: Shorter Lives, Poorer Health, Figure 1-1 (data from World Health Organization), by S. Woolf and L. Aron, 2013, National Research Council and Institute of Medicine; Vital Signs, High Blood Pressure and Cholesterol, by Centers for Disease Control, figure data from National Vital Statistics System and U.S. Census Bureau, www.cdc.gov/vitalsigns/CardiovascularDisease/.

connect ACTIVITY

For many years, medical practitioners prescribed hormone replacement therapy (HRT) for postmenopausal women to relieve the symptoms of menopause, lower the risk of osteoporosis (bone thinning), and reduce the risk of CVD. The belief in the benefits of estrogen was so strong that at one point, nearly one in three postmenopausal women was on HRT. Research has now shown that HRT actually increases rather than decreases the risk of heart attack, stroke, and breast cancer. HRT is still prescribed as a treatment for the symptoms of menopause and prevention of osteoporosis, but these benefits must now be weighed against an individual woman's risk for CVD.[22]

Testing and Treatment

People with no symptoms of CVD are usually not tested for evidence of disease; instead, the focus is on screening for risk factors such as hypertension, cholesterol levels, and family health history. An exception is people in certain occupations, such as airline pilots or truck drivers, whose sudden incapacity would place other people at risk. People may also be screened for signs of CVD before surgery, and the American College of Sports Medicine recommends that an exercise stress test be performed on men older than age 40 and women older than age 50 if they are sedentary and about to begin an exercise program.

For people with a family history of sudden death or symptoms suggestive of CVD, such as shortness of breath, dizziness, chest pain on exertion, weakness, numbness or neurologic problems, physical examination and diagnostic tests can determine whether CVD is present and the extent of the problem. If CVD is found, a variety of steps can be taken, from lifestyle changes, to medication, to surgery.

Diagnostic Testing for Heart Disease Several tests can evaluate heart function and determine if underlying disease is present. An **electrocardiogram** (ECG or EKG), a record of the electrical activity of the heart as it beats, can detect abnormal rhythms, inadequate blood flow (possibly due to ischemia or heart attack), and heart enlargement. An **echocardiogram** (or echo), an ultrasound test that uses sound waves to visualize the heart structure and motion, can detect structural abnormalities in the valves, arteries, and heart chambers; the thickness of the muscle walls; and how well the heart pumps. An **exercise stress test** evaluates how well the heart functions with exercise.

electrocardiogram
Record of the heart's electrical activity as it beats.

echocardiogram
Diagnostic test for a heart attack in which sound waves are used to visualize heart valves, heart wall movement, and overall heart function.

exercise stress test
Procedure that evaluates how well the heart functions with exercise.

Diagnostic Testing for Stroke At the hospital, a CT scan or an MRI can generate images of the brain and blood flow and determine whether a stroke has occurred. These tests can also show whether a stroke has been caused by a blockage or by a hemorrhage. Further testing may be done to find the source of the blockage. The carotid arteries, the large arteries on the sides of the neck that supply blood to the brain, are examined to see if they are blocked with atherosclerotic plaques. If so, part of a plaque may have broken off and caused an embolism blocking a blood vessel in the brain.

Management of Heart Disease Multiple categories of medications can be used in the treatment of heart disease. There are medications that help control heart rhythm (anti-arrhythmics), dilate the coronary arteries and reduce angina (anti-anginals), decrease blood clotting (anti-coagulants), and dissolve blood clots during a heart attack (thrombolytics). Other medications, such as anti-hypertensives, cholesterol-lowering medications, and antiplatelet medications, are used to control risk factors and reduce the chance of developing heart disease or a recurrence of heart disease.

When a heart attack occurs, emergency treatment is critical. The effectiveness of treatment depends on the length of time between the first symptoms and the reestablishment of blood flow to the heart muscle. Thrombolytics are most effective when given within the first hour after a heart attack.

Every day thousands of people have heart surgery; there are many different types of surgery, depending on the underlying problem. For structural abnormalities, surgeons can repair or replace heart valves, close septal defects (holes) that allow blood to flow abnormally, reposition arteries and veins that are attached incorrectly, and repair aneurysms in the aorta. If the problem is related to abnormal electrical conduction through the heart, a cardiologist can destroy a small amount of heart tissue in an area that is disturbing the flow of electricity or can implant a defibrillator into the chest that will automatically shock the heart if a life-threatening arrhythmia develops. Also, often as a last resort, a surgeon can replace a damaged heart completely with a heart from a donor. If the underlying abnormality is related to coronary artery disease, a surgeon can reopen the vessel with angioplasty, in which a balloon catheter (a thin plastic tube) is threaded into a blocked or narrowed artery and inflated to stretch the vessel open again; a *coronary stent,* a springy framework that supports the vessel walls and keeps the vessel open, is often permanently placed in the artery to prevent it from closing again. Another surgical option is **coronary artery bypass grafting**, usually just called *bypass.* A healthy blood vessel is taken from another part of the body, usually the leg, and grafted to the coronary arteries to allow a bypass of blood flow around a narrowed vessel.

coronary artery bypass grafting Surgical procedure in which a healthy blood vessel is taken from another part of the body and grafted to the coronary arteries to allow a bypass of blood flow around a narrowed vessel.

Management of Stroke If a stroke is found to be thrombotic (caused by a blockage) and there is no evidence of bleeding in the brain, thrombolytic medications can be administered to dissolve the clot and restore blood flow to the brain. Thrombolytic medications must not be given if the stroke is hemorrhagic, because they can cause increased bleeding. Aspirin and other anticlotting medications can be used after a thrombotic stroke to reduce the risk of another stroke. Treatment for hemorrhagic stroke depends on the underlying cause of the bleed. Surgery is sometimes necessary to control bleeding and decrease pressure in the brain. Control of blood pressure and other risk factors is important for all people who have a stroke, whether thrombotic or hemorrhagic.

Rehabilitation is an important component of treatment for stroke. If an area of the brain is damaged or destroyed, the functions that were controlled by that part of the brain will be impaired. Rehabilitation consists of physical therapy (to strengthen muscles and coordination), speech therapy (to improve communication and eating), and occupational therapy (to improve activities of daily living and job retraining if appropriate). Progress and return of functions vary by individual. Some people recover fully within a few days to weeks, while others are left with long-term impairment.

Areas of Interest for Future CVD Research

Factors that promote cardiovascular health or that contribute to cardiovascular disease are not fully understood, and some people with heart disease have none of the risk factors

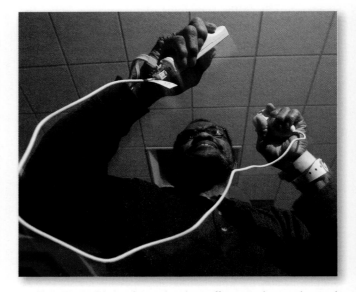

■ About two-thirds of people who suffer a stroke survive and require rehabilitation. When a stroke has caused muscle weakness or paralysis, therapy focuses on regaining use of impaired limbs, improving coordination and balance, and developing strategies for bypassing deficits.

discussed so far. Researchers are constantly trying to identify additional risk factors. A few promising areas are the following:

- Low levels of vitamin D are increasingly associated with heart disease, diabetes, hypertension, and obesity.

- High blood levels of homocysteine, an amino acid, have been associated with increased risk of cardiovascular disease.

- Metabolic syndrome, a condition that can precede the development of Type-2 diabetes, is associated with significantly increased risk of CVD.

- Inflammation is well established as a factor in all stages of atherosclerosis.

- High levels of C-reactive protein, a protein in the blood, are associated with increased risk for coronary heart disease.

- Infections appear to promote atherosclerosis and may cause atherosclerotic plaques to break free and block arteries.

- Lower birth weight is associated with higher risk of CVD later in life.[23–26]

DIABETES

Diabetes is the most common disorder of the endocrine or metabolic system and the seventh leading cause of death in the United States. Rates of all forms of diabetes are increasing nationally and globally. In the United States alone, 19.7 million people have been diagnosed with diabetes (8.3 percent of the adult population), 8.2 million have diabetes but are undiagnosed, and another 87 million are at high risk of developing diabetes in the next 10 years. Rates of diabetes have doubled every 15 years since the 1950s.[3]

There are different types of diabetes, but all result in elevated blood glucose levels due to a disruption in the production or use of insulin. Figure 14.7 illustrates the basic relationships between glucose, insulin, and glucose uptake by cells.

In a healthy person, increased glucose in the blood after a meal triggers the release of insulin from the pancreas. Molecules of insulin bind to cells around the body and facilitate the uptake of glucose into cells, which use it for energy or store it. When levels of blood glucose drop, the pancreas stops releasing insulin, so that blood glucose levels are maintained in a healthy range, typically between 80 and 120 milligrams per deciliter (mg/dL), depending on time since the last meal. Problems at any stage of the process can cause blood glucose levels to rise to abnormal levels. Long-term exposure to elevated levels of glucose is toxic, leading to damage

---

diabetes
Metabolic disorder in which the production or use of insulin is disrupted, so that body cells cannot take up glucose and use it for energy, and high levels of glucose circulate in the blood.

Normal
Insulin binds to receptors on the surface of a cell and signals special transporters in the cell to transport glucose inside.

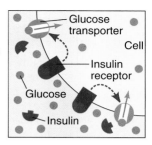

Type 1 diabetes
The pancreas produces little or no insulin. Thus, no signal is sent instructing the cell to transport glucose, and glucose builds up in the bloodstream.

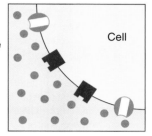

Type 2 diabetes
The pancreas produces too little insulin and/or the body's cells are resistant to it. Some insulin binds to receptors on the cell's surface, but the signal to transport glucose is blocked. Glucose builds up in the bloodstream.

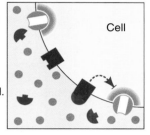

figure 14.7 **Insulin and glucose uptake.**
A healthy person's body releases a normal amount of insulin from the pancreas after meals. As shown in the first diagram, molecules of insulin bind to cells and facilitate the uptake of glucose into cells, which use it for energy or store it. Type-1 diabetes and Type-2 diabetes disrupt this process, as shown in the second and third diagrams.

to blood vessels and, as a result, kidney failure, blindness, nerve damage, and cardiovascular disease. In addition, people with diabetes are at increased risk from infectious diseases with higher rates of complications from influenza, pneumonia, and skin infections. They also experience more dental problems and more complications in pregnancy.[27,28]

Type-1 Diabetes

Type-1 diabetes is caused by the destruction of insulin-producing cells in the pancreas by the immune system. When the cells are destroyed, insulin cannot be produced and body cells cannot take up glucose. Levels of glucose circulating in the blood rise rapidly while cells are starving. Insulin must be provided from an external source to keep blood glucose levels under control and to allow the cells to use it. For people with Type-1 diabetes, insulin is necessary for survival and must be supplied every day.

The onset of Type-1 diabetes usually occurs before age 20, though it can occur at any age (see the box, "Stacy: Living with Type-1 Diabetes"). Symptoms include dry mouth, frequent urination, extreme thirst, rapid weight loss, fatigue,

Stacy: Living with Type-1 Diabetes

Stacy was diagnosed with Type-1 diabetes during her sophomore year of high school. Her older brother had diabetes, so she wasn't completely surprised when she developed symptoms. With her family's help, she learned how to inject insulin, manage her blood sugar levels, and monitor her meals. When she first got to college, she maintained the same habits she had developed at home. She checked her blood glucose levels in the morning when she woke up, between classes, before she commuted home from campus in the evening, and before bed. She ate well, counted carbohydrates, exercised, and adjusted her insulin as needed. She was able to maintain and monitor her blood glucose levels as well as her diet and activity. This made her diabetes a manageable condition.

During her second quarter, she got a job to help ease the financial burden of college for her family. The busy schedule meant less time: she grabbed toast and tea for breakfast, was less consistent in the timing of lunch and dinner, and found she was staying up late doing homework and not making time for the gym. She stopped checking her blood sugar as regularly, occasionally not checking it for days at a time. And because she wasn't sure of her blood sugar levels, she stopped injecting her insulin regularly.

One day leaving class, Stacy felt so exhausted that she stumbled to a nearby bench and slumped down on it. She felt nauseous and light-headed, and when a friend asked her if she was okay, she was unable to answer coherently. Her friend called 911, and paramedics took her to the emergency room. There, the nurses immediately recognized the fruity smell on her breath and checked her blood sugar level. It was more than three times higher than normal. Stacy was hospitalized and treated for hyperglycemia and dehydration. She was monitored for two days and then allowed to check out.

After this episode, Stacy went home for a week to regain her equilibrium. She saw her endocrinologist and diabetes care team, and they recommended that she start using an insulin pump. The pump would provide a constant low level of insulin and would allow her to give extra doses with meals. In addition, when she checked her blood sugar, her pump could calculate and administer the correct amount of insulin. Stacy returned to school feeling more confident about managing her diabetes. The new system allowed her to continue focusing on her academics and job and, with a little additional teaching, improve her glucose control.

- Do you have any health conditions or concerns that affect your daily life? If so, what measures do you have to take to manage them?

- Have you had the experience of sacrificing your health to meet academic deadlines or participate in social activities? If so, how can you balance choices, commitments, and your body's needs to maintain a healthy lifestyle?

connect ACTIVITY

and blurred vision. Type-1 diabetes is probably caused by a combination of genetic, autoimmune, and environmental factors (such as viruses or dietary triggers). Rates of Type-1 diabetes have increased in the past 20 years, but Type-1 continues to make up only an estimated 5 to 10 percent of all diabetes cases. This type is not associated with obesity, and there are no known ways to prevent it at this time.[27]

Type-1 diabetes must be treated with insulin replacement. Frequent monitoring of blood glucose levels and the use of insulin pumps or self-injected insulin multiple times a day have significantly improved blood glucose control and can prevent or reduce risk of long-term complications. In addition, dietary education is important, as balancing carbohydrate intake with insulin requirements becomes important for stable control of blood sugar. A balance must be maintained between too high glucose levels (and increased risk for long-term complications) and too low glucose levels (and increased risk for loss of consciousness, seizure, or death). Physical activity is an important component of Type-1 diabetes control and reduction in long-term complications.

Type-2 Diabetes

In Type-2 diabetes, the production of insulin by the pancreas is initially normal, but over time the insulin receptors in body cells become insulin resistant (less able to respond to insulin). Cells cannot take up some of the glucose, and blood glucose levels rise. The pancreas initially responds by increasing production of insulin, but eventually it cannot keep up. Type-2 diabetes accounts for 90 to 95 percent of all cases of diabetes. It is the type that has been rapidly increasing in parallel with rising rates of overweight and obesity levels.[27]

Risk Factors Type-2 diabetes appears to have both genetic and environmental components. Historically, Type-2 diabetes was almost unheard of in people below 20 years of age. Now, 1 in 2,500 children and adolescents between the ages of 10 and 19 in the United States has diabetes. Rates are rising quickly, especially in racial and ethnic minority groups. African Americans, Native Americans, Hispanic Americans, and some Asian Americans have higher rates of diabetes than the general population and are at greater risk for complications. Visceral fat, as indicated by abdominal circumference, and lack of physical activity appear to be strong indicators of risk. Age is also a risk factor. The onset of Type-2 diabetes is usually gradual. Symptoms include excessive thirst, frequent urination, and fatigue; rarely, symptoms include nausea, vomiting, and confusion.

Prediabetes is diagnosed when fasting blood glucose levels are between 100 and 126 mg/dL. (Normal fasting blood glucose is under 100.) In this condition, cells are starting to have a problem in the uptake and utilization of glucose. An estimated 38 percent of U.S. adults (87 million Americans) have prediabetes. Nearly half (40 to 50 percent) of these people will go on to develop Type-2 diabetes, which is diagnosed when blood glucose levels are higher than 126 mg/dL.

Dietary changes, exercise, and weight loss can prevent or delay the onset of diabetes. The risk of progression to diabetes is significantly reduced with 7 percent weight loss, especially if the weight loss occurs through lifestyle modification. Increasingly medications are also being used to reduce the risk of progression to full diabetes.[27–29]

A set of conditions known as *metabolic syndrome* also significantly increases the risk for developing diabetes and other health complications. Although several criteria have been identified, the condition is commonly diagnosed when three of the following five risk factors are present:

- Fasting glucose level ≥ 100.

- HDL cholesterol <40 in men or <50 in women.

- Triglycerides ≥ 150.

- Waist circumference ≥ 40 inches (102 cm) for men or ≥ 35 inches (88 cm) for women.

- Systolic blood pressure ≥ 130 and diastolic blood pressure ≥ 85.

An estimated 34 percent of adult Americans have metabolic syndrome, but prevalence varies by ethnic and racial group. For men, prevalence is 25.3 percent in Blacks, 33.2 percent in Mexican Americans, and 37.2 percent in Whites. For women, prevalence is 38.8 percent in Blacks, 40.6 percent in Mexican Americans, and 31.5 percent in Whites.[3,30] It is important to identify and address metabolic syndrome because of the high risk of progressing to diabetes and cardiovascular complications. Recommendations for treating metabolic syndrome include increasing physical activity, losing weight, and making dietary changes; medications are often recommended as well.

- Tom Hanks announced in 2013 that he has Type-2 diabetes. He had had high blood sugar for 20 years, which predisposed him to diabetes. In his case, large fluctuations in weight—gaining 30 pounds in 1992 for *A League of Their Own,* dropping that weight and more for *Philadelphia* the next year, and losing 50 pounds in 2000 for *Cast Away*—may also have contributed to developing the disease.

Detection and Treatment Screening for diabetes can detect early stages of the disease, identify prediabetes, and prevent progression of prediabetes to diabetes (see the box, "Preventing Type-2 Diabetes"). At present, the U.S. Preventive Services Task Force (USPTF) recommends diabetes screening for pregnant women and people with elevated blood pressure, for whom diabetes would further increase the risk of CVD. However, the American Diabetic Association recommends broader screening to include anyone over age 45 as well as younger people who have a BMI greater than 25 and another risk factor (physical inactivity; family history of diabetes; racial/ethnic status as African American, Latino American, Native American, or Asian and Pacific Islander; high blood pressure; or high lipids).[31] Screening involves a blood test to look at fasting glucose level.

Treatment for Type-2 diabetes includes lifestyle modification (improving diet, increasing physical activity, losing weight), oral medications, and, eventually, for some, insulin replacement. Exercise is especially important because it can improve HDL levels and increase the number of insulin receptors on cells, which enhances the body's ability to use insulin; it also helps prevent prediabetes from progressing to diabetes. Long-term control of both Type-1 and Type-2 diabetes is monitored by a blood test called the hemoglobin A1c test, and the closer the blood glucose is to the normal range, the lower the risk of complications.

Gestational Diabetes

The hormonal changes of pregnancy can affect how the body responds to insulin. In 2 to 10 percent of pregnancies, the pregnant woman develops gestational diabetes (diabetes of pregnancy). Risk factors for gestational diabetes are similar to those for Type-2 diabetes but also include pregnancy after age 35, family history of gestational diabetes, and a personal history of diabetes in a prior pregnancy or a large infant in a prior pregnancy.

Women are usually screened for gestational diabetes early in pregnancy. Detection and treatment are important to reduce the risk of complications for both mother and child. For most women, glucose levels return to normal after delivery, but for 5 to 10 percent, diabetes becomes an ongoing condition. In addition, a woman with a history of gestational diabetes is at significant risk of developing diabetes in the next 10 to 20 years.[3,32]

Preventing Type-2 Diabetes

The prevention of chronic diseases requires identification and understanding of their causes, just as the prevention of infectious diseases requires identification of the pathogens that cause them. Identifying the causes is more difficult with chronic diseases, however, because the diseases take years to develop and they are multi-determined—that is, they are caused by the interaction of multiple factors. Public heath efforts typically focus on three levels of prevention, identified as primary, secondary, and tertiary prevention.

Primary prevention efforts are public health interventions that target the underlying causes of a disease and attempt to mitigate or remove them: an unhealthy diet, hypertension, tobacco use. Prevention efforts are taken prior to the development of risk factors. This is a highly cost-effective form of prevention because it eliminates or reduces risk factors. For Type-2 diabetes, an example of primary prevention is nutrition and exercise programs for elementary-school children.

Secondary prevention efforts take place as soon as possible after development of risk factors and prior to the appearance of symptoms. For Type-2 diabetes, examples of secondary prevention are educational campaigns about the benefits of weight loss and programs to encourage adults to have their blood glucose levels monitored regularly.

Tertiary prevention efforts focus on reducing complications of a disease once it has manifested or reversing the effects of the disease to restore function. Tertiary prevention tends to be the most expensive and invasive stage of public health intervention;

it is more expensive to treat disease and prevent further complications than it is to prevent onset of the disease. For Type-2 diabetes, tertiary prevention includes regular screenings for nerve damage, kidney function, eye problems, and heart disease. It can also involve adopting lifestyle changes, like getting a membership at a gym and switching to a healthier diet.

Primary prevention is the most cost-effective approach to decreasing the incidence of chronic diseases. In addition, because many chronic diseases share underlying risk factors, primary prevention can reduce the risk of more than one disease. For example, physical inactivity and obesity are risk factors for CVD, diabetes, and cancer, and smoking is a risk factor for CVD, lung diseases, and cancer. Another advantage of primary prevention is that it starts early, when lifestyle habits are being formed. Behaviors adopted early in life are more likely to continue and become lifelong patterns.

Type-2 diabetes, like other chronic diseases, is a very serious illness—but it is also one of the easiest to prevent and control. Even those with a genetic predisposition can control their risk of developing the disease. In support of prevention efforts, the Centers for Disease Control runs the National Diabetes Prevention Program, a research-based lifestyle-change program that reduced the risk of developing Type-2 diabetes by 58 percent in people at high risk for diabetes. If you are at risk or just want to increase your awareness, you can learn more about this program at the CDC website.

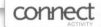

Sources: "National Diabetes Prevention Program," 2012, Centers for Disease Control and Prevention, www.cdc.gov/diabetes/prevention/about.htm; "Diabetes Public Health Resource," 2012, Centers for Disease Control and Prevention, www.cdc.gov/diabetes/consumer/prevent.htm.

CHRONIC LUNG DISEASES

Chronic lung diseases, also known as chronic lower respiratory diseases, are the third leading cause of death in the United States. The two most common forms of chronic lung disease are asthma and chronic obstructive pulmonary disease (COPD), which includes chronic bronchitis and emphysema. All of these diseases impair the ability to breathe.

Although they are all characterized by airway obstruction and shortness of breath, they have different causes and treatments. Genetic factors play a larger role in asthma than in COPD, and both are triggered by smoking, infection, and pollution. Asthma can have an allergic component and often appears in childhood. COPD is more typical in older adults.

The Respiratory System

When you breathe, air travels down your trachea and enters your lungs through airways called bronchial tubes, or bronchi. The bronchi carry the air through a series of smaller and smaller branching airways (bronchioles) into the alveoli, tiny round air sacs. The alveoli are surrounded by capillaries, tiny blood vessels, where gas exchange takes place. Oxygen in the air passes through the walls of the air sacs

into the blood in capillaries, and carbon dioxide moves from the capillaries into the air sacs. The carbon dioxide is pushed back through the bronchioles and exhaled, and the oxygen travels through the bloodstream to body cells (Figure 14.8). Healthy lungs are elastic and stretchy; the alveoli work like tiny balloons—they fill when you breathe in and deflate when you breath out.

Asthma

Asthma is the most common chronic lung condition, and rates have been increasing in the last few decades (see the box, "Why Do More People Have Asthma, and What Can Be Done About It?"). Nearly 25 million people in the United States live with this condition, which often starts in childhood. Although asthma cannot be cured, symptoms can usually be controlled by avoiding triggers and using medications, so people can live normal, active lives. Deaths from asthma are rare but do occur; they are usually associated with poor control of the disease.[33]

In asthma, the lining of the airways becomes inflamed and swollen, narrowing the airway passage, and excess mucus is produced, further obstructing the flow of air. In addition,

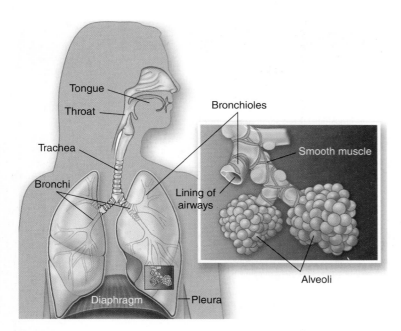

figure 14.8 **The respiratory system.**

the smooth muscles that encircle the bronchioles become tight or go into spasm, constricting the airways. The inflammation, obstruction, and constriction cause the symptoms of asthma—wheezing, coughing, chest tightness, and shortness of breath. For a person with asthma, the airways are chronically inflamed; an asthma attack (also called a flare or an exacerbation) occurs when the inflammation increases and airways become further constricted. Some people with asthma have very mild intermittent symptoms, often in response to specific triggers. Other people have persistent, chronic symptoms that affect their daily life.

Risk Factors and Triggers The causes of asthma are not completely understood, but they appear to involve both genetic and environmental factors. For people with an underlying genetic predisposition, asthma attacks can occur in response to multiple triggers. Viral infections are associated with 50 to 75 percent of adult wheezing episodes. In particular, influenza virus can lead to serious exacerbations of asthma and an increased risk of complications. Bacteria may be the trigger for another 5 to 10 percent of flares. Inhaled irritants—such as smoking or exposure to secondhand smoke, wood smoke, and air pollution—can trigger an attack and exacerbate underlying airway inflammation and muscle spasm. Air pollution can be a major issue, especially in urban areas and poor communities. Other irritants can include perfumes, hair spray, paint fumes or other chemicals.

Allergies are a common trigger; allergens can include animal dander, dust mites, cockroach droppings, mold, and various foods and food additives. Asthma attacks can also be triggered by strenuous physical exercise, cold air, and strong emotions. Other conditions that have been associated with worsening symptoms include obesity, acid reflux (heart

burn), sleep apnea, stress, and chronic sinus infections or nasal congestion. Between 3 and 5 percent of adults can also have an exacerbation triggered by use of aspirin or nonsteroidal anti-inflammatory medications (such as ibuprofen).[33,34]

Detection and Treatment Asthma is typically diagnosed when a person complains of shortness of breath, prolonged coughing, or coughing with certain activities. A health care provider will listen to the lungs and may hear wheezing as the air moves in and out through narrowed airways. A lung function test can be used to see how quickly and with how much force the person can blow air out of the lungs, which is influenced by how large or small the airways are. Diagnostic categories include intermittent asthma, in which a person has discrete episodes of symptoms but no symptoms in between; mild persistent asthma, in which someone has symptoms a few times a week but not daily; moderate asthma, in which daily symptoms limit some normal activity; and severe asthma, in which daily symptoms place extreme limits on normal activity.

Treatment is based on diagnostic category and how often someone is having symptoms. Long-term control also involves avoiding common triggers, such as tobacco smoke, allergens, and air pollution. Because of the increased risk of complications associated with influenza virus, people with asthma are considered a priority group to receive an annual flu shot and a one-time pneumonia shot. When exercise is a trigger, people are encouraged to continue exercising but use medication to control symptoms before or during exercise.

Quick-relief medications, called bronchodilators, can be used during an asthma attack to reduce symptoms immediately. These medicines, delivered through an inhaler, cause the smooth muscles lining the bronchioles to relax, opening the airways. Long-term control can be achieved by using a different medicine, usually an inhaled steroid that works locally within the bronchioles to reduce inflammation, opening the airways and making the smooth muscle less reactive.[35] These medications reduce the need for quick-relief medicines, reduce the frequency of asthma attacks, and reduce chronic coughing or shortness of breath. They are not for use during an asthma attack.

Because asthma is an inherently variable disease with relapses and remissions, management is an active process and self-care is critical. A person with asthma has to monitor symptoms, such as frequency of coughing or degree of shortness of breath, and use quick-acting medications to respond rapidly to exacerbations. Understanding what is likely to trigger an episode and attempting to avoid or decrease exposure to triggers is also critical. A person with asthma should develop an Asthma Control Plan available through the Centers for Disease Control and Prevention[36] and always carry a quick-acting inhaler.

Starting the Conversation

Why Do More People Have Asthma, and What Can Be Done About It?

Q: Do you have asthma, or do you know someone who does? If so, what activity limits does the disease impose?

The prevalence of asthma has been increasing in the United States, and it has been increasing disproportionately among children, women, poor people, and African Americans. These demographic disparities have persisted despite improvements in outdoor air quality and decreases in cigarette smoking and exposure to secondhand smoke.

In 2011, the CDC reported that the prevalence of asthma among Americans had increased by more than 12 percent between 2001 and 2009. More than 8 percent of the population—1 in 12 people—now suffer from the symptoms of asthma—shortness of breath, wheezing, coughing, and chronic airway inflammation. The prevalence of asthma is higher among children (9.6 percent) than across the whole population and highest among poor children (13.5 percent) and among non-Hispanic Black children (17.0 percent). More boys than girls have asthma, but more women than men have it.

Causes for this increase in asthma prevalence, and for the demographic disparities, are not entirely clear. Among the possible factors identified by researchers are genetic predisposition, allergies, health risk factors like smoking and obesity, and exposure to pollutants, both indoor and outdoor. Many studies have found associations between exposure to air pollution and acute exacerbation of asthma symptoms. For example, one study, published in 2012, looked at the disparity in asthma prevalence, ranging from 3 percent to 18 percent, in neighborhoods in New York City. Researchers measured levels of combustion by-products both inside homes and in children's exhalations and found a correlation between higher rates of asthma and exposure to environmental pollutants, particularly

diesel truck exhaust. Where the density of truck routes was higher, so was the prevalence of asthma.

Another study, also conducted in New York City (where asthma rates are among the highest in the nation), looked at differences in environmental conditions between midtown Manhattan and the South Bronx, which are about 4 miles apart. Rates of hospital admissions for asthma in the Bronx are roughly twice those in Manhattan. Researchers noted the presence in the Bronx of 20 waste transfer facilities, where diesel garbage trucks from all over the city congregate; a major wholesale produce market, where 12,000 trucks move in and out daily; and a network of major highways. Schools, playgrounds, and homes are all located within a few blocks of these pollution sources.

Residents in more affluent areas are able to wield the political power necessary to keep highways and waste transfer facilities out of their neighborhoods. Those in poorer areas bear the burden not just of pollution but of the disease caused by pollution.

Given these realities, are there actions that communities can take to ease the burden of air pollution for people with asthma—and everyone else? As described in Chapter 9, one step that many colleges and universities have taken to improve air quality for all is to go smoke-free.

Whatever the underlying causes of asthma, it is certain that air pollution, whether caused by trucks or tobacco, exacerbates asthma's acute symptoms and increases their severity—making life miserable for the growing number of Americans who suffer from the disease.

Q: Where does your campus stand on the smoke-free movement? Where do you stand on it?

Q: What are your thoughts about the disparities in prevalence of asthma, with children, particularly minority children, being more affected?

Sources: "Domestic Airborne Black Carbon and Exhaled Nitrous Oxide in Children in New York City," by A. G. Cornell et al., 2012, *Journal of Exposure Science and Environmental Epidemiology, 22,* pp. 258–266; "Asthma in the United States: Growing Every Year," 2012, Centers for Disease Control and Prevention, www.cdc.gov/vitalsigns/Asthma; "South Bronx Environmental Policy Study: Final Report of NYU School of Medicine Research," by G. D. Thurston, A. Spira-Cohen, and L. C. Chen, 2007, http://graphics8.nytimes.com/packages/pdf/nyregion/20081002_SOM.pdf; "Smoke and Tobacco Free U.S. and Tribal Colleges and Universities," 2014, American Nonsmokers Rights' Foundation, www.no-smoke.org/pdf/smokefreecollegesuniversities.pdf.

Chronic Obstructive Pulmonary Disease

In contrast to asthma, chronic obstructive pulmonary disease (COPD) tends to develop as people experience cumulative damage to their airways and alveoli over time and is usually diagnosed in middle or older aged adults. COPD is a leading cause of disability and the third leading cause of death in the United States. There are two components to COPD: chronic bronchitis and emphysema. Most people have both components.

In chronic bronchitis, there is persistent inflammation of the bronchioles, which causes the airway walls to thicken and the airway passages to narrow; there is also excess secretion

of mucus, which obstructs airflow. A person with this disorder has bronchial congestion and a chronic cough. Smokers with chronic bronchitis have an increased risk for lung cancer.

In emphysema, the alveoli become less stretchy and elastic, and the walls between alveoli are damaged or destroyed, creating less space for air exchange. It becomes harder for the lungs to take up oxygen and expel carbon dioxide. A person with emphysema is breathless and has to gasp for air. The disease puts a strain on the heart, increasing the risk for heart disease.

The primary cause of COPD is smoking. Exposure to other lung irritants, such as secondhand smoke, air pollution, and inhaled chemicals or dust, can also contribute to these diseases. Symptoms often begin gradually, progress slowly and can eventually make activities of daily living, such as cooking or getting dressed, difficult. They include an ongoing cough, shortness of breath, wheezing, and chest tightness. Because these symptoms resemble those of asthma, a health care provider performs lung function testing to determine the cause of the symptoms. Treatment can improve symptoms and slow the progression but cannot cure the disease. Inhaled bronchodilators and inhaled steroids are again the mainstay of treatment. At later stages, supplemental oxygen may be necessary; sometimes lung surgery and even lung transplantation are performed. The principal way to prevent COPD is not to start smoking and to quit as soon as possible if you have already started.

PREVENTING CHRONIC DISEASES

As scientists learn more about the progressive nature of chronic diseases like CVD, diabetes, and lung disease, the significance of early prevention becomes clearer. Adopting healthy lifestyle habits now, regardless of your age or current health status, is the best way to reduce your risk of developing chronic disease in the future.[37] Complete the Personal Health Portfolio for this chapter to assess your cardiovascular health.

Strategies for preventing chronic diseases are included throughout this chapter. Here is a quick review:

- Eat a heart-healthy diet.
- Avoid overweight and obesity.
- Don't smoke, and avoid secondhand smoke.
- Be physically active.
- Limit alcohol consumption.
- Maintain healthy blood pressure levels.
- Maintain healthy lipid levels.
- Maintain healthy blood glucose levels.
- Manage stress, and take care of your mental, emotional, and social health.

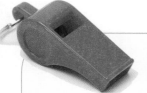

You Make the Call

Screening for Cardiovascular Disease in Athletes: How Much Is Enough?

Did you play sports in high school? Are you on a college team, or do you participate in intramural activities? Do you exercise vigorously on your own? If so, you should be aware that sudden cardiac arrest is the most common cause of death in young athletes (those younger than age 35). Vigorous exercise is a trigger for lethal arrhythmias in athletes with unrecognized heart disease, typically congenital disease. On average, only 11 percent of athletes will survive a sudden cardiac arrest—a worse outcome than might be expected, given their age, fitness level, and the fact that many of these events are witnessed. The low survival rates may be due to the underlying congenital disease, the exertion at the time of arrest, or slow recognition by bystanders of what has happened. These low survival rates highlight the critical importance of early recognition of underlying disease.

The American Heart Association (AHA) recommends preparticipation screening of athletes with a medical history and a physical exam. However, debate has ensued as to whether this is enough.

In 1979, Italy started a national program that added electrocardiogram (ECG) screening to the traditional screening. The addition of ECG identified many asymptomatic athletes whose conditions would have gone unrecognized by traditional screening. Since adding ECG screening, the incidence of sudden cardiac death among athletes in Italy has been reduced by 90 percent. The European Society of Cardiology (ESC) and the International Olympic Committee (IOC) thus adopted similar recommendations.

If you played sports in high school, you may or may not have participated in a screening physical prior to sports participation. This is because there is no national mandate in the United States regarding screening standards for high school athletes. And yet, 65 percent of sudden death in athletes occurs in high school students.

On the college level, there are no requirements for intramural sports teams or other school-affiliated teams, such as ultimate Frisbee teams. However, the National College Athletic Association (NCAA) has recently mandated a preparticipation evaluation for all Division I, II, and III athletes. The traditional evaluation involves a visit to a health care provider for screening

Continued…

Concluded...

questions concerning an athlete's personal and family history and a physical exam, with findings suggestive of heart disease prompting further evaluation. This screening has limitations because 60 to 80 percent of athletes have no symptoms, many have no family history of CVD or don't know their family history, and results of physical exams are normal in many people with congenital heart problems.

Some health experts think the United States should add ECG screening as a national preparticipation requirement for high school and college athletes, pointing to the healthy young people whose lives would be saved. A prohibiting factor is cost: if national screening were adopted, an estimated 10 million athletes would require screening at a theoretical cost of $2 billion dollars a year or approximately $330,000 for each athlete detected with cardiac disease. Another problem is the number of false-positive results that would occur—abnormal ECG findings in athletes who do not have underlying cardiac disease. An estimated 10 percent of results could be false positives. These athletes would have to go through the stress of an additional workup and temporary disqualification from their sport.

In a 2009 review, the American Heart Association (AHA) did not recommend the addition of ECG screening for American athletes. The AHA concluded that a national screening program would not be practical given the financial resources, staffing, and logistics that would be required. However, the AHA did recognize that, at present, we do not have full knowledge of how many young athletes die per year of sudden cardiac arrest and thus called for a national mandatory reporting system for sudden cardiac deaths in young competitive athletes.

Proponents of the additional ECG screening argue that any measures that save the lives of otherwise healthy young adults are worth the time and money invested. Opponents respond that such measures are unrealistic and impractical at this time. What do you think?

Pros

- Because survival rates from sudden cardiac arrest are very low, prevention is critical.
- Although it may be expensive and result in some false positives, the ECG is a straightforward, noninvasive test, and further evaluation is done with another noninvasive test, the echocardiogram.
- Italy demonstrated the will to save lives by adding ECG screening to its other athletic screening requirements. If a small country like Italy can institute such screening, a large, wealthy country like the United States should be able to do so, too.
- Cost should not be a factor when the lives of otherwise healthy young adults are at stake.

Cons

- The high rate of false positives from ECGs means that many athletes would be unnecessarily sidelined from their sports while awaiting further evaluation.
- Because of its larger population and geographical size, the United States cannot do ECG screening with the same ease as Italy or other European countries. The United States does not have the infrastructure (staffing, finances) to support a national program adding ECG screening.
- There isn't even a national requirement for the traditional screening (personal history, family history, and physical exam) in the United States right now. Thus, it is unrealistic to talk about adding an ECG requirement.

connect
ACTIVITY

Source: "Sudden Deaths in Young Competitive Athletes: Analysis of 1866 Deaths in the United States, 1980–2006," by B. J. Maron, J. J. Doerer, T. S. Hess, et al., 2009, *Circulation, 119* (8), pp. 1085–1092. "Cardiac Screening Before Participation in Sports," 2013, *New England Journal of Medicine, 369,* pp. 2049–2053; "Sudden Cardiac Death Screening in Adolescent Athletes: An Evaluation of Compliance With National Guidelines," by N. L. Madsen, J. A. Drezner, and J. C. Salerno, 2013, *British Journal of Sports Medicine, 47,* pp. 172–177.

In Review

What is cardiovascular disease?
The disease process underlying most forms of CVD is atherosclerosis, a condition in which the arteries become clogged and blood flow is restricted, causing heart attack, stroke, or peripheral vascular disease. A disturbance in the electrical signals controlling the heartbeat can cause an arrhythmia (disorganized beating) and sudden cardiac arrest. Other forms of CVD are hypertension (high blood pressure), congestive heart failure, heart valve disorders, rheumatic heart disease, congenital heart disease, and cardiomyopathy (disease of the heart muscle). A stroke occurs either when a blood vessel serving the brain is blocked or when a blood vessel in the brain ruptures.

What is diabetes?
Diabetes is the most common disorder of the endocrine or metabolic system and results in elevated blood glucose levels due to a disruption in the production or use of insulin. Type-1 diabetes typically starts in childhood, and Type-2 diabetes develops later and has genetic and lifestyle causes such as overweight and obesity. Without tight control and treatment, diabetes can lead to blindness, kidney failure, foot and leg amputations, and heart disease.

What is asthma?
Asthma is a condition in the lungs where inflammation and muscle spasm lead to narrowing of the airways and symptoms of difficulty breathing, wheezing, chest tightness, shortness of breath and coughing. The symptoms any one person experiences with asthma can drastically differ. Common triggers include viral infections, pollution, tobacco, allergies, and exercise. Symptoms can be controlled with medications but do not cure the disease.

What is chronic obstructive pulmonary disease?

Chronic obstructive pulmonary disease (COPD) is a progressive destructive process in the lungs that tends to develop as people get older in response to a lifetime accumulation of exposure to lung irritants that damage the airways and alveoli. There are two main forms of COPD—chronic bronchitis and emphysema. The main risk factor for COPD is tobacco use or exposure to other lung irritants (such as secondhand smoke, air pollution, inhaled chemical or dust exposure). Symptoms often begin gradually and progress slowly. Medications can reduce symptoms but not cure the disease.

What are the best ways to protect against the diseases discussed in this chapter?

The seven health behaviors and risk factors—smoking status, healthy BMI, healthy diet, participation in physical activity, and healthy levels of blood pressure, blood glucose, and total cholesterol—identified as being important for ideal cardiovascular health are actually key factors in reducing risk for all chronic diseases. Starting early and trying to maintain ideal cardiovascular health throughout life will protect against heart disease, stroke, chronic lung disease, and diabetes.

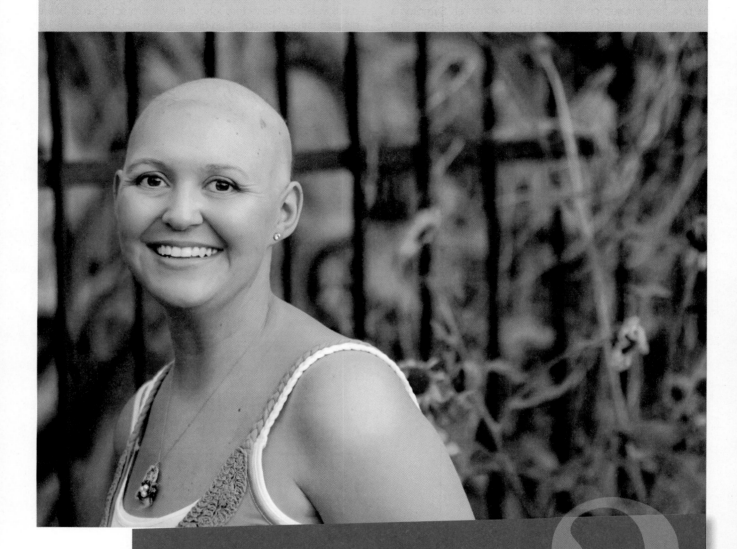

Ever Wonder...

- how to reduce your risk of skin cancer?

- what cancer screening tests you or your parents should be getting?

- if someone who gets cancer can ever be fully cured?

ancer is the second leading cause of death in the United States. In the past, people with cancer often hid their diagnosis; the word *cancer* was not used even in obituaries. Today, with greater understanding of this complex condition, cancer patients are diagnosed earlier and have higher survival rates, better prospects for a cure, and more social support. Although there is still much to learn, there is cause for optimism.

The American Cancer Society (ACS) projected an estimated 1.66 million new cancer cases in 2013 and more than 580,350 deaths from cancer, about 1,600 per day. Cancer causes about 25 percent of all deaths in the United States, with lung cancer the leading killer among both men and women. The four most common cancers—lung, colon, breast, and prostate—combined account for nearly half of all cancer deaths (Figure 15.1).[1] In this chapter, we provide an overview of the many forms cancer takes and the steps you can follow to reduce your risk of developing this disease.

WHAT IS CANCER?

Cancer is a condition characterized by the uncontrolled growth of cells. It develops from a single cell that goes awry, but a combination of events must occur before the cell turns into a tumor. The process by which this occurs is called *clonal growth*, the uncontrolled replication of a single cell that produces thousands of copies of itself. With 30 billion cells in a healthy person, the fact that one out of three people develops cancer is not surprising; what is surprising is that two out of three people do not.

cancer
Condition characterized by the uncontrolled growth of cells.

Healthy Cell Growth

Healthy cells have a complicated system of checks and balances that control cell growth and division. From the start, beginning with the single-celled fertilized egg, cells develop in contact with other cells, sending and receiving messages about how much space is available for growth. Healthy cells in solid tissues (all tissues except the blood) require the presence of neighboring cells. This tendency to stick together serves as a safety mechanism, discouraging cells from drifting off and starting to grow independently.

Healthy cells divide when needed to replace cells that have died or been sloughed off. Each time a cell divides, there is a possibility that a mutation, an error in DNA replication, will occur. Mutations are always occurring randomly, but the risk of mutations is increased by exposure to certain substances, such as tobacco smoke, radiation, and toxic chemicals. Certain mutations may start the cell on a path toward cancer.

Estimated New Cases*		Estimated Deaths	
Male	**Female**	**Male**	**Female**
Prostate 238,590 (28%)	Breast 232,340 (29%)	Lung & bronchus 87,260 (28%)	Lung & bronchus 72,220 (26%)
Lung & bronchus 118,080 (14%)	Lung & bronchus 110,110 (14%)	Prostate 29,720 (10%)	Breast 39,620 (14%)
Colon & rectum 73,680 (9%)	Colon & rectum 69,140 (9%)	Colon & rectum 26,300 (9%)	Colon & rectum 24,530(9%)
Urinary bladder 54,610 (6%)	Uterine corpus 49,560 (6%)	Pancreas 19,480 (6%)	Pancreas 18,980(7%)
Melanoma of the skin 45,060 (5%)	Thyroid 45,310 (6%)	Liver & intrahepatic bile duct 14,890 (5%)	Ovary 14,030 (5%)
Kidney & renal pelvis 40,430 (5%)	Non-Hodgkin lymphoma 32,140 (4%)	Leukemia 13,660 (4%)	Leukemia 10,060(4%)
Non-Hodgkin lymphoma 37,600 (4%)	Melanoma of the skin 31,630 (4%)	Esophagus 12,220 (4%)	Non-Hodgkin lymphoma 8,430 (3%)
Oral cavity & pharynx 29,620 (3%)	Kidney & renal pelvis 24,720 (3%)	Urinary bladder 10,820 (4%)	Uterine corpus 8,190 (3%)
Leukemia 27,880 (3%)	Pancreas 22,480 (3%)	Non-Hodgkin lymphoma 10,590 (3%)	Liver & intrahepatic bile duct 6,780 (2%)
Pancreas 22,740 (3%)	Ovary 22,240 (3%)	Kidney & renal pelvis 8,780 (3%)	Brain & other nervous system 6,150 (2%)
All sites 854,790 (100%)	All sites 805,500 (100%)	All sites 306,920 (100%)	All sites 273,430 (100%)

*Excludes basal and squamous cell skin cancers and in situ carcinoma except urinary bladder.

figure 15.1   **Leading sites of new cancer cases and deaths, 2013 estimates.**
Source: American Cancer Society. *Cancer Facts and Figures 2013.* Atlanta: American Cancer Society. www.cancer.org/acs/groups/content/@epidemiologysurveilance/documents/document/acspc-036845.pdf.

Specific safety mechanisms are designed to correct genetic mutations and destroy cells with mutations. As one safety mechanism, enzymes within the nucleus of each cell scan the DNA as it replicates, looking for errors. If an error is detected, the enzyme repairs it, or the cell destroys itself. As another safety mechanism, cells are programmed to divide a certain number of times, and then they become incapable of further division. The immune system also helps watch for cells that are not growing normally and destroys them.

A special protective mechanism exists for **stem cells**. These are cells that did not differentiate into specific cell types (e.g., nerve cells, skin cells, bone cells) during prenatal development. Instead, they retain the ability to become different cell types, and they are capable of unlimited division. A small number of stem cells are present within most tissue types, where they are needed to replace lost or damaged cells.

Because stem cells, unlike regular cells, do not have a predetermined number of cell divisions, they pose a risk for cancer. As a safety mechanism, they are located deep within tissues, where they are protected from factors that increase the risk of genetic mutations, such as exposure to the sun, chemicals, and irritation.

Cancer Cell Growth

Cancer starts from a single cell that undergoes a critical genetic mutation, either as a result of an error in duplication or in response to a **carcinogen** or radiation. This *initiating event* must be in a location in the cell's DNA that alters the functioning of a growth-controlling safety mechanism and allows a cell to evade one of the restraints placed upon healthy cells. To become a cancer, however, it must escape all the control mechanisms. Usually this process requires a series of 5 to 10 critical mutations within the cell's genetic material. It may take many years for these changes to progress to cancer, or they may never do so.

In time, perhaps a period of years, another mutation, such as one in an **oncogene** (a gene that drives cell growth regardless of signals from surrounding cells), may allow the cell line to divide

stem cells
Undifferentiated cells capable of unlimited division that can give rise to specialized cells.

carcinogen
Cancer-causing substance or agent in the environment.

oncogene
Gene that drives a cell to grow and divide regardless of signals from surrounding cells.

tumor
Mass of extra tissue.

benign tumor
Tumor that grows slowly and is unlikely to spread.

malignant tumor
Tumor that is capable of invading surrounding tissue and spreading.

metastasis
Cancer that has spread from one part of the body to another.

carcinomas
Cancers that arise from epithelial tissue.

sarcomas
Cancers that originate in connective tissue.

leukemias
Cancers of the blood, originating in the bone marrow or the lymphatic system.

lymphomas
Cancers that originate in the lymph nodes or glands.

forever rather than follow its preprogrammed number of divisions. A condition of cell overgrowth, called *hyperplasia,* develops at the site, and some cells may become abnormal, a condition called *dysplasia.* Eventually, a mass of extra tissue—a **tumor**—may develop.

A **benign tumor** grows slowly and is unlikely to spread. Benign tumors can be dangerous, however, if they grow in locations where they interfere with normal functioning and cannot be completely removed without destroying healthy tissue, as in the brain. A **malignant tumor** is capable of invading surrounding tissue and spreading. Malignant cells do not stick together as much as normal cells, and as the tumor grows, some cancer cells may break off, enter the lymphatic system or the bloodstream, and travel to nearby lymph nodes or to distant sites in the body. At a new site, the cancerous cell can grow and become a secondary tumor, or **metastasis**. When a cancer spreads from one part of the body to another, it is said to have *metastasized.*

Classifying Cancers

Cancers are classified according to the tissue in which they originate, called the *primary site.* If a cancer originates in the cells lining the colon, for example, it is considered colon cancer, even when it metastasizes to other, secondary sites. The most common sites of metastases are the brain, liver, and bone marrow.

When a cancer is still at its primary site, it is said to be *localized.* When it has metastasized, it is referred to as *invasive.* The greater the extent of metastasis, the poorer the *prognosis* (likely outcome).

Cancers are staged at time of diagnosis—a process that helps guide treatment choices and predict prognosis. The stage of disease is a description of how far the cancer has spread. One common staging system uses five categories (stages 0–IV). Stage 0 is also called cancer *in situ,* an early cancer that is present only in the layer of cells where it began. Stage I cancers are generally small and localized. Stages II and III are locally advanced and may or may not involve local lymph nodes. Stage IV cancers have metastasized to distant sites.

Types of Cancer

Different tissues of the body have different risks for cancer, due in part to their different rates of cell division. Four broad types of cancer are distinguished, based on the type of tissue in which they originate. **Carcinomas** arise from *epithelial tissue,* which includes the skin, the lining of the intestines and body cavities, the surface of body organs, and the outer portions of the glands. Epithelial tissue is frequently shed and replaced. From 80 to 90 percent of all cancers originate in epithelial tissues—including most lung, colon, breast, and prostate cancers. **Sarcomas** originate in *connective tissue,* such as bone, tendon, cartilage, muscle, or fat tissues. **Leukemias** are cancers of the blood and originate in the bone marrow or the lymphatic system. **Lymphomas** originate in the lymph nodes or glands.

Who's at Risk?

Cancer affects people of all races and ethnicities, but disparities in *incidence* (number of new cases) and *mortality* (number of deaths) between population groups are striking, as the graphs in this box show. Multiple factors contribute to these disparities, but most are believed to be attributable to socioeconomic differences in risk of exposure to carcinogens and barriers to early cancer detection and treatment.

Take a look at the graphs. Which groups have the highest incidence of cancer, and for which types are they most at risk? Compare the incidence rates to the mortality rates. Which populations' members are more likely to survive the different types of cancer? Why do you think that is the case?

Cancer Incidence and Death Rates* by Site, Race, and Ethnicity†, U.S., 2005–2009

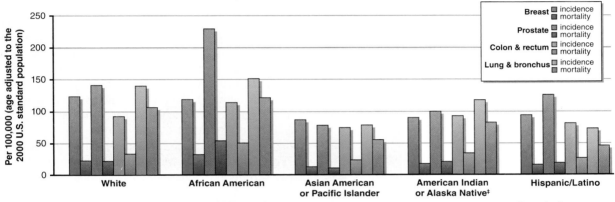

* Per 100,000, age adjusted to 2000 U.S. standard population. † Race and ethnicity categories are not mutually exclusive; persons of Hispanic/Latino origin may be of any race. ‡ Data based on Contract Health Service Delivery Area counties.

Source: "Cancer Facts and Figures 2013," American Cancer Society, 2013, www.cancer.org/acs/groups/content/@epidemiology surveillance/documents/document/acspc-036845.pdf.

connect
ACTIVITY

RISK FACTORS FOR CANCER

Because some cancers occur as a result of random genetic mutations, there is an element of chance in the development of the disease. Other cancers are associated with inherited genetic mutations. Still others occur as a result of exposure to carcinogens. Some such exposures can be limited by lifestyle behaviors, such as using sunscreen and avoiding tobacco, but others are beyond individual control and require the involvement of local authorities, the larger society, or even the international community, as in the case of air pollution (see the box, "Cancer Mortality and Risk Factor Disparities").

Risk factors are associated with a higher incidence of a disease but do not determine that the disease will occur. For example, if you smoke, you are 23 times more likely to develop lung cancer than a nonsmoker. Smoking does not guarantee you will get lung cancer, but your risk, relative to that of a nonsmoker, is greater. Conversely, if you do not smoke, you still may get lung cancer, but your risk is much lower than that of a smoker. The most significant risk factor for most cancers is age. Advancing age increases the risk for cancer; 77 percent of all cancers occur in people aged 55 or older.[1]

Family History

A family history of cancer increases an individual's risk. Examining your family health tree can help you understand whether you have an increased risk for any cancers. Family history does alter some cancer screening recommendations, such as when to start screening, how frequently to have screenings repeated, and what types of tests to have performed. However, genes are not the entire story. Only 5 percent of all cancers are due to an inherited genetic alteration. Most cancers result from damage to genes from environmental exposures and lifestyle behaviors that accumulate during our lifetime. Social determinants of health—including socioeconomic and cultural factors—are also influential.

Lifestyle Factors

Some environmental agents, carcinogens, have a direct impact on a cell, causing an initial genetic alteration that can lead to cancer. Other agents, called *cancer promoters,* have a less direct effect, enhancing the possibility that a cancer will develop if an initiating event has already occurred in a cell.

341

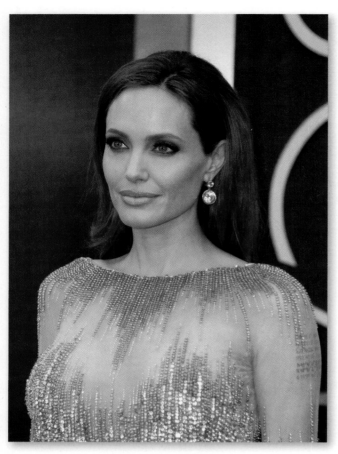

■ A family history of cancer can indicate that a person may have a genetic predisposition to the disease, especially if the cancer occurred in a first-degree relative (like a parent) at an early age. After Angelina Jolie learned she had inherited a defective BRCA1 gene, which is linked to breast and ovarian cancer, she had a preventive double mastectomy in 2013. Her mother, grandmother, and aunt had all died of breast or ovarian cancer.

Tobacco Use Tobacco use is the leading preventable cause of cancer in the United States. It is responsible for 30 percent of all cancer deaths and 87 percent of all lung cancer deaths.[1]

Tobacco use increases the risk of cancers of the mouth, throat, lung, and esophagus by directly exposing them to the chemicals in tobacco smoke. It also increases the risk of other cancers, including bladder, pancreas, stomach, liver, kidney, and bone-marrow cancers, because other chemicals from tobacco are absorbed into the bloodstream and travel to distant sites. Individual risk from tobacco use depends on the age at which the person starts smoking, the number of years the person smokes, and the number of cigarettes smoked per day. "Light" and "low tar" cigarettes and cigars have the same level of risk as "regular" cigarettes; it is no longer legal to use these terms in cigarette labels.

Smokeless tobacco products increase risk for oral, esophageal, and pancreatic cancers.[1]

Nutrition and Physical Activity Poor nutrition and lack of physical activity are the second most important contributors to cancer risk for the general population. Dietary patterns rich in foods such as fruits, vegetables, and whole grains that are naturally high in antioxidants and other phytochemicals appear to decrease the risk for many cancers, including lung, colon rectal, breast, stomach, and ovarian cancers. (See Chapter 5 for more on how antioxidants protect against cell damage.) Many fruits, vegetables, and whole grains are also high in dietary fiber, which some research has linked to reduced risk of colon cancer and possibly to reduced risk of breast, rectal, pharyngeal, and stomach cancers. Plant-based diets are recommended for the many ways by which they many reduce the risk for cancer.

Only 6 percent of college students report eating the recommended five or more servings of fruits and vegetables per day.[2] Although fruits and vegetables can have trace amounts of pesticides and herbicides, which can be toxic in high amounts, there is no evidence currently that the amounts in foods outweigh the proven benefits of consuming fruits and vegetables. To encourage people to eat fruits and vegetables, the National Cancer Institute has partnered with the non-profit Produce for Better Health Foundation in the "Fruits and Veggies—More Matters" public health initiative (www.fruitsandveggiesmorematters.org/).[3]

To date, there is no clear evidence that taking supplements of individual antioxidants reduces cancer risk as much as eating healthy whole foods. In fact, high-dose supplements of beta-carotene (an antioxidant found in fruits and vegetables) and vitamin E (an antioxidant and essential fat-soluble vitamin) have been shown to increase the risk of developing some cancers. Your best strategy is to choose a balanced diet rich in foods from a variety of plant sources.

Certain food preparation techniques may also increase the risk of cancer. Cooking meats at high temperatures, such as when grilling, frying, or broiling, may produce chemicals that increase risk for colon cancer. Processed meats, which are high in nitrites, appear to increase risk for colorectal, prostate, and stomach cancers. However, food irradiation, a practice commonly used with meats and spices to reduce risk of infectious disease contamination, has not been shown to increase cancer risk. Also, despite earlier reports to the contrary, studies have *not* shown an increase in cancer risk associated with the artificial sweeteners saccharin and aspartame.[4]

Exercise is directly linked to a reduction in risk of breast and colon cancers, though its effect on other cancers is less clear. The benefits of exercise on cancer risk go beyond exercise's impact on weight. Exercise improves body functions; for example, it increases the rate at which food travels through the intestines, thus reducing the bowel lining's exposure to potential carcinogens. Appropriate exercise after a cancer diagnosis and during treatment can also help people feel better, eat better, and recover faster. Decreasing sedentary activity, such as sitting, is most likely another important way to reduce cancer risk.[4]

Overweight and Obesity Overweight and obesity increase the risk of developing many types of cancer as well as the risk of dying from cancer once it occurs. Overweight and obesity not only make it harder to detect cancers at an early stage but also delay diagnosis and may make treatment more difficult.

Although it is not clear how fat cells contribute to an increased risk of cancer, several pathways are possible. Fat cells produce hormones, some of which (such as estrogen) are linked to cancer. Fat cells may trigger an immune and inflammatory reaction, alter insulin production, or release proteins that trigger cell growth, all of which may contribute to the development of cancer. Fat cells may also accumulate more environmental toxins. Maintaining a healthy BMI throughout your lifespan is another way to reduce your cancer risk.[1,4,5]

Alcohol Consumption and Cancer Risk Consumption of more than one alcoholic drink a day for women and two drinks a day for men increases the risk for cancers of the mouth, throat, esophagus, liver, breast, and possibly pancreas. Regular intake of just a few drinks per week may increase risk of breast cancer. Alcohol and tobacco used together amplify the risk for cancer and are associated with a greater risk than is either one alone. Total alcohol consumption, not the type of alcohol, is what matters; wine, beer, and hard liquor all increase risk.[1,4]

Social and Economic Factors

Although the number of new cases of cancer and the number of deaths from cancer are reported by gender, age, race, and ethnicity, more complex factors such as income, education, geographical location, housing, and cultural beliefs are believed to be stronger indicators of risk. These socioeconomic factors, or *social determinants of health,* influence risk behaviors (such as tobacco use), exposure to environmental carcinogens (such as housing proximity to highways or industrial sites), access to health care, and quality of health care.

People who are unemployed, who are poor, who live in rural areas, or who are underinsured or uninsured are at greater risk for developing cancer and dying from it. They may have less access to safe areas for physical activity and less access to nutritious foods. They may not be able to afford cancer screening tests, or they may not have access to physicians or clinics that provide screening. Getting recommended tests in a timely way increases the likelihood that a cancer will be detected or diagnosed at an earlier, more treatable stage. When cancers are detected at later stages, chances of survival are lower.

Public policy and community programs to reduce disparities in exposure to risk factors have been discussed in previous chapters. In attempts to reduce socioeconomic barriers to screening and early detection, the Centers for Disease Control has implemented a number of programs. For example, the National Breast and Cervical Cancer Early Detection Program provides access for low-income, uninsured, and underserved women to breast and cervical cancer screening, including clinical breast exams, Pap tests, mammograms, and further diagnostic testing or treatment as necessary. The Colorectal Cancer Control Program provides access for low-income and under- or uninsured men and women aged 50 to 64 to screening for colorectal cancer. In addition, the Affordable Care Act of 2010 includes provisions to make cancer prevention tools more accessible to underserved segments of the population.

Environmental Factors

Some cancers are caused by exposure to carcinogens in the environment. Some are more easily avoidable than others.

Sunlight and Other Sources of Ultraviolet Radiation Ultraviolet (UV) radiation, the rays of energy that come from the sun (and from sun lamps and tanning beds), can damage DNA but doesn't have enough power to penetrate deep into the body. Two types of UV come from the sun (and sun lamps and tanning beds): ultraviolet B (UVB) and ultraviolet A (UVA). UVB rays are more likely to cause sunburns and have long been associated with skin cancers. UVA rays tend to pass deeper into the skin and are now believed to cause skin cancer and premature aging of the skin.

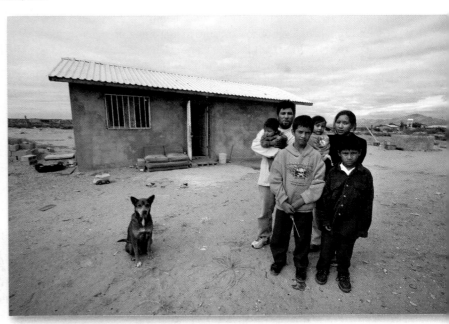

■ Being poor and living in a rural locale are risk factors for cancer. This low-income family living in the desert has less access to well-paying jobs, health insurance, health information, and health care services, including cancer screening tests, than a more affluent family living in an urban environment.

The risk for the two milder forms of skin cancer, basal cell and squamous cell carcinomas, is cumulative; the more UV exposure over the years, the higher the risk. The risk for melanoma, the most dangerous form of skin cancer, appears to be related more to the timing and number of sunburns. Sunburns that occur during childhood seem to be the most dangerous, and the more sunburns, the greater the risk. Indoor tanning poses as great a risk of skin cancer as outdoor sunbathing.

People who live close to the equator or in areas affected by the hole in the ozone layer have a higher risk of developing skin cancers. The ozone layer of the atmosphere protects the earth from the sun's damaging UV rays, but it is being disrupted by chemical pollution and is thinning over Antarctica and southern portions of the globe. Australia has one of the highest rates of skin cancer in the world, presumably because of this environmental condition.[6,7]

Other Forms of Radiation It has been proven that ionizing radiation can cause thyroid and bone marrow cancers, and it has been associated with other types of cancer depending on the location and level of exposure. An estimated 82 percent of ionizing radiation comes from natural sources, such as radon (a naturally occurring radioactive gas in the ground in certain regions of the world), cosmic rays, and release from soil and rocks. The other 18 percent is from human-made sources, such as medical X-rays, nuclear medicine, tobacco products, building materials, and television and computer screens. In contrast, exposure to non-ionizing radiation, including visible light, infrared radiation, microwaves, and radio waves, has not been considered a health risk. However, some concerns are now being raised about possible effects of long-term exposure to non-ionizing radiation (see the box, "Do Cell Phones Cause Cancer?").[8–12]

Residents in many parts of North America are exposed to low levels of radon in their homes, particularly homes with basements. In regions known to have high levels of radon in the ground, testing of homes is recommended. A ventilation system can be installed if the level of radon is high.

Nuclear fallout is another environmental source of radiation. Survivors of nuclear bomb explosions and tests have high levels of cancer, particularly cancers of the bone marrow and thyroid. The nuclear reactors used in power plants have not been shown to emit enough ionizing radiation to place surrounding communities at risk. However, accidental releases of radioactive gases from the nuclear power plants in Chernobyl, Ukraine, in 1986 and in Fukushima, Japan, in 2011 contaminated the area for miles around them and are responsible for cancers in people exposed to radiation and radioactive debris.

In medical settings, radiation is used in the treatment of cancers and in diagnostic imaging. The high-dose radiation for cancer treatment has been shown to increase the risk for leukemia and thyroid and breast cancers years later. Lower levels of radiation are used in diagnostic X-rays and CT scans, but exposure can accumulate in people who need many tests. To reduce risk, the number of medical procedures using radiation should be minimized as much as possible, especially in children.[8,10]

Chemical and Physical Carcinogens Many substances in the environment have been associated with different forms of cancer. Environmental carcinogens include metals (such as arsenic, mercury, and lead), natural fibers (such as asbestos and silica), combustion by-products (including motor vehicle exhaust, diesel exhaust, and soot), solvents (benzene, toluene), polychlorinated biphenyls (PCBs), and pesticides. Your exposure to environmental carcinogens varies depending on where you live, where you work, what your hobbies and recreational activities are, and what you eat, among other factors. Exposures are higher and rates of cancer are higher in cities, farming states, industrial areas, and near hazardous waste sites.[13–15]

Infectious Agents Some viruses are known to cause cancer. Human papillomavirus (HPV) is linked to cancers of the cervix, anus, vagina, penis, mouth, and more recently lungs and skin. The hepatitis B and C viruses are associated with liver cancer. Certain strains of Epstein-Barr virus, which causes mononucleosis, are associated with Hodgkin's lymphoma, non-Hodgkin's lymphoma, and some stomach cancers. Human immunodeficiency virus (HIV) suppresses the immune system and allows several types of cancer to develop.[16–20]

The only bacterium linked to cancer thus far is *Helicobacter pylori,* which causes a chronic irritation of the stomach lining and is associated with stomach ulcers and an increased risk of stomach cancer. Newer studies also suggest it may increase risk for colon, pancreatic, and potentially lung cancer.[21,22]

COMMON CANCERS

Since 1930, changes have occurred in the rates of different cancers in the United States (Figure 15.2). The most dramatic change in overall rates can be seen for lung cancer. The significant increase in lung cancer for both sexes is believed to be the result of increased rates of smoking. Rates of smoking increased among women about 20 to 30 years after they increased in men, and there has been a corresponding increase in lung cancer among women.

Lung Cancer

The leading cause of cancer death for both men and women in the United States and the second most commonly diagnosed cancer is lung cancer. In 1987, lung cancer overtook breast cancer as the leading cause of cancer death for American women. However, the incidence rates are declining for men and women.[1]

The leading risk factor for lung cancer is the use of tobacco products in any form. A genetic link has been identified that makes people more likely to become addicted to tobacco, makes it harder to quit, and increases the risk of lung cancer.[23–25] Other risk factors are exposures to

Starting the Conversation

Do Cell Phones Cause Cancer?

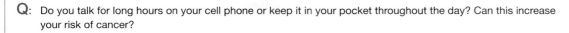

Q: Do you talk for long hours on your cell phone or keep it in your pocket throughout the day? Can this increase your risk of cancer?

In 2011, the International Agency for Research on Cancer listed radiofrequency electromagnetic fields (EMF) as a "possible human carcinogen." Because cell phones emit radiofrequency EMF and there are 5.5 billion cell phone subscribers worldwide, the question of whether radiofrequency fields cause cancer is a pressing one.

The electromagnetic spectrum ranges from low-energy static electric and magnetic fields to high-energy ultraviolet radiation, X-rays, and gamma rays. At the high end of the spectrum, the radiation has enough energy to displace electrons from atoms—creating free radicals, or "ionized particles," that can disrupt DNA and cell function. Lower frequencies of radiation ("non-ionizing" radiation) carry less energy. Visible light, infrared radiation, radiofrequency radiation, and microwaves are all types of non-ionizing radiation.

The safety of cell phones is first a question of whether non-ionizing radiation can have harmful effects on humans. You do not need to look to research to prove to yourself that non-ionizing radiation can have an effect on the human body. Simply turn on your microwave for two minutes to heat your dinner and you prove that focused, high-level exposure to microwave radiation causes a lot of heat. Cell phones' radiofrequency radiation has slightly less energy and substantially less intensity than microwaves, and the further the phone is from your body, the lower the exposure.

So the next question is whether long-term exposure to radiation at the radiofrequency level—such as that emitted from cell phones—can cause problems. This is where the data get tricky. Many studies have investigated whether there is a link between cell phones and human health. None have shown conclusive evidence of a strong link, and most have not even been able to show a connection. Animal studies and laboratory studies have not been able to confirm a carcinogenic effect. However, a few studies have shown a possible association between some brain tumors and high cell phone use and between childhood leukemia and radiofrequency-radiation exposure in the home. Current conclusions are that radiofrequency-radiation exposure is clearly not a strong carcinogen because, if it were, at least some of the studies would have found that. However, because of the inconsistencies, it remains possible that radiofrequency radiation may be a weak carcinogen. More data are needed before we can be absolutely certain that it is not and that long-term exposure is not harmful.

From computers to cell phones to remote controls, all populations are now exposed to increasing amounts of non-ionizing radiation, and the levels will continue to increase as technology advances. In addition, the length of time people are exposed is increasing as children are starting to use cell phones at younger and younger ages.

Q: Given that exposure decreases the further you are from your cell phone, would you change how often or how you use your phone based on the available data?

Q: Would you allow your children (or future children) to use cell phones? At what age?

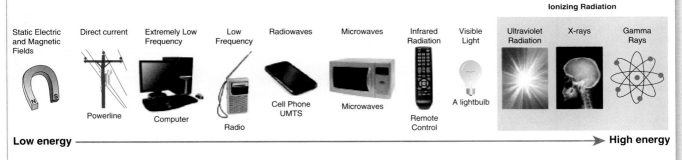

■ The electromagnetic spectrum

Sources: "Non-Ionizing Radiation, Part 2: Radiofrequency Electromagnetic Fields," 2013, *IARC Monographs on the Evaluation of Carcinogenic Risks in Humans, 102,* http://monographs.iarc.fr/ENG/Monographs/vol102/index.php; "Next Steps after the 2011 IARC Review," by J. M. Samet, K. Straif, J. Schuz, and R. Saracci, 2014, *Epidemiology, 25* (1), pp. 23–27; "Cancer Risks Related to Low-Level RF/MW Exposures, Including Cell Phones," by S. Szmigielski, 2013, *Electromagnetic Biology and Medicine, 32* (3), pp. 273–280; "Swedish Review Strengthens Grounds for Concluding that Radiation from Cellular and Cordless Phones Is a Probable Human Carcinogen," by D. L. Davis, S. Kesari, C. L. Soskolne, et al., 2013, *Pathophysiology, 20* (2), pp. 123–129; "Electric and Magnetic Fields," National Institute of Environmental Health Sciences, 2013, *Health and Education,* www.niehs.nih.gov/health/topics/agents/emf/.

carcinogenic chemicals, arsenic, radon, asbestos, radiation, air pollution, and environmental (secondhand) tobacco smoke. Recently, experts determined that dietary supplements containing beta-carotene, a form of vitamin A, further increase the risk for lung cancer in people who smoke.

Reducing risk factors, especially exposure to tobacco smoke and environmental tobacco smoke, is the first line of defense against this disease.

Signs and symptoms of lung cancer include coughing, blood-streaked sputum, chest pain, difficulty breathing, and

bronchoscopy
Procedure in which a fiber-optic device is inserted into the lungs to allow the health care provider to examine lung tissue for signs of cancer.

colon polyps
Growths in the colon that may progress to colon cancer.

flexible sigmoidoscopy
Procedure in which a fiber-optic device is inserted in the colon to allow the health care provider to examine the lower third of the colon for polyps or cancer.

colonoscopy
Procedure in which a fiber-optic device is inserted in the colon to allow the health care provider to examine the entire colon for polyps or cancer.

double-contrast barium enema
Test for colon polyps or cancer in which contrast material is inserted into the colon and X-rays are taken of the abdomen, revealing alterations in the lining of the colon if polyps or cancer is present.

recurrent lung infections. Unfortunately, symptoms do not appear in most people until the disease is advanced. There is currently no routine screening test recommended for lung cancer, but many organizations have begun to recommend low-dose computerized tomography (LDCT) to screen high-risk, heavy smokers (or former smokers) for lung cancer; this has been shown to reduce lung cancer mortality by 20 percent.[25]

If symptoms suggest lung cancer and an abnormality is found on an X-ray or CT scan, the diagnosis is confirmed by a biopsy, performed either by surgery or by **bronchoscopy**. People with small tumors that can be removed surgically have the best prognosis. For more advanced cancers or for people who are unable to tolerate surgery, radiation or a combination of radiation and chemotherapy is used. If the cancer has spread to distant sites, radiation and chemotherapy can be used for *palliative care* (care provided to give temporary relief of symptoms but not to cure the cancer). The one-year survival rate for lung cancer is 43 percent, and the five-year survival rate is 16 percent.[1]

Colon and Rectal Cancer

The third leading cause of cancer death and the third most commonly diagnosed cancer is colon and rectal cancer. During the 1990s, the incidence of colon and rectal cancer declined in the United States along with the number of deaths from the disease. The decrease is believed to be due to improved screening, detection, and removal of **colon polyps** before they become cancer.[1]

The most important risk factor for colorectal cancer is age. More than 90 percent of colorectal cancers are diagnosed in people over age 50. A personal or family history of colon polyps or inflammatory bowel disease also increases risk, as does a family history of colorectal cancer, especially in a first-degree relative. Other factors associated with an increased risk for colon and rectal cancer include smoking, alcohol use, obesity, physical inactivity, a diet high in fat or red or processed meat, and inadequate amounts of fruits and vegetables. Higher dietary intake of milk, and calcium may reduce risk of colon cancer. Higher serum levels of vitamin D, daily aspirin, and hormone replacement therapy may reduce the risk for colon and rectal cancer.[1]

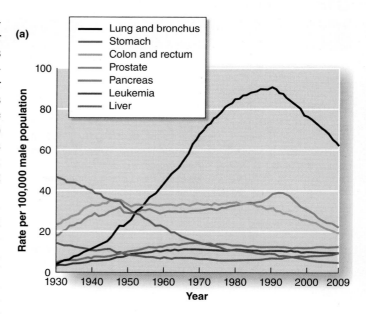

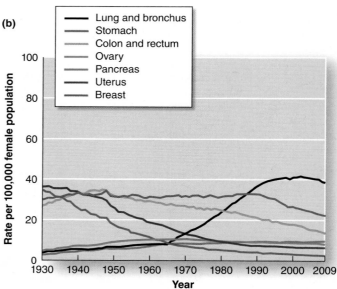

figure 15.2 **Cancer death rates by site, 1930–2009: (a) death rates for men; (b) death rates for women.**
Source: American Cancer Society Surveillance Research, using data from U.S. Mortality Data Volumes 1930–2009, National Center for Health Statistics, Centers for Disease Control and Prevention, 2013.

Warning signs of colorectal cancer include a change in bowel movements, change in stool size or shape, pain in the abdomen, and blood in the stool. The signs do not usually occur until the disease is fairly advanced. Screening tests can enhance early detection of polyps or cancer. Four techniques allow "visualization" of the colon. In a **flexible sigmoidoscopy**, a thin, flexible fiber-optic tube is inserted into the rectum and moved through the lower third of the colon. In a **colonoscopy**, a longer scope is used and the entire colon is viewed (Figure 15.3). If a polyp is found, it can be biopsied or removed during the procedure. In a **double-contrast barium enema**, the colon

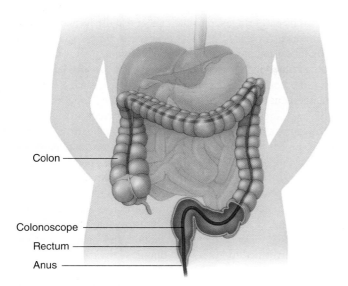

Colon

Colonoscope

Rectum

Anus

figure 15.3   Colonoscopy.
A colonoscopy allows the entire colon to be examined and facilitates the removal of growths, such as polyps, that may become cancerous.
Source: Fit & Well: Core Concepts and Labs in Physical Fitness and Wellness, 8th ed., by T. Fahey. Copyright © 2009 The McGraw-Hill Companies. Reprinted by permission of The McGraw-Hill Companies, Inc.

is partially filled with a contrast material and then X-rays are taken. A colon cancer or polyp will alter the lining of the colon and can be seen. In **CT colonography** (or virtual colonoscopy), a CT scanner is used to take multiple pictures of the colon and can detect polyps or cancer.[26]

Several other tests can screen for colon cancer but are not as good at detecting polyps. These include the fecal occult blood test, the stool immunochemical test, and the stool DNA test. The first two screen for trace amounts of blood, which can signal a cancer or a bleeding polyp, which is rare. The DNA test looks for changes in DNA known to be related to colon cancer.

The American Cancer Society recommends that people of average risk start colorectal cancer screening at age 50. For people with higher than average risk (e.g., someone who has a close family member with colon cancer or polyps), earlier and more frequent screening with colonoscopy is usually recommended.[1,26]

Surgery is the most common treatment for colon and rectal cancer; it can cure the cancer if it has not spread. Chemotherapy and/or radiation is added if the cancer is large or has spread to other areas. The one-year survival rate for all stages of colorectal cancer is 84 percent; the five-year survival rate is 64 percent.[1,25]

Breast Cancer

The second leading cause of cancer death in women and the most commonly diagnosed non-skin cancer in women is breast cancer. Breast cancer occurs in men as well as women, but it is much less common. For example, an estimated 232,340

cases were expected in women and 2,240 cases were expected in men in the United States in 2013.[1]

There are both controllable and noncontrollable risk factors for breast cancer. Among the noncontrollable factors are early onset of menarche (first menstruation), late onset of menopause, family history of breast cancer in a first-degree relative, older age, and higher socioeconomic class. A mutation in the BRCA1 or BRCA2 (BReast CAncer) gene is associated with an increased risk of breast cancer. These mutations are very rare in the general population, but people in families with a strong family history of breast or ovarian cancer may want to discuss testing with a genetic counselor. Although inherited susceptibility accounts for only 5 to 10 percent of all breast cancer cases, having these genes confers a lifetime risk of developing the disease ranging from 35 to 85 percent.

Controllable risk factors for breast cancer include never having children or having a first child after age 30, being obese after menopause, taking hormone replacement therapy, and drinking more than two alcoholic beverages a day. Breastfeeding, engaging in moderate or vigorous exercise, and maintaining a healthy body weight are all associated with decreased risk of breast cancer.

Early stages of breast cancer have either no symptoms or changes that may be detected only by a mammogram. Symptoms of later stages include a persistent lump; swelling, redness, or bumpiness of the skin; and change in nipple appearance or discharge. Breast pain or tenderness is common in women without cancer and is usually not a cause for concern; more likely explanations are hormonal changes, infection, or breast cysts, which are rarely cancerous.

Breast cancer can be detected at an early stage by a mammogram, a low-dose X-ray of the breast. The effectiveness of mammography in detecting cancer depends on several factors, including the size of the cancer, the density of the breasts, and the skills of the radiologist. Although mammograms cannot detect all cancers, they have been shown to decrease the number of women who die from breast cancer.

The American Cancer Society (ACS) and the National Cancer Institute (NCI) recommend annual mammograms for all women aged 40 and older. In 2009, the U.S. Preventive Services Task Force (USPSTF) ignited a controversy when it recommended changing this recommendation, citing the anxiety and cost associated with false positives (an abnormal finding when a woman does not have breast cancer). It recommended that women begin screening through mammograms at age 50 and that women younger than 50 talk with their doctors about their risk for breast cancer and the value of mammography based on their individual risk factors. The ACS, NCI, and similar institutions have remained firm in their recommendations that mammograms begin at age 40, and insurance companies continue to cover the procedure for women 40 and older.[27–31]

Another screening technique for breast cancer is the breast exam. The American Cancer Society recommends that women in their 20s and 30s have a clinical breast exam

CT colonography
Screen for colon polyps or cancer using a CT scanner.

(CBE) performed by a health care provider every three years and that women over 40 have a breast exam performed by their health care provider annually near the time of their mammogram. The ACS also suggests that, beginning in their 20s, women be told about the benefits and limitations of performing a breast self-exam (BSE) every month (see the box, "Breast and Testicular Self-Exams"). The ACS considers it acceptable for women to choose not to do self-exams or to do them only occasionally. The Preventive Services Task Force recommended in 2009 that women not perform breast self-exams but instead be on the lookout for any changes in their breasts during the course of daily activities.[28,30,32]

Any suspicious lumps, changes, or mammogram findings that are suggestive of cancer are typically followed by a biopsy so that cells or tissues can be evaluated under the microscope, the only way to make a definitive diagnosis. There are several noncancerous causes of lumps in the breast; in younger women, a lump is much more likely to be caused by a cyst or a benign tumor called a fibroadenoma. Other screening tools, including ultrasound and magnetic resonance imaging (MRI), are sometimes used to help determine whether a lump or abnormality is cancerous; they are also used for screening in high-risk women.

Surgery is usually the first line of treatment for breast cancer, either a *lumpectomy* (removal of the tumor and some breast tissue around) or a *mastectomy* (removal of the entire breast). One or more lymph nodes under the arm on the affected side are usually tested to determine whether the cancer has spread from the breast. Radiation, chemotherapy, and hormonal-inhibition therapy are frequently used in the treatment of breast cancer.

The five-year survival rate for all stages of breast cancer is 90 percent. For cancer that is localized (no lymph node involvement), it is 98 percent; for cancer that has spread regionally (only local lymph node involvement), it is 84 percent; and for cancer that has distant metastases, it is 24 percent.[1]

Prostate Cancer

The second most common cause of cancer death in men and the most commonly diagnosed cancer in men is prostate cancer. The incidence of prostate cancer is significantly higher among Black men than White men, as is the death rate. The number of diagnosed cases of prostate cancer increased in the early 1990s, probably as a result of better screening, and has leveled off since 1998. Death rates declined during the same period, although death rates for Black men remain twice as high as those for White men.[1]

The most important risk factor for prostate cancer is age. More than 60 percent of prostate cancer cases are diagnosed in men aged 65 and older. Other risk factors include a family history of prostate cancer, being Black, and possibly having a high animal-fat or full-fat dairy diet. The risk of dying from prostate cancer appears to increase with increasing body weight. Lycopene, an antioxidant found in red and pink fruits and vegetables, may reduce risk. Vitamin E and selenium supplementation does not appear to reduce risk.[1]

In its early stages, prostate cancer usually has no signs or symptoms. Advanced prostate cancer can be associated with difficulty urinating, pain in the pelvic region, pain with urination, or blood in the urine. These symptoms can also be caused by more common, noncancerous conditions, such as benign enlargement of the prostate gland and bladder infections.

Two screening tests are available to detect prostate cancer. One is a *digital rectal exam,* in which a health care provider inserts a gloved finger into the rectum and palpates the prostate gland. The other is the *prostate-specific antigen (PSA) test,* a blood test that detects levels of a substance made by the prostate (prostate-specific antigen) that are elevated when certain conditions are present, including benign prostate enlargement, infection, and prostate cancer. If the PSA level is high, a rectal ultrasound and prostate biopsy can be performed to assess and diagnose the cause.

At present, it is unclear whether the benefits of screening tests for prostate cancer—earlier detection of cancer when it is most treatable—outweigh the negatives. As with mammography, screening tests for prostate cancer can produce false positives, requiring invasive follow-up tests. Sometimes, fast-growing prostate cancers do not elevate PSA levels, causing a false negative result from a PSA test. On the other hand, some prostate cancers grow very slowly and would not actually lead to an earlier death. The treatment of these cancers can sometimes cause more harm and undesirable side effects than if they were left untreated. The American Cancer Society (ACS) recommends that all men discuss with their health care providers whether they should have a digital rectal exam and PSA screening annually

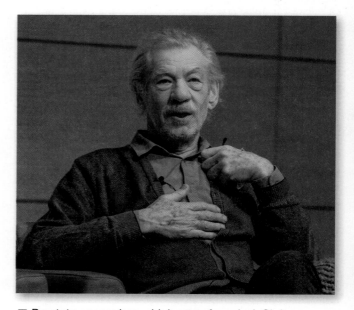

■ Prostate cancer has a high rate of survival. Sir Ian McKellen was diagnosed with prostate cancer almost a decade ago and has chosen the course of "watchful waiting" instead of surgery or radiation. He told the press, "When you have got it, you monitor it and you have to be careful it doesn't spread. But if it is contained in the prostate, it's no big deal."

Action Skill-Builder

Breast and Testicular Self-Exams

Whether you are a woman or a man, the point of conducting regular self-exams is the same: to get to know your body and to recognize any change that could be cancerous, such as the development of a lump or swelling. If you notice any kind of a change during your self-exam, see your health care provider right away for an evaluation. In many cases, changes do not turn out to be cancerous, but detecting cancer early increases your chance of survival. Frequent self-exams are not recommended, however, because research has not shown that they reduce the risk of dying from breast or testicular cancer.

Breast Exam

☐ The best time to do your exam is a few days after your period when the breast tissue is least tender. If you no longer menstruate or have very irregular periods, do the exam on the same day every month.

☐ Lie down and put a pillow under your right shoulder. Place your right arm behind your head.

☐ Use the finger pads of your three middle fingers on your left hand to feel for lumps or thickening in your right breast. Use overlapping dime-sized circular motions of the finger pads to feel the breast tissue.

☐ Use three different levels of pressure—light, medium, and firm—to feel all the breast tissue. Use each pressure level

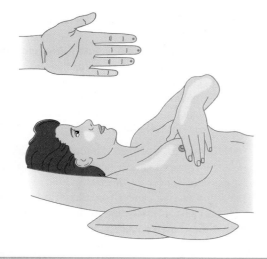

to feel the breast tissue before moving on to the next spot. If you're not sure how hard to press, talk with your health care provider. A firm ridge in the lower curve of each breast is normal.

☐ Move around the breast in an up-and-down pattern starting at an imaginary line drawn straight down your side from the underarm and move across the breast to the middle of the chest (breast bone).

☐ Don't just check for lumps. Look for skin irritation or dimpling, nipple pain or retraction, redness or scaliness of the nipple or skin, or a discharge other than breast milk. Most of the time, these changes are not cancer.

☐ Repeat the exam on your left breast, using the finger pads of the right hand and moving the pillow under your left shoulder.

☐ While standing in front of a mirror with your hands pressing firmly down on your hips, look at your breasts for any changes of size, shape, contour, or dimpling. (Pressing down on your hips contracts the chest wall muscles and enhances any breast changes.)

☐ Examine each underarm while sitting up or standing and with your arm only slightly raised so you can easily feel in the area.

Testicular Self-Exam*

☐ Stand in front of a mirror. Look for any changes or swelling on the skin of the scrotum.

☐ Examine each testicle with both hands. Place your index and middle fingers under the testicle with the thumbs placed on top. Roll the testicle gently between the thumbs and fingers. It's normal for one testicle to be slightly larger than the other.

☐ Find the epididymis, the soft, tubelike structure behind the testicle that collects and carries sperm. If you are familiar with this structure, you won't mistake it for a suspicious lump.

☐ Cancerous lumps are usually found on the sides of the testicle but also can appear on the front.

☐ If you find a lump, see your doctor right away. Testicular cancer is highly curable, especially when it's detected and treated early. In almost all cases, testicular cancer occurs in only one testicle, and men can maintain full sexual and reproductive function with the other testicle.

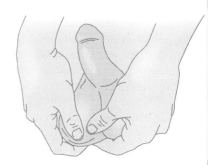

starting at age 50; the ACS also recommends that Black men and men with a family history of prostate cancer begin having this discussion at age 45.[1]

Treatment for prostate cancer depends on the stage of the cancer and the man's age and other health conditions. In its early stages and in younger men, prostate cancer is usually treated with surgery (removal of the prostate gland) and radiation, sometimes in combination with chemotherapy, and hormonal medication, which blocks the effects of testosterone and can cause tumors to shrink. Later stages are treated with chemotherapy, radiation, and hormonal medication. Radiation is sometimes administered by the implantation of radioactive seeds, which destroy cancer tissue and leave normal prostate tissue intact. A breakthrough treatment that received approval in 2010—the use of a vaccine to fight advanced prostate cancer—stimulates a patient's immune system to respond to the cancer cells. Although not expected to cure the disease, it does appear to prolong life.[33]

The five-year survival rate for all stages of prostate cancer is nearly 100 percent. In studies that follow prostate cancer for more than five years, the survival rate decreases to 98 percent at 10 years and to 91 percent at 15 years.[1]

Cancers of the Female Reproductive System

Cancer can develop anywhere in the female reproductive system but occurs most frequently in the cervix, uterus, and ovaries.

Cervical Cancer The incidence of cervical cancer and the number of related deaths have declined sharply in the past several decades as a result of improved detection and treatment of precursor lesions, primarily by means of the Pap test.

As described in Chapter 13, cervical cancer is closely related to infection with certain strains of the human papillomavirus (HPV). However, although HPV infection is common in women, the majority of women never develop cervical cancer. Persistent infection and progression to cancer are influenced by other factors, such as tobacco use, immunosuppression, multiple births, early sexual activity, multiple sex partners, socioeconomic status, and nutritional status. Currently two vaccines are available and reduce the risk of HPV infection, as described in Chapter 13.

In its early stages, cervical cancer usually does not cause any symptoms. Warning signs of more advanced cancer include abnormal vaginal discharge or abnormal vaginal bleeding. Pain in the pelvic region can be a late sign of cervical cancer.

Early detection through the Pap test has significantly reduced the rates of cervical cancer and mortality. The Pap test, recommended for all women over age 21, is performed as part of a pelvic exam (see the box, "Changing Pap Test Guidelines"). A small sample of cells is collected from the cervix with a swab or brush, placed on a slide or into a liquid suspension, processed, and then examined under the microscope to detect cells that may be abnormal. Pap tests are good but not perfect, occasionally giving either a false negative or a false positive. HPV tests can be used with liquid Pap suspensions to identify HPV strains and are particularly helpful if the Pap results are unclear.

Treatment for cervical cancer involves removing or destroying precursor cells. Invasive cervical cancer is treated with a combination of surgery, local radiation, and chemotherapy. Overall, the five-year survival is 68 percent, but the rate is 91 percent if the disease is localized.[1]

Uterine Cancer

Also called *endometrial cancer,* uterine cancer usually develops in the endometrium, the lining of the uterus. Uterine cancer is diagnosed more often in White women than in Black women, but the death rate among Black women is nearly twice the rate among White women. Black women tend to have more advanced cancer when they are diagnosed, perhaps as a result of having less access to health care.

The risk for uterine cancer is related to a woman's exposure to estrogen, so factors that increase estrogen—such as obesity and estrogen replacement therapy without progesterone—increase risk. Other factors associated with increased risk include young age at menarche, late-onset menopause, irregular ovulation, and infrequent periods. Pregnancy and oral contraceptives reduce the risk of uterine cancer.

Warning signs of uterine cancer include abnormal uterine bleeding (spotting between periods or spotting after menopause), pelvic pain, and low back pain. Pain is usually a late sign of uterine cancer. Uterine cancer is frequently detected at an early stage in postmenopausal women because of vaginal bleeding.

If uterine cancer is diagnosed, a *hysterectomy*—surgical removal of the uterus—is usually performed. Depending on the stage of cancer, other treatment methods may also be used, including radiation, chemotherapy, and hormonal therapy. Overall, the five-year survival rate is 82 percent.[1]

Ovarian Cancer The leading gynecological cause of cancer death and the fifth overall cause of cancer death in women is ovarian cancer. Ovarian cancer has a low rate of survival because most cases are not diagnosed until they have spread beyond the ovaries. If ovarian cancer is diagnosed early, the survival rate is as high as 92 percent. However, the overall one-year survival rate is 75 percent and the five-year survival rate is 44 percent.

Public Health Is Personal

Changing Pap Test Guidelines

The Pap test, widely used since the 1940s, is credited with the dramatic reduction in number of deaths from cervical cancer, which was once the leading cause of cancer death for women in the United States. Doctors performing Pap tests looked for any abnormal cell changes in the cervix, and if they found abnormal cells, they removed them. Although the cause of cervical cancer was not known, the Pap test provided a highly effective screening tool for it.

However, scientists, health care professionals, and public health officials came to the conclusion that Pap test guidelines were too stringent, leading doctors to overdiagnose and overtreat precancerous symptoms. In turn, anxious patients underwent needless emotional, physical, and financial tolls after they opted for invasive and costly treatments. Often, those treatments were unnecessary, and sometimes they were harmful, causing a higher risk for future miscarriage.

Prior to November 2009, women had been advised to start getting cervical cancer screenings—Pap tests—at age 18 or within three years of becoming sexually active, but no later than age 21. They were advised to have the test every year up until age 30, and then every two to three years. In November 2009, new recommendations were issued: women should not begin getting Pap tests until age 21, should then have them every two years until age 30, and should have them every three years after age 30. In March 2012, revised, "final" recommendations advised that testing should not begin until age 21, regardless of sexual history, and should be done every three years until age 30 and then every three to five years until age 65.

These changes were made in response to research findings that called into question the usefulness of earlier and more frequent screenings. Health organizations and agencies regularly review the latest research and new biotechnology and update their recommendations when the evidence suggests a change is needed. In this case, the American Cancer Society, the American Congress of Obstetricians and Gynecologists, the U.S. Preventive Services Task Force, and several other organizations separately or jointly issued revised guidelines for Pap testing based on clear clinical findings.

Meanwhile, scientists have been trying to learn the cause of cervical cancer. In the 1980s, researchers proposed a causal link between cervical cancer and the human papillomavirus (HPV), and years of investigation and clinical trials confirmed that virtually all cases of cervical cancer are caused by strains of HPV. More recently, it was found that although HPV infection is very common in young, sexually active women, most women clear the infection within 18 to 24 months. Thus, even if they have early cervical cell abnormalities, in most cases, the cells revert to normal on their own. Furthermore, it often takes 10 years or more for HPV to develop into cervical cancer, so if abnormal cells are detected when a woman is in her 20s, there is still time to treat them. New technology allows for HPV testing, so screening can now identify women who have ongoing active, high-risk strains of HPV.

It is now the consensus that for otherwise healthy women, screening at less frequent intervals and starting later prevents cervical cancer just as well as earlier, more frequent testing, with less negative side effects. The combination of Pap and HPV testing in women 30 and older allows for identification of cellular changes and ongoing high-risk HPV infection. If there is no evidence of either, screening intervals can increase to every five years. HPV testing is not recommended for women in their 20s because so many women at that age will have evidence of active HPV, which in the majority of them will resolve on its own without treatment. Screening start time and intervals are different for women with a history of cervical cancer, HIV, or other conditions that weaken the immune system.

Public policy guidelines like these are intended to promote consistent practices by doctors across the country, based on the latest and best research. Doctors, in turn, rely on official recommendations to guide their practices, even though they may be reading the research themselves. Thus, findings from research conducted over the past few decades affects what happens today when a woman goes for an annual gynecological exam. The doctor may decide that a Pap test is not necessary, even if the woman previously had one annually, and healthy women under the age of 21 should not be screened at all.

Sources: "New Guidelines for Cervical Cancer Screening," 2013, Patient Education Fact Sheet, The American College of Obstetricians and Gynecologists, www.acog.org/For_Patients/Search_FAQs/documents/New_Guidelines_for_Cervical_Cancer_Screening.

Between 90 and 95 percent of women with ovarian cancer have no risk factors. The strongest risk factor is a family history of breast or ovarian cancer in a first-degree relative, especially if the BRCA1 or BRCA2 gene is involved. Women with either of these genetic mutations have a 20 to 60 percent chance of developing ovarian cancer. Risk is also increased in women with a personal history of breast, colon, or endometrial cancer. In addition, tobacco use and being overweight increase risk. Factors that reduce risk include oral contraceptive pills, pregnancy, and breastfeeding. Avoidance of postmenopausal hormone replacement therapy may also reduce risk. Women with the BRCA1 or BRCA2 gene mutation may consider more aggressive measures to reduce risk, including removal of the ovaries and fallopian tubes.

The early stages of ovarian cancer have few signs or symptoms. At later stages, a woman may notice swelling of the abdomen, bloating, or a vague pain in the lower abdomen. Several blood tests have been evaluated for use as a screening tool, and another potential screening tool is a pelvic ultrasound, in which sound waves are used to visualize the ovaries and show whether they are enlarged or contain a mass. At present, however, no screening test has been shown to decrease mortality, so currently there is no recommended screen. A screen to increase early detection would be beneficial, given the improved survival with early diagnosis.[34,35]

A "bimanual exam," in which a health care provider feels the uterus and ovaries with two gloved fingers in the vagina and a hand on the lower abdomen, occasionally detects ovarian cancer but usually only when the disease is advanced.

Treatment for ovarian cancer depends on the stage at diagnosis. Typically, all or part of the ovaries, uterus, and fallopian tubes are surgically removed, and lymph nodes are biopsied to determine whether the cancer has spread. Chemotherapy and radiation may then be recommended. Treatment options currently under investigation include vaccinations, targeted drugs, and immunotherapy.[34]

Skin Cancer

The three forms of skin cancer are basal cell carcinoma, squamous cell carcinoma, and melanoma. An estimate 3.5 million cases of basal cell and squamous cell cancers occur each year in the United States (exact figures are difficult to know because skin cancer is not a reportable disease). Most of these are curable, although both types can be disfiguring and, if ignored, sometimes fatal. Melanoma is a less common form of skin cancer but more likely to be fatal. Skin cancers occur in all racial and ethnic groups, but they are more common in people with lighter skin colors.

All forms of skin cancers are linked directly to ultraviolet light exposure—both UVA and UVB.[36] The most effective way to reduce risk for skin cancer is to limit UV exposure, both from the sun and from UV lights in tanning salons. To limit UV exposure from the sun, in order of importance, stay out of the sun during midday (10:00 a.m. to 4:00 p.m.), wear protective clothing (including a hat to shade the face and neck, long sleeves, and long pants), use a broad-spectrum sunscreen with a **sun protective factor (SPF)** of 15 or higher (see the box, "Sunscreen and Other Sun Protection Products"), and wear sunglasses that offer UV protection. Tanning beds and sun lamps should be avoided. Parents should be particularly vigilant about protecting their children from the sun, and babies under 6 months of age should be kept out of the sun altogether.

sun protective factor (SPF) Measure of the degree to which a sunscreen protects the skin from damaging UV radiation from the sun.

Melanoma Because it is capable of spreading quickly to almost any part of the body, melanoma is a particularly dangerous form of cancer. Rates of melanoma have increased over the past 30 years, especially in young White women and older White men.

The risk of melanoma is greatest for people with a personal history of melanoma, a large number of moles (especially those that are large or unusual in shape or color), or a family member with melanoma (see the box, "Maggie: A Case of Skin Cancer"). The risk is greater in people with fair skin and sun sensitivity (burning easily). The rate in Whites is 23 times higher than the rate in Blacks, but the disease does occur in Blacks. Although it can occur on any part of the body, melanoma is directly related to sun exposure, especially intermittent, acute UV exposure, as from sunlight (sunburns) or UV light in tanning salons. Exposure during childhood or adolescence may be particularly dangerous.

Melanomas usually develop in pigmented, or dark, areas on the skin. Signs suggestive of melanoma are changes in a mole: a sudden darkening or change in color, spread of color outward into previously normal skin, an irregular border, pain, itchiness, bleeding, or crusting. You can monitor your skin for these signs by using the "ABCDE" test for melanoma (Figure 15.4).

Early detection of skin cancer is usually the result of individuals' monitoring their own skin and visiting a health care provider for evaluation of any changes or progressive growth. The American Cancer Society recommends that people have a skin exam (visual inspection of the skin all over the body) as part of a regular physical examination every three years between ages 20 and 40 and annually after age 40.

Treatment for melanoma begins with surgically excising (cutting out) and doing a biopsy of any suspicious lesions. If melanoma is confirmed, a larger area of surrounding skin is removed, which improves the chance of survival. Chemotherapy and immunotherapy can be added for advanced

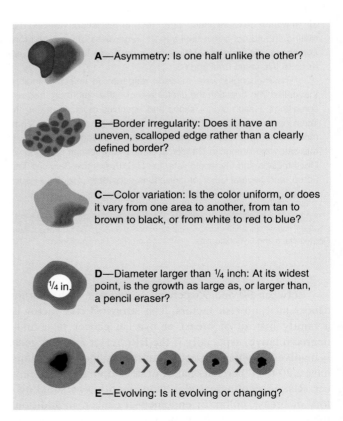

figure 15.4   The ABCDE evaluation of moles for melanoma.
Source: "What to Look For: The ABCDEs of Melanoma," 2014, American Academy of Dermatology, www.aad.org/spot-skin-cancer/understanding-skin-cancer/how-do-i-check-my-skin/what-to-look-for.

Consumer Clipboard

Sunscreen and Other Sun Protection Products

Sun exposure is the most preventable risk factor for skin cancers. Sunscreens can reduce the damaging effects of UV radiation. Historically, sunscreens protected primarily against UVB exposure, long known to cause sunburns and skin damage and to be associated with skin cancer. Data now indicate that UVA exposure also causes skin cancer, in addition to aging (wrinkling and sagging) and other skin damage. UVA penetrates the skin more deeply than UVB and is responsible for tanning.

Look for the SPF (sun protective factor or sunburn protective factor) number.
SPF indicates the amount of time you can stay in the sun without burning compared to how long you could stay if you weren't wearing the sunscreen. An SPF of 15 means that a person can stay out in the sun 15 times longer than he or she could without sunscreen before a sunburn would occur. Only sunscreens with an SPF of 15 or greater can claim to reduce risk of skin cancer and early skin aging. A pending proposal will limit the maximum SPF protection to "50+" as values above 50 have not shown additional advantage.

Look for "broad spectrum" on the label.
A sunscreen may be labeled broad spectrum only if it provides protection against UVA and UVB radiation. Ingredients such as titanium dioxide, zinc oxide, Mexoryl, and Helioplex reduce UVA exposure.

Look for a sunscreen that is "water resistant."
Water resistance labeling tells you how long you can expect to get protection while swimming or sweating; 40 or 80 minutes is standard.

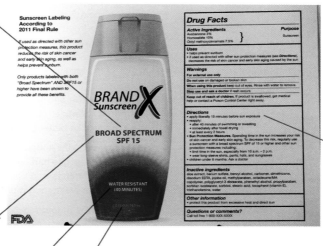

Apply sunscreen liberally to all sun-exposed areas.
Most people do not apply enough sunscreen. An average-sized adult in a swimsuit needs about 1 ounce, or a shot glass, of sunscreen for one application. If applied properly, you could easily use a whole bottle of sunscreen in one day at the beach or pool. Avoid sunscreen powders and sprays.

Avoid combination products unless you really need them.
Combination products, such as sunscreen and insect repellent, reduce the effect of SPF by up to one-third. When using a combination product, use one with a higher SPF and reapply it more frequently.

Reapply early and often, as directed on the bottle.
Sunscreen should be applied at least 20 to 30 minutes before going outside—it takes that long for sunscreen to be absorbed. It should also be reapplied frequently, at least every two hours and after swimming or sweating. Apply even on cloudy days or when behind glass, such as in a car—80 percent of UVA rays still get through.

Don't rely on sunscreen alone.
Consider it your last defense. Decrease UV exposure by limiting time in the sun and wearing protective clothing. The protectiveness of clothing varies. Hats typically offer an SPF between 3 and 6; summer-weight clothing has an SPF of about 6.5; newer sun-protective clothing can have an SPF of up to 30+.

Sources: "FDA Sheds Light on Sunscreen," 2012, U.S. Food and Drug Administration, www.fda.gov/ForConsumers/ConsumerUpdates/ucm258416.htm; "Sunscreen," 2013, U.S. Food and Drug Administration, www.fda.gov/Drugs/ResourcesForYou/Consumers/BuyingUsingMedicineSafely/Understanding Over-the-CounterMedicines/ucm239463.htm.

stages. The overall five-year survival rate for melanoma is 91 percent; if the melanoma is diagnosed at an early stage, the five-year survival rate is 98 percent.[1]

Basal Cell and Squamous Cell Carcinomas Sun-exposed areas of the body are susceptible to basal cell and squamous cell cancers. People at high risk include those with fair skin; blonde, red, or light brown hair; blue, green, or hazel eyes; and freckles and moles. Other risk factors are cumulative sun exposure and age, with rates increasing after age 50. However, both types are increasing among younger people.

The signs of a basal cell cancer include new skin growth; a raised, domelike lesion with a pearl-like edge or border; or a sore that bleeds and scabs but never completely heals. The signs of a squamous cell cancer include a red, scaly area that does not go away; a sore that bleeds and does not heal; or a raised, crusty sore. Squamous cell cancers often develop from a precancerous spot called an actinic keratosis, a red, rough spot that develops in a sun-exposed area.

Early detection of basal and squamous cell cancers involves monitoring the skin and having any persistent changes evaluated. The American Cancer Society recommends the same skin exams for these cancers as for melanoma. Treatment usually involves local removal and destruction of the cancer by surgery, heat, or freezing; radiation therapy is sometimes an option.[1]

Testicular Cancer

Although testicular cancer accounts for only 1 percent of all cancers in men, it is the most common malignancy in men 20 to 35 years of age. The incidence of testicular cancer has nearly doubled worldwide over the past 40 years. It is not clear why this increase is occurring, but some researchers

Life Stories

Maggie: A Case of Skin Cancer

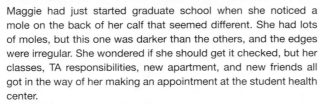

Maggie had just started graduate school when she noticed a mole on the back of her calf that seemed different. She had lots of moles, but this one was darker than the others, and the edges were irregular. She wondered if she should get it checked, but her classes, TA responsibilities, new apartment, and new friends all got in the way of her making an appointment at the student health center.

Maggie grew up in southern California and had spent a lot of her childhood outside. As a kid, she swam on her school swim team and played tennis. As a teenager, she and her friends went to the beach almost every weekend during the summer. Sometimes they used sunscreen, and sometimes they didn't. One time, Maggie got such a bad sunburn on her back that her mom took her to the doctor, who shook his head looking at the open blisters weeping down her back.

In college, Maggie occasionally went to a local tanning salon during the spring when she wanted to start wearing shorts and a bathing suit. Several of her friends went too, and all of them acquired a healthy-looking tan while other students retained their winter pallor. Maggie heard warnings about tanning, but she liked the look.

A month after she first noticed the mole on her calf, Maggie saw that it had gotten larger and had some red and purple coloring in it. She looked up moles and skin cancer on the Internet and felt alarmed enough by what she read to make an appointment at the health center to get it checked. The doctor agreed that it looked a bit different and said she wanted to remove it and do a biopsy. The mole was removed easily and sent for pathology.

A week later, Maggie received a call from the doctor, saying that the mole was in fact cancerous, a melanoma. Maggie was shocked and could hardly understand what the doctor was saying, but she did hear that the cancer was caught at an early stage and the procedure had completely removed it. The doctor wanted her to come back in for a follow-up appointment, to remove extra skin around the area to make sure that there were no remaining cancer cells and to check her other moles. As she hung up the phone, Maggie felt a mixture of concern and relief, and she resolved to take better care of her skin in the future.

- Why do you think Maggie continued going to the tanning salon even though she had heard warnings about the dangers? Have you done things that you knew could put your health at risk? What was your thought process in making those choices?

- What kinds of information or education would be more effective in deterring people from making unhealthy choices or encouraging them to make healthy choices?

connect ACTIVITY

---

speculate that it could be due to fetal exposure to higher levels of estrogen during prenatal development as a result of environmental toxins. Because of improved treatment methods, however, the survival rate has increased. In the United States, testicular cancer occurs nearly five times more often in White men than in Black men. Rates for men of Hispanic, Asian, and Native American backgrounds fall between those for White and Black men.[37,38]

The risk for testicular cancer is 3 to 17 times higher in men with a history of an undescended testicle (one of the testes fails to descend into the scrotum and is retained in the abdomen or inguinal canal). However, only 7 to 10 percent of men diagnosed with testicular cancer have a history of this condition. Other risk factors include a family history of testicular cancer, a personal history of testicular cancer in the other testicle, abnormal development of the testes, and infertility or abnormal sperm.[37,38]

Warning signs of testicular cancer include a painless lump on the testicle and swelling or discomfort in the scrotum. Testicular cancer is usually detected by an individual, often during a testicular self-exam. Back pain and difficulty breathing can develop in the later stages after cancer metastasizes.

Most testicular cancers are detected by men or their partners even without formal screening programs. Therefore formal screening is not recommended, but men should be familiar with their bodies (see the earlier box, "Breast and Testicular Self-Exams"). If a lump is detected, an ultrasound is performed, and if the ultrasound suggests cancer, a biopsy is performed to confirm the diagnosis.

Testicular cancer is treated with surgery to remove the testicle; depending on the stage of disease, radiation or chemotherapy may be needed as well. Testicular cancer is highly treatable, with 95 percent of cases at all stages being cured. The cure rate is 99 percent if the cancer is diagnosed at an early stage. Even in a man with a late-stage diagnosis and extensive metastases, testicular cancer can be cured. Among those who have been successfully treated for testicular cancer are figure skater Scott Hamilton, cyclist Lance Armstrong, ice hockey player Brandon Davidson, comedian Tom Green, and football punter Josh Bidwell.[37,38]

Oral Cancer

Cancers that develop in the mouth or the pharynx (the back of the throat), which can involve the lips, tongue, gums, or throat, are classified as oral cancers. The rate of new cases had been declining since the 1980s, and death rates have been decreasing. Oral cancers are twice as common in men as in women.[1]

The major risk factor for oral cancers is tobacco use (smoking cigarettes, cigars, or a pipe or using smokeless tobacco); high levels of alcohol consumption further increase the risk. Human Papilloma Virus (HPV) is a newly recognized risk factor, perhaps due to improved techniques for detecting the virus; it has been found to be associated with 62 percent of mouth and throat cancers.[39] This large percentage of HPV-associated cancers may also be due to increasing rates of oral sex.

Early signs of oral cancer include a sore in the mouth that does not heal or bleeds easily; a lump or bump that does not go away or that increases in size; or a patch of redness or whiteness along the gums or skin lining the inside of the cheeks. Late signs of oral cancer can include pain or difficulty swallowing or chewing.

Oral cancers are usually detected by a doctor or dentist, or the individual may notice a sore that does not heal. A biopsy is necessary to confirm the diagnosis. Treatment usually starts with surgery to remove as much as possible of the cancer, along with local radiation. If the cancer is advanced, chemotherapy can be added. The five-year survival rate for all stages of oral cancer is 62 percent.[1]

Leukemia

Leukemia is a group of cancers that originate in the bone marrow or other parts of the body where white blood cells form. Leukemia is the overproduction of one type of white blood cell, which prevents the normal growth and function of other blood cells and can lead to increased risk of infection, anemia, and bleeding. The American Cancer Society estimated 48,610 new cases of leukemia in 2013 and 23,720 deaths.[1]

Risk factors include cigarette smoking and exposure to certain chemicals, particularly benzene, a chemical found in gasoline products and in cigarette smoke. Ionizing radiation can increase the risk for several types of leukemia; people who survive other cancers are at risk for developing leukemia as a result of radiation treatment. Infection with human T-cell leukemia/lymphoma virus (HTLV-1) can increase the risk of leukemia and lymphoma, another cancer of the white blood cells.

Symptoms of leukemia include fatigue, increased incidence of infection, and easy bleeding and bruising. They often occur because healthy white blood cells, red blood cells, and platelets are unable to perform their functions. These symptoms can appear suddenly in acute leukemia, but in chronic leukemia, they may appear gradually.

Because the symptoms are fairly nonspecific, early detection of leukemia can be challenging. There is no recommended screening test, but a health care provider can diagnose leukemia with a blood test or bone marrow biopsy if symptoms are present. The most effective treatment is chemotherapy. Therapy can also include blood transfusion, antibiotics, drugs to boost the function of healthy blood cells, and drugs to reduce the side effects of chemotherapy. Bone marrow transplantation can be effective for certain types of leukemia. Survival rates vary tremendously based on type of leukemia and range from 25 percent to 82 percent at five years.[1]

Lymphoma

Cancers that originate in the lymph system, part of the body's immune system, are called lymphomas. There are two main types: Hodgkin's lymphoma (about 12 percent of

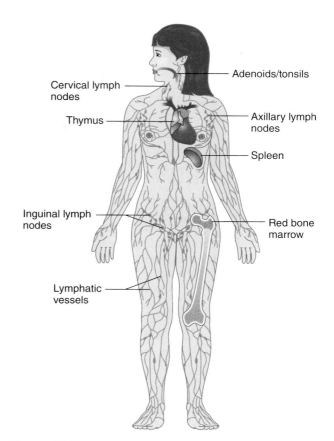

figure 15.5 The lymph system.
Structures include the lymph nodes and lymph vessels, the adenoids/tonsils, the thymus gland, the spleen, and the bone marrow. Clusters of lymph nodes can occur anywhere along the lymphatic vessels. Prominent areas include the neck (cervical lymph nodes), armpits (axillary lymph nodes), and groin (inguinal lymph nodes).

all lymphomas) and non-Hodgkin's lymphoma (about 88 percent). Lymphomas can start almost anywhere, since the lymph system exists throughout the body (Figure 15.5). Rates of lymphoma are nearly twice what they were 40 years ago, but they have stabilized since 1998. Non-Hodgkin's lymphoma is more common in older populations, with an average age at diagnosis in the 60s. Hodgkin's lymphoma usually presents during adolescence and the young adult years.[1]

Factors that increase risk for lymphoma include infections, medications, or genetic changes that weaken the immune system. HIV infection explains some of the increase in lymphoma rates in recent decades. Radiation, herbicides, insecticides, and some chemical exposures also increase risk. The bacterium *H. pylori* increases risk for stomach lymphoma. However, the majority of people with lymphoma do not have clearly identified risk factors.

Symptoms of lymphoma depend on where it originates. A swollen lymph node is a common presentation, but the majority of swollen lymph nodes are not due to lymphoma. If the lymphoma originates in the thymus, it can cause a cough or shortness of breath; in the abdomen, it can cause swelling or pain. Other general symptoms associated with lymphoma include weight loss, fever, drenching night sweats, and severe itchiness.

Diagnosis is made by a biopsy of the swollen lymph node or other tissue. Imaging studies, such as chest X-rays, CT scans, and MRIs, are important to determine if and how far the lymphoma has spread. Treatment often includes a combination of surgery, chemotherapy, and radiation. It can sometimes involve immunotherapy or bone marrow transplant. The five-year survival rate for Hodgkin's and non-Hodgkin's lymphoma is 85 and 68 percent, respectively.[1]

CANCER SCREENING

Early detection is the key to successful treatment of cancer, and **screening tests** are the key to early detection. Cancer screening involves trying to identify risk factors, precancerous lesions, or undetected cancers in an asymptomatic person. An ideal screening test would always detect precursors or cancer at an early, treatable stage and never produce a false negative or false positive result.

screening test
Test given to a large group of people to identify a smaller group of people who are at higher risk for a specific disease or condition.

Unfortunately, no screening test meets the ideal. Screening recommendations for breast, colon, prostate, uterine, testicular, cervical and lung cancers are summarized in the box, "Cancer Detection Guidelines." No screening recommendations exist for some cancers, including ovarian cancers, because to date, no test has been shown to improve detection without increasing harm.

Genetic screening can also be done to assess cancer risk. At this time, it is being reserved for members of high-risk families, that is, families with multiple members with cancer. Complete the Personal Health Portfolio for this chapter to assess your personal risk and protective factors.

■ Michael C. Hall of the TV show *Dexter* announced in January 2010 that he had been undergoing treatment for Hodgkin's lymphoma. Later that year he was reported to have fully recovered. The five-year survival rate for Hodgkin's lymphoma is 84 percent.

CANCER TREATMENTS

Surgery is the oldest treatment for cancer; newer options include chemotherapy, radiation, biological therapies, bone marrow transplantation, and gene therapy.[40]

Surgery

Surgery remains a mainstay in the diagnosis and treatment of cancer. When a cancer is detected early and is small and localized, surgery can cure it, as when an *in situ* cancer of the breast is removed via a lumpectomy. Sometimes an organ affected by cancer can be removed surgically without threatening life, as in the case of prostate or testicular cancer. Certain cancers are unlikely to spread widely, such as a basal cell carcinoma, and surgery often cures these cancers as well. If a cancer has spread, surgery may still be performed as part of the treatment.

Chemotherapy

Chemotherapy is a drug treatment administered to the entire body to kill any cancer cells that may have escaped from the local site to the blood, lymph system, or another part of the body. More than 50 chemotherapy medicines have been developed; different combinations are used for different cancers. All chemotherapeutic drugs operate by a similar mechanism—they interfere with rapid cell division. Because cancer cells divide more rapidly than normal cells, they are more vulnerable than healthy cells to destruction by chemotherapy.

Other normal tissues that divide rapidly are also harmed by chemotherapy, including the hair, stomach lining, and white blood cells. The timing and dosage must be carefully adjusted so the drugs kill cancer cells but do not damage normal cells beyond repair.

Radiation

Radiation causes damage to cells by altering their DNA; it can be used to destroy cancer cells with minimal damage to surrounding tissues. Radiation is a local treatment that can be used before or after surgery or in conjunction with chemotherapy. It can also be used to control pain in patients with cancer that cannot be cured.

Biological Therapies

Biological therapies enhance the immune system's ability to fight cancer (an approach called

Cancer Detection Guidelines

Regular physical exams should include examinations for cancers of the thyroid, oral cavity, skin, lymph nodes, testes, and ovaries. Special tests for certain cancer sites are recommended as outlined here. Talk with your physician about your and your family's health history to determine your specific screening needs.

Breast Cancer

- Yearly mammograms starting at age 40 and continuing for as long as a woman is in good health.*

- A clinical breast exam as part of a periodic health exam, about every one to three years for women in their 20s and 30s and every year for women 40 and over.

- Women should know how their breasts normally feel and report any change promptly to their health care providers. Breast self-exam is an option for women starting in their 20s.

- High-risk women—because of their family history or certain other factors—should be screened with an MRI in addition to mammograms.

Colon and Rectal Cancer

Beginning at age 50, both men and women at *average risk* should be screened with one of the following tests:

Tests that find polyps and cancer (preferred if these tests are available to you)

- Flexible sigmoidoscopy every five years**
- Colonoscopy every 10 years
- Double-contrast barium enema every five years**
- CT colonography (virtual colonoscopy) every five years**

Tests that mainly find cancer

- Fecal occult blood test (FOBT) every year***
- Fecal immunochemical test (FIT) every year***
- Stool DNA test, interval uncertain**

All positive tests should be followed up with colonoscopy. Screening should begin earlier if high risk (a personal or family history of colon polyps or colon cancer, a personal history of chronic inflammatory bowel disease, or a family history of a hereditary colorectal cancer syndrome).

Cervical Cancer

- Women should begin cervical cancer screening when they are 21 years old. Women aged 21 to 29, should be screened with a Pap test every three years. They should not receive HPV testing.

- Women age 30 to 65 should be screened every five years with a Pap test and HPV testing. If HPV testing is unavailable, a Pap every three years is acceptable.

- Women age 65 and older who have had regular Pap testing and normal results should no longer be tested.

- Women who have certain risk factors, such as diethylstilbestrol (DES) exposure before birth; HIV infection; weakened immune system due to organ transplant, chemotherapy, or chronic steroid use; or treatment for cervical precancers or cancer, may need to be screened more frequently.

Endometrial (Uterine) Cancer

- At the time of menopause, all women should be informed about the risks and symptoms of endometrial cancer and strongly encouraged to report any unexpected bleeding or spotting to their doctors. Some women—because of their history—may need to consider having a yearly endometrial biopsy.

Lung Cancer

- Men and women aged 55 to 74 who are high risk for lung cancer due to being current or former smokers with a 30-pack/year history should receive low-dose CT screening.

Prostate Cancer

- Starting at age 50, men should talk to their physician about the pros and cons of testing so they can decide if testing is the right choice for them. Black men and men who have a father or brother who had prostate cancer before age 65 should have this talk with their physician by age 45. Men who decide to be tested should have the prostate-specifics antigen (PSA) blood test with or without a rectal exam. How often a man is tested will depend on his PSA level.

*As discussed in the "Breast Cancer" section of this chapter, ACS continues to recommend start at age 40; USPSTF now recommends start at age 50 with discussion of earlier start.
**Colonoscopy should be done if test results are positive.
***For FOBT or FIT as a screening test, the take-home multiple-sample method should be used. An FOBT or FIT done during a digital rectal exam in the doctor's office is not adequate for screening.

Sources: "American Cancer Society Guidelines for the Early Detection of Cancer," reprinted by permission of the American Cancer Society, Inc., from www.cancer.org. All rights reserved.

immunotherapy) or reduce the side effects of chemotherapy. One kind of immunotherapy is a vaccine that can be developed after a person has been diagnosed with a cancer. Administering the vaccine can boost the person's immune response to the cancer and may help prevent a recurrence. Vaccines for several types of cancers, including melanoma and cancers of the breast, colon, ovary, and prostate, are in use or development. Vaccines can also be used to prevent cancer, as in the case of the HPV vaccine for cervical cancer.

immunotherapy
Administration of drugs or other substances that enhance the ability of the immune system to fight cancer.

Medications can also be used to boost the immune response. Such drugs as interleukin-2, herceptin, and interferon-alpha are used to treat some cancers. Immunotherapy also includes boosting the immune system with social support, whether in the form of friends, family, or cancer support groups. Prolonged cancer survival is associated with good support systems.

Bone Marrow Transplantation

Bone marrow transplantation was initially used for cancer of the white blood cells (leukemia, lymphoma). Now it is sometimes used for other cancers when healthy bone marrow cells are killed by high doses of chemotherapy. This treatment approach is controversial for some types of cancer because of complications from high-dose chemotherapy and the high risk of infection. Additionally, data have not conclusively shown a significantly improved survival rate for some cancers.

Gene Therapy and Genetic Testing

Gene therapy could be used in several different ways to improve cancer treatment. It is still in the clinical-trials stage at this time. In theory, mutated genes could be replaced with functional genes, decreasing the risk that cancer would occur or stopping a cancer that had started to develop. Genes could be inserted into immune cells to increase their ability to fight cancer cells.[40]

Genetic testing may also become important in cancer treatment. It could allow physicians to predict more accurately how a cancer will behave, which chemotherapy drugs will work best against it, and which patients will benefit from chemotherapy.

Clinical Trials

Studies designed by researchers and physicians to test new drugs and treatment regimens are known as *clinical trials.* Participants in clinical trials are patients with cancer who enroll both in the hopes of finding a better treatment for their own cancer and in the interest of furthering cancer research in general.

Once enrolled in the study, participants are usually randomly assigned to either a group receiving a new drug or a group receiving the standard treatment. In rare situations, usually when there is no effective standard treatment, one group of patients may receive a placebo (a "sugar pill" that has no effect). If cancer is advancing in a patient who is receiving the placebo, he or she may be switched to the group receiving the drug. For more information about new and ongoing clinical trials, visit the website of the National Cancer Institute.

Complementary and Alternative Medicine

The role of complementary and alternative medicine (CAM) in cancer treatment is currently a hot topic for research. Cancer patients and survivors use CAM practices at higher rates than the general population as an adjunct to standard treatment options, often with the goal of reducing the side effects of cancer or cancer treatment, speeding recovery, improving pain control, and increasing chances of survival. At present, data do not support the role of CAM instead of standard treatments because CAM practices have not been shown to *cure* cancers.

Ginger and acupuncture have been shown to reduce treatment-associated nausea and vomiting; acupuncture may reduce cancer pain or surgical pain. Massage, yoga, and mindfulness meditation techniques can help relieve stress, anxiety, depression, and pain; massage and yoga may reduce cancer-related fatigue; meditation and mindfulness practices may boost immune function. Qigong may reduce pain and increase activity. Hypnosis may reduce pain, nausea, and vomiting.

Most herbal, vitamin, and mineral supplements have limited evidence showing benefit, and there is concern they may interact with cancer treatments and thus should be used with caution and under the guidance of a cancer treatment doctor. In particular, supplementation with vitamin E and beta carotene is associated with increased risk of prostate and lung cancer, respectively. Instead, experts recommend a healthy, balanced diet.[41,42]

LIVING WITH CANCER

As a result of improved screening and treatment, cancer is no longer seen as a death sentence; rather, it is seen in many cases as a chronic disease that can be managed. In the United States, the survival rate for all stages and types of cancer combined is 68 percent. Many cancers are now curable or controllable, and cancer survivors often return to a healthy life. An estimated 14 million people living in the United States have a history of cancer.[1]

As a chronic disease, however, cancer does change the way a person lives his or her life. If you or a friend or family member receives a diagnosis of cancer, many issues will arise that you probably have never had to deal with before. Here are some suggestions that may help in this difficult time:

■ Participate in decisions about your treatment and care to the greatest extent possible, or ask the person with cancer how much he or she wants to be involved in treatment decisions. Maintaining a sense of control is associated with better health outcomes.

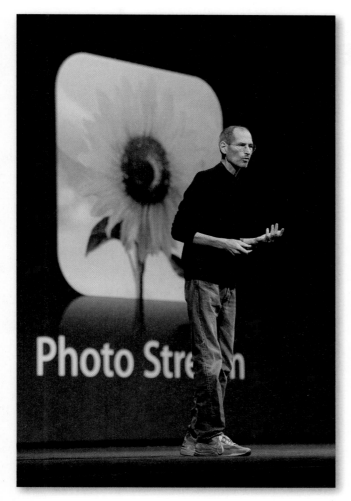

- Apple founder Steve Jobs publicly acknowledged that he had been diagnosed with neuroendocrine pancreatic cancer in 2004. Doctors removed a cancerous tumor from his pancreas, and he expressed optimism about his overall health. Over the next several years, though, his health appeared to waver, and in 2011, he stepped down as Apple CEO. He died on October 5, 2011, of what doctors reported was a recurrence of the pancreatic cancer. Pancreatic cancer is particularly deadly, with a one-year survival rate of about 20 percent.

- Be an informed consumer. Gather information about your cancer (or your family member's cancer). If you have questions, write them down and ask your health care provider at the next appointment. Make sure you are comfortable with the health team's technical expertise and emotional support.

- Consider how you will interact with family members, friends, and acquaintances. With whom will you share

the diagnosis and when? Who will provide you with emotional support? If you need assistance, who might help with tasks, such as driving to appointments, cooking meals, or shopping? If you have a friend or family member with cancer, consider your strengths and what you can offer—perhaps a day spent helping in the garden or taking a child on an outing.

- Consider school or work obligations. You may have to take time off for treatment, and you may experience job discrimination. The Rehabilitation Act and the Americans with Disabilities Act are two federal laws that protect cancer patients. Your health insurance provider cannot drop you even if you leave your job (although your rates may go up and you may have to pay for it yourself).

- Enlist support. A cancer support group can offer information, teach coping skills, and give you a place to voice your concerns and share your experiences. You can find support groups through your health care team, church, or community or on the Internet.

- Know what physical changes are likely to occur. Your sense of identity may be affected, as you adapt to the changes in your health or appearance. As a support person, remembering the "whole" person and not just focusing on the cancer-related changes can be helpful.

- If you or your partner is about to start a treatment that affects your future fertility and you want to have children, consider the possibility of sperm or egg donation and freezing.

- If you have spiritual beliefs or practices, they can be an important part of life now. Research suggests that people with a sense of spirituality have a better quality of life while living with cancer than those who are not spiritual.

- Coping with a cancer diagnosis and treatment can be exhausting. Supporting someone with cancer can also lead to burnout. In either situation, it is important not to think about the cancer all the time. Caregivers should try not to feel guilty about enjoying life and activities. They also need to be able to ask for help so that they can remain supportive in the long run.

Important discoveries in the areas of cancer biology, genetics, screening, and treatment have transformed the face of cancer. Greater knowledge of risk factors has led to more effective prevention strategies. Mortality is declining, survival rates are rising, and the quality of life for those with cancer is improving. The future holds great promise for continuing progress.

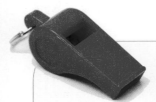

You Make the Call

What Do You Do With Conflicting Health Recommendations?

In the late 1990s, the Centers for Disease Control (CDC) began to report a rise in cases of rickets, a vitamin D deficiency disease not seen for decades. Rickets causes bone softening and deformities in children and bone loss and fractures in adults. The reason for the resurgence of the crippling disease was, in part, avoidance of sun exposure by parents who were protecting their children from the risks of sunburn and future skin cancer, as recommended by health experts. The story of vitamin D deficiency versus risk of skin cancer points to the complexity of current health advisories.

Vitamin D is an essential micronutrient. It is needed for the development and maintenance of bones and teeth and a healthy immune system. Higher levels are associated with lower rates of colon, prostate, breast, esophageal, and pancreatic cancers and improved survival among melanoma patients. Lower levels are associated with multiple health problems, including reduced calcium absorption, osteoporosis (thinning of the bones), autoimmune disorders, and an increased risk of heart disease. Extreme vitamin D deficiency causes rickets.

The body's major source of vitamin D is sunlight. Exposure to sunlight, specifically UVB, triggers synthesis of vitamin D in skin cells. In some areas of the United States, an estimated 20 to 30 percent of people have moderate to severe vitamin D deficiency, mostly because of lack of sun exposure. Studies have also found that between 40 and 70 percent of adolescents have low levels of vitamin D. Risk is greatest in northern latitudes, in individuals who are homebound, and in people with dark skin. Anything that diminishes sun exposure increases the chance of vitamin D deficiency.

At the same time that sun exposure is needed for vitamin D synthesis, it is also the most dangerous risk factor for skin cancer. To reduce the risk of skin cancer, including melanoma, people are advised to avoid being in the sun between 10 a.m. and 4 p.m., to stay in the shade, to wear protective hats and clothing, and to use sunscreen. A sunscreen with an SPF of 15 absorbs 99 percent of the UVB radiation in sunlight, reducing the risk for sunburn and skin cancer—but it also decreases the synthesis of vitamin D by 99 percent.

How do we balance these conflicting health recommendations? The Recommended Daily Allowance for vitamin D is 400 international units (IUs). How long do you have to be in the sun to get that amount? Recommendations vary from 10 to 15 minutes of sun exposure without sunscreen twice a week to 30 minutes outside per day.

Vitamin D can also be obtained from a few foods, including salmon, mackerel, sardines, cod liver oil, and some fortified milks, yogurts, and cereals. Vitamin D is available in the form of a supplement; however, a large review of Vitamin D supplementation did not show any change in risk of overall mortality. Nevertheless, the Institute of Medicine recommends 200 IUs of vitamin D a day for people under age 50 and 400 to 600 IUs for people over age 50. The National Osteoporosis Foundation recommends that postmenopausal women take 800 to 1,000 IUs per day. Some data suggest that these recommendations may be too low—it may be that all people need up to 1,000 IUs per day.

At present, there is no routine recommendation to check vitamin D levels in the general public. Thus, according to some experts, it makes sense to get sun exposure to ensure that adequate amounts of this micronutrient are being obtained. Others disagree. What do you think?

PROS

- Sunlight is a natural way to get the vitamin D we need.
- The benefits of a moderate amount of sun exposure outweigh the risk of skin cancer.
- Even if sun exposure increases the risk of skin cancer, adequate levels of vitamin D reduce the risk of other kinds of cancer and improve survival for people with melanoma—the worst kind of skin cancer.

CONS

- Sun exposure is linked directly to skin cancer—the most common form of cancer—and avoiding time in the sun is recommended by the CDC, the American Cancer Society, and other leading health organizations.
- You can get vitamin D from other, safer sources, including some fish and vitamin supplements.
- Sun exposure causes skin damage and premature aging. It's an irresponsible health behavior choice to spend time in the sun without sunscreen.

connect ACTIVITY

Sources: "Is Vitamin D Deficiency a Major Global Public Health Problem?" by C. Palacios and L. Gonzalez, 2013, *Journal of Steroid Biochemistry and Molecular Biology, S0960-0760* (13), 00233-1; "Vitamin D and Adolescents: What Do We Know?" by N. Stoffman and C. M. Gordon, 2009, *Current Opinion in Pediatrics, 21* (4), pp. 465–471; "Vitamin D Supplementation for Prevention of Mortality in Adults," by G. Bjelakovic, L. Gluud, et al., 2011, *Cochrane Database Systematic Review, 6* (7), CD007470.

In Review

What is cancer?
Cancer, the second leading cause of death in the United States, is a condition characterized by an uncontrolled growth of cells, which develop into a tumor and have the potential to spread to other parts of the body.

What causes cancer?
Cancer can be caused by random genetic mutations, a genetic predisposition, or exposure to carcinogens. Usually a combination of innate and environmental factors is involved. Risk factors include a family history of cancer; lifestyle factors like tobacco use, poor nutrition, overweight and obesity, physical inactivity, and alcohol consumption; and environmental factors like exposure to UV radiation, infectious agents, and chemical and physical carcinogens.

What are the most common cancers?
The leading cause of cancer death for both men and women is lung cancer, and the third leading cause for both men and women is colorectal cancer. The second leading cause of cancer death for women is breast cancer and for men, prostate cancer. Cancers of the female reproductive system include cervical, uterine, and ovarian cancer. Testicular cancer, though rare, is the most common cancer among young men. Two types of skin cancer, basal cell and squamous cell carcinomas, are highly curable, but melanoma is an aggressive and dangerous form of skin cancer. Oral cancer is associated with tobacco and alcohol use. Leukemia is a cancer of the blood cells, and lymphoma is a cancer that arises in the lymph system.

How is cancer detected and treated?
Many cancers can be detected early by screening tests like mammograms; for other cancers, no test has been shown to improve detection, and symptoms appear only when the cancer is advanced. The traditional treatment is surgery to remove the cancer; other treatments include chemotherapy, radiation, biological therapies, bone marrow transplantation, and, in the clinical-trial phase, gene therapy. Some complementary and alternative therapies, such as acupuncture, yoga, and meditation, can give relief from cancer pain or the side effects of cancer treatment. Millions of people have survived cancer and live with it as a chronic condition.

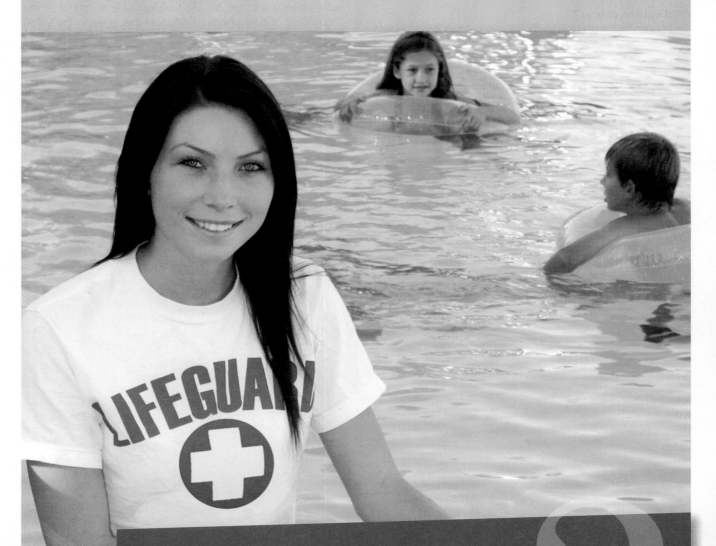

16 Injury and Violence

Ever Wonder...

- how to do the Heimlich maneuver?

- if listening to loud music on your MP3 player can damage your hearing?

- if campus communication systems have been improved since the shootings at Virginia Tech?

nintentional injuries are injuries that are not purposely inflicted,[1] in contrast to intentional injuries like homicides, assaults, and rapes. Unintentional injuries are the fifth leading cause of death for Americans overall and the leading cause of death for children and adults between the ages of 1 and 39. Intentional injuries are usually associated with violence; although they account for fewer deaths than unintentional injuries, they also take a toll on Americans every year, physically, psychologically, and materially.

INJURY: CREATING SAFE ENVIRONMENTS

Public health experts avoid the term *accident* in referring to **unintentional injuries**, because it implies that injury is a chance occurrence or an unpreventable mishap over which individuals have no control.[1] The term *unintentional injuries* implies that injuries are preventable if people adopt behaviors that promote safety and if society does its part in reducing environmental hazards. Examples of safety-promoting behaviors are wearing safety belts in cars, keeping medications in locked cabinets out of the reach of children, and having working smoke detectors in the home.

The leading cause of unintentional-injury death for Americans of all ages is motor vehicle crashes, followed by poisoning, falls, choking, and drowning. The leading causes of injury death vary by age and by ethnicity and race. For example, for infants under 1 year of age, the leading cause of injury death is suffocation; for children aged 1 to 14, the second leading cause (after motor vehicle crashes) is drowning; and for individuals aged 15 to 54, the second leading cause (after motor vehicle crashes) is poisoning, typically from drugs.

Similarly, for Blacks and people of Hispanic background, the second leading cause of death is poisoning, whereas for non-Hispanic Whites and all other groups, it is falls. Vehicle-related death rates for American Indians and Alaska Natives are more than twice those for Whites and almost twice those for Blacks.[2]

Across all groups, more males than females die from unintentional injuries from birth to age 80. For males, the greatest number of injury deaths occur at age 21, and totals remain high until the early 50s; for females, the greatest number of injury deaths occur after age 75.[1,2]

Motor Vehicle Safety

Motor vehicle deaths in the United States reached a peak in 2005. They declined from 2005 to 2011, but in 2012 they increased by about 5.3 percent.[3]

Factors Contributing to Motor Vehicle Crashes About 85 percent of motor vehicle crashes are believed to be caused by **improper driving**, or driving behaviors such as speeding, failing to yield

the right of way, disregarding signals and stop signs, making improper turns, and following too closely. Speeding is especially dangerous; it is a major factor in most fatal crashes. Speed-related crashes decrease with driver age.[3,4] Other factors contributing to motor vehicle crashes include driver inattention, aggressive driving, alcohol-impaired driving, and environmental hazards.

Defensive driving can help you reduce your risk of injury by people who drive improperly. Defensive driving means anticipating potential hazards by keeping your eyes on other drivers and monitoring changing environmental conditions.

The National Highway Traffic Safety Administration (NHTSA) estimates that at least 9 people are killed and more than 1,060 are injured every day in crashes involving distracted drivers.[5] The three main types of distraction are visual (taking eyes off the road), manual (hands off wheel), and cognitive (mind off what person is doing). Drivers under age 20 are the most likely to be involved in distraction-related crashes.

Electronic devices such as smart phones, navigation systems, and iPods visually and cognitively, and sometimes manually distract drivers from safely operating a vehicle. Talking on a cell phone and sending text messages are major sources of distraction; almost 70 percent of drivers aged 18 to 64 text, and 31 percent read e-mail or send text messages while driving. But, by the time you type "R u home yet" on your smartphone, you have increased your risk for a potential fatal accident by 2,300 percent (see Figure 16.1). Talking on a cell phone increases your risk fourfold; putting on makeup, threefold; and eating or drinking, twofold.[5,6] Studies have found that it is not using the phone that causes distraction as much as shifting attention to the conversation and away from driving.[4] As the number of distracting devices inside cars increases, more states are passing legislation to limit the use of electronic devices in motor vehicles (see the box, "Cell Phones and Driver Distraction").

Drowsiness is another source of driver inattention. Drowsiness reduces awareness of your surroundings, impairs judgment, and slows reaction time. The NHTSA conservatively estimates that 2.5 percent of fatal crashes and 2 percent of injuries are caused by drowsy driving. Cognitive impairment for someone who is awake for 18 straight hours is equivalent to a 0.5 blood alcohol content.[7,8] And, as you learned in Chapter 4, 24 straight hours is equivalent to a 0.010 BAC. If you start to feel drowsy while driving, it is best to pull over until you

unintentional injuries Injuries that are not purposefully inflicted.

improper driving The cause of most motor vehicle crashes, including speeding, failing to yield right-of-way, following too closely, and passing on a yellow line.

defensive driving Responsible driving that anticipates potential hazards and monitors changing environmental conditions.

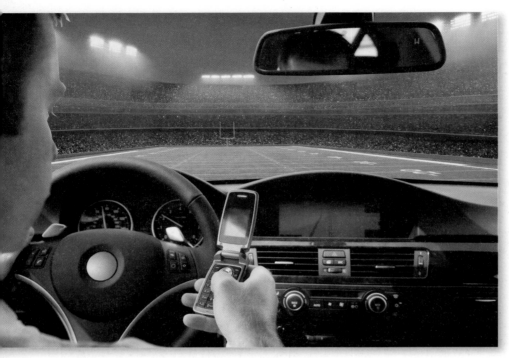

figure 16.1 **Typical distance covered while texting.**
The average driver looks away from the road for 5 seconds when texting. At a speed of 55 miles per hour, a vehicle covers about 400 feet—more than the length of a football field, including the end zones, during those 5 seconds.

Any drugs that induce dizziness, light-headedness, nausea, drowsiness, fatigue, nervousness, or fuzzy thinking make driving dangerous.

Environmental hazards account for less than 5 percent of vehicle crashes, but when combined with human error, they account for 27 percent. Environmental hazards can be natural, such as snow, ice, wind, poor visibility, or glare, or of human origin, such as construction zones, broken-down cars on the side of the road, or drunk drivers. To reduce the number and lethality of injuries that occur as a result of environmental factors, states and local communities use such measures as ice-melting chemicals, crash cushions, breakaway signs and light poles, and median barriers and guard rails.[11]

Approaches to Motor Vehicle Safety One approach to motor vehicle safety is testing cars to make sure they meet NHTSA standards. All cars sold in the United States must pass a test that measures the effectiveness of the vehicle's structural design in preventing occupants from being ejected, trapped, burned, or crushed in a 30-mph (miles per hour) collision. The test also determines a vehicle's ability to absorb, control, or reduce crash impacts on occupants.[12]

Another approach is designing effective restraint systems and increasing the likelihood that people will use them. Every 14 seconds, an adult in the United States is treated in

are fully rested or change drivers. Opening the window, turning up the radio, and turning down the air conditioner are not effective in preventing drowsy-driving accidents.

The NHTSA estimates that two-thirds of all traffic fatalities are associated with overly aggressive driving behavior.[3] An aggressive driver is someone who tailgates, speeds, runs red lights, changes lanes without signaling, and makes illegal turns. Aggressive driving can escalate into *road rage,*[9] an extreme form of aggressive driving that may occur when a driver becomes enraged at another driver. People who experience this kind of uncontrolled anger need to seek help in managing their anger.

Alcohol is involved in a large proportion of car crashes, including fatal crashes. About 3 in 10 Americans are involved in an alcohol-related crash at some point in their lives.[10] Alcohol slows reaction time and impairs perception, judgment, and motor coordination. To reduce alcohol-related traffic fatalities, many states require repeat drunk-driving offenders to install interlock devices in their vehicles. If the device detects that a driver's blood alcohol concentration is above a certain level, usually 0.02, it prevents the vehicle from starting. Additionally, the violation information can be sent directly from the device to state law enforcement officials.

Many drugs other than alcohol impair the ability to drive safely. They include illicit drugs such as marijuana and heroin, prescription drugs, and over-the-counter drugs such as sleep aids. Driving safely requires mental alertness, clear vision, physical coordination, and the ability to react quickly.

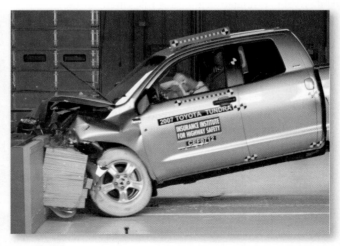

■ A federal program in place since 1979 rates cars for crash safety on a five-star scale. Starting in 2012, a new program added an overall safety rating that combines scores from front-end, side, and rollover tests.

Starting the Conversation

Cell Phones and Driver Distraction

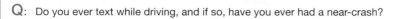

Q: Do you ever text while driving, and if so, have you ever had a near-crash?

Safety advocates around the world believe that texting while driving is a dangerous distraction. In 2009, President Obama issued an executive order prohibiting federal employees from texting while driving on government business or using government equipment. Additionally, the Federal Motor Carrier Safety Administration banned commercial vehicle drivers from texting while driving. As of 2014, 13 states and the District of Columbia had banned the use of handphones when operating a vehicle, and 32 states and the District of Columbia ban texting. So, why all the fuss? What evidence is there to support such swift revocation of one's right to text and drive?

Studies by the Virginia Tech Transportation Institute (VTTI) determined the risk of a crash or near-crash for various cell phone tasks compared to the risk during nondistracted driving, shown in this table:

Cell Phone Task	Risk of Crash/Near-Crash
In light vehicles and cars	
Dialing a cell phone	2.5 times as high
Talking on or listening to a cell phone	1.3 times as high
Reaching for an object	1.4 times as high
In heavy vehicles and trucks	
Dialing a cell phone	5.9 times as high
Talking on or listening to a cell phone	1.0 times as high
Using or reaching for an electronic device	6.7 times as high
Text-messaging	23.2 times as high

The conclusion from this study was that texting should be banned in moving vehicles for all drivers. Headset cell phone systems are not substantially safer than handheld cell phones.

Voice-activated systems make it possible to dictate and send messages without typing and to have incoming messages read aloud to you. Although voice activation is less risky, it still causes cognitive distraction. This technology will likely lead states to revisit their texting laws. Although the National Transportation Safety Board has recommended a federal ban on driver use of portable electronic devices when operating a vehicle, research suggests that this will not be a successful response. Education and legislation have failed to decrease the problem of distracted driving due to the difficulty of strictly enforcing such laws. Safety experts believe that technology is the solution. Handheld electronic devices, for example, could be rendered inoperable whenever the vehicle is in motion or the transmission shift lever is engaged. Opponents argue that this technology is a violation of personal freedom and increases the consumer cost for vehicles and electronic devices.[6] What do you think?

Q: Should texting while driving be banned?

Q: Should states allow texting if drivers are using mobile phone devices that allow them to send and receive messages vocally?

Sources: "New Data from VTTI Provides Insight into Cell Phone Use and Driving Distraction," Virginia Tech Transportation Institute, 2009, www.vtnews.vt.edu/articles/2009/07/2009-571.html; "Distracted Driving Laws." Governors Highway Safety Association. www.ghsa.org/html/stateinfo/laws/cellphone_laws.html.

the emergency room for injuries sustained from a vehicle crash.[13] Still, nearly one in seven adults does not wear a seat belt on every trip. Seat belts cut in half the risk of being seriously injured or killed in a vehicle crash.[14]

States have either primary or secondary enforcement laws for seat belt use. Primary laws allow law enforcement officers to pull vehicles over and issue tickets solely because drivers and passengers are not wearing seat belts. Secondary laws allow tickets to be issued only if the vehicle operator has been pulled over for violating another law. States with primary enforcement laws have a 9 percent higher seat belt usage than states with secondary enforcement laws.[14]

Because many people resisted using safety belts when they were first installed in cars, public information campaigns, incentive programs, and seat belt reminder systems in vehicles were introduced to encourage usage; most of these measures had little effect. Mandatory safety belt laws have proved more effective; today, 49 states and the District of Columbia have such laws in place (New Hampshire requires seat belt use by those under 18 only).

Air bags—fabric cushions that instantly inflate during a collision—are a kind of **passive restraint** that protects front-seat passengers from impact with the interior of the vehicle in a crash. Generally, sensing devices in the dashboard inflate air bags at impacts of 12 mph or more. The bags deflate seconds after the impact.

Motor vehicle crashes are the leading cause of death for children under age 4.[11,15] Infants and children need to be secured in child seats placed in the backseat and anchored by the vehicle's safety belts. Infants and toddlers should not ride in the front seats of cars with air bags because air bags can deploy with enough force to cause severe head and neck injuries in very young children. For maximum protection, children aged 13 and under should always ride in the back seat.

passive restraint
A safety device that does not require vehicle occupants to engage it.

Infants should ride in carriers in which they are in a semi-reclining position facing the rear of the car. The Academy of Pediatrics recommends that children in car seats should not face forward until after their second birthday at the earliest. Children under 2 are 75 percent less likely to die or sustain serious injury in a crash when using a rear-facing child restraint. The five-point harness, which runs across the child's shoulders and hips and buckles between the legs, should be used until the child weighs more than 85 pounds. The harness can be used in booster mode until the child exceeds 120 pounds. Booster seats should also be used until children are at least 4 feet tall.[15]

Pet Restraints The American Society for the Prevention of Cruelty to Animals (ASPCA) recommends that people use restraints for dogs and cats to prevent injury to the pet, driver, or passengers. Only one in six people use animal restraints such as harnesses or pet vehicle seats or pet carriers. Unrestrained pets can distract a driver, and they can cause serious injury to the driver and passengers in the event of an accident. If thrown during a 30-mile-per-hour crash, an 80-pound Labrador retriever will exert 2,400 pound of force on whatever it strikes. Some states are considering a law that will fine drivers who do not restrain their dogs or cats.

Motorcycle Safety Motorcyclists are about 5 times more likely than passenger car occupants to die in a motor vehicle crash and about 26 times more likely to be injured.[1] Contributing factors in these crashes are lack of proper training, distraction, alcohol, and environmental conditions (weather, roadway surface, equipment malfunction). The Motorcycle Safety Foundation (MSF) has a program called the Rider Education and Training System that promotes lifelong learning for motorcyclists (you can visit the website at www.msf-usa.org). However, the MSF reports that about 65 percent of all collisions between motorcycles and other types of vehicles are precipitated by a vehicle operator other than the motorcyclist, usually because the driver failed to see the motorcycle.

Wearing a helmet reduces a motorcyclist's risks of both fatal injury and traumatic brain injury. A study by the NHTSA found that about half of unhelmeted riders suffered a head injury in a crash, compared with about 35 percent of those wearing a helmet.[16] Despite these safety benefits, most motorcyclists choose not to wear helmets, unless state law requires it.[16,17] Only 12 percent of college students report wearing a helmet all of the time.[18]

Bicycle Safety

Collisions between bicycles and motor vehicles result in many deaths and nonfatal disabling injuries. A successful bicycle safety program combines the use of safety equipment with injury-reducing behaviors. Three important considerations are making sure your bicycle fits you properly, wearing a helmet, and employing safe cycling practices. Only 11 percent of college students report wearing a helmet all of the time and about 6 percent most of the time.[18]

The biggest safety problem for bicyclists is making themselves visible to other vehicle operators. Reflective tape, brightly colored cycling clothes and safety vests, portable leg or arm lights, and headlights are effective for making riders more visible. Air-powered horns can add another dimension to safety.

Bicycles are considered vehicles, and riders must follow all traffic laws that apply to cars, including stopping at traffic lights and stop signs and signaling before turning.

Pedestrian Safety

In the next 24 hours in the United States, 12 pedestrians will be killed and about 460 people will be treated in emergency rooms for pedestrian-related injuries.[19] About one out of every six pedestrian deaths occurs in a hit-and-run incident. About 45 percent of pedestrian deaths occur when pedestrians enter or cross streets, and 10 percent occur when pedestrians are walking in the roadway. A few times every year, a bicyclist strikes and kills a pedestrian.[20]

The pedestrian fatality rate for men is about twice that for women, and the rate of nonfatal pedestrian injuries is also higher for men. The pedestrian fatality rate for Blacks is almost twice that for Whites, and for American Indians and Native Alaskans it is nearly three times as high. Safety experts believe this difference can be partly attributed to the fact that members of these groups generally walk more than Whites because they own fewer cars. Children and older pedestrians are also especially vulnerable to being injured or killed by a car.[1,19]

To increase your safety as a pedestrian at night, carry a flashlight and wear retro-reflective clothing. Many vehicles have a beeping alarm that is activated when the vehicle is backing up; pay attention to them. Some newer vehicles have sensor alarms that can detect small children and animals within a few feet behind them. Many safety experts are calling for such alarms to be standard equipment on all vehicles.

Pedestrians texting, e-mailing, or talking on their smartphone are vulnerable to inattention blindness. Surprisingly, research suggests that listening to music does not cause cognitive distraction and may actually increase attention awareness. The NHTSA cites drunk walking as another problem. In 2011, 35 percent of the pedestrians killed had a BAC of 0.8.[21–23] Half of these fatalities were pedestrians aged 25 to 34. Anti-drunk driving programs now include drunk walking.

■ Safety equipment for skateboarding includes wrist guards, knee and elbow pads, and a helmet. About 50,000 skateboarding injuries are treated in hospital emergency rooms each year.

Recreational Safety

Injuries occur in a wide variety of recreational activities and sports, such as football, basketball, soccer, swimming, skateboarding, snowboarding, inline skating, and many others. Wearing the right safety equipment and clothing for the activity significantly reduces the risk of injury. Anyone engaging in a sport or recreational activity should refrain from drinking alcohol beforehand.

All-Terrain Vehicle Safety The Consumer Product Safety Commission estimates that there are nearly 600 ATV-related deaths and 100,000 injuries every year caused by rollovers, excessive speed, falls, and collision with stationary objects. Children under the age of 16 are one-third of those who are killed and injured on ATVs. To confront the problem, states are passing laws to mandate helmet use and restrict ATV use by age. They are also opening ATV parks that provide groomed trails for a fee.[24]

Pocket Bike Safety Miniature motorcycles called pocket bikes have become popular among children and young adults. However, there are many safety concerns about pocket bikes, including the difficulty of riders being seen by motorists, poor braking mechanisms, sluggish throttles, and excessive noise. Many states have prohibited the use of pocket bikes on streets and public property because they lack key safety features like turn signals and mirrors. Riders should be aware of the laws in their state regarding pocket bike use on public property. Safety guidelines include purchasing a bike that has mirrors and turn signals; wearing a helmet, elbow and knee pads, gloves, and shoes when riding; and riding only in the daytime and in good weather.[25]

■ Water safety means always wearing a personal flotation device, or life jacket, when in or on the water. For children, parental supervision is also essential.

Water Safety Overall, about nine people drown every day in the United States; 80 percent of them are male.[2] More than one-third of adults are unable to swim the length of a pool 24 yards long.[26] More than half of all drowning victims are White non-Hispanic males, but Black males have the highest drowning rate per 100,000 persons. Drowning rates increase for Blacks through childhood and then peak between ages 15 to 19 years. Drowning rates for Hispanics increase substantially at 15 to 19 years, and then peak between the ages of 20 to 24 years.[26]

About half of drownings occur in natural water settings, such as lakes, rivers, and the ocean, or occur in boating incidents. Of boating drownings, more than 80 percent of the victims were not wearing a life jacket.[27] Life jackets, or **personal flotation devices (PFDs)**, are essential protection for anyone participating in boating or another recreational activity on the water, including water-skiing and riding jet-skis. PFDs are made of buoyant material; various types have been designed for different watercraft. Check with your local jurisdiction for rules and regulations governing PFDs for your recreational activity.

personal flotation device (PFD)
Life jacket worn while participating in water sports.

If you are on a boat that turns over, stay with the boat, where you are more likely to be spotted and rescued, rather than trying to swim to shore. If you are close to shore, however, and immediate rescue is unlikely, attempting to swim to shore may be your best option.[27]

Alcohol is a principal factor in deaths associated with water recreation activities. Many states have laws covering intoxication by people operating boats that are comparable to those covering intoxication by drivers of motor vehicles.

Rock Climbing Safety Indoor rock-climbing walls have become very popular at fitness and recreation centers, both on college campuses and in communities. Their popularity has resulted in significant increases in emergency room visits due to fractures, dislocations, sprains, strains, and lacerations, though concussions and other head injuries rarely occur. The National Electronic Injury Surveillance System (NEISS) estimates that there are about 2,300 climbing-related injuries treated at emergency centers each year. Attention to safety equipment, environmental protections, and climbing instruction are needed to lower the risk of injury.[28]

Home Safety

Although more deaths occur each year in motor vehicle crashes than in any other category of unintentional injury, the highest number of injuries occurs in the home. In fact, nearly 40 percent of all disabling injuries occur in the home.[1] The primary causes of home injuries and deaths are falls, fires, poisonings, and choking and suffocation.

Falls Falls are responsible for more open wounds, fractures, and brain injuries than any other cause of injury.[1] They are the most common cause of injury visits to the emergency room for two groups: young children and older adults.

About 70 deaths occur each year when children fall out of windows.[1] Other injuries occur when babies roll off beds or young children fall down stairs. Parents can lower the risk of fall-related injuries by supervising their children, buying products that promote safety (such as nonslip rugs), and modifying the home (e.g., installing gates at the top of stairs and guards on windows).

Older adults have the highest rate of injury and death from falls of any age group. Falls account for one-third of the deaths from unintentional injuries among older adults.[1] Older adults are more susceptible to falls than are younger people because of medical problems, changes in skeletal composition, poor balance, limited vision, muscular weakness, and effects of medications. Environmental factors like slippery floors, loose rugs, and poor lighting also make falls more likely.[1]

Fires On average in the United States, one person dies in a fire every 158 minutes, and someone is injured in a fire every 31 minutes. Most victims die from smoke or toxic gases, not burns. Of all fire-related deaths and injuries, 65 to 85 percent occur in homes. About 50 percent of the homes in which a fire fatality occurred did not have smoke detectors.[29]

To help avoid injury from fire in the home, your home should have at least one smoke detector on every level, placed on the ceiling or on a wall 6 to 12 inches from the ceiling. Smoke detectors are either battery-operated or powered by household current with a battery backup. Batteries in battery-powered detectors should be replaced every 6 to 12 months. Research indicates that young children are not easily roused from deep sleep by the sound of a smoke alarm, but they are roused by the sound of their mother's voice calling their names. Smoke alarms are available that can be programmed for this purpose.

Home fire extinguishers are intended to knock down a fire long enough to allow the occupants to escape; most discharge their extinguishing agent for only about 30 seconds.[30] Many extinguishers contain a multipurpose dry chemical and are labeled ABC, meaning they can be used on any type of fire. They can be purchased in hardware stores. Many commercial buildings have sprinkler systems, and most states require sprinkler systems in newly constructed apartments, condominiums, and other multifamily dwellings.[30]

The 2008 federal Campus Fire Safety Right-to-Know Act was implemented to increase fire awareness on college campuses. This act provides current and prospective students and their families with the right to access fire safety records of their college. The information in these records includes the number of fires and the cause of each fire, the number of injuries and deaths related to each fire, the value of property damage caused by each fire, and the number of mandatory, supervised fire drills.

Poisonings A poison is any substance harmful to the body that is ingested, inhaled, injected, or absorbed through the skin.[31] Poisoning can be intentional or unintentional. Intentional poisonings (to commit suicide) account for about 18 percent of poisoning incidents. About half of all unintentional poisoning deaths are from drug overdoses. Prescription drug overdoses now account for as many deaths as cocaine and heroin combined. Alcohol poisoning accounts for a small percentage of poisoning deaths, but some poisoning deaths are caused by alcohol in combination with other drugs. Native Americans have the highest unintentional poisoning death rate, followed by Whites and Blacks.[31]

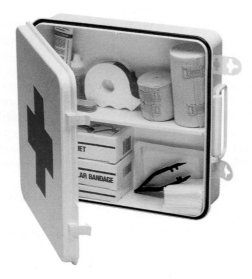

■ To operate an ABC fire extinguisher, remove the locking pin, point the nozzle at the base of the fire, squeeze the handle, and use a sweeping motion as the extinguisher discharges. Although they discharge for less than a minute, even small fire extinguishers can give people time to escape a fire.

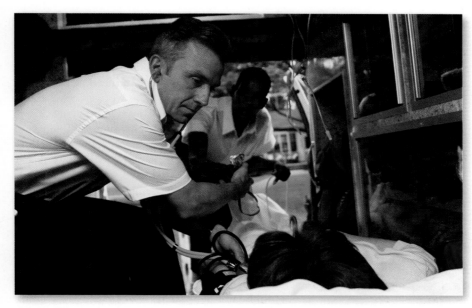

■ According to the CDC, more than 50 people die from unintentional drug overdoses every day in the United States. The rate of lethal overdoses has increased dramatically in the past 10 years, making poisoning the second leading cause of unintentional death.

Children are especially vulnerable to accidental poisoning in the home. The most common cause of poisoning in children is ingestion of household products. All such products should be kept well out of the reach of children and stored in a locked cupboard or one with childproof safety latches. Federal law requires that many of these products be sold in containers with child-resistant caps.[32] Lead in paint and in plastic toys is especially dangerous for young children because it is invisible and odorless.[33]

Another poisoning hazard in the home is gases and vapors, such as carbon monoxide and natural gas. More than 400 people die and 20,000 go to the emergency room each year in the United States from carbon monoxide poisoning.[34] Carbon monoxide is a major component of motor vehicle exhaust; to avoid poisoning by this lethal gas, never leave your car engine running in a closed garage. Natural gas is used to operate many home appliances, such as furnaces, stoves, and clothes dryers. Although natural gas is odorless, producers add a gas with an odor so that leaks can be detected. If you smell gas, check to see if the gas is turned on but not lit on a stove burner or other appliance; if you cannot find the source of the leak, leave the area and call your utility company.

If you or someone you are with has been poisoned, seek medical advice and treatment immediately.[35] Signs that a person has ingested or inhaled a poisonous substance include difficulty breathing or speaking, dizziness, unconsciousness, foaming or burning of the mouth, cramps, nausea, and vomiting. Prolonged exposure to low levels of carbon monoxide produces flulike symptoms. In all cases of toxic contamination or poisoning, call 911, your local poison control center, or the national poison control hotline (1-800-222-1222).

Carbon monoxide alarms are recommended for in-home use. An alarm should be installed in the hallway by every bedroom.

Choking Death rates for choking are highest in children under 4 years of age and adults over 65 years of age. Rates soar in adults over 75 years of age. Most choking emergencies occur when a piece of food or a swallowed object becomes lodged in the throat, blocking the tracheal opening and cutting the oxygen supply to the lungs. Muscles in the trachea may spasm and wrap tightly around the object.[1]

A person whose airway is obstructed may gasp for breath, make choking sounds, clutch the throat, or look flushed and strained. If a person's airway is only partially blocked, he or she may cough forcefully. Do not slap someone on the back if he or she is coughing; usually the coughing will clear the obstruction. If the person continues to have difficulty breathing, the coughing is shallow, or the person is not coughing or cannot talk or breathe, a rescue technique such as the **Heimlich maneuver** is needed (see the box, "The Heimlich Maneuver").

Heimlich maneuver Technique used to help a person who is choking.

Temperature-Related Injuries Each year, scores of people die from excessive heat, particularly older adults and people with weak hearts. The danger is highest for people 75 years of age and older. High temperatures can be exacerbated by high humidity, which prevents the evaporation of perspiration from the skin and makes it difficult for the body to control its core temperature.

On average, 38 children in the United States die of hyperthermia in vehicles each year.[36] These children may have been forgotten or unintentionally left in the vehicle by an adult, or they may have been playing in an unattended vehicle. About 10 percent of these deaths occur in situations involving alcohol, drugs, or neglect.[36] Temperatures inside vehicles can quickly reach dangerous levels. Child hyperthermia deaths in vehicles can occur when the ambient temperature outside is as low as 70°F. It takes only 10 minutes for temperatures inside cars to rise by 20 degrees. In less than 15 minutes, the child's temperature can reach 104 degrees, at which point internal organs shut down. Death occurs at 107 degrees.

Children should never be left in a vehicle, even if the windows are down, or be allowed to play in an unattended vehicle, and adults should establish a "look back before

Action Skill-Builder

The Heimlich Maneuver

The Heimlich maneuver (also referred to as abdominal thrusts) is used to dislodge an object blocking the airway of a person who is choking. To perform this maneuver, follow these four steps:

1. Stand behind the person and put your arms around his or her waist.

2. Make a fist with one hand and place the thumb side of your fist against the victim's upper abdomen, just below the rib cage and above the navel.

3. Grasp your fist with your other hand and thrust upward. Do not squeeze the rib cage. Confine the force of your thrust to your hands.

4. Repeat the upward thrusts until the object is expelled.

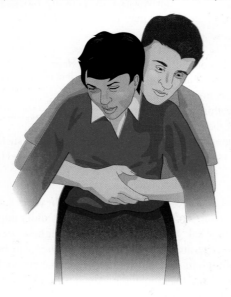

The Heimlich Institute provides special instructions for rescuing infants adults and yourself. For details, visit its website at www.heimlichinstitute.org.

you leave" policy every time they vacate a vehicle. A large stuffed animal may be placed in the front seat as a visual reminder that a child is in the back car seat. Placing needed objects such as a purse or cell phone next to the car seat is another prevention strategy.

Excessive cold is dangerous as well and can lead to hypothermia, a condition in which body temperature drops to dangerously low levels. If you are with someone who is experiencing hypothermia, seek medical treatment immediately.

Excessive Noise Exposure to loud noise can damage hearing and lead to permanent hearing loss. Loud noise destroys hair cells at the nerve endings in the inner ear. These tiny hair cells translate sound vibrations into electrical currents that go to the brain. Some **noise-induced hearing loss (NIHL)** is inevitable and irreversible as we age, so we should protect our hearing from additional, avoidable damage.[37]

Common sources of excessive environmental noise are machinery, power tools, traffic, airplanes, and construction. Loud music is also a hazard (see the box, "MP3 Players and Hearing Loss"). When you listen to loud music for a prolonged period, you experience a "temporary threshold shift" that makes you less sensitive to high volumes. In effect, the ears adapt to the environment by anesthetizing themselves.

Early symptoms of hearing loss include ringing or buzzing in the ears; difficulty understanding speech, especially in noisy settings; and a slight muffling of sounds. More serious symptoms include dizziness, discomfort, and pain in the ears. People who listen to loud music should have their hearing tested periodically because hearing loss can be unnoticeable until damage is extensive.

noise-induced hearing loss (NIHL) Damage to the inner ear, causing gradual hearing loss, as a result of exposure to noise over a period of years.

Concussions A concussion is a type of traumatic brain injury caused by a blow or jolt to the head (a whiplash causing the head to move violently forth and back). Concussion forces twist and break the long, slender axons of brain cells. Blood vessels break on the surface of the brain or near the brain surface. Concussions are graded by level of severity: grade 1: confusion lasting less than 15 minutes; grade 2: confusion and amnesia lasting longer than 15 minutes; and grade 3: brief unconsciousness and more serious amnesia. A second-impact concussion (a second blow to the head within hours, days, or weeks of the initial concussion before the brain has fully healed) can cause additional damage.

Early symptoms of a concussion include confusion, disorientation, memory loss, headaches, nausea, and vision changes. Later symptoms include memory disturbances, poor concentration, irritability, sleep disturbances, personality changes, and fatigue. Concussions in collision sports, such as football, causing damage to the brain's white matter have been linked to depression, amyotrophic lateral sclerosis (Lou Gehrig disease), Parkinson's disease, Alzheimer's disease, and suicidal thoughts. Wearing a helmet in such activities as bicycling and skiing reduce the risk of head injury by 60 percent.[38,39]

Adults with concussions should seek medical help if they have a headache that gets worse and does not go away, weakness, numbness, decreased coordination, repeated vomiting or nausea, or slurred speech. If you are checking symptoms in someone else, seek medical assistance if one of the person's pupils is more dilated than the other or if he or she seems very drowsy or cannot be awakened, has convulsions or seizures, cannot recognize places or people, gets more

Consumer Clipboard

MP3 Players and Hearing Loss

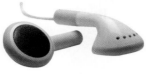

Noise-induced hearing loss is usually a gradual process that can take 10 to 20 years, but people who listen to music at high volume through headphones have been found to have advanced hearing loss beyond their years. Manufacturers have developed different kinds of headphones to reduce risk of hearing loss. "Isolator" earphones sit deeper in the ear canal and block out external sound so that volume does not have to be cranked up so high; "supra-aural" headphones sit on top of the ears and deliver sound at lower decibel level. However, researchers have found that it is not so much the type of earphone that makes a difference in hearing loss as it is the volume level. Ultimately, it is up to you, and not your headphones, to protect your hearing.

Noise levels are measured in decibels (dB): the higher the dB level, the louder the noise. Noise levels from portable media players can reach 115 to 125 dB. Exposure to 125 dB for just one hour can cause permanent hearing loss, as can repeated exposure to 115 dB for half a minute per day. If you have listened to music at the highest volume for even a few seconds, or if you have felt pain in your ears from loud music, you may already have experienced some hearing damage. The following table classifies noise along a continuum from faint to painful and can help you determine whether your music is too loud:

Classification	dB	Example
Faint	30 to 39	Whisper (30 dB)
Moderate	40 to 60	Clothes dryer (40 dB)
Very loud	61 to 90	Blow-dryer (80 to 90 dB)
Extremely loud	91 to 119	Chain saw (110 dB)
Painful	120 or higher	Siren (120 dB)

Protect your hearing by avoiding prolonged exposure to sounds above 85 dB. Here are some ways to listen to your music without endangering your hearing:

- The 60 percent/60-minute rule—using MP3 players at volume levels no more than 60 percent of maximum and no more than one hour a day.

- Turn it down if (1) it's loud enough to prevent normal conversation, (2) it causes ringing in your ears, (3) you have trouble hearing for a few hours after exposure, or (4) the person next to you can hear the music from your headphones.

Sources: "Researchers Recommend Safe Listening Levels for iPod," Hearing Loss Web, 2006, www.hearinglossweb.com/Medical/Causes/nihl/mus/safe.htm; "Prevent Tech-Related Hearing Loss," by G. Hughes, 2006, http://tech.yahoo.com/blog/hughes/35.

---

confused or agitated, displays unusual behavior, or loses consciousness. Someone who has had a concussion should get sufficient rest and should not return to moderate or vigorous activity until cleared by a health care professional.

Providing Emergency Aid

You can help provide care for other people who have been injured or are in life-threatening situations if you learn first aid and emergency rescue techniques. **Cardiopulmonary resuscitation (CPR)** is used when someone is not breathing and a pulse cannot be found. It traditionally consists of mouth-to-mouth resuscitation to restore breathing, accompanied by chest compressions to restore heartbeat. Unfortunately, bystanders provide CPR only 20 to 30 percent of the time when needed, largely out of apprehension of placing their mouth on someone else's mouth. In 2008, the American Heart Association (AHA) announced that *hands-only CPR*— with chest compressions only—is just as effective for sudden cardiac arrest as standard CPR with mouth-to-mouth breathing. However, mouth-to-mouth resuscitation should still be used for children and for adults who suffer from a lack of oxygen caused by near-drowning, carbon monoxide poisoning, or drug overdose.[40] Check the AHA's website (www.americanheart.org) for the latest guidelines.

The American Heart Association (AHA) recommends training for performing CPR. However, even without training, the AHA states that on average any attempt to perform CPR is better than no attempt. Many organizations offer classes, including the AHA and the American Red Cross. Check your community or campus resource center for information on where to take a class in first aid or rescue technique.[40]

cardiopulmonary resuscitation (CPR) Technique used when a person is not breathing and a pulse cannot be found; differs from pulmonary resuscitation by including chest compressions to restore heartbeat.

Work Safety

Safety in the workplace improved steadily throughout the 20th century as a result of occupational laws and advances in safety technology. The part of the body most frequently injured is the back, accounting for 24 percent of total injuries.[1]

Improper lifting of heavy objects is a major cause of back injury. When you are lifting an object, bend your knees and hips and lower your body toward the ground, keeping your back as upright as you can. Keep your feet about shoulder-width apart. Grasp the object and lift it gradually with straight arms, using your leg muscles to stand up. Put the object down by reversing these steps.

Although not necessarily related to work, another common source of back pain is carrying a heavy backpack. Backpacks should, when filled, weigh no more than 10 to 20 percent of a person's body weight and should have wide, padded shoulder straps, a waist strap, and a padded back to distribute weight and enhance comfort. Carry heavier items in the center of your backpack.

Extensive computer use can cause strain not only on the back but on the neck, arms, hands, and eyes. If your body is not properly aligned while you are using your computer (Figure 16.2), you may end up with irritated or pinched nerves, inflamed tendons, or headaches. The average human head weighs 10 pounds in a neutral position (ears straight above shoulders). The pressure on your spine doubles for every inch you tilt your head forward. For example, if you are looking at your smartphone or tablet on your lap, your neck is supporting what feels like 20 or 30 pounds. This forward tilt can cause muscle strain, disc hernias, and pinched nerves. If neck strain continues over time, your neck spine support can flatten or reverse the natural curve of your neck. Bending your neck and hunching your shoulders can also reduce your lung capacity by 30 percent. To experience this decrease, take a deep breath in a slumped position; then, straighten up and take a deep breath again. The loss of lung capacity can lead to vascular diseases due to insufficient oxygen delivery to body organs. To avoid neck strain keep your feet flat on the floor, roll your shoulders back, and keep your ears directly over your shoulders. Docking stations, headsets, and wrist guards are effective mobile support devices. The Text Neck Institute has a mobile app that provides an electronic warning if your phone is not at a safe viewing angle. In addition to maintaining good posture, take breaks every 20 minutes, stand up, roll your shoulders, and go for a short walk to improve blood flow.[41]

When motions and tasks are repeatedly performed in ergonomically incorrect ways, injuries to the soft tissues, known as **repetitive strain injuries**, can occur. A common repetitive strain injury is **carpal tunnel syndrome (CTS)**, the compression of the median nerve in the wrist caused by certain repetitive uses of the hands, including working at the computer, playing video games, and text-messaging. The median nerve is located inside a "tunnel" created by the carpals (wrist bones) and tendons in the hand (Figure 16.3). When the tendons

repetitive strain injuries
Injuries to soft tissues that can occur when motions and tasks are repeatedly performed in ergonomically incorrect ways.

carpal tunnel syndrome (CTS)
Compression of the median nerve in the wrist caused by certain repetitive uses of the hands.

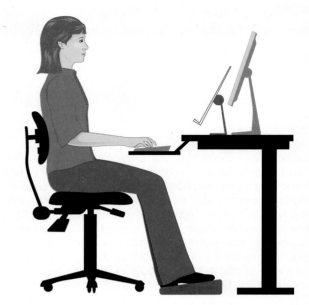

figure 16.2   **Proper workstation setup.**
Your hips should be slightly higher than your knees, and your feet should be flat on the floor or on a footrest slightly in front of your knees. Your monitor should be an arm's length away from you, and your eyes should be level with the top of the screen. When you type, your wrists should be in a neutral position, tilted neither up nor down.

become inflamed through overuse or incorrect use, they compress the median nerve. The symptoms of CTS are numbness, tingling, pain, and weakness in the hand, especially in the thumb and first three fingers. Symptoms are often worse at night, when pain can radiate up into the shoulder.

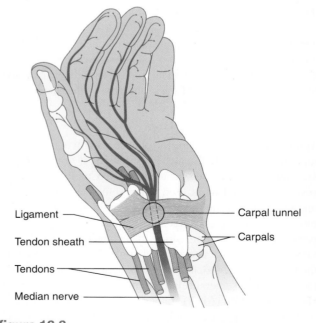

Ligament

Tendon sheath

Tendons

Median nerve

Carpal tunnel

Carpals

figure 16.3   **Carpal tunnel syndrome (CTS).**
Source: From *Core Concepts in Health*, 10th ed., by P. Insel and W. Roth. Copyright © 2006 by The McGraw-Hill Companies. Reprinted by permission of the McGraw-Hill Companies, Inc.

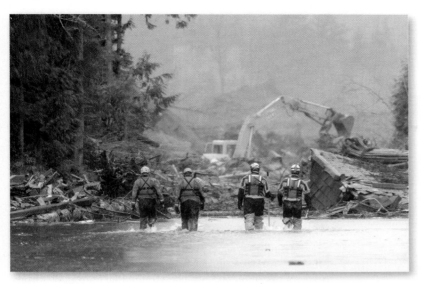

■ Major disasters, like the 2014 mudslide near Oso, Washington, require the coordinated responses of federal and local governments and aid organizations.

The first steps in addressing this condition are correcting ergonomic problems in the workstation, taking frequent breaks from repetitive tasks, and doing exercises that stretch and flex the wrists and hands. If symptoms persist, a physician should be consulted.

Natural Disasters

A *disaster* is defined as sudden event resulting in loss of life, severe injury, or property damage. Disasters can be caused by humans, as in the case of terrorist attacks, or by natural forces, such as tornadoes, hurricanes, floods, wildfires, and earthquakes. For example, in March 2011, a magnitude 9.0 earthquake followed by a tsunami with waves reaching 130 feet ravaged Japan and caused a nuclear power plant disaster. The earthquake moved the main island of Japan 8 feet east and shifted the Earth on its axis by several inches. When natural disasters occur on this scale, governments and international aid organizations have to provide the assistance and relief that people need to recover. Individuals can help themselves by preparing as much as they can for the types of disasters that are likely to occur where they live (e.g., tornadoes in the Midwest or hurricanes on the East Coast). The National Center for Environmental Health (part of the CDC) provides detailed information on preparedness for all types of events, including natural disasters and severe weather emergencies. Visit its website at www.cdc.gov/nceh.

VIOLENCE: WORKING TOWARD PREVENTION

More than many of the other health topics discussed in this text, violence is a societal issue. **Violence** is defined as the use of force or the threat of force to inflict intentional injury, physical or psychological, on oneself or another person. Murder, robbery, and **assault** are all violent crimes, but violence also occurs in association with child abuse, sexual harassment, suicide, and several other kinds of conduct. Although violent acts are committed by individuals, the causes of violence are rooted in social and cultural conditions. This does not mean that people who commit violent crimes are not held accountable for their actions—they are. In fact, the United States incarcerates a larger proportion of its population than does any other nation.

It does mean that taking action to reduce violence is difficult to do as an individual, unlike deciding to improve one's diet or get more exercise. What you as an individual can do about violence falls into two categories: knowing how to reduce your own risk of encountering violence and working to create safer communities and to prevent violence in society. To assess how well you protect yourself from encountering violence, answer the questions in this chapter's Personal Health Portfolio.

Rates of violent crime in the United States are similar to those in many other developed countries, except in one area—homicide, especially homicide committed with a firearm. The number of firearm homicides is higher in the United States than in any other country; it is almost 15 times higher than in Canada.[42] Most experts attribute this difference to the ready availability of firearms in the United States.[43]

violence
Use of force or the threat of force to inflict intentional injury, physical or psychological, on oneself or another person.

assault
Attack by one person on another using force or the threat of force to intentionally inflict injury. Aggravated assault is an attack that causes bodily injury, usually with a weapon or other means capable of producing grave bodily harm or death. Simple assault is an attack without a weapon that causes less serious physical harm.

What Accounts for Violence?

Age and sex are among the most reliable risk factors for violence.[44] The typical offender is a young male between the ages of 14 and 24. Forty-four percent of those arrested for violent crimes in the United States are under 25 years of age. Men are much more likely to commit a violent act than women. Women do commit violent acts, but they are often in self-defense.

Being a member of a minority group is a significant risk factor for violence. Although Blacks make up 12 percent of the population, they are nearly half (47 percent) of all homicide victims.[44] Similarly, Blacks account for 52 percent of homicide offenders. Thirty-seven percent of those arrested for violent crimes are Black, 60.5 percent are White, and the remainder are Native American, Asian, or Pacific Islander. (People of Hispanic ethnic origin are included in the racial categories "Black" and "White" in these statistics.)

Like risk factors for mental illness, risk factors for violence occur at the levels of the society, the family, and the individual. Risk factors at the societal and cultural levels—social determinants of health—include poverty, poor schools, disorganized neighborhoods, use of alcohol and drugs, availability of guns, exposure to media violence, and lack of economic, educational, and employment opportunities. Violence is also more common on college campuses than in the general population, perhaps because of the transient nature of the community. Risk factors at the family level include child abuse, substance abuse or criminal activity by family members, lack of positive role models, and chaotic family organization.

Risk factors at the individual level include biological factors such as genetics, brain structure, brain chemistry, and medical disorders; low intelligence; certain personality traits, such as aggressiveness and poor impulse control; and a history of previous criminal or antisocial behavior. Other individual risk factors include attention deficit disorder and hyperactivity in children, deficits in cognitive and social cognitive functioning, poor behavior control, and early antisocial and aggressive behaviors. Conversely, protective factors, which buffer young people from the effects of risk factors, include high IQ, a positive social orientation, and involvement in school activities. No single factor is sufficient to explain why violence occurs or why levels of violent crime rise or decline in different time periods.

Violence on the College Campus

In 2007, a student at Virginia Polytechnic Institute and State University shot and killed 27 students and 5 faculty members and wounded 16 more. The on-campus killing spree, the worst shooting incident by a single gunman in U.S. history, stunned the nation. Many people believe college campuses are safe havens and that violence rarely occurs on them.[45] Unfortunately, this is not true. Seventeen percent of college students report being a victim of violence or harassment in the previous year.[18] Regardless of whether the campus has distinct boundaries or is an urban campus within a city, colleges confront the same types of societal and violence issues that occur in almost any city in the nation. The U.S. Department of Education provides data on the safety of college campuses. To find out about your campus, visit www.ope.ed.gov/security.

Since the Virginia Tech shooting, college campuses have improved the ways they communicate with students and faculty during an emergency—by e-mail, phone messages, text messages, and siren and/or verbal warnings from communication towers. At some campuses, freshman orientation includes signing up for campus e-mail and phone alerts. Some schools also use social networking sites like Facebook and Twitter to distribute safety alerts. All of these measures

speed up the distribution of information and the likelihood that students will receive it.

The U.S. Department of Education collaborated with the U.S. Secret Service and the Federal Bureau of Investigation to explore the prevalence of violent incidents on college campuses and to identify perpetrators and potential perpetrators. They looked at data filed under the 1990 Jeanne Clery Disclosure of Campus Security Policy and Crime Statistics Act, which was named for Jeanne Clery, a 19-year-old student at Lehigh University, who was raped and murdered in her residence hall in 1986. The act requires all colleges and universities that participate in Title IV federal financial aid programs to collect and disclose information about crimes committed on or near campus. The most common campus crimes reported are burglary, motor vehicle theft, and aggravated assault. Other crimes tracked include homicides, sex offenses, robbery, and arson.[45] Investigators also looked at perpetrators' motivations. They found that current or former relationships between the perpetrator and victim were the predominant trigger for violent acts, followed by retaliation for specific actions (see Figure 16.4).

A 1992 amendment to the Clery Act, the Campus Sexual Assault Victims' Bill of Rights, requires college administrators to provide justice, medical treatment, and psychological counseling for crime victims and survivors. They must inform victims of the outcomes of disciplinary action and of their options to notify law enforcement and to change their academic and living situations. This law also requires colleges to promote educational awareness programs about sexual assault and to facilitate reporting of sexual assaults. Amendments in 2008 protect victims and whistleblowers against retaliation.

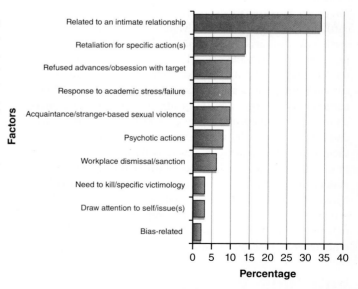

figure 16.4 **Factors that motivated or triggered direct assaults.**

Source: "Campus Attacks: Targeted Violence Affecting Institutions of Higher Education," Table 7, by U.S. Secret Service, U.S. Department of Education, and Federal Bureau of Investigation, April 2010, www.secretservice.gov/ntac/CampusAttacks041610.pdf.

Hazing **Hazing** is defined as "any action taken or situation created intentionally, whether on or off fraternity premises, to produce mental or physical discomfort, embarrassment, or ridicule." According to the National Collegiate Athletic Association (NCAA), four out of every five college students are subjected to some form of hazing in their college years. Ninety-five percent of these students do not report the hazing incident to college officials.[46,47] Hazing is typically imposed as an initiation rite or a requirement for joining an organization, usually a fraternity, sorority, or athletic team. Hazing activities have included kidnapping, alcohol chugging, forced swallowing of food and nonfood items, sleep deprivation, beatings, and calisthenics to the point of exhaustion. Deaths have occurred as a result of hazing, most often fraternity hazing. A common cause is alcohol poisoning.

Hazing is illegal in many states and may be either a misdemeanor or a felony, depending on the state and the severity of the offense. Parents whose children have died in these senseless incidents have filed wrongful death suits against both colleges and fraternities. Stop-hazing.org and hazingprevention.org are websites providing useful information on hazing prevention.

Free Speech vs. Hate Speech **Hate speech**—defined as verbal, written, or symbolic acts that convey a grossly negative view of particular persons or groups based on their gender, ethnicity, race, religion, sexual orientation, or disability[48]—is a troublesome phenomenon on many college campuses. Its intent is to humiliate or harm rather than to convey ideas or information, and it has the potential to incite violence. Epithets, slurs, taunts, insults, and intimidation are common modes of hate speech; posters, flyers, letters, phone calls, e-mail, websites, and even T-shirts are media by which the message is distributed.

Some schools have adopted speech codes that require civility in discourse for all campus community members. Some of these codes have been struck down by the courts as a violation of First Amendment rights. According to the rulings, hate speech must be proven to inflict real, not trivial, harm before it can be regulated. The U.S. Supreme Court has made it clear that colleges and universities cannot suppress speech simply because it is offensive. For this reason, many colleges and universities have adopted conduct codes that regulate certain actions associated with hate speech but not the speech itself.

Sexual Violence

Sexual violence includes not just rape but also sexual harassment, stalking, and other forms of forcible or coercive sexual activity.

Sexual Assault and Rape **Sexual assault** is any sexual behavior that is forced on someone without his or her consent. At the least, the victim is made to feel uncomfortable and intimidated; at the worst, he or she is physically and emotionally harmed.[49] Sexual assault includes forced sexual intercourse (rape), forced sodomy (oral or anal sexual acts), child molestation, incest, fondling, and attempts to commit any of these acts. Another category of victimization is called **sexual coercion**, defined as imposing sexual activity on someone through the threat of nonphysical punishment, promise of reward, or verbal pressure rather than through force or threat of force.

According to various studies, 25 to 60 percent of men (15 to 25 percent of college men) have engaged in sexual assault and coercive sexual behavior.[50] The causes of this behavior are complex and probably include personality traits in the perpetrator as well as situational factors, including time and place of assault, use of alcohol and other drugs, and the relationship between victim and perpetrator.

In the general population, 1 in 6 women experience rape or attempted rape at some time in their lives, and 1 in 33 men experience rape or attempted rape.[50,51] More than half of rape and sexual assault victims are under the age of 18, and one in five is under the age of 12.[49] When a victim is younger than the "age of consent," usually 18, the perpetrator can be charged with **statutory rape** whether there was consent or not. An estimated 20 percent of college women experience rape or attempted rape during their college years; for college men, the number is about 6 percent.[50,52] First-year college women are at highest risk for sexual assault during the first few weeks of their first semester (discussed further in "The Red Zone").[52]

Only 25 to 50 percent of all rapes are reported to the police, and among college students, 95 percent of rapes go unreported to law enforcement or college administrators. There are many reasons rapes are not reported.[51] Victims may be embarrassed or traumatized, may not be sure that what happened qualifies as rape, may think they won't be believed, may blame themselves or feel guilty, may be afraid because they had been drinking or using drugs, or may not want to identify someone they know as a rapist (see the box, "Heather: A Case of Sexual Assault").

Relatively few rapes are *stranger rapes,* that is, rapes committed by someone unknown to the victim. In about 60 percent of rapes and sexual assaults, the victim knows the perpetrator.[49] In 40 percent of cases, the perpetrator is a friend or an acquaintance; *acquaintance rape* can be committed by

hazing
Actions taken to cause mental or physical discomfort, embarrassment, or ridicule in individuals seeking to join an organization.

hate speech
Verbal, written, or symbolic acts that convey a grossly negative view of particular persons or groups based on their gender, ethnicity, race, religion, sexual orientation, or disability.

sexual assault
Any sexual behavior that is forced on someone without his or her consent.

sexual coercion
The imposition of sexual activity on someone through the threat of nonphysical punishment, promise of reward, or verbal pressure rather than through force or threat of force.

statutory rape
Sexual intercourse with someone under the "age of consent," usually 18, whether consent is given or not.

Heather: A Case of Sexual Assault

Heather was a freshman in her first semester at a large university a few hundred miles from the midsize city where she grew up. During Welcome Week, her R.A. put up some flyers around her dorm floor about sexual assault, but Heather didn't stop to read them. One night during the second week of classes, Heather and her roommates attended an off-campus party where there were several kegs. She got very drunk and left her friends to hang out with a cute and funny junior, Tom, and continued to drink for the next hour until she started to feel like she was going to be sick. She thought Tom was being helpful when he showed her to a bedroom at the house where he said she could rest until she felt better. But once they were in the room alone, Tom started kissing her. She tried to turn away, but she was too drunk to resist him or say anything. He then sexually forced himself on her.

When she realized what had happened the next day, she tried to forget about it. But over the next week, she found herself unable to concentrate on her classes. She was worried she might be pregnant or have gotten an STD. She cycled through feeling guilty for getting so drunk, angry at Tom, and embarrassed. She went back and forth about whether she had really been raped that night.

Heather didn't have many people to talk to because it was only the second week of school, but one of her high school friends who was a year ahead of her was a sophomore at the same school. Heather texted her and they met up at Keisha's apartment. Heather was nervous about sharing something so personal, but Keisha quickly jumped in and said that something similar had happened to her during freshman year. Heather told her how she felt embarrassed, angry, and confused about whether she had been raped. Keisha reminded her that Tom should have stopped when she turned away from him and didn't return his advances. If she didn't report the incident, she asked, how many other girls would Tom do this to? Keisha also explained that because Heather was 18, her parents would not find out unless she told them herself.

Keisha encouraged Heather to report the incident, but she also warned her about the school administration, which she felt had not handled her own report well. She had been made to sign a gag order that threatened the possibility of suspension if she violated it—and technically she was violating it by telling her story to Heather. Keisha advised Heather to contact the Rape Victim Advocacy Program (RVAP), which Keisha had done only after her bad experience with the campus administration. Heather did so, and RVAP listened to her story and advised her about what to do next, which included filing sexual assault charges against Tom, making an appointment with an off-campus counselor, and getting pregnancy and STD tests at the campus clinic.

- Did it matter that Heather was intoxicated? Should juries be allowed to use intoxication as a deliberation factor in rape cases?

- What is your college's policy on reporting sexual assaults? Do you think the policy is appropriate? Why or why not?

- What support systems does your community have in place for survivors of sexual assault?

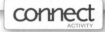

connect
ACTIVITY

a classmate, coworker, or someone else casually known to the victim. *Date rape,* sexual assault by a boyfriend or someone with whom the victim has a dating relationship, is a type of acquaintance rape. About 90 percent of campus assaults are committed by someone the victim knows. About 18 percent of rapes and sexual assaults are committed by the victim's intimate partner or husband.[49,50] Many states now allow rape charges to be brought by a woman against her husband.

Acquaintance-rape survivors are more likely to have consumed alcohol or drugs before the assault, possibly reducing their awareness of signs of aggression in the rapist or their ability to respond to violence.[49] Sexual predators also use so-called date rape drugs, including rohypnol, gamma hydroxybutyrate (GHB), ketamine, and Ecstasy, to incapacitate their victims. These drugs typically have no color, smell, or taste, so they can be difficult to detect if mixed into a drink. Date rape drugs are very potent, and they take effect quickly—from a few minutes to half an hour. Effects can include physical and cognitive distortion, blackouts, and loss of memory. These effects can inhibit one's ability to say no to sexual advances or fight back if a sexual assault occurs.

Recommendations for protection against date rape drugs include getting your drink directly from the bartender and watching your drink being made in bars or clubs, never leaving your drink unattended or turning your back on your table, and not accepting open drinks from those you do not trust. A test kit called Drink Safe Technology can detect the presence of date rape drugs in drinks; its drink testing strips or coasters change color when they come in contact with a date rape drug.

The Red Zone The *red zone,* a term drawn from a campus sexual assault violence prevention program, is the period of time at college when female students are at greatest risk for sexual assault. The zone includes the first few days or weeks of the initial fall semester as female students transition from the security of their parents' home to a less restrictive lifestyle on campus, which often includes binge drinking. For second-year females, the zone encompasses the entire first semester, when many make the move from campus housing to sororities or off-campus apartments.[53]

Counseling centers, student affairs offices, and public safety centers at colleges and universities use web-based and print media to warn female students about the red zone. Although sexual assault is a serious health problem on many college campuses, college students sometimes prefer to call these assaults "unwanted sex" and not sexual assaults. The reluctance to view these events as assaults is likely due to the victim being acquainted with her assailant.

These safety tips for college students from the Rape, Abuse, and Incest National Network (RAINN) are particularly important for the red zone times:[54]

- Trust your instincts. If you feel unsafe in any situation, go with your gut.

- Avoid being alone or isolated with someone you don't know well.

- Get to know your surroundings and learn well-lit routes to your residence.

- Don't put information about your whereabouts on your Facebook page or in your voicemail message.

- Form a buddy system when you go out. Arrive and leave with friends, and check in with each other throughout the evening. If you suspect a friend has been drugged, call 911.

- Always lock your door, and don't let strangers into your room.

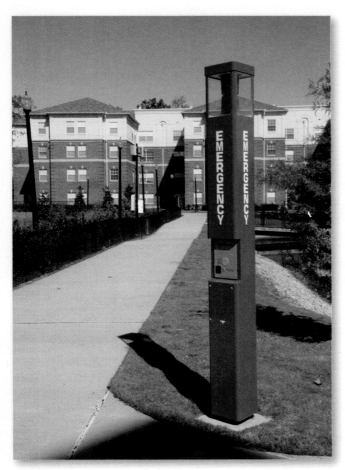

- Many college campuses have emergency phones that students can use to call for help from campus security officers if they feel in danger.

- Practice safe drinking. Don't accept drinks from people you don't know, watch while your drink is being prepared, and don't leave your drink unattended.

- Don't go out alone at night. If you'll be walking home at night, arrange to walk with a friend or in a group, or use the campus security escort system, if there is one.

Male Rape In about 1 to 2 percent of completed and attempted rapes in the United States, the victim is male. Like women, men are reluctant to report that they have been raped. They may feel embarrassed or ashamed, or they may not want to believe they have been raped.[49]

Law enforcement personnel, medical personnel, and social service agencies may be less supportive of male rape victims than of female rape victims because of similar misperceptions and misinformation.[49] The law is clear, however, on defining forced penetration as rape or sodomy. Male rape victims require the same level of medical treatment, counseling, and support as female victims.

Effects of Rape Rape is a crime about dominance, power, and control. For many victims, the effects of rape can be profoundly traumatic and long lasting. Physical injuries usually heal quickly, but psychological pain can endure.

Victims often experience fear, anxiety, phobias, guilt, nightmares, depression, substance abuse, sleep disorders, sexual dysfunctions, and social withdrawal. They may develop rape-related post-traumatic stress disorder, experiencing flashbacks and impaired functioning. Between 4 and 30 percent of victims contract an STD from the rape, and many worry that they may have been infected with HIV.[55] Some state laws now mandate HIV testing of an alleged rapist if the victim requests it.

Many victims blame themselves for the rape, and our society tends to foster self-blame. Myths about rape include the false beliefs that women or men who are raped did something to provoke it, put themselves in dangerous situations and so deserved it, or could have fought off their attacker. The fact is that no matter what a person does, nobody ever has the right to rape.

What to Do If You Are Raped There is no one way to respond to rape that works in all cases, and authorities recommend that you do whatever you need to do and can do to survive. No matter how you respond, remember that your attacker is violating your rights and committing a crime; rape is not your fault.

After the rape, seek help as soon as you can. If you choose to call the police, there is a better chance that the perpetrator will be brought to justice and will be prevented from raping others. The police will probably take you to the hospital, where you will be given a rape exam and treated for your injuries. You should also contact your local Rape Victim Advocacy Program (RVAP) or the Rape, Abuse and Incest National Network (RAINN). These organizations can inform you of your rights under the Campus Sexual Assault

Victims' Bill of Rights and provide advocate support during campus and local law enforcement investigations.

Rape counseling is critical to your recovery from the attack. Talking about the rape, either one-on-one with a rape counselor or in a rape survivors' support group, can help you come to terms with your reactions and feelings. Rape crisis hotlines, such as the RAINN hotline (800-656-HOPE), are available when you need immediate help, although research suggests an increasing reluctance among young people to use the phone to discuss sexual assault. It takes time to recover from rape, so be patient and take care of yourself.

Culture of Secrecy Crime statistics under the Clery Act are supposed to be pulled from diverse campus programs and centers and local law enforcement agencies. However, an investigative report by the Center for Public Integrity (CPI) suggests that colleges and universities are underreporting sexual assaults as required by the act. This gap in reporting is largely caused by loopholes in the systematic collection of sexual assault data. Licensed mental health counselors and pastoral counselors are exempt under confidentiality provisions by the Family Education Reporting Protection Act. Many of these counselors are housed in rape victim advocacy programs, student health centers, and hospitals. When victims seek help from these types of counselors and not the police, their assaults are not reported.[56,57]

More troublesome are controversial policies used by some colleges and universities to investigate sexual assault reports.[57] Some rely on mediation procedures whereby the alleged perpetrator and alleged victim meet with a college administrator who serves as a mediator to resolve the situation. Both the Department of Justice and the Department of Education explicitly discourage the use of mediation without legal representation to resolve sexual assault complaints. Moreover, sexual assault charges are potentially felony counts that should not be subjected to informal investigations. According to the CPI, college female victims who come forward with a sexual assault complaint also often feel betrayed by gag policies.[58] Victims of sexual assault are advised to contact an advocacy group like RVAP or RAINN, which can ensure that their rights are being upheld, in addition to contacting the police.

Preventing Sexual Violence Rape prevention efforts need to include efforts to change the environment that promotes violence against women. Rape prevention involves creating a culture and a community in which sexual violence is not tolerated. Changing social and cultural norms can be a slow process, but programs like Take Back the Night and the Green Dot Strategy have taken on this challenge.

The Green Dot Violence Prevention Strategy, a program that began in the United Kingdom and is now appearing on U.S. college campuses, seeks to reduce and prevent power-based personal violence,

child sexual abuse Any interaction between a child and an adult or an older child for the sexual gratification of the perpetrator.

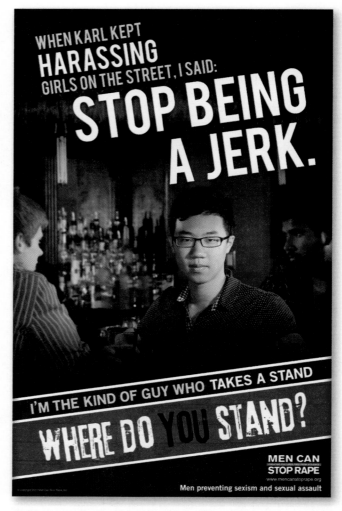

■ The organization Men Can Stop Rape takes a nontraditional approach to sexual violence prevention, emphasizing healthy masculinity and redefining male strength.

including sexual violence, domestic violence, dating violence, stalking, child abuse, elder abuse, and bullying. Rather than focusing on victims or perpetrators, as many campaigns do, it focuses on bystanders. Green Dot aims to mobilize the vast majority of the population who consider violence unacceptable and move them from passive bystanding to engagement and action. The Green Dot strategy addresses individual factors (such as shyness and lack of assertiveness), interpersonal factors (such as peer pressure and the well-known "bystander effect," in which everyone assumes someone else will act), community factors (training influential members of the community to model new behaviors), and societal factors (addressing cultural norms about the acceptability of violence).

Child Sexual Abuse Any interaction between a child and an adult or an older child for the sexual gratification of the perpetrator is defined as **child sexual abuse**. This definition includes intercourse, fondling, and viewing or taking pornographic pictures. Rates of child sexual abuse are difficult to verify because many cases go unreported. One study estimated that one in five children experiences some form of maltreatment: about 1 percent were victims of sexual assault, 4 percent were victims of neglect, 9 percent were victims of physical abuse, and 12 percent were victims of emotional abuse.[59] African American, American Indian, Alaska Native, and multiracial children have higher rates of victimization than White children.[59] Children are most frequently abused between ages 9 and 11.[60] Girls are sexually abused three times as often as boys.[60] The abuse is usually committed by a family member or other person known to the family. **Incest**, sexual activity between family members, is a particularly traumatic form of child sexual abuse because of the profound betrayal of trust involved.

Victims of sexual abuse usually suffer long-term effects, including anxiety, depression, post-traumatic stress disorder, and sexual dysfunctions. The seriousness of these problems is influenced by the frequency of abuse, the kind of sexual abuse, the child's age when the abuse began, the child's relationship with the abuser, the number of perpetrators, the victim's sex, and the perpetrator's sex.

Child sexual abusers may or may not be pedophiles. A pedophile is a person who is sexually attracted to children. Individuals who are not pedophiles and abuse or molest children are more likely to be opportunists with psychological problems and poor impulse control.

Federal laws were passed in the 1990s requiring convicted sex offenders to register their names and addresses with the local police department. These laws were then amended to require police departments to notify schools, day care centers, and youth groups about moderate- and high-risk sex offenders in the community. In addition, names, addresses, and photos of registered sex offenders are now available to the public on the Internet. In 2005, many states passed laws prohibiting sex offenders from living close to where children gather, mandating lifetime GPS monitoring, and requiring that "sex offender" be printed on offenders' driver's license or license plate. In 2006, the Adam Walsh Child Protection and Safety Act established a national DNA database and registry that includes GPS monitoring, a longer period of registration, increased penalties for failure to register, and longer mandatory minimum sentences.

The proliferation and severity of federal and state sex offender laws have begun to evoke a backlash. Several civil rights groups, including Human Rights Watch, have objected that the laws are overbroad, unconstitutional, and counterproductive. Some sex offenders have been unable to find housing in familiar areas and have had to locate in rural areas, where there is less access to mental health services and jobs. Experiencing stigmatization, ostracism, and isolation destabilizes offenders further and makes it more likely they will commit another crime. Many child safety experts and rape prevention advocates argue that the laws should be limited in scope and duration. They also argue that more money should be spent on prevention and treatment programs rather than registration, tracking, and notification programs.

Pedophiles and other sex offenders have found a community on the Internet, where they exchange stories and buy and sell child pornography. Sexual predators also contact children through social networking sites and gaming sites. The sites themselves, however, are pursuing technologies that can protect users from potential abuses, identifying offenders and deleting them from the site. There is also a push for state and federal laws that will require these sites to protect users under age 18 through age identity verification and parental consent.[61] In 2012, for example, New York State, in cooperation with major tech and game companies, purged 3,500 sex offenders from various online gaming networks. A similar number of offenders had been deleted from Facebook and MySpace by New York in a 2009 initiative. Some opponents to these controls argue that there is no simple way to screen for sexual predators, identify underage users masquerading as adults, or ensure that underage users have parental permission.

Sexual Harassment   **Sexual harassment** includes two types of situations: (1) a person in a position of authority, such as an employer or a teacher, offering benefits for sexual favors or threatening retaliation for the withholding of sex, and (2) suggestive language or intimidating conduct that creates a hostile atmosphere and interferes with a person's work or academic performance.

Of all sexual harassment claims, 95 percent result from actions that create a hostile environment.[62] A hostile environment can be created by visual images (e.g., sexually explicit photos), language (e.g., jokes, derogatory comments, obscene e-mails), or behavior (e.g., inappropriate touching). An American Association of University Women study found that 62 percent of college women and 61 percent of college men had been verbally or physical sexually harassed while in college (see the box, "A Profile of Sexual Harassment on Campus"). Only about 7 percent reported this harassment to university officials.[63] One-third of the college women felt afraid, and 18 percent of women and 11 percent of men were disappointed in their college experience due to sexual harassment.[63] Under federal regulations, colleges and universities are liable for sexual harassment perpetrated by their faculty or staff, regardless of whether the advance is accepted or rejected.

Differentiating between sexual harassment and flirting depends on three factors: (1) whether the behavior is by someone who has power over the offended person that limits his or her ability to object for fear of reprisal, (2) whether the behavior puts pressure on the offended person, and (3) whether the offended person wants to end the interaction.

incest
Sexual activity between family members.

sexual harassment
Behavior in which a person in authority offers benefits for sexual favors or threatens retaliation if sexual favors are withheld, or sexually oriented behavior that creates an intimidating or hostile environment that interferes with a person's work or academic performance.

Who's at Risk?

A Profile of Sexual Harassment on Campus

A study by the American Association of University Women found that as many men as women are sexually harassed on college campuses. Women are most likely to be harassed by one man (58 percent) or a group of men (48 percent). Men may be harassed by one man (37 percent), one woman (33 percent), or by a group of men (21 percent) or a group of both men and women (23 percent). For 13 percent of the respondents, the harasser was anonymous—someone spreading rumors verbally or online. As the following graphs show, LGBT students are more likely to be harassed than straight students, and White students are more likely than Black or Latino students to be the targets of sexual harassment. What are the likely effects of sexual harassment on the educational experience? What are the likely gender differences on educational experiences?

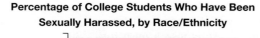

Percentage of College Students Who Have Been Sexually Harassed, by Race/Ethnicity

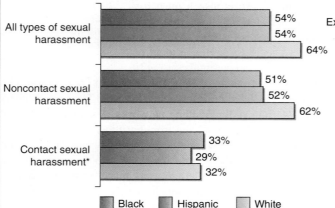

All types of sexual harassment: 54%, 54%, 64%

Noncontact sexual harassment: 51%, 52%, 62%

Contact sexual harassment*: 33%, 29%, 32%

■ Black ■ Hispanic ■ White

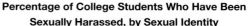

Percentage of College Students Who Have Been Sexually Harassed, by Sexual Identity

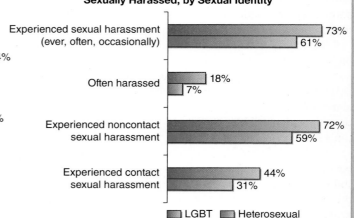

Experienced sexual harassment (ever, often, occasionally): 73%, 61%

Often harassed: 18%, 7%

Experienced noncontact sexual harassment: 72%, 59%

Experienced contact sexual harassment: 44%, 31%

■ LGBT ■ Heterosexual

*For contact sexual harassment, there are no statistically significant differences by race/ethnicity.
Note: Differences between Black and Hispanic populations are not statistically significant for any category.
A minority of respondents (9.7 percent) chose a category other than Black, White, or Hispanic—such as Asian or Pacific Islander, mixed racial background, or other race—or declined to answer; those respondents are not shown in the graphs.

connect ACTIVITY

Source: *Drawing the Line: Sexual Harassment on Campus*, Figures 4 and 5, by Catherine Hill and Elena Silva, 2005, American Association of University Women Education Foundation, www.aauw.org/resource/drawing-the-line-sexual-harassment-on-campus/.

Gender and culture differences complicate the situation. For example, men are more likely than women to misperceive friendliness as sexual interest.

If you have experienced sexual harassment, keep a written record of all incidents of harassment, including the date, time, place, people involved, words or actions, and any witnesses. If you can, speak up and tell your harasser that the behavior is unacceptable to you. If you do not feel comfortable confronting the harasser in person, consider doing so by letter.

If confrontation does not change the harasser's behavior, complain to a manager or supervisor. If that person does not respond properly to your complaint, consider using your organization's internal grievance procedures. Most colleges have an administrative office where students can report incidents of sexual harassment and a procedure for doing so. Legal remedies are also available through your state Human Rights Commission and the Federal Equal Employment Opportunity Commission.

stalking
Malicious following, harassing, or threatening of one person by another.

Stalking and Cyberstalking Another form of potentially dangerous conduct is **stalking**, in which a person repeatedly and maliciously follows, harasses, or threatens another person. Women are four times as likely as men to be victims of stalking; it is estimated that 1 in 6 heterosexual women, 1 in 3 bisexual women, and 1 in 19 men have been stalked at some point during their lifetime.[49,64] About 7 percent of women and 4 percent of men report being stalked during their college years.[18]

The harassment typically includes surveillance at work, school, or home; frequent disturbing telephone calls; vandalism of the target's property; physical encounters; and attempts to get the victim's family and friends to aid the stalker. Targets of stalkers live in constant fear.

Many states have passed laws to protect individuals who are being stalked, but in some cases it is difficult to arrest and prosecute stalkers without violating their rights, such as the right to be present in a public place. If you plan to report a stalker to the police, keep a written record of all dates, times, locations, witnesses, and types of incidents (personal encounters, telephone calls, e-mails).

Cyberstalking is the use of electronic media to pursue, harass, or contact another person who has not solicited the contact.[65] Online stalkers may send threatening, harassing, sexually provocative, or other unwanted e-mails to the target or attack or impersonate the person on bulletin boards or in chat rooms. College students need to be particularly cautious about Facebook stalking. New additions to Facebook include potential stalking sites such as Secret Admirers' page and Confessions page. Laws against cyberstalking are in place in some states, but prosecution is hampered by Internet protocols that preserve anonymity as well as by the Constitution's protection of free speech. If you are experiencing this kind of harassment, you can contact the stalker's Internet service provider (ISP) and complain about its client; the company will often take action to try to stop the conduct.

Family and Intimate Partner Violence

Violence in families can be directed at any family member, but women, children, and older adults are the most vulnerable. Violence between intimate partners is called **intimate partner violence** or **domestic violence**.

Family Violence Family violence is a broad term that includes several forms of violence and abuse, including child abuse and elder abuse.

Maltreatment of a child, or **child abuse**, includes physical abuse, sexual abuse, emotional abuse, and neglect. It occurs in all cultural, ethnic, and socioeconomic groups, with the highest rates of abuse occurring among the poorest children and among those who are disabled.[66] The highest number of victims are among newborns and infants, who are the most fragile, followed by teenagers.

Abusive parents often lack the emotional resources to cope with the stress of childrearing; they may not be knowledgeable about normal child development and have unrealistic expectations of their children. Some may have been abused themselves as children. Social determinants like unemployment, poverty, and isolation, as well as alcohol or drug abuse, can be contributing factors. When a case of child abuse comes to light, the abusive parent or guardian is usually removed from the home to keep the child safe. Therapy typically focuses on the abuser but includes all family members.[66]

Maltreatment of an older adult, or **elder abuse**, can include physical abuse (slapping, bruising), sexual abuse, emotional abuse (humiliating, threatening, intimidating), financial abuse (illegal or improper exploitation of funds), and neglect (abandonment, denial of food or health-related services). The abuser is usually a family member, often an adult child, who is taking care of an aging parent or other elderly relative. Interventions for elder abuse include counseling and support groups for caregivers; battered women's services tailored to the needs of older women; family counseling that attempts to improve relationships within the family; and community services such as Meals on Wheels, home health programs, and elder day care.

Intimate Partner Violence Intimate partner violence, or domestic violence, is defined as abuse by a person against his or her partner in an intimate relationship. This definition includes the intentional use of fear and humiliation to control another person. About 30 percent of heterosexual women, 36 percent of lesbians, 55 percent of bisexual women, 26 percent of heterosexual men, 24 percent of gay men, and 27 percent of bisexual men report being slapped, pushed, or shoved by an intimate partner at some point in their lifetime. Severe intimate partner violence has been reported by one in four heterosexual women, 29 percent of heterosexual men, one in three lesbians, one in two bisexual women, 14 percent of bisexual men, and 16 percent of gay men.[49] Twelve percent of college women and 7 percent of college men report being in an abusive relationship.[18]

Cycle of Abuse Domestic violence is usually characterized by a cycle of abuse, a recurring pattern of escalating violence. Typically, tension builds up in the relationship until there is a violent outburst, followed by a "honeymoon" period in which the abuser is contrite, ashamed, apologetic, and nonviolent.[60] Often, the abuser begs his or her partner for forgiveness and promises it will never happen again. Unless the abuser gets help, however, the violence does recur and the cycle repeats itself, almost always becoming more severe (Figure 16.5). If the couple is heterosexual, the pattern is sometimes referred to as **battered woman syndrome**, but it can occur in any relationship, including gay and lesbian partnerships.

Research indicates that men who batter are more likely to abuse drugs and alcohol, suffer from mental illness, and have financial problems.[60] Most women who are battered eventually leave their abusive relationships, but they may make several attempts before they succeed. Battered women's shelters provide a safe haven where the woman and her children cannot be found by the abuser. They provide housing, food, and resources to help the woman start a new life. When shelters aren't available, private homes are sometimes available as safe houses, and churches, community centers, and YWCAs may also offer temporary facilities.[60]

Dating Violence Dating violence is widespread. According to a 2011 survey, 43 percent of college women report having experienced violent or abusive dating

cyberstalking
Use of electronic media to pursue, harass, or contact another person who has not solicited the contact.

intimate partner violence or domestic violence
Violence between two partners in an intimate relationship.

child abuse
Maltreatment of a child; can be physical, sexual, or emotional abuse or neglect.

elder abuse
Maltreatment of an older adult; can be physical, sexual, emotional, or financial abuse or neglect.

battered woman syndrome
Cycle of abuse in an intimate relationship, characterized by escalating tension, a violent episode, and a period of lowered tension and nonviolence.

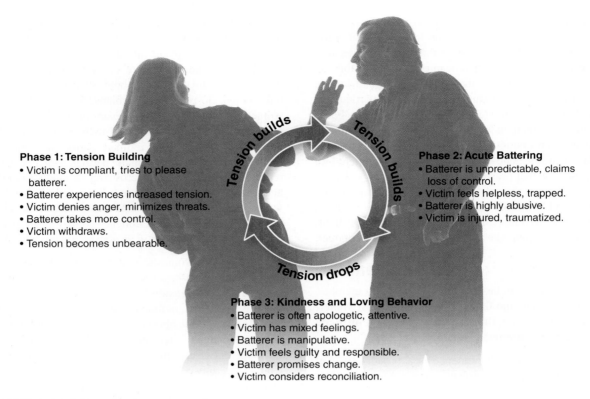

Phase 1: Tension Building
- Victim is compliant, tries to please batterer.
- Batterer experiences increased tension.
- Victim denies anger, minimizes threats.
- Batterer takes more control.
- Victim withdraws.
- Tension becomes unbearable.

Phase 2: Acute Battering
- Batterer is unpredictable, claims loss of control.
- Victim feels helpless, trapped.
- Batterer is highly abusive.
- Victim is injured, traumatized.

Phase 3: Kindness and Loving Behavior
- Batterer is often apologetic, attentive.
- Victim has mixed feelings.
- Batterer is manipulative.
- Victim feels guilty and responsible.
- Batterer promises change.
- Victim considers reconciliation.

figure 16.5   Cycle of domestic violence.

behaviors, and 22 percent report actual physical abuse, sexual abuse, or threats of violence.[67] Fifty-two percent of college women report knowing a friend who experienced an abusive relationship, including physical, sexual, digital, verbal, or controlling abuse, and 38 percent said they would not know how to help someone in an abusive relationship.[67] In response to these findings, a teen dating violence prevention organization called Break the Cycle teamed up with the National Dating Abuse Helpline to launch an initiative called Love Is Respect (www.loveisrespect.org). This initiative targets college students and provides resources to address abusive dating relationships.[67]

hate crime
Crime motivated by bias against the victim's ethnicity, race, religion, sexual orientation, or disability.

Studies show that individuals at risk for dating violence are more likely than others to have been sexually assaulted, to have peers who have been sexually victimized, and to accept dating violence. Perpetrators are more likely than others to abuse alcohol or drugs, to have adversarial attitudes toward others, to have sexually aggressive peers, and to accept dating violence.[68]

Resources for Survivors of Intimate Partner Violence If you are concerned that someone you know may be in an abusive relationship, try talking to the person about the nature of the relationship and giving him or her information about resources available in your community. Encourage the person to maintain contact with friends and family members while getting support to leave the relationship and begin building a new life.[60] As described in the previous sections, help is available from social service agencies, educational programs, hotlines, shelters, advocacy organizations, and informational books and packets provided by national, state, and local organizations.

Hate Crimes and Terrorism

Violence can occur where there are high levels of stress, bias, and perceived injustice. In most cases, however, multiple risk factors are present; very often, the perpetrator of violence is psychologically disturbed.

Hate Crimes A **hate crime** is a crime motivated by bias against the victim's ethnicity, race, religion, sexual orientation, or disability. Hate crimes tend to be excessively brutal, are frequently inflicted at random on people the perpetrators do not know, and are often committed by multiple perpetrators.[69]

Most states have laws against hate crimes, as does the federal government. Many colleges and universities have policies prohibiting hate crimes and harassment of individuals in targeted groups, as well as programs that promote cultural knowledge and diversity.[69] Because hate crimes against lesbian, gay, bisexual, and transgender (LGBT) persons have increased on campuses in recent years, many colleges and universities have specific policies forbidding violence directed toward LGBT students.[69] The Matthew Shepard Act was passed to expand federal hate crime law to include crimes motivated by a victim's actual or perceived gender, sexual orientation, or gender identity. Colleges also report what is called biphobia—shunning of bisexual students by support groups for gay and lesbian students. This shunning has led bisexual students to form their own support group organizations.

Terrorism **Terrorism** is a form of violence directed against people or property, including civilian populations, for the purpose of instilling fear and engendering a sense of helplessness. Often, terrorist acts are committed in supposed furtherance of political or social aims. For many Americans, the September 11, 2001, attacks on the World Trade Center in New York City and the Pentagon in Washington, DC, remain the most traumatizing events of their lives.

In response to the September 11 attacks, the U.S. government created the Department of Homeland Security to prevent and guard against future attacks and the Homeland Security Advisory System, a color-coded warning system, to alert citizens of the likelihood of attack. In 2005, Congress passed a counterterrorism measure called the Real ID Act, establishing minimum standards for driver's licenses and state-issued ID cards, and in 2007, Congress passed the John Doe provision as part of the renewal of the Homeland Security bill, protecting people who report suspicious activity from being sued by those they report.

The December 25, 2009, attempted bombing of a jetliner over Detroit by a would-be terrorist who was hiding plastic explosives in his underwear led the Transportation Safety Administration (TSA) to accelerate plans for deploying more than 450 full-body scanners at U.S. airports. Full-body scanners are designed to uncover what may not be found by a pat-down search or by metal detectors. Opponents to full-body scanners claim they are a violation of privacy rights. Moreover, scanners cannot detect items hidden in body cavities, a common ploy used by drug smugglers and one that terrorist organizations may also try to exploit. Opponents of body scanners recommend the use of more aggressive behavioral profiling, bomb-sniffing dogs, machines that detect the scent of explosives, and heat sensors to increase airline security.

New iris screening technology that can snap a person's iris in one second from a few feet away is being developed for passenger scanning. Some safety experts believe that by 2020 most people will be processed automatically at airports by matching iris scans against databases. Privacy experts are concerned that the database could be hacked, resulting in stolen identities.

terrorism
Violence directed against persons or property, including civilian populations, for the purpose of instilling fear and engendering a sense of helplessness.

Some terrorism prevention practices used by the FBI and Homeland Security are facing scrutiny as possibly violating Fourth Amendment privacy rights, for example, phone monitoring and use of domestic drones for surveillance. Is this information needed for prevention of domestic terrorism? What do you think?

Preventing Violence

Although protecting yourself from terrorism is difficult, there are ways you can limit your risks in life; to assess how well you protect yourself from unsafe situations, complete this chapter's Personal Health Portfolio activity at the end of the book. At the same time, self-protection measures must be part of a more comprehensive approach that addresses violence at the societal level. Current efforts to curb violence focus primarily on arresting and imprisoning offenders. Strategies are also needed that prevent violence before it occurs—that is, interventions that change the social conditions underlying violence.

The Role of Guns: Facilitating Violence

Guns contribute to the lethality of any incident involving violence. The Second Amendment to the U.S. Constitution protects the right of citizens to "keep and bear arms," a right that was important in colonial times but that may not be as important today. The gun industry—along with its powerful lobby and many clubs, organizations, and individual enthusiasts—defends

■ Some people still suffer from symptoms of post-traumatic stress disorder as a result of the terrorist attacks of September 11, 2001, including individuals who weren't there but viewed the events on television.

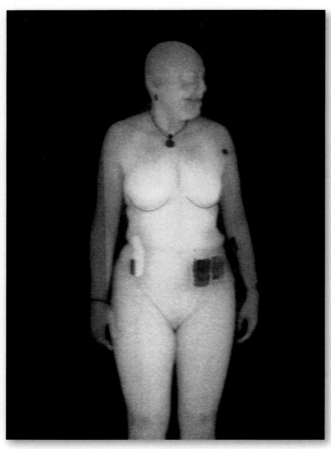

■ The X-rays that are used in backscatter scanners can "see" through clothing. They can detect weapons, dangerous substances, and explosives that might be missed by a metal detector or pat-down search.

manufacturers point out that gun owners frequently do not use the locks, and Congress has concluded that locks are effective only with children younger than age 6.[70,71] For more about such efforts, see the box, "Curbing Gun Violence."

In the wake of the mass shooting at Sandy Hook Elementary School, the Obama administration commissioned the Institute of Medicine and the National Research Council to analyze the research on gun violence. Its key conclusions favor neither pro-gun-control nor pro-gun advocates:

■ The U.S has more fire-arm related homicides than any other industrialized country, and 19.5 times higher than other high-income countries.

■ Overall, violent crime rates, including homicides, have declined in the past 15 years.

■ There are 300 million guns in the United States, but only 100 million are handguns that are used in more than 87 percent of violent crimes.

■ Since 1983 there have been 78 events in which four or more people were killed by a single shooter, resulting in 547 fatalities (compared with 335,000 gun deaths of individuals between 2000 and 2010).

■ Gun suicide is a bigger problem than gun homicide.

■ Most people who own guns say it makes them feel safer.

■ Denying guns to people under restraining orders saves lives.

■ Guns are used for self-defense often and safely.[72]

Among organizations that support the right to bear arms is the organization Students for Concealed Carry on Campus (SCCC), which advocates changing federal and state laws and college policies to allow gun-licensed college students to carry concealed handguns on campus. The organization argues that students may need handguns for self-defense in the event of a shooting incident and will feel safer if allowed to carry concealed guns on campus. The organization also points out that concealed handguns are legal in most states at virtually any locale—at movie theaters, offices, and shopping malls, to name just a few. Opponents argue that allowing concealed guns on campus would result in a "Wild West" environment.[73] The American Association of State Colleges and Universities strongly opposes laws that would allow concealed guns on campus. Currently, 12 colleges allow people to carry concealed handguns on campus.

Three-D printers, also called additive manufacturing, may revolutionize gun manufacturing. It promises an easy way to bypass gun control restrictions. As sturdier and cheaper 3-D printers become available, websites devoted to gun design

the right of Americans to own guns with minimal restrictions. Some laws are in place regulating gun sales, such as computerized background checks on persons seeking to buy guns, though the U.S. Supreme Court has deemed unconstitutional more severe restrictions, as when it overturned Washington, DC's ban on handguns in 2009. Some colleges are now being challenged for providing personal information about student behavior and academic performance to local law enforcement agencies when they apply for gun permits. Many legal experts view this practice as a violation of the Federal Education Rights and Privacy Act.

Proponents of gun control support banning the sale of assault guns to private individuals and other measures, including waiting periods for gun purchases, licensing of guns, and restrictions on access to guns by young people.[70] They also support the design of safer guns, such as guns with trigger locks, although gun

Public Health Is Personal

Curbing Gun Violence: A Public Health Perspective

The 2012 mass shootings at Sandy Hook Elementary School in Newtown, Connecticut, and in a theater in Aurora, Colorado, reenergized efforts of pro-gun control advocates to pass strict gun access laws at the federal level. However, these horrific shootings provided only a temporary refocusing on the nation's burden of gun violence. Within the year following the Sandy Hook massacre, there were 14 school shootings resulting in multiple injuries and deaths. Every day in the United States, about 85 people die and many more are injured by guns.

President Obama remarked that the day of the Newtown shooting "was the worst day of my presidency. Something fundamental in the United States has to change." President Obama's aggressive gun-control plan called for closing background check loopholes, banning assault weapons and high-capacity magazines, and improving mental health services.

Skeptics argue that there are already laws making it illegal to sell a gun to a felon and for a felon to buy a gun. However, these laws do not prevent felons, and nonfelons, from killing innocent people. There are more guns in the United States than there are people. How can new federal laws control more than 300 million guns? The answer is enforcement of existing laws and not new laws.

State gun-control laws exhibit wide disparity. California bans the selling of assault weapons. Texas and Kansas do not require gun dealers to apply for gun licenses. Missouri and Idaho hardly regulate gun purchases. After the Sandy Hook shooting, some states pursued more restrictive gun laws and other states proposed expanding gun rights to arm law-abiding citizens, including allowing students to carry concealed guns on college campuses and arming teachers. Personal preferences and regional partisan politics have thwarted federal attempts to confront the patchwork of state laws.

Some health professionals have called for a broader public health perspective, saying that the causes of gun violence are sociocultural, educational, behavioral, and product safety issues that transcend gun ownership rights. A comprehensive, multidimensional strategy can be designed based on the successful campaigns that targeted smoking, unintentional poisonings, and motor vehicle deaths. For example, a substantial new tax on firearms could provide an endowment to benefit those harmed by gun violence, to fund campaigns to increase gun safety, and to assist in the identification of high-risk individuals. Decreasing depictions of gun violence in movies, television programs and video games may help protect children from permissive gun violence. Product changes to promote gun safety are also needed. The priority is reducing gun violence and not compromising Second Amendments rights for gun owners. This distinction, which emphasizes sensible safety policies, may not succumb to regional partisan politics.

Sources: "Curing Gun Violence: Lesson From Public Health Successes," by D. Mozaffarian, D. Hemenway, and D. Ludwig, 2013, *Journal of the American Medical Association, 309* (6), pp. 551–552; "A Systematic Plan for Firearms Law Reform," by K. L. Record and L. O. Gostlin, 2013, *Journal of the American Medical Association, 309* (12), pp. 1231–1232; "Search for Ways to Reduce Gun Violence Spurred by Toll of Recent Shootings," by M. Mitka, 2013, *Journal of the American Medical Association. 309* (8), pp. 755–756.

are expected to proliferate. There is nothing illegal about making guns at home as long as they do not violate the 2003 Undetectable Firearms Act. High-powered weapons, such as machine guns, and those that are not detectable by airport scanners are not legal.

The Trayvon Martin shooting in Florida has raised questions about state "stand your ground" laws, which are self-protection rather than gun laws. Most state self-protection laws have three components: (1) law-abiding residents may employ defensive force, including deadly force, if someone breaks into their residence or occupied vehicle; (2) if attacked, people may use deadly force to prevent death or great bodily harm to themselves; and (3) if the defensive force is permitted by law, the person using it is immune from civil or criminal action. Opponents to state self-protection laws have labeled them as "shoot first" laws. Stand your ground laws are likely to be extensively challenged in judicial proceedings.

The use of guns in suicides is a serious public health problem. Handguns are the most common means of suicide, and suicides using guns are fatal 85 percent of the time. Each year, more than 38,000 Americans commit suicide, and there are 1,000 to 1,500 murder-suicides per year. Most of these suicides are associated with mental illness. Suicide rates are particularly increasing for middle-aged Americans. Although guns are used in more than half of suicides, health experts are divided on whether stricter gun control would decrease the number of suicides.[74]

The Role of Media and Entertainment: Glorifying Violence Violent acts occur much more frequently in movies and television shows than they do in real life.[75] Repeated exposure to violence may also lead to habituation and **desensitization**, a raised threshold for reaction to violence and a loss of compassion. Repeated exposure to graphic images of violence also feeds the appetite for more intense violence.[75]

The American Academy of Pediatrics and five other prominent medical groups concluded in 2000 that there is a connection between violence in mass media and increases in both acceptance of aggressive attitudes and aggressive behavior in children. The entertainment industry maintains that these studies demonstrate only possible associations between media violence and aggression. Media defenders warn that attempts at regulation would border on censorship.

In response to this information, communities have organized boycotts of products of companies

desensitization
Raised threshold of reaction to violence and a loss of compassion.

that sponsor violent and sexually explicit programs. Parents can use blocking technologies to keep their children from seeing selected television programs and Internet sites. The entertainment industry also regulates itself, primarily to avoid government regulation.[75] The National Association of Theater Owners, for example, has promised to enforce the movie ratings system vigorously.

The Role of Communities and Campuses: Promoting Safety   Common sense suggests that safe physical environments are less conducive to criminal activity than are rundown environments. Communities where neighbors look out for one another, as with neighborhood watch programs, are less inviting to criminals. Communities also have to support social changes that enhance economic and social stability.[76] To bring about change, communities have used strategies such as cleaning up trash and graffiti and fixing broken windows, providing organized leisure activities and mentoring programs for youth, encouraging parent involvement in school activities, supporting low-income housing to curb an exodus of middle-income residents of all races, and increasing police presence in high-risk areas.[77,78] Some large cities like New York City and Philadelphia are using a practice called "stop and frisk" to confront violence and crime. This practice is being challenged as a violation of privacy rights under the Fourth Amendment, but city officials are vigorously defending stop and frisk as an effective law enforcement practice; see the box, "Should Stop-and-Frisk Laws Be Legal?"

College campuses have an important role to play in the prevention of violence, especially sexual violence. Prevention efforts in this area are undergoing major changes on many college campuses, which are moving away from awareness programs to broad community-based strategies that target the underlying issues surrounding sexual violence.[78] The organization Men Can Stop Rape sponsors a Campus Strength Program that helps students develop and support healthy masculinity and consider the ways men can be allies of women. The Mentors in Violence Prevention Program

takes a "bystander approach" to violence prevention in communities and schools, like that of Green Dot discussed earlier in the chapter. In this model, men are not viewed as potential perpetrators and women are not viewed as potential victims; the focus is on both as bystanders who can confront abusive peers and support abused peers. The American College Health Association has developed a sexual assault prevention toolkit that promotes gender equality, healthy relationships, healthy sexuality, and civility on campus.

Individuals who want to take action against violence have a variety of options, from volunteering at women's shelters to supporting public policies that address the root causes of violence in our society. Keeping a sense of perspective about violence is important, however. Some observers have suggested that Americans live in a media-driven "culture of fear," frightened by overblown accounts of crime, drugs, and violence.[79] The key is to take media portrayals of violence with a grain of salt while using your common sense to keep yourself safe.

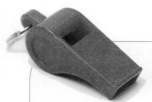

You Make the Call

Should Stop-and-Frisk Laws Be Legal?

Racial profiling is defined as the consideration of race, ethnicity, or national origin by an officer deciding when and how to intervene in an enforcement action. It profiles certain types of individuals who are more likely to perpetrate a crime. Law enforcement justifies profiling as an essential strategy to prevent criminal activity. Racial profiling becomes controversial when officers stop, question, and search African Americans, Hispanic Americans, and other racial minorities disproportionately based solely on their race and ethnicity. The issue is whether the profiling is based on stereotypes or reasonable suspicion. If based on stereotypes, racial profiling is seen as discrimination and a violation of a citizen's Fourth Amendment rights.

New York's stop-and-frisk program is a profiling strategy that was ruled unconstitutional in 2013 by a federal district judge. This decision has caused tension as to liberty versus

Continued...

Concluded...

public safety. New York's stop-and-frisk program is based on the 1968 Supreme Court decision in *Terry v. Ohio* that allowed law enforcement to detain a person based on "reasonable suspicion" that he or she might be about to commit a crime. Prior to the *Terry* decision, police officers had to use "probable cause" to stop, question, and search someone, which required a greater deal of certainty than reasonable suspicion. Legal justifications for a stop include appearing not to fit the time or place, matching the description on a "wanted" flyer, acting strangely or aggressively, loitering, running away or engaging in furtive movements, and being present in a crime scene area (particularly a high-crime area).

A frisk is invasive because it requires contact by the officer with the suspect, so it is used only to detect concealed weapons or contraband. If evidence can be felt under the suspect's clothing, the evidence can be seized by the officer, referred to as the "plain feel" doctrine. Legal justifications for a frisk include concerns for the safety of the officer and others, suspicion the suspect is armed and dangerous, suspicion the suspect is about to commit a crime in which a weapon is commonly used, the officer is alone and backup has not arrived, the number of suspects and their physical size, the behavior and emotional state of the suspect(s), evasive answers by the suspect to an officer's questions, and time of day and location.

Does the stop-and-frisk program go too far?

Crime rates in the United States have declined since the early 1990s. Criminologists have not been able to definitively explain why crime has decreased. Their theories include changing demographics, "hot-spot" policing strategies in crime-prone areas, life-saving medical practices, and eliminating low-income high rises. Law enforcement and public officials in New York, however, believe the answer is the use of "Terry stops," which established a lower threshold for legally searching citizens for weapons or contraband. But "Terry stops" are not legal if used to disproportionately discriminate by race, ethnicity, or national origin. The federal district judge ruled that New York City was deliberately indifferent to police officers illegally targeting minority residents,

although she did not strike down New York's stop-and-frisk tool for law enforcement. The judge required the tool be revised to not discriminate against minorities. New York public officials refused to do so and the judge then appointed an outside monitor to oversee sweeping changes in stop-and-frisk. New York public officials continue to argue that stop-and-frisk is legal and justified because minorities commit more crimes; African Americans, for example, make up 13.6 percent of the U.S. population but commit 40.2 percent of all crime. The district judge emphasized that this logic was flawed because the people stopped were overwhelmingly innocent and not criminals. The city appealed her ruling, but a new mayor came to office in January 2014 and, unlike his predecessor, agreed to the judge's reforms.

So, what do you think? Is stop-and-frisk a viable tool used by police to prevent crime? Or is it another example of racial profiling that violates the Fourth Amendment rights of citizens?

Pro

- African Americans and Hispanics account for a significantly disproportionate amount of crime.
- Stop-and-frisk reduces crime by scaring criminals into thinking they may be stopped and frisked at any time.
- When used appropriately, the stop-and-frisk tool benefits all citizens of race, ethnicity and national origin.
- There are fewer legal requirements for security personnel's "pat-down" searches at airports than for police departments, so why should police departments be singled out?

Cons

- White serial child molesters and rapists are less likely to be stopped than people of color.
- Stop-and-frisk is used by police departments to meet unwritten quotas that reward officers with promotions.
- Tools that promote illegal stops and searches alienate the police department from the community it serves.
- Stop-and-frisk is a form of racial profiling that continues to be a prevalent and egregious form of discrimination.

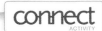

Sources: When the Police Stop and Frisk You on the Street, *Legal Zoom,* www.legalzoom.com/us-law/privacy/when-can-police-stop; "Is 'Stop and Frisk' Legal?" by J. Reynolds, http://lawenforcementtoday.com./2013/07/28/is-%80%9cstop-and-frisk%e2%80%9d-1; "Racial Profiling," *Encyclopedia.com,* www.encyclopedia/com/topic/Racial_Profiling.aspz; "Mayor Says City Will Settle Suits on Stop-and-Frisk Tactics," by B. Weiser and J. Goldstein, January 30, 2014, *New York Times,* http://www.nytimes.com/2014/01/31/nyregion/de-blasio-stop-and-frisk.html?_r=0.

In Review

How does injury affect personal health?

Unintentional injuries are the fifth leading cause of death in the United States and the leading cause of death for children and adults aged 1 to 39. Public health experts believe that injuries are preventable if people adopt behaviors that promote safety and if society takes steps to reduce environmental hazards.

What are the leading causes of injury-related death?

The top cause for all age groups is motor vehicle crashes, followed by falls, poisoning, choking, and drowning. Common

causes vary by age and race/ethnicity, but males are more likely than females to die from unintentional injuries across all groups until age 80.

How does violence affect personal health?

Many people, especially members of minority groups, are the victims of violence and of violent crimes, which include homicide, assault, robbery, and rape. Compared with other developed countries, the United States has higher rates of homicide, especially homicide committed with a firearm.

What forms does violence take in our society?

Males between the ages of 14 and 24 are the most like to commit acts of violence. Crimes on college campuses include assaults, rapes, and very rare but high-profile mass shootings. Sexual violence includes sexual assault and rape, child sexual abuse, sexual harassment, and stalking and cyberstalking. Family violence includes child and elder abuse, intimate partner violence, and dating violence. Violence against strangers often takes the form of hate crimes or terrorism, which is intended to create fear and helplessness in the general public.

What are strategies to prevent violence?

Individuals can learn how to reduce their risk of encountering violence, and they can work to create safer communities and campuses and to prevent violence in society. Some public health professionals advocate reducing gun violence through a multidimensional strategy like the campaigns against smoking and drunk driving. The public can oppose the glorification of violence in the media through boycotts and monitoring what their children are watching. Communities can support neighborhood watch programs and upkeep of common areas. Many types of violence-prevention programs can be used on college campuses.

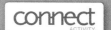
Are you wondering how you are doing in regard to your overall health and well-being? This is the first of a series of self-assessment activities that are included in this text. Your Personal Health Portfolio, the final product of all activities, will be a collection of documents that explore your strengths and challenges. It will represent a snapshot of your health and self-reflections throughout the course.

This first portfolio activity is centered on an adaptation of a well-studied assessment tool (the Rand Corporation's Short Form 36) that will help you take a general look at components of your physical and mental health.

Read each question carefully and circle the point value corresponding to your answer.

PHYSICAL FUNCTIONING

The following items are about activities you might do during a typical day. Does your health now limit you in these activities? If so, how much?

	Yes, limited a lot	Yes, limited a little	No, not limited at all
1. Vigorous activities, such as running, lifting heavy objects, participating in strenuous sports	0	50	100
2. Moderate activities, such as moving a table, pushing a vacuum cleaner, bowling, or playing golf	0	50	100
3. Lifting or carrying groceries	0	50	100
4. Climbing several flights of stairs	0	50	100
5. Climbing one flight of stairs	0	50	100
6. Bending, kneeling, or stooping	0	50	100
7. Walking more than a mile	0	50	100
8. Walking several blocks	0	50	100
9. Walking one block	0	50	100

LIMITATIONS DUE TO PHYSICAL HEALTH

During the past month, have you had any of the following problems with your work or other regular daily activities as a result of your physical health?

	Yes	No
1. Cut down the amount of time you spent on work or other activities	0	100
2. Accomplished less than you would like	0	100
3. Were limited in the kind of work or other activities you did	0	100
4. Had difficulty performing work or other activities (e.g., it took extra effort)	0	100

LIMITATIONS DUE TO EMOTIONAL PROBLEMS

During the past month, have you had any of the following problems with your work or other regular daily activities as a result of any emotional problems (such as feeling depressed or anxious)?

	Yes	No
1. Cut down the amount of time you spent on work or other activities	0	100
2. Accomplished less than you would like	0	100
3. Didn't do work or other activities as carefully as usual	0	100

ENERGY/FATIGUE

These questions are about how you feel and how things have been going for you during the past month. For each question, give the one answer that comes closest to the way you have been feeling. How much of the time during the past month . . .

	All of the time	Most of the time	A good bit of the time	Some of the time	A little of the time	None of the time
1. Did you feel full of pep?	100	80	60	40	20	0
2. Did you have a lot of energy?	100	80	60	40	20	0
3. Did you feel worn out?	0	20	40	60	80	100
4. Did you feel tired?	0	20	40	60	80	100

EMOTIONAL WELL-BEING

These questions are about how you feel and how things have been going for you during the past month. For each question, give the one answer that comes closest to the way you have been feeling. How much of the time during the past month . . .

	All of the time	Most of the time	A good bit of the time	Some of the time	A little of the time	None of the time
1. Have you been a very nervous person?	0	20	40	60	80	100
2. Have you felt so down in the dumps that nothing could cheer you up?	0	20	40	60	80	100
3. Have you felt calm and peaceful?	100	80	60	40	20	0
4. Have you felt downhearted and blue?	0	20	40	60	80	100
5. Have you been a happy person?	100	80	60	40	20	0

SOCIAL FUNCTIONING

1. During the past month, to what extent has your physical health or emotional problems interfered with your normal social activities with family, friends, neighbors, or groups? (Circle one number.)

Not at all	100
Slightly	75
Moderately	50
Quite a bit	25
Extremely	0

2. During the past month, how much of the time has your physical health or emotional problems interfered with your social activities (like visiting with friends, relatives, etc.)? (Circle one number.)

All of the time	0
Most of the time	25
Some of the time	50
A little of the time	75
None of the time	100

PAIN

1. How much bodily pain have you had during the past month? (Circle one number.)

None	100
Very mild	80
Mild	60
Moderate	40
Severe	20
Very severe	0

2. During the past month, how much did pain interfere with your normal work (including both work outside the home and housework)? (Circle one number.)

Not at all	100
A little bit	75
Moderately	50
Quite a bit	25
Extremely	0

GENERAL HEALTH

1. In general, you would say your health is

Excellent	100
Very good	75
Good	50
Fair	25
Poor	0

How TRUE or FALSE is *each* of the following statements for you?

	Definitely true	Mostly true	Don't know	Mostly false	Definitely false
2. I seem to get sick a little easier than other people.	0	25	50	75	100
3. I am as healthy as anybody I know.	100	75	50	25	0
4. I expect my health to get worse.	0	25	50	75	100
5. My health is excellent.	100	75	50	25	0

SCORING

Add up your scores from each section and divide by the number of questions in the section to obtain an average score. The highest possible score in each section is 100.

PHYSICAL FUNCTIONING

____ + ____ + ____ + ____ + ____ + ____ + ____ + ____ + ____ = ____ ÷ 9 = ____
  1   2   3   4   5   6   7   8   9   raw score   average

LIMITATIONS DUE TO PHYSICAL HEALTH

____ + ____ + ____ + ____ = ____ ÷ 4 = ____
  1   2   3   4   raw score   average

LIMITATIONS DUE TO EMOTIONAL PROBLEMS

____ + ____ + ____ = ____ ÷ 3 = ____
  1   2   3   raw score   average

ENERGY/FATIGUE

____ + ____ + ____ + ____ = ____ ÷ 4 = ____
  1   2   3   4   raw score   average

EMOTIONAL WELL-BEING

____ + ____ + ____ + ____ + ____ = ____ ÷ 5 = ____
  1   2   3   4   5   raw score   average

SOCIAL FUNCTIONING

____ + ____ = ____ ÷ 2 = ____
  1   2   raw score   average

PAIN

____ + ____ = ____ ÷ 2 = ____
  1   2   raw score   average

GENERAL HEALTH

____ + ____ + ____ + ____ + ____ = ____ ÷ 5 = ____
  1   2   3   4   5   raw score   average

Your scores can be interpreted in the following manner. Mark an X where your score falls on the continuum for each section. Recognize that the behaviors exist on a continuum with low scores indicating areas of concern and higher scores indicating healthier behaviors/feelings.

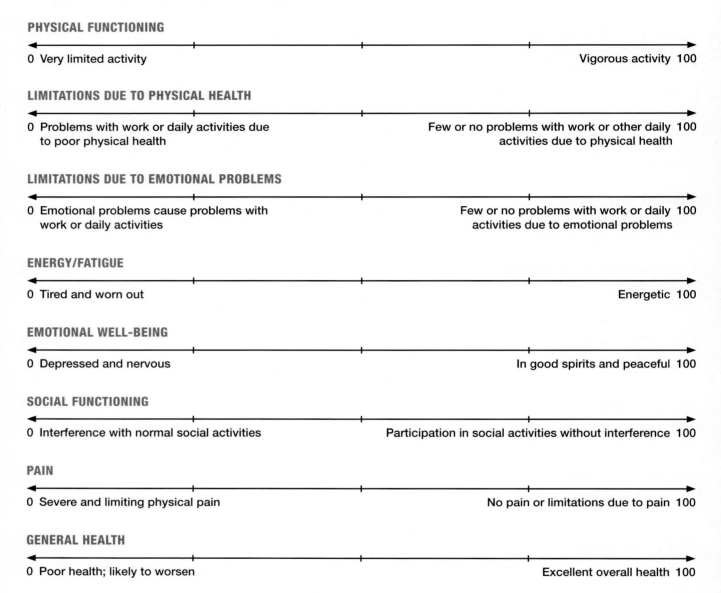

PHYSICAL FUNCTIONING

0 Very limited activity   Vigorous activity 100

LIMITATIONS DUE TO PHYSICAL HEALTH

0 Problems with work or daily activities due   Few or no problems with work or other daily 100
   to poor physical health   activities due to physical health

LIMITATIONS DUE TO EMOTIONAL PROBLEMS

0 Emotional problems cause problems with   Few or no problems with work or daily 100
   work or daily activities   activities due to emotional problems

ENERGY/FATIGUE

0 Tired and worn out   Energetic 100

EMOTIONAL WELL-BEING

0 Depressed and nervous   In good spirits and peaceful 100

SOCIAL FUNCTIONING

0 Interference with normal social activities   Participation in social activities without interference 100

PAIN

0 Severe and limiting physical pain   No pain or limitations due to pain 100

GENERAL HEALTH

0 Poor health; likely to worsen   Excellent overall health 100

Source: Adapted from the 36-Item Short Form Health Survey developed from the Medical Outcomes Study. Copyright © the RAND Corporation. RAND's permission to reproduce the survey is not an endorsement of the products, services, or other uses in which the survey appears or is applied.

CRITICAL THINKING QUESTIONS

1. Look over your total scores. In what areas do you have high scores—reflecting healthier behaviors and feeling? In what areas do you have lower scores—reflecting possible areas of concern?

2. In areas of higher scores, what helps you maintain healthy behaviors? Consider your personal knowledge about what it means to be healthy and your attitudes and beliefs. Then consider factors in your environment that support healthy patterns—consider how you are supported by friends and family, your school community and living situation, institutions to which you belong, and local or national policies.

3. In areas of lower scores, what are some of the barriers that make improvement difficult for you? As with your strengths, consider each level in the ecological model of health.

4. Finally, consider if there are areas in which you would like to make changes. What would these changes look like? How ready are you to make changes? What steps would you take to start the change process? If you are ready, complete a behavior change contract (see next activity).

This general quality of life assessment is a starting point for exploring your health. In areas where your scores are at the lower or higher end of the continuum, you may already have a sense of what factors contribute to your concerns or strengths. As you continue through each chapter, you will be asked to complete portfolio activities that will help you explore in greater detail factors that influence your general health and well-being. Keep this portfolio activity in mind. Come back and revisit it throughout the term. See if you think differently about various factors in your life as you learn more.

Personal Health Portfolio

Chapter 1
Behavior Change Contract

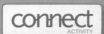

Behavior I want to change: _____

My goal: _____

_____

Remember that your goal should be SMART: specific, measurable, attainable, realistic, and time-bound.

I will achieve my goal by _____ .
                                date

Along the way, I will create a series of smaller, incremental goals to help me reach my overall goal:

Incremental goal 1: _____ Target date: _____

Incremental goal 2: _____ Target date: _____

Incremental goal 3: _____ Target date: _____

Benefits associated with this behavior change:

- _____
- _____
- _____

Barriers I expect to encounter:

- _____
- _____
- _____

Strategies for overcoming these barriers:

- _____
- _____
- _____

Signature: _____ Date: _____

Witness signature: _____ Date: _____

1. How important is this change to you?

  not very important   **very important**

2. How confident are you that you can make this change?

  not confident   **very confident**

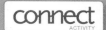
A family health tree is a diagram of your family's health history over several generations. As such, it can provide important clues to the genes you have inherited from your parents, grandparents, and ancestors. Constructing a family health tree has three broad steps: (1) mapping the family structure, (2) recording family information, and (3) finding family relationships. Refer to the model provided in Figure 1.7 as you construct your own family health tree. You can use the template provided on the next page, or create one online at www.hhs.gov/familyhistory (which can be printed).

1. Begin with yourself and your immediate family. Then add your cousins, your aunts and uncles, your grandparents, and as many other relatives as you can. The more generations and individuals you include, the more useful your tree will be.

2. When placing children beneath their parents, begin with the oldest on the left. Connect adopted or foster children to their parents with a dotted line to indicate that no biological relationship exists.

3. If a person is deceased, draw an X in the square and write his or her date of death (or age at death) and the cause of death. If a woman has had a miscarriage or stillbirth, indicate that with an X in the square of the deceased child. Because some genetic conditions are more common in certain ethnic groups, include the ethnicity of each person in the oldest generation you include.

4. Now add as much health-related information as you know for each person. Include major diseases or health conditions, such as diabetes, osteoporosis, cancer, heart disease, and so on, and person's age when diagnosed. Also include surgeries, allergies, mental health problems, and any genetic or chromosomal disorders, such as Down syndrome.

5. Once you have gathered all the information, analyze your family health tree by completing the Critical Thinking Questions. You may want to take your family health tree to your physician or a genetic counselor for a professional opinion on your health risks. He or she may recommend that you modify certain lifestyle behaviors (such as diet or exercise) or have particular screening tests (such as an early test for cancer). You may want to have your physician keep a copy of your family health tree in your medical file for future reference. You may also want to share what you have found out, as well as your physician's recommendations, with your siblings and other family members.

CRITICAL THINKING QUESTIONS

1. What are your family's strengths? Consider such things as longevity, fitness, mental well-being, etc.

2. What are the patterns of disease or illness in your family? Are there certain diseases that appear frequently? Does the pattern suggest a possible genetic link? What lifestyle factors may have contributed to illness in your family? How might the environments in which your relatives lived have contributed to illness?

My Family Health Portrait

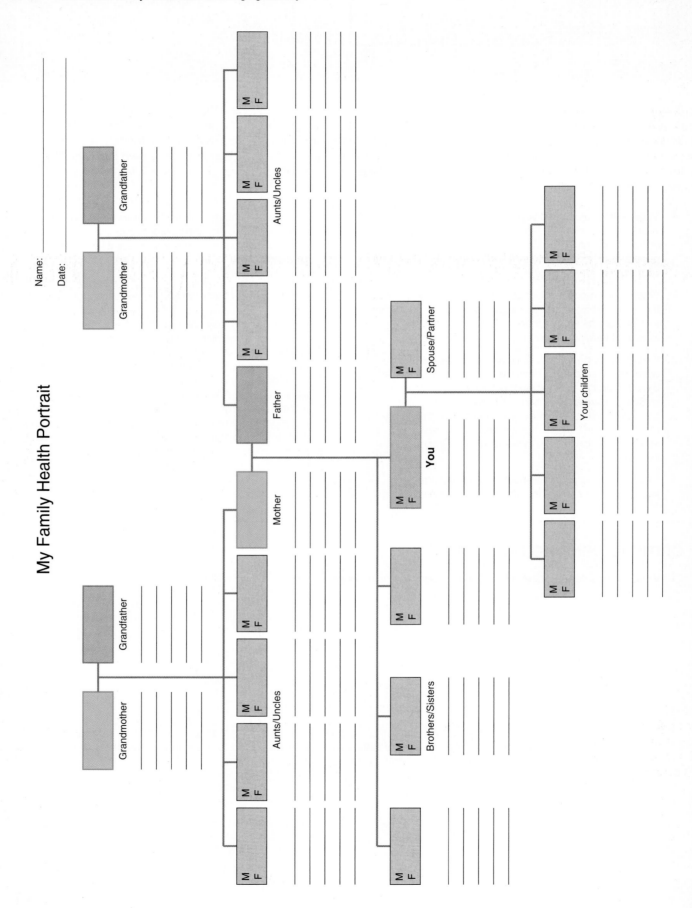

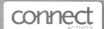
Resilience is described as the ability to regain equilibrium or recover when faced with adversity. Individuals who are resilient are often more self-confident, recognizing their strengths and abilities. For those people whose resilience is low, failures and setbacks are a drain on their energy and motivation, and they are more prone to depression and other mental disorders. Resilience is also important in dealing with stress. Resilient people have the perseverance to deal with stressors in positive ways and rebound more quickly after stressful events.

Take some time and complete the Resilience Scale to gain a better understanding of your ability to respond during times of adversity. Circle the number to the right of each statement that best reflects your feelings. If you are neutral or undecided on a particular item, select 4.

		Strongly disagree				Strongly agree		
1. When I make plans, I follow through with them.	1	2	3	4	5	6	7
2. I usually manage one way or another.	1	2	3	4	5	6	7
3. I am able to depend on myself more than anyone else.	1	2	3	4	5	6	7
4. Keeping interested in things is important to me.	1	2	3	4	5	6	7
5. I can be on my own if I have to.	1	2	3	4	5	6	7
6. I feel proud that I have accomplished things in life.	1	2	3	4	5	6	7
7. I usually take things in stride.	1	2	3	4	5	6	7
8. I am friends with myself.	1	2	3	4	5	6	7
9. I feel that I can handle many things at a time.	1	2	3	4	5	6	7
10. I am determined.	1	2	3	4	5	6	7
11. I seldom wonder what the point of it all is.	1	2	3	4	5	6	7
12. I take things one day at a time.	1	2	3	4	5	6	7
13. I can get through difficult times because I've experienced difficulty before.	1	2	3	4	5	6	7
14. I have self-discipline.	1	2	3	4	5	6	7
15. I keep interested in things.	1	2	3	4	5	6	7
16. I can usually find something to laugh about.	1	2	3	4	5	6	7
17. My belief in myself gets me through hard times.	1	2	3	4	5	6	7
18. In an emergency, I'm someone people can generally rely on.	1	2	3	4	5	6	7
19. I can usually look at a situation in a number of ways.	1	2	3	4	5	6	7
20. Sometimes I make myself do things whether I want to or not.	1	2	3	4	5	6	7
21. My life has meaning.	1	2	3	4	5	6	7
22. I do not dwell on things that I can't do anything about.	1	2	3	4	5	6	7
23. When I'm in a difficult situation, I can usually find my way out of it.	1	2	3	4	5	6	7
24. I have enough energy to do what I have to do.	1	2	3	4	5	6	7
25. It's okay if there are people who don't like me.	1	2	3	4	5	6	7

SCORING

Add up your numbers for each question. Your score will be between 25 and 175.

Score: _____

146 or more: Your score indicates moderately high/high levels of resilience. You are optimistic and see your life as having purpose. Although you have had your share of rough times, you are confident that you can handle future obstacles.

126–145: Your score indicates moderately low/moderate resilience. You have many characteristics of resilience, but you may not be satisfied with all areas of your life. You can move forward with your life, but without enthusiasm. Work to strengthen your resilience and you will have an easier time dealing with the ups and downs of life.

125 or below: Your score indicates low resilience. You may be going through some hard times right now and lack confidence about your ability to get through them. Although your score is on the low end, that doesn't mean you don't have any resilience. If you work to strengthen it, you will make a positive change in your life.

The first critical step in taking the scale is self-awareness. You can then assess how you might want to build on strengths and work on areas of weakness.

Source: The Resilience Scale, by Gail Wagnild and Heather M. Young. © 2009. Used by permission. Scoring adapted from *The Resilience Scale User's Guide,* by Gail M. Wagnild and Heather M. Young. 2009. The Resilience Center, P.O. Box 313, Worden, Montana 59088.

CRITICAL THINKING QUESTIONS

1. Analyze your score. Was it higher or lower than you expected? What areas of strength or weakness do you see?

2. It has been suggested that when you face adversity and find a way to recover you actually gain confidence for the next time you face a very difficult situation. Think back to your own adolescence. Was it easy? Or did you face issues related to building friendships, becoming comfortable with your body, or participating in sexual activity? How have your past experiences contributed to your resilience today?

3. What people or circumstances have influenced your resilience? Consider your parents, other family members, and friends and the community in which you were raised. Describe your social support network and other factors that might contribute to your bouncing back (being resilient) when facing adversity.

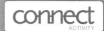
One important aspect of well-being is your perceived meaning in life. Do you believe you have a meaningful life? Are you interested in personal growth and developing your own values?

Researchers believe that there is a relationship between finding meaning in life and a person's well-being. As you search to uncover the meaning in your life, the first step in the process is increasing your self-awareness about your sense of meaning and purpose.

There are two subscales in the questionnaire. The first, Presence of Meaning, measures how meaningful people perceive their life to be. The second, Search for Meaning, measures how actively people are seeking to discover or augment the level of meaningfulness they experience in life.

PRESENCE OF MEANING

	Absolutely untrue			Can't say true or false			Absolutely true	
1. I understand my life's meaning.	1	2	3	4	5	6	7
2. My life has a clear sense of purpose.	1	2	3	4	5	6	7
3. I have a good sense of what makes my life meaningful.	1	2	3	4	5	6	7
4. I have discovered a satisfying life purpose.	1	2	3	4	5	6	7
5. My life has no clear purpose.	7	6	5	4	3	2	1

SEARCH FOR MEANING

	Absolutely untrue			Can't say true or false			Absolutely true	
1. I am looking for something that makes my life feel meaningful.	1	2	3	4	5	6	7
2. I am always looking to find my life's purpose.	1	2	3	4	5	6	7
3. I am always searching for something that makes my life feel significant.	1	2	3	4	5	6	7
4. I am seeking a purpose or mission for my life.	1	2	3	4	5	6	7
5. I am searching for meaning in my life.	1	2	3	4	5	6	7

SCORING

Add up your numbers for each section. Scores will range from 5 to 35.

Presence of Meaning score: _____

Search for Meaning score: _____

If you scored **above** 24 on Presence and also **above** 24 on Search, you feel your life has a valued meaning and purpose, yet you are still openly exploring that meaning or purpose. You likely are satisfied with your life, are somewhat optimistic, experience feelings of love frequently, and rarely feel depressed. You are probably somewhat active in spiritual activities, and you tend not to value pursuing sensory stimulation as much as others. You are generally certain of, and occasionally forceful regarding, your views and supportive of having an overall structure in society and life. People who know you would probably describe you as conscientious, thoughtful, easy to get along with, somewhat open to new experiences, and generally easygoing and emotionally stable.

If you scored **above** 24 on Presence and **below** 24 on Search, you feel your life has a valued meaning and purpose, and you are not actively exploring that meaning or seeking meaning in your life. One might say that you are satisfied that you've grasped what makes your life meaningful, why you're here, and what you want to do with your life. You probably are satisfied with your life, are optimistic, and have healthy self-esteem. You frequently experience feelings of love and joy and rarely feel afraid, angry, ashamed, or sad. You probably hold traditional values. You are usually certain of, and often forceful regarding, your views and likely support structure and rules for society and living. You are probably active in and committed to spiritual pursuits. People who know you would probably describe you as conscientious, organized, friendly, easy to get along with, and socially outgoing.

If you scored **below** 24 on Presence and **above** 24 on Search, you probably do not feel your life has a valued meaning and purpose, and you are actively searching for something or someone that will give your life meaning or purpose. You are probably not always satisfied with your life. You may not experience emotions like love and joy that often. You may occasionally, or even often, feel anxious, nervous, or sad and depressed. You are probably questioning the role of spirituality in your life, and you may be working hard to figure out whether there is a God, what life on Earth is really about, and which, if any, religion is right for you. People who know you would probably describe you as liking to play things by ear or "go with the flow" when it comes to plans, occasionally worried, and not particularly socially active.

If you scored **below** 24 on Presence and also **below** 24 on Search, you probably do not feel your life has a valued meaning and purpose and are not actively exploring that meaning or seeking meaning in your life. You may not always be satisfied with your life, or yourself, and you might not be particularly optimistic about the future. You may not experience emotions like love and joy that often. You may occasionally, or even often, feel anxious, nervous, or sad and depressed. You probably do not hold traditional values and may be more likely to value stimulating, exciting experiences, although you are not necessarily open-minded about everything. People who know you would probably describe you as sometimes disorganized, occasionally nervous or tense, and not particularly socially active or especially warm toward everyone.

Sources: Adapted from "The Meaning in Life Questionnaire: Assessing the presence of and search for meaning in life," by M. F. Steger, P. Frazier, S. Oishi, and M. Kaler, 2006, *Journal of Counseling Psychology, 53,* pp. 80–93; "Understanding the search for meaning in life: Personality, cognitive style, and the dynamic between seeking and experiencing meaning," by Michael F. Steger, Todd B. Kashdan, Brandon A. Sullivan, and Danielle Lorentz, April 2008, *Journal of Personality, 76,* pp. 197–227.

CRITICAL THINKING QUESTIONS

1. Analyze your scores for each scale. Were they higher or lower than you expected? What areas of strength do you see? Where is there room for growth?

2. Think about the environmental factors in your life, like your friends, family, school, and community. How do they affect your pursuit of meaning in life?

3. After having taken this assessment and considered the results, do you want to be able to find more meaning in your life? If so, what are some actions you can take to begin this process?

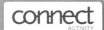
Part 1 Sleep Diary

A sleep diary can help identify habits that interfere with quality sleep. The diary can also be a source of valuable information if you need to consult a medical professional about sleep. Use the sleep diary on the following page to track your sleep for seven days. You may want to keep it close to your bed so that you will remember to fill it out before you go to sleep and when you awake.

Part 2 Do You Have Symptoms of a Sleep Disorder?

Ask yourself the following questions:

- Do you have trouble falling asleep three nights a week or more?
- Do you wake up frequently during the night?
- Do you wake up too early and find it difficult to get back to sleep?
- Do you wake up unrefreshed?
- Do you snore loudly?
- Are you aware of gasping for breath or not breathing while you are sleeping, or has anyone ever told you that you do this?
- Do you feel sleepy during the day or doze off watching TV, reading, driving, or engaging in daily activities, even though you get eight hours of sleep a night?
- Do you have nightmares?
- Do you feel unpleasant, tingling, creeping sensations in your legs while trying to sleep?

If you answer yes to any of these questions, it is possible that you are suffering from a sleep disorder. The first step to take is to make sure you have good sleep habits and practices, as described in Chapter 4. If you are doing everything you can to ensure a good night's sleep, consult your physician. He or she may refer you to a sleep disorder specialist.

Sources: Part 1: "Weekly Sleep Diary," Helpguide, www.helpguide.com. Part 2: Adapted from National Sleep Foundation, 2004, www.sleepfoundation.org.

CRITICAL THINKING QUESTIONS

1. Analyze your sleep over the week. What was the average number of hours you slept for the five weekday nights? What was the average number of hours you slept on the weekend? Discuss the factors (individual and environmental) that affected the duration or quality of your sleep. For example, perhaps you slept worse on the days you drank Pepsi after dinner, or perhaps you slept worse on the weekend because your neighbors had a noisy party. Conversely, perhaps you slept well because you didn't play video games before going to sleep or because your partner goes to sleep and wakes up at the same time you do.

2. In Part 2, did you answer yes to any of the questions? If so, do you think you need to see your doctor about your sleep quality?

3. Overall, do you think you are meeting your sleep needs? Why or why not? If you are not meeting your sleep needs, what are some things you can do to change this?

SLEEP DIARY

	Day 1 Date:	Day 2 Date:	Day 3 Date:	Day 4 Date:	Day 5 Date:	Day 6 Date:	Day 7 Date:
Daytime Activities & Pre-Sleep Ritual (Fill in each night before going to bed)							
Exercise What did you do? When? Total time?							
Naps When? Where? How long?							
Alcohol & Caffeine Types, amount and when							
Feelings Happiness, sadness, stress, anxiety; major cause							
Food & Drink (Dinner/snacks) What and when?							
Medications or Sleep Aids Types, amount and when							
Bedtime Routine Meditation/ Relaxation? How long?							
Bed Time							
Sleeping & Getting Back to Sleep (Fill in each morning)							
Wake-up Time							
Sleep Breaks Did you get up during the night? If so, what did you do?							
Quality of Sleep & Other Comments							
Total Sleep Hours							

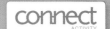
For this activity, you will use the USDA's online MyPlate SuperTracker, located at www.supertracker.usda.gov First, complete the free registration in order to use the site. Once you have your profile set up, you can use the "Food Tracker" tool to evaluate the quality of your diet.

Part 1

Complete the food log below, recording all the food you eat and drink in one full day. Make sure to include everything you drink—water, soft drinks (even diet), coffee, alcohol, and so on. List the foods you eat and drink and the serving size (1/2 apple, 2 cups of pasta, 24 oz. Diet Mountain Dew, etc.).

Day/Date: _____

Food/Drink item	Serving size/Amount

Part 2

Now enter the information from your food log in the "Food Tracker" section of the MyPlate SuperTracker (go to www.supertracker.usda.gov, complete the free registration, and click on "Food Tracker"). Also, use "My Top 5 Goals" as part of your portfolio report. Your report should identify diet areas that you meet and areas in which improvement is needed. You can also click on "My Reports" to view trends in your diet over time. Use these reports as part of your portfolio to see where you are meeting your goals and to identify diet areas that need improvement.

CRITICAL THINKING QUESTIONS

1. Analyze how well your food intake for the day matches up to your MyPlate recommendations. Did you meet your recommendations for milk, meat and beans, vegetables, fruits, and grains?

2. Now analyze your food intake in terms of calories, fat, fiber, sugar, sodium, and cholesterol (click on "Nutrient Intake Report" to get your average intake of nutrients). How did you do in nutrient intake? What nutrients did you get enough of? What nutrients do you need more of?

3. Based on your analysis in the first two questions, do you think you need to make any dietary changes? Why or why not? If you do need to make changes, what specific dietary modifications do you need to make and how can you realistically achieve them? Consider both behavioral and environmental strategies.

4. Consider how the ecological model of health and wellness (pages 3–4) relates to your own life. Describe the specific behavioral and environmental factors that make it easier or more difficult for you to reach your goals of eating healthfully.

You may want to analyze your diet for a few more days—or even longer—to get a better idea of how well your diet is meeting your nutritional needs. Make a note of your login for MyPlate SuperTracker as you will be using the site again for the Personal Health Portfolio activity in Chapter 6.

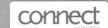
For this activity, you will use the USDA's online MyPlate SuperTracker, located at www.supertracker.usda.gov. You will need to complete the free registration in order to use the site, or log in with the user name and password you created in the Chapter 5 Portfolio activity. The physical activity tracker provides an online assessment tool that will help you evaluate your daily physical activity.

Part 1

Complete the activity log below, noting all your activity over a period of 24 hours, including time spent sleeping, watching TV, and so on.

Day/Date: _____

Activity	Duration

Part 2

Now enter the information from your activity log in the "Physical Activity Tracker" section of MyPlate SuperTracker [go to www.supertracker.usda.gov, complete the free registration (if you have not already done so), and click on the "Physical Activity Tracker"]. Search for and select the activities you recorded in your log, enter a duration for each, and check off the days on which you did each activity. Click the "Add" button. When you finish entering your activities, review your physical activity profile for the week on the right side of the screen. You can also click on "MyReports" at the top of the page to see if your weekly physical activities measure up to the Physical Activity Guidelines for Americans.

CRITICAL THINKING QUESTIONS

1. What is your weekly total for moderate intensity equivalent (MIE) minutes? Note that every minute of vigorous exercise counts as two minutes of moderate activity. Light activity and activity of less than 10 minutes in duration do not count as MIE minutes. Did you meet your weekly total for muscle-strengthening days?

2. As mentioned in Chapter 6, walking is an excellent lifestyle physical activity for health. Walking to public transportation, like the bus or the subway, can be an easy way to accumulate the weekly recommended amount of physical activity. How do you get to and from campus (and around your campus itself) and to your job if you have one? What factors affect how much you are or aren't able to incorporate walking into your daily activity? For example, perhaps you are taking this class online and thus don't have to leave the house to attend class. Or perhaps your part-time job as a dog walker means you walk for two hours five days a week.

3. If you did not meet the Physical Activity Guidelines for Americans, what are some things you can do to increase your daily physical activity?

4. Think about your neighborhood or community. Does it facilitate physical activity, or does it present barriers to physical activity? For example, can you and your neighbors walk to the local grocery store? Is there a park nearby where you can walk or play sports? If your community does not encourage physical activities, what needs to change?

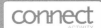
You can *estimate* your daily energy needs by (1) determining your basal metabolic rate (BMR) and (2) determining your energy expenditure above BMR from physical activity. Combining the two numbers gives you an estimate of your total energy requirement. This will require fine-tuning based on your body composition, metabolism, and activity and is intended as a start.

1. First, estimate your BMR, the minimum energy required to maintain your body's functions at rest. Begin by converting your weight in pounds to weight in kilograms. Then multiply by the BMR factor, which is estimated at 1.0 calorie/kg/hour for men and 0.9 for women. Then multiply by 24 hours to get your daily energy needs from BMR.

   • Let's look at Gary, a 30-year-old, 180-pound man.

$$\frac{180 \text{ lb}}{2.2 \text{ lb/kg}} = 82 \text{ kg}$$

   82 kg   1 calorie/kg/hour = 82 calories/hour

   82 calories/hour   24 hours/day = 1,968 calories/day

   Gary's BMR—the energy he uses every day just to stay alive—is 1,968 calories.

   • Now let's look at Lisa, a 24-year-old, 115-pound woman.

$$\frac{115 \text{ lb}}{2.2 \text{ lb/kg}} = 52 \text{ kg}$$

   52 kg   0.9 calorie/kg/hour = 47 calories/hour

   47 calories/hour   24 hours/day = 1,128 calories/day

   Lisa's BMR is 1,128 calories per day.

   • Now calculate your own BMR.

   Your weight in lbs _____ /2.2 lb/kg = _____ kg

   _____ kg   1 (men) = _____ calories/hour

   _____ kg   0.9 (women) = _____ calories/hour

   _____ calories/hour   24 hours/day = _____ calories/day

2. Next, estimate your voluntary muscle activity level. The following table gives approximations according to the amount of muscular work you typically perform in a day. To select the category appropriate for you, think in terms of muscle use, not just activity.

Lifestyle	BMR factor
Sedentary (mostly sitting)	0.4–0.5
Lightly active (such as a student)	0.55–0.65
Moderately active (such as a nurse)	0.65–0.7
Highly active (such as a bicycle messenger or an athlete)	0.75–1

A certain amount of honest guesswork is necessary. If you have a sedentary job but walk or bicycle to work every day, you could change your classification to lightly active (or even higher, depending on distance). If you have a moderately active job but spend all your leisure time on the couch, consider downgrading your classification to lightly active. Competitive athletes in training may actually need to increase the factor above 1.

   • Let's assume that Gary works in an office. He does walk around to talk to coworkers, go to the cafeteria for lunch, make photocopies, and do other everyday activities. We'll assess his lifestyle as sedentary but on the high side of activity for that category, say 0.5. To estimate Gary's energy expenditure above BMR, we multiply his BMR by this factor:

   1,968 calories/day   0.50 = 984 calories/day

   • Let's assume that Lisa works as a stock clerk in a computer store. She spends a lot of time walking around and sometimes lifts fairly heavy merchandise. She doesn't own a car and rides her bike several miles to and from work each day and also for many errands, so she's at the high end of moderately active, say 0.7. To estimate Lisa's energy expenditure above BMR, we multiply her BMR by this factor:

   1,128 calories/day   0.70 = 790 calories/day

Note that although Lisa is much more active than Gary, she uses less energy because of her lower body weight.

   • Now calculate your own estimated energy expenditure from physical activity.

   _____ calories/day   BMR factor _____
       = _____ calories/day

3. To find your total daily energy needs, add your BMR and your estimated energy expenditure.

   - For Gary, this is

     1,968 calories/day + 984 calories/day
     = 2,952 calories/day

   - For Lisa, it is

     1,128 calories/day + 790 calories/day
     = 1,918 calories/day

   Because several estimates are used in this method, total daily energy needs should be expressed as a 100-calorie range roughly centered on the final calculated value, which would be about 2,900–3,000 calories/day for Gary and about 1,870–1,970 calories/day for Lisa.

   - Now calculate your total daily energy needs.

     BMR calories/day _____
     + physical activity calories/day _____
     = _____ total calories/day

   Finally, compare your daily energy needs with your daily calorie intake. You may want to refer to question 2 from the Chapter 7 Portfolio activity, where you recorded your calorie intake for one day.

   Your daily energy needs: _____

   Your daily calorie intake: _____

Remember, if you want to lose weight, you need to take in less energy than you use up. You can shift the balance by increasing your activity level or decreasing your food intake. Moderate changes in both intake and activity level are the safest way to lose weight.

CRITICAL THINKING QUESTIONS

1. How do your calorie needs and calorie intake match up? Are you balancing your needs with your intake, or is one higher than the other? Do you need to make any changes to your calorie intake and/or your energy expenditure?

2. What factors influence how well you are able to balance your food intake and energy expenditure? Consider your taste in food and its cost and convenience. Also consider the factors that influence your ability to get daily physical activity, such as your available leisure time, your community's walkability and safety, availability of recreation areas, affordability of the campus gym or local gyms, etc.

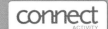
The goal of this activity is to help you think about your self-esteem and body image. Consider the following statements and then circle the response indicating how strongly you agree or disagree with each of them.

1. On the whole I am satisfied with myself.	Strongly agree	Agree	Neutral	Disagree	Strongly disagree
2. I have a number of good qualities.	Strongly agree	Agree	Neutral	Disagree	Strongly disagree
3. I am able to do things as well as most other people.	Strongly agree	Agree	Neutral	Disagree	Strongly disagree
4. I have done things I am proud of.	Strongly agree	Agree	Neutral	Disagree	Strongly disagree
5. I wish I had more respect for myself.	Strongly agree	Agree	Neutral	Disagree	Strongly disagree
6. I feel more in control when I restrict the food I eat.	Strongly agree	Agree	Neutral	Disagree	Strongly disagree
7. I consistently compare myself to others.	Strongly agree	Agree	Neutral	Disagree	Strongly disagree
8. I make sure to exercise if I have eaten too much.	Strongly agree	Agree	Neutral	Disagree	Strongly disagree
9. I would agree to cosmetic surgery if it were free.	Strongly agree	Agree	Neutral	Disagree	Strongly disagree
10. I am anxious about how people perceive or judge me.	Strongly agree	Agree	Neutral	Disagree	Strongly disagree
11. I eat to make myself feel better when I am sad, upset, or lonely.	Strongly agree	Agree	Neutral	Disagree	Strongly disagree
12. I often skip meals to lose weight.	Strongly agree	Agree	Neutral	Disagree	Strongly disagree

CRITICAL THINKING QUESTIONS

Consider your responses and answer the following questions.

1. Statements 1 through 5 relate to self-esteem. How do you think you do in regard to your self-esteem? What areas do you feel are your strengths? How are you supported in maintaining high self-esteem? Are you supported by family, friends, academics, sports, or other institutions?

2. In areas of lower self-esteem, what are some of the factors that make it difficult or contribute to feelings of self-doubt? Are there areas that you could strengthen or change? Are there ways that family, friends, or community could help you?

3. Statements 6 through 12 relate to body image. Your responses here are probably linked to your responses to the self-esteem statements. What areas appear to be your strengths? What factors support them?

4. Are there areas of concern for you in your body image responses? How might factors in your environment be contributing to these concerns? Is there anything you would like to change or could change in your environment to reduce the impact of these factors?

Note: This activity is not intended to diagnose eating disorders. The intent is to help you think about the factors discussed in the chapter and apply them to your life.

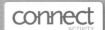
Drinking alcohol is not necessarily bad for you. What does matter is how much you drink and how it affects your life. This Portfolio activity will help you explore the place of alcohol in your life.

Part 1 Track Your Consumption

Recall as best you can your alcohol consumption during the past week (do not include today).

Date	Situation (people, place) or trigger (incident, feelings)	Type of drink(s)	Amount	Consequence (what happened?)

Now track your alcohol consumption for the next week, starting with today.

Date	Situation (people, place) or trigger (incident, feelings)	Type of drink(s)	Amount	Consequence (what happened?)

Part 2 Assess Your Consumption

Using the drink sizes from Figure 9.1 in your text or from www.rethinkingdrinking.niaaa.nih.gov, answer the following questions:

1. On any one day in the past two weeks, have you ever had

   Men: more than 4 drinks? Yes _____   No _____

   Women: more than 3 drinks? Yes _____   No _____

2. On average, how many days a week did you drink alcohol?

_____ Days

3. On average, how many drinks did you have over the past two weeks?

_____ Drinks

Source: Rethinking Drinking, National Institute on Alcohol Abuse and Alcoholism, 2009, NIH Publication No. 09-3770.

CRITICAL THINKING QUESTIONS

1. If you consume alcohol, are you a low-risk drinker or an at-risk drinker? Recall that low-risk drinking means no more than 14 drinks per week and no more than 4 drinks on any one day for men. For women, it means no more than 7 drinks per week and no more than 3 drinks on any one day. Drinks above these levels are considered at risk.

2. What were the situations and triggers that affected your decision to drink or not drink on various days? For example, if you ended up drinking more on one day than you had intended to, what led you to overindulge? If you did not drink at all during the two weeks, were you ever tempted to, or does your environment make the decision not to drink an easy one?

3. What are some reasons why you may want to make a change in your alcohol consumption? What are some of the barriers to making this change? How will you overcome these barriers?

4. What policies are in place at your campus to prevent or control excessive drinking? Are these policies effective?

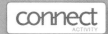
If you wonder whether you are becoming dependent on a drug, complete the following assessment. These questions refer to your use of drugs other than alcohol. Circle the letters of the answers which best describe your use of the drug(s) you use most. Even if none of the answers seems exactly right, pick the one(s) that come closest to being true. If a question does not apply to you, leave it blank.

1. How often do you use drugs?
   - (0) a. never
   - (2) b. once or twice a year
   - (3) c. once or twice a month
   - (4) d. every weekend
   - (5) e. several times a week
   - (6) f. every day
   - (7) g. several times a day

2. When did you last use drugs?
   - (0) a. never used drugs
   - (2) b. not for over a year
   - (3) c. between 6 months and 1 year ago
   - (4) d. several weeks ago
   - (5) e. last week
   - (6) f. yesterday
   - (7) g. today

3. I usually start to use drugs because:
   (Circle all that are true for you.)
   - (1) a. I like the feeling
   - (2) b. to be like my friends
   - (3) c. to feel like an adult
   - (4) d. I feel nervous, tense, full of worries or problems
   - (5) e. I feel sad, lonely, sorry for myself

4. How do you get your drugs?
   (Circle all that are true for you.)
   - (1) a. use at parties
   - (2) b. get from friends
   - (3) c. get from parents
   - (4) d. buy my own
   - e. other (please explain)

   _____

5. When did you first use drugs?
   - (0) a. never
   - (1) b. recently
   - (2) c. after age 15
   - (3) d. at ages 14 or 15
   - (4) e. between ages 10 and 13
   - (5) f. before age 10

6. What time of day do you use drugs?
   (Circle all that apply to you.)
   - (1) a. at night
   - (2) b. afternoons
   - (3) c. before or during school or work
   - (4) d. in the morning or when I first wake
   - (5) e. I often get up in my sleep to use drugs

7. Why did you first use drugs?
   (Circle all that apply to you.)
   - (1) a. curiosity
   - (2) b. parents or relatives offered
   - (3) c. friends encouraged me
   - (4) d. to feel more like an adult
   - (5) e. to get high

8. Who do you use drugs with?
   (Circle all that are true for you.)
   - (1) a. parents or relatives
   - (2) b. brothers or sisters
   - (3) c. friends own age
   - (4) d. older friends
   - (5) e. alone

9. What effects have you had from drugs?
   (Circle all that apply to you.)
   - (1) a. got high
   - (2) b. got wasted
   - (3) c. became ill
   - (4) d. passed out
   - (5) e. overdosed
   - (6) f. freaked out
   - (7) g. used a lot and next day didn't remember

10. What effect has using drugs had on your life?
    (Circle all that apply.)
    - (0) a. none
    - (2) b. has interfered with talking to someone
    - (3) c. has prevented me from having a good time
    - (4) d. has interfered with my schoolwork
    - (5) e. have lost friends because of drug use
    - (6) f. has gotten me into trouble at home
    - (7) g. was in a fight or destroyed property
    - (8) h. has resulted in an accident, an injury, arrest, or being punished at school for using drugs

11. How do you feel about your use of drugs?
    (Circle all that apply.)
    - (0) a. no problem at all
    - (0) b. I can control it and set limits on myself
    - (3) c. I can control myself, but my friends easily influence me
    - (4) d. I often feel bad about my drug use
    - (5) e. I need help to control myself
    - (6) f. I have had professional help to control my drug use

12. How do others see you in relation to your drug use?
    (Circle all that apply to you.)
    - (0) a. I can't say or no problem with drug use
    - (2) b. when I use drugs, I tend to neglect my family or friends
    - (3) c. my family or friends advise me to control or cut down on my drug use
    - (4) d. my family or friends tell me to get help for my drug use
    - (5) e. my family or friends have already gone for help for my drug use

Source: "The Adolescent Drug Involvement Scale," by D. P. Moberg and L. Hahn, 1991, *Journal of Adolescent Chemical Dependency 2*(1), pp. 75–88.

SCORING

Add up the point values of your responses. For questions where you circled multiple answers, add the highest point value of your answers.

Score: _____

The higher your score, the more serious your level of drug involvement is. Plot your score on the continuum below.

0 No dependence   Severe dependence 69

CRITICAL THINKING QUESTIONS

1. Reflect on your score. What do your responses indicate about your drug use?

2. Is there anything in your environment that makes it easy or difficult to control or limit your drug use?

3. In what direction are you moving on the continuum—toward increased dependence, toward decreased dependence, or holding steady? Do you need to make any changes to your substance use? If so, what?

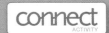
Good communication is vital to keeping your relationships healthy. However, bad communication habits—like avoiding discussing difficult subjects—are easy to fall into. This assessment will help you determine how well you are communicating with your partner. If you aren't currently in an intimate relationship, take this assessment with a close friendship in mind. Communication is important in all relationships—intimate or not.

Read each question and choose the response that reflects how you think or respond the majority of the time. Think about what you actually do or believe as opposed to what you "know" you should do or believe.

1. Do you believe that disagreements or arguments are
   a. harmful and negative for a relationship or
   b. helpful and positive for a relationship

2. Do you believe that your partner should
   a. know what you are thinking and feeling or
   b. hear what you are thinking and feeling

3. Do you
   a. drop hints about your concerns in the relationship or
   b. get right to the point when discussing a concern in the relationship

4. Do you tell your partner
   a. what you don't like about him or her and your relationship or
   b. what you like about him or her and your relationship

5. Do you
   a. withdraw from a conflict or conversation with your partner or
   b. stay around until there is a resolution of the conflict or conversation

6. Do you
   a. hint at what you want or don't want from your partner or
   b. state clearly what you want and don't want

7. Do you
   a. interrupt your partner's conversation or
   b. wait until your partner has finished stating his or her thoughts and ideas

8. Do you
   a. blame your partner or others for your relationship problems or
   b. acknowledge and accept your part in your relationship problems

9. Were your parents
   a. poor communicators or
   b. good communicators

Source: "Communication Assessment. How Well Do You Communicate? Nine Questions and Analysis," by Steven Martin and Catherine Martin, The Positive Way®, from www.positive-way.com/communication.htm.

Turn over the page to score your responses and view feedback for each question.

SCORING

The answer "b" to all questions indicates more effective communication. The more "b's" you have, the better you're doing. The "a's" indicate an opportunity to improve.

Here is why "b" is the better answer for each question:

1. Intimacy and conflict go hand in hand. If you want real intimacy with your mate, then there will be real conflict. People just don't agree on everything at all times. How you handle the resulting disagreements is more important than whether or not you have them. The most successful couples work through their disagreements and conflicts together and develop a stronger relationship as a result of that teamwork.

2. No one is a mind reader, and it is really impossible for your partner to know what you are thinking and feeling no matter how long you have known each other. It is important that you agree to *say* what is important and to *talk* until you both agree that you *understand*.

3. Dropping hints wastes your time and your partner's time, and it usually leads to misunderstanding and disappointment. Get right to the point so your partner won't have to guess what your concerns are in the relationship. State how you feel by using "I" statements instead of "you" statements.

4. Concentrating on what you like about your mate and your relationship will lead to a more positive relationship. If you concentrate on the things you don't like, it's easy to overlook the good things. Negativity breeds negativity, which then makes communication and problem solving more difficult. Use positive elements of the relationship as a foundation upon which to learn and grow.

5. Communication requires two people. Issues will remain unsettled unless you and your partner agree to communicate. We recommend that you agree to communicate with the guidelines of *understanding, kindness, honesty,* and *respect* as ground rules. These guidelines will serve to reduce tension and remind you both that you are on the same team. As a couple, agree to your own discussion rules, which can include such things as *time-outs* for cooling off or thinking.

6. Most of us don't pick up on hints, so don't expect your partner to guess what you do or don't want. Make clear and direct statements. Follow the guidelines of *understanding, kindness, honesty,* and *respect*. These guidelines make it easier to state your desires in a positive way and are more likely to be understood and well received.

7. Successful communication requires good listening. No one wants to be interrupted while speaking. We all want our feelings and thoughts to be heard, valued, and understood. Listen for understanding. Rephrase what you have heard your partner say, and then ask if this is correct. Save your side of the discussion until you have validated your partner's feelings. Validating your partner's feelings and thoughts is the key to success.

8. Blame fuels the fire of disagreement. Most of the time we believe that our position is acceptable and tend to blame the other person for any misunderstanding rather than seeing our own flaws in communicating. Analyze your part in fueling a problem, and avoid blaming others. Be responsible for your role in the relationship.

9. We tend to learn by example. If your parents were poor communicators, more than likely you have learned and now act out some ineffective ways of communicating. These habits may seem quite comfortable to you even if they are not working. It is up to you to learn new positive ways to communicate. Be persistent and practice until they become habit.

CRITICAL THINKING QUESTIONS

1. How did you do on the assessment? Discuss your strengths and any areas for improvement.

2. Think more about your parents' communication. Why did you respond the way you did to question 9? How did they handle conflict? Do you see yourself following any of their habits, good or bad?

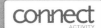
As you learned in Chapter 12, many contraception options are available to you. This activity will help you determine which contraceptive method best fits your needs. You may also want to discuss your options and decisions with your primary care physician, especially since many methods require a prescription.

Part 1 Your Partner's and Your Preferences

	Yes	No
1. I am sure I do not want children at this time.		
2. My partner and I are in a monogamous relationship with no concerns about sexually transmitted diseases.		
3. I want a method that I can control myself.		
4. My partner or I am good at remembering to take medication daily.		
5. My partner or I am willing to visit a physician or clinic to get birth control.		
6. My partner or I like sexual spontaneity and don't want to have to worry about contraception right before sex.		
7. Using birth control is not acceptable within my moral and/or religious belief system.		

Part 2 Your Sexual Behavior

	Yes	No
1. I sometimes have sex after using alcohol or drugs.		
2. I sometimes hook up with people I don't know well.		
3. I am in a relatively new relationship or have more than one partner.		
4. I have not discussed with my partner his/her prior sexual history or history of sexually transmitted diseases.		

Part 3 Risk Factors

Do any of the following apply to you (if you are a female) or your partner (if you are a male)?	Yes	No
1. Over age 35 and a smoker		
2. Liver disease, blood clots, breast cancer		
3. Personal history of migraine headaches		
4. Family history of blood clots, stroke, heart attack		

Interpretation

Part 1

Question 1. Yes responses: If you do not want children at any time in the future, permanent sterilization may be the best option. However, if your goal is to delay children for several years, you may want a reliable reversible contraceptive, such as an IUD or birth control pills.

Question 2. Yes responses: You do not need to use condoms or other barrier methods to provide STD protection. Hormonal methods are an option for you.

Question 3. Yes responses: If you are male, the male condom and vasectomy will allow you to take full responsibility for contraception. If you are female, tubal ligation, hormonal contraception, and barrier methods (excluding the male condom) will all allow you to take full responsibility for contraception.

Question 4. Yes responses: Birth control pills would be an effective option for you since they need to be taken daily. The vaginal ring and the transdermal patch, which must be changed every month, are other options.

Question 5. No responses: Contraceptive methods that can be purchased over the counter include male and female condoms and the contraceptive sponge.

Question 6. Yes responses: You may benefit from hormonal contraception such as an IUD or a contraceptive implant that does not require any action at the time of sex. However, if you are at risk for STDs, you will still need to use a barrier method like a condom, even if you would prefer not to.

Question 7. Yes responses: Your options are fertility awareness–based methods if you are sexually active or abstinence. Withdrawal may be another option, but keep in mind that many do not consider this to be a real contraceptive method.

Part 2

If you answered yes to the majority of questions in this section, condom use is an important part of your contraceptive needs. Hooking up and alcohol and drug use all increase the risk for sexually transmitted diseases. However, these behaviors also make it less likely that you will actually use a condom or other barrier method at the time of intercourse, so it is also recommended that women use a reliable contraceptive to prevent pregnancy that does not require action at the time of intercourse (like birth control pills or the vaginal ring).

Part 3

These factors increase the risk of side effects from hormonal contraceptives. If you answered yes to any of these questions, you and your partner may want to consider a barrier contraceptive or permanent contraception, depending on your future plans.

See the Consumer Clipboard box on page 262 for an overview of specific contraceptive methods.

CRITICAL THINKING QUESTIONS

1. Based on your responses, what type of contraception would be best for you? Are you using this method currently? Why or why not?

2. What factors in your environment influence your sexual decision making and contraception use? Consider your partner pattern and your social network.

3. Is there anything you would like to change in this area of your life? If so, consider making a behavior change plan and decide what your first steps would be.

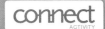
Vaccination, screening, and good hygiene habits are all ways to prevent the spread of infectious disease. Complete the following activity to see how well you are keeping yourself and others from contracting an infectious disease.

Part 1 Immunizations

Collect your immunization records. If you do not have a copy of your records, start by asking your parents or guardians. If they do not have records, check with your doctor. Your state health department may also have a program to track childhood vaccines. Record your immunizations in the table below.

Vaccine	Type of vaccination	Date	Location (doctor's office and doctor name, health clinic, etc.)
Tetanus, diphtheria, pertussis (TdaP)			
Human papillomavirus (HPV)			
Varicella			
Zoster			
Measles, mumps, rubella (MMR)			
Influenza			
Pneumococcal, polysaccharide			
Hepatitis A			
Hepatitis B			
Meningococcal			

Part 2 STD Risk

1. Are you sexually active?

   ☐ Yes   ☐ No

2. If yes, have you ever been tested for sexually transmitted diseases?

   ☐ Yes   ☐ No   ☐ N/A

3. Have you had a new partner since you were last tested?

   ☐ Yes   ☐ No   ☐ N/A

Part 3 Basic Hygiene Practices

1. Do you wash your hands with soap and warm water regularly before preparing food or eating, after using the toilet, and prior to touching your face?

   ☐ Most of the time   ☐ Sometimes   ☐ Rarely

2. Do you shower after exercise?

   ☐ Most of the time   ☐ Sometimes   ☐ Rarely

3. Do you share personal items (clothes, towels, etc.) with others?

   ☐ Often   ☐ Sometimes   ☐ Rarely

CRITICAL THINKING QUESTIONS

1. Compare your vaccine record to the immunization recommendations in Figure 13.5. Are you current on all your vaccination recommendations? If not, which ones do you need to get?

2. Find two sites in your community where you can go to obtain vaccinations. List the name, address, and phone number of each.

3. Based on your responses to Part 2 and based on the recommendations discussed in the section on STDs in Chapter 13, do you need to get tested for STDs?

4. Find two sites in your community where you can get tested for STDs. List the name, address, and phone number of each.

5. Do you have health insurance that covers vaccinations and/or STD testing? If so, do the facilities you listed in questions 2 and 4 accept your insurance? How much do uninsured patients have to pay out-of-pocket for vaccinations and STD testing at the facilities you listed in questions 2 and 4?

6. Based on your responses to Part 3, evaluate your basic hygiene habits. Is there anything in your environment or community that makes it easier or harder to practice good habits? Where is there room for improvement?

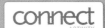
Your behaviors, blood pressure, cholesterol levels, and family history are factors that determine your risk for cardiovascular disease. Complete this assessment of the seven components of ideal cardiovascular health to find out what your risk is in each of these areas.

Part 1 Your Lifestyle

1. Do you avoid tobacco smoking, or if you have smoked, did you quit at least a year ago?	Yes	No
2. Do you exercise at least 150 minutes at moderate intensity or 75 minutes at vigorous intensity each week?	Yes	No
3. Are you at a healthy body weight (as defined by a BMI between 18.5 and 24.9)?	Yes	No
4. How healthy is your diet?		
a. Are you in energy balance (not gaining or losing weight, unless appropriate based on BMI)?	Yes	No
b. Do you eat at least four to five servings of fruits and vegetables a day?	Yes	No
c. Do you eat at least two 3.5 oz servings of fish a week?	Yes	No
d. Do you eat at least three 1 oz servings of fiber-rich whole grains per day?	Yes	No
e. Is your sodium intake less than 1,500 mg per day?	Yes	No
f. Do you limit sugar-sweetened beverages to less than 450 calories per week?	Yes	No
g. Do you eat least four servings of nuts, legumes, and seeds per week?	Yes	No
h. Do you limit servings of processed meats to two or fewer servings per week?	Yes	No
i. Do you limit saturated fat to less than 7 percent of total energy intake?	Yes	No

SCORING

Add up your number of "yes" answers and "no" answers. Congratulations for your "yes" answers! These are areas where you have developed strong patterns to promote cardiovascular health. Pay attention to your "no" answers. These are areas you should address now to promote general cardiovascular health.

_____ "Yes" responses

_____ "No" responses

Part 2 Clinical Parameters

If you do not have this information on hand, you may be able to obtain it by visiting your student health center or your primary care physician. A blood test will be necessary to determine your cholesterol levels.

1. Is your blood pressure < 120/80 mm Hg?	Yes	No	Don't know
2. Is your total cholesterol < 200 mg/dl?	Yes	No	Don't know
3. Is your HDL cholesterol > 60 mg/dl?	Yes	No	Don't know
4. Is your fasting blood glucose (sugar) < 100 mg/dl?	Yes	No	Don't know

SCORING

Add up your number of "yes" answers and "no" answers. Congratulations again for any "yes" answers! These additional parameters promote cardiovascular health. "No" answers in this section mean you may have developed risk factors for cardiovascular disease already. It is even more important for you adopt and maintain the heart-healthy behaviors listed in Part 1. You may also want to seek help from a health professional to explore other options that will help reduce your risk. If you didn't know the responses to these questions, have your blood pressure checked the next time you visit a physician (and write down the numbers) and ask for a blood test to determine your cholesterol levels.

_____ "Yes" responses

_____ "No" responses

Part 3 Your Noncontrollable Factors

1.	Do any of your first-degree relatives (mother, father, sister, brother, child) have a history of heart disease or stroke?	Yes	No
2.	Do any of your first-degree relatives have a history of diabetes?	Yes	No
3.	Do any of your first-degree relatives have a history of high blood pressure?	Yes	No
4.	Do any of your first-degree relatives have a history of high cholesterol?	Yes	No

Any "yes" answers are red flags for your own health. If you haven't already, talk with your primary care physician about your family history. Health issues in family members can suggest a genetic predisposition to cardiovascular disease or risk factors. In addition, it can suggest patterns of behavior within your family of origin that increase risk.

CRITICAL THINKING QUESTIONS

1. Reflect on your responses to Part 1. What good lifestyle habits do you have? Where is there room for improvement? Are there ways you could incorporate change into your usual routines?

2. What are your unique characteristics that make it easy or difficult to practice heart-healthy behaviors? Consider such factors as acquired food tastes, cooking skills, money, physical attributes, or tobacco addiction.

3. What characteristics of your environment may be contributing to your behaviors? Consider your access to foods or exercise facilities, family and peer behaviors, campus policies, and other characteristics.

4. How might your family have influenced your own behavior patterns? Think about activity levels and food consumption patterns within your family. Think about where they live and what role their environment plays in their lives. Think about their occupations and hobbies—how do they impact your family members' lifestyle and habits?

5. Overall, how would you rate your cardiovascular health? Why?

6. Consider the relationship between risk factors for cardiovascular health and other chronic diseases. Do you see any risk factors for diabetes or lung disease in the assessment you just completed?

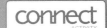
The more risk factors you have for a particular cancer, the greater the likelihood that you will develop that cancer. In the lists below for six common cancers—lung, colon, breast, prostate, cervical, and melanoma—check any risk factors and protective factors that apply to you. The more risk factors you check, the more important it is that you adopt healthy lifestyle behaviors and have regular screening tests. The final section lists general protective factors against cancer. There is no score.

Lung cancer risk factors

____ Age greater than 40 (median age at diagnosis: 71)

____ Family history of lung cancer

____ Smoking cigarettes

____ Smoking cigars

____ Exposure to environmental tobacco smoke

____ Exposure to air pollution

____ Exposure to workplace chemicals

____ Fewer than three servings of vegetables per day

____ Fewer than three servings of fruit per day

Colon cancer risk factors

____ Age greater than 50 (median age at diagnosis: 71)

____ Family history of colon cancer

____ Overweight

____ More than one serving of red meat per day

____ Fewer than three servings of vegetables per day

____ More than one alcoholic drink per day

____ Less than 30 minutes of physical activity per day

____ Having inflammatory bowel disease for 10 years or more

Lower risk associated with:

____ Taking a multivitamin with folate every day

____ Taking birth control pills for at least 5 years

____ Taking postmenopausal hormones for at least 5 years

____ Taking aspirin regularly for more than 15 years

____ Having regular screening tests

Breast cancer risk factors

____ Age greater than 40 (median age at diagnosis: 61)

____ Female sex

____ Family history of breast cancer

____ Jewish ethnicity, especially Ashkenazi descent

____ Overweight

____ Fewer than three servings of vegetables per day

____ More than two alcoholic drinks per day

____ Having had hyperplasia (benign breast disease)

(Breast cancer, continued)

Longer exposure to estrogen:

____ Early age at menarche

____ Older age at birth of first child

____ Older age at menopause

____ Fewer than two children

____ Breastfeeding for less than one year combined for all pregnancies

____ Currently taking birth control pills

____ Taking postmenopausal hormones for 5 years or more

Prostate cancer risk factors

____ Age greater than 55 (median age at diagnosis: 68)

____ Family history of prostate cancer

____ Five or more servings per day of foods containing animal fat

____ Having had a vasectomy

____ African American ethnicity

Lower risk associated with:

____ Asian ethnicity

____ At least one serving per day of tomato-based food

Cervical cancer risk factors

____ Older age (median age at diagnosis: 48)

____ Smoking cigarettes

____ Having had sex at an early age

____ Having had many sexual partners

____ Having had an STD, especially HPV

____ Having given birth to two or more children

Lower risk associated with:

____ HPV vaccination

____ Using a condom or diaphragm on every occasion of sexual intercourse

____ Having regular Pap tests

Melanoma risk factors

____ Older age (median age at diagnosis: 59)

____ Family history of melanoma

____ Light-colored hair and eyes

____ Having had severe, repeated sunburns in childhood

____ Exposure to ultraviolet radiation

____ Taking immunosuppressive drugs (for example, after organ transplant)

Lower risk associated with:

____ Protecting the skin from the sun

____ Regular self-examination of the skin

General protective factors

____ Maintaining a healthy weight

____ Living a physically active lifestyle

____ Consuming a balanced diet with at least five servings of fruit and vegetables a day

____ Limiting alcohol consumption (no more than two drinks a day for men and one for women)

____ Avoiding tobacco

____ Having health insurance

Source: Adapted from "Your Disease Risk," Harvard Center for Cancer Prevention, www.yourdiseaserisk.harvard.edu.

CRITICAL THINKING QUESTIONS

1. For which cancers do you have protective factors?

2. For which cancers do you have risk factors?

3. What factors can you change to lower your cancer risk? Consider your environment and your individual behaviors.

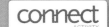
Violence is a serious health problem on many college and university campuses. Many students who survive violent encounters are left with permanent physical and emotional scars. The purpose of this activity is to help you assess how well you protect yourself from becoming a victim of violence. Consider the following statements and decide whether each one is always, sometimes, or never true for you.

General safety considerations	Always	Sometimes	Never
I am aware of my surroundings.			
I tell someone where I'm going whenever I leave home.			
I'm careful about giving personal information or my daily schedule to people I don't know.			
I vary my daily routine and walking patterns.			
If I walk at night, I walk with others.			
Auto safety	**Always**	**Sometimes**	**Never**
I look in the backseat before I get in my car.			
I look around before parking, stopping, or getting into or out of my car.			
I keep my car doors locked at all times.			
I have a plan of action in case my car breaks down.			
I scan ahead of me and behind me, with my mirrors, for potential dangers.			
I avoid dangerous, high-risk places whenever possible.			
If hit from behind, I drive to the nearest police station or well-lit, populated area, motioning for the person who hit me to follow.			
If I notice anyone loitering near my car, I go straight to a safe place and call the police.			
I never hitchhike.			
ATM safety	**Always**	**Sometimes**	**Never**
I avoid using ATMs at night.			
I try to take someone with me when I use an ATM.			
I look for suspicious people or activity before entering or driving into an ATM area.			
I do not write my personal identification number on any paper I carry with me.			
I take all my ATM and credit card receipts with me to avoid leaving behind personal information.			

Violence, rape, and homicide	Always	Sometimes	Never
I carefully limit my alcohol intake at parties.			
I do not drink alcohol on a first date.			
I refuse to be with anyone who seems violent.			
I do not allow anyone to strike me.			
I don't stay around anyone who has a gun and is drinking alcohol or using other drugs.			
I break off any relationship that is verbally or physically abusive.			
Ramps and parking lots	**Always**	**Sometimes**	**Never**
I park in well-lit areas.			
I avoid walking down ramps in parking lots if there are other options.			
I keep my arms as free as possible when walking to my car.			
I check the backseat of my car before getting in.			
Public transportation	**Always**	**Sometimes**	**Never**
While waiting for transportation, I am aware of my immediate surroundings.			
While waiting for transportation, I place myself so that I am protected from behind.			
I hold items under my arm so that they will be difficult to grab.			
While riding on buses or trains, I look aware and alert.			

SCORING

Give yourself 3 points for each "Always" answer, 2 points for each "Sometimes," and 0 points for each "Never."

Score: _____

90–99	You are probably safe as long as you continue to follow these precautions.
80–89	You may need to reexamine some of your habits and make changes to improve your safety.
79 or less	You may need to make significant changes in your habits to improve your safety.

Source: Adapted from *Wellness: Concepts and Applications,* 5th ed., by D. J. Anspaugh, M. H. Hamrick, and F. D. Rosato. Copyright © 2005 The McGraw-Hill Companies. Reprinted by permission of The McGraw-Hill Companies.

CRITICAL THINKING QUESTIONS

1. Based on your responses to the questions, what is your risk level? Where are there areas for improvement? What are key changes that you can make to lower your risk in these areas?

2. What is your overall perception of the safety of your college campus? What are a few ways your campus and overall community can improve on safety?

Chapter 1

1. Thaler, R. H., & Sunstein, C. R. (2008). *Nudge: Improving decisions about health, wealth and happiness.* New Haven, CT: Yale University Press.

2. Preamble to the Constitution of the World Health Organization as adopted by The International Health Conference. New York, 19–22 June, 1946; signed on 22 June 1946 by the representatives of 61 States (Official Records of the WHO, No. 2, p. 100) and entered into force on 7 April 1948.

3. Lindstrom B, & Eriksson M. (2005). Salutogenesis. *Journal of Epidemiology of Community Health, 59,* 440–442.

4. Bravernan, P., Egerter S., & Williams, D. R. (2011). The social determinants of health: Coming of age. *Annual Review of Public Health. 32,* 381–398.

5. Rudolph, L., Caplan, J., Ben-Moshe, K., & Dillon, L. (2013). *Health in all policies: A Guide for state and local governments.* Washington, DC and Oakland, CA: American Public Health Association and Public Health Institute.

6. Christakis, N. A., &. Fowler, J. H. (2007). The spread of obesity in large social network over 32 years. *New England Journal of Medicine, 357,* 370–379.

7. Burt, R. S., Kilduff, M., & Tasselli, S. (2013). Social network analysis: Foundations, frontiers on advantage. *Annual Review of Psychology, 64,* 527–547.

8. Green, E. D. Guyer, M. S., & National Human Genome Research Institute. (2011, February). Charting a course for genomic medicine from base pairs to bedside. *Nature, 470,* 204–213.

9. Wright, M. W., & Bruford, E. A. (2011). Naming "junk": Human non-protein coding RNA (ncRNA) gene nomenclature. *Human Genomics 5* (2), 90–98.

10. U.S. Department of Energy Genome Research Programs. (2008, June). Genomics and its impacts on science and society: The human genome project and beyond. www.ornl.gov/hgmis/publicat/primer/.

11. Kilpinen, H., and Dermitzakis, E. T. (2012). Genetic and epigenetic contribution to complex traits. *Human Molecular Genetics, 21*(1), 24–28.

12. U.S. Department of Health and Human Services. (n.d.). Surgeon General's family health history initiative. www.hhs.gov/familyhistory/.

13. Simons-Morton, B., McLeroy, K. R., & Wendel, M. L. (2012). *Behavior theory in health promotion practice and research.* Burlington, MA: Jones and Bartlett Learning.

14. Green, L. W. & Kreuter, M. W. (2005). *Health promotion planning: An educational and ecological approach.* New York: McGraw-Hill.

15. Robinson L. M., & Vail, S. R. (2012). An integrative review of adolescent smoking cessation using the Transtheoretical Model of Change. *Journal of Pediatric Health Care. 26* (5), 336–345.

16. Berkman, N. D., et al. (2011). Low health literacy and health outcomes: An updated systematic review. *Annals of Internal Medicine, 155* (2), 97–107.

17. U.S. Department of Health and Human Services, Office of Disease Prevention and Health Promotion. (2010). *National action plan to improve health literacy.* Washington, DC: Author.

18. Zikmund-Fisher, B. J., et al. (2010). Risky feelings: Why 6% risk does not always feel like 6%. *Patient Education and Counseling, 81* (1), S87–S93.

19. Friel, S., Ackerman, M., Hancock, T., et al. (2011). Addressing the social and environmental determinants of urban health equity: Evidence for action and a research agenda. *Journal of Urban Health, Bulletin of the New York Academy of Medicine, 88* (5), 860–874.

20. CIA. *The world fact book.* www.cia.gov/library/publications/the-world-factbook/geos/us.html.

21. U.S. Department of Health and Human Services. (2013). *Healthy People 2020.* www.healthypeople.gov/hp2020.

22. U.S. Census Bureau. (2010). *December 2010 current population survey.* http://2010.census.gov/2010census/about/.

23. U.S. Department of Health and Human Services, Office of Minority Health. (2005). *What is cultural competency?* www.omhrc.gov/templates/browse.aspx?lvl=2&lvlID=11.

24. Mead, H., Cartwright-Smith, K., Jones, C., Ramos, C., et al. (2008, March). *Racial and ethnic disparities in U.S. health care: A chartbook.* New York: The Commonwealth Fund.

25. LaVeist, T. A., Gaskin, D., & Trujillo, A. J. (2011, September). *Segregated spaces, risky places: The effects of racial segregation on health inequalities.* Washington, DC: Joint Center for Political and Economic Studies. www.jointcenter.org/sites/default/files/upload/research/files/Segregated%20Spaces-web.pdf.

26. Fry, R., & Taylor, P. (2012, August 1). The rise of residential segregation by income. *Pew Research Center.* www.pewsocialtrends.org/2012/08/01/the-rise-of-residential-segregation-by-income.

27. Crowder, K., Pais, J., & South, S. J. (2012). Neighborhood diversity, metropolitan constraints, and household migration. *American Sociological Review, 77* (3), 325–353.

28. National Research Council and Institute of Medicine. (2013). *U.S. health in international perspective: Shorter lives, poorer health. panel on understanding cross-national health differences among high-income countries,* eds. S. H. Woolf and L. Aron, Committee on Population, Division of Behavioral and Social Sciences and Education and Board on Population Health and Public Health Practice, Institute of Medicine. Washington, DC: The National Academies Press.

Chapter 2

1. National Institute of Mental Health. (2008). The numbers count. *Mental Disorders in America.* www.nimh.nih.gov.

2. Gable, S., & Haidt, J. (2005). What (and why) is positive psychology? *Review of General Psychology, 9* (2), 103–110.

3. Peterson, C., & Seligman, M. (2004). *Character strengths and virtues: A handbook and classification.* Washington, DC: American Psychological Association.

4. Boehm, J., Peterson, C., Kivimaki, M., & Kubzansky, L. (2011). A prospective study of positive psychological well-being and coronary heart disease, *Health Psychology, 30* (3), 259–267.

5. Seligman, M. (1998). *Learned optimism: How to change your mind and your life.* New York: Basic Books.

6. Rasmussen, H., & Scheier, M. (2009). Optimism and physical health. *Annals of Behavioral Medicine, 37,* 239–256.

7. Kahneman, D. (2011). *Thinking fast and slow.* New York: Farrar, Straus and Giroux.

8. Morse, G. (2012). The science behind the smile. *Harvard Business Review, 90* (1/2), 84–90.

9. Wallis, C. (2005, January 17). The new science of happiness. *Time, 165* (3), A2–A9.

10. Seligman, M. (2002). *Authentic happiness.* New York: Simon and Schuster.

11. Goleman, D. (2006). *Emotional intelligence: Why it can matter more than IQ* (10th ed.). New York: Bantam Books.

12. Sternberg, R.J. (1996). *Successful intelligence: How practical and creative intelligences determine success in life.* New York: Simon and Schuster.

13. Rivers, S., Brackett, M.A., Omori, M., Sickler, C., Bertoli, M., Salovey, P. (2013). Emotion skills as a protective factor for risky behaviors among college students. *Journal of College Student Development, 54* (2), 172–183.

14. Mancini, A., Griffin, P., & Bonanno, G. (2012). Recent trends in treatment of prolonged grief. *Current Opinion in Psychiatry, 25* (1), 46–51.

15. Moss, E., & Dobson, K. (2006). Psychology, spirituality and end of life care: An ethical integration. *Canadian Psychology, 47* (4), 284–299.

16. Harvard Health Publications. (2012). Can you die of a broken heart? *Harvard Heart Letter* (blog). www.health.harvard.edu/blog-extra/can-you-die-of-a-broken-heart.

17. Bonanno, G. (2009). *The other side of sadness: What the new science of bereavement tells us about life after loss.* New York: Basic Books.

18. Jabr, F. (2013). The newest edition of Psychiatry's "bible", the DSM 5, *Scientific American* January 28.

19. Kubler-Ross, E. (1997). *On death and dying.* New York: Simon and Schuster.

20. Mueller, P.S., Plevak, D.J., & Rummans, T.A. (2001). Religious involvement, spirituality, and medicine: Implications for clinical practice. *Mayo Clinic Proceedings, 76* (12).

21. American Psychiatric Association. (2000). *Diagnostic and statistical manual of mental disorders* (5th ed.). Washington, DC: American Psychiatric Association.

22. Howard, P.J. (2006). *The owners manual for the brain: Everyday applications for mind-brain research* (3rd ed.). Austin, TX: Bard Press.

23. Epstein, R. (2007, April 18). The myth of the teenage brain. *Scientific American Mind, 18* (2), 55–64.

24. Andreasen, N. (1984). *The broken brain.* New York: Harper and Row, Perennial Library.

25. Seligman, M., Steen, T., Park, N., & Peterson, C. (2005). Positive psychology progress: Empirical validation of interventions. *American Psychologist, 60* (5), 410–421.

26. Hansen, H., Donaldson, Z., Link, B., Bearman, P., Hopper, K., Bates, L., Cheslack-Postava, K., Harper, K., Holmes, S., Lovasi G., Springer, K., Teitler, J. (2013). Independent review of social and population variation in mental health could improve diagnosis in DSM revisions, *Health Affairs* (Millwood) 32 (5)984–993.

27. *Medscape.* (2013). Multispeciality DSM 5 news and perspectives, May.

28. Jabr, F. (2013). The newest edition of Psychiatry's "bible", the DSM 5, *Scientific American* January 28.

29. National Institute of Mental Health. (2011). Panic disorder. In *Anxiety disorders.* www.nimh.nih.gov/health/publications/anxiety-disorders/panic-disorder.shtml.

30. National Institute of Mental Health. (2009). What is schizophrenia? *Schizophrenia.* www.nimh.nih.gov/health/publications/schizophrenia/what-is-schizophrenia.shtml.

31. American College Health Association. (2011). *National college health assessment, spring.* Baltimore: American College Health Association.

32. Recognizing the warning signs of suicide. (2012). *Depression Health Center.* WebMD. www.webmd.com/depression/guide/depression-recognizing-signs-of-suicide.

33. American Academy of Child and Adolescent Psychiatry. (2009).

Facts for families, self-injury. www.aacap.org/cs/root/facts_for_families/selfinjury_in_adolescents.

34. American College Health Association. (2013). *American College Health Association–National College Health Assessment II: Reference Group Executive Summary Fall 2012.* Hanover, MD: ACHA.

35. Whitlock, J., Eckenrode, J., & Silverman, D. (2006). Self-injurious behavior in college populations. *Pediatrics, 117* (6), 1939–1948.

36. Barlow, D., Bullis, J., Comer, J., Ametaj. A. (2013). Evidence based psychological treatments: an update and a way forward, *Annual Review of Clinical Psychology*, 9, 1–27.

37. Agency for Healthcare Research and Quality. (2008). Antidepressant prescriptions climb by 16 million. *AHRQ News and Numbers.* http://archive.ahrq.gov/news/nn/nn072408.htm.

38. U.S. Food and Drug Administration. (2004). Public health advisory, Suicidality in children and adolescents being treated with antidepressant medications. www.fda.gov.

39. Olfson, M., & Marcus, S.C. (2008). A case control study of antidepressants and attempted suicide during early phase treatment of major depressive disorders. *Journal of Clinical Psychiatry, 69* (3), 425–432.

40. National Institute of Mental Health. (2012). Antidepressant medications for children and adolescents, Information for parents and caregiver. www.nimh.nih.gov/health/topics/child-and-adolescent-mental-health/antidepressant-medications-for-children-and-adolescents-information-for-parents-and-caregivers.shtml.

41. Sammons, M.T. (2009). Writing a wrong: Factors influencing the overprescription of antidepressants to youth. *Professional Psychology: Research and Review, 40* (4), 327–329.

42. U.S. Food and Drug Administration. (2007). FDA proposes new warnings about suicidal thinking, behavior in young adults who take antidepressant medications (press release).

43. Begley, S. (2010, February 8). The depressing news about antidepressants. *Newsweek, 155* (6), 34.

44. Hegerl, U., Schhonknecht, P., & Mergl, R. (2012). Are antidepressants useful in the treatment of minor depression: A critical update of the current literature. *Current Opinion in Psychiatry, 25* (1), 1–6.

45. American Psychological Association. (2014, February 11). *Stress in America: Are teens adopting adults' stress habits?* www.apa.org/news/press/releases/stress/2013/stress-report.pdf.

46. Schmidt, M., & Schwabe, L. (2011). Splintered by stress. *Scientific American Mind, 22* (4), 22–29.

47. Blonna, R. (2011). *Coping with stress in a changing world* (5th ed.). New York: McGraw-Hill.

48. Benson, H. (1993). The relaxation response. In D.P. Goleman & J. Gurin (Eds.), *Mind-body medicine: How to use your mind for better health* (pp. 233–257). Yonkers, NY: Consumer Reports Books.

49. Kiecolt-Glaser, J. (2002). Psychoneuroimmunology: Psychological influences on immune function and health. *Journal of Consulting and Clinical Psychology, 70,* 537–547.

50. Benson, H. (2006). *Stress management: Techniques for preventing and easing stress.* Cambridge, MA: Harvard Medical School Press.

51. Charles, S., Piazza, J., Mogle, J., Sliwinski, M., Almeida, D. (2013). The wear and tear of daily stressors on mental health, *Psychological Science, 24* (5) 733–741.

52. Friedman, M., & Rosenman, R.H. (1982). *Type A behavior and your heart.* New York: Fawcett Books.

53. Williams, R. (1991). *The trusting heart: Great news about Type A behavior.* New York: Random House.

54. Chida, Y., & Steptoe, A. (2009). The association of anger and hostility with future coronary heart disease: A meta analytic review of prospective evidence. *Journal of the American College of Cardiology, 53,* 936–946.

55. Barnett, M.D., Ledoux, T., Garcini, L.M., & Baker, J. (2009). Type D personality and chronic pain; Construct and concurrent validity of the DS 14. *Journal of Clinical Psychology in Medical Settings, 16,* 194–199.

56. Beutel, M., et al. (2012). Type D personality as a cardiovascular risk marker in the general population: Results from the Gutenberg health study. *Psychotherapy and Psychosomatics, 81,* 108–117.

57. Compare, A., Bigi, R., Orrego, P.S., Proietti, R., Grossi, E., Steptoe, A. (2013). Type D personality is associated with the development of stress cardiomyopathy following emotional triggers, *Annals of Behavioral Medicine, 45,* (3) 299–307.

58. Kobasa, S.O. (1984, September). How much stress can you survive? *American Health,* 71–72.

59. Maddi, S. (2002). The story of hardiness: Twenty years of theorizing, research and practice. *Consulting Psychology: Practice and Research, 54* (3), 175–185.

60. Holmes, T., & Rahe, R. (1967). The social readjustment rating scale. *Journal of Psychosomatic Research, 11,* 213–218.

61. Segerstrom, S.C., & Miller, G.E. (2004). Psychological stress and the human immune system: A meta-analytic of 30 years of inquiry. *Psychological Bulletin, 130* (4), 610–630.

62. Greenberg, J. (1984). A study of the effects of stress on college students: Implications for school health education. *Health Education, 15,* 11–15.

63. Greenberg, J. (1981). A study of the stressors in the college student population. *Health Education, 12,* 8–12.

64. American Psychological Association. (2009, November). *Stress in America 2009.* www.apa.org/news/press/releases/stress/2009/stress-exec-summary.pdf.

65. Gleick, J. (2000). *Faster: The acceleration of just about everything.* New York: Vintage Books.

66. Expedia.com. (2011). Vacation deprivation study. http://media.expedia.com/media/content/expus/graphics/other/pdf/vacation-deprivation-fact-sheetnov2011.pdf.

67. Kraft, U. (2006, June–July). Burned-out. *Scientific American Mind, 17* (3), 28–33.

68. Pines, A.M. (1993). Burnout: An existential perspective. In W.B. Schaufeli, C. Maslach, & T. Marek (Eds.), *Professional burnout: Recent developments in research and practice.* Philadelphia: Taylor and Francis.

69. Pennebaker, R. (2009, August 30). The mediocre multitasker. *New York Times,* The Week in Review, p. 5.

70. Shay, J. (1996, July–August). Shattered lives. *Family Therapy Networker, 20* (4), 46–54.

71. Ong, A.J., Fuller-Rowell, T., & Burrow, A.L. (2009). Racial discrimination and the stress process. *Journal of Personality and Social Psychology, 96,* 1259–1271.

72. Pascoe, E.A., & Richman, L.S. (2009). Perceived discrimination and health: A meta-analytic review. *Psychological Bulletin, 135* (4), 531–554.

73. Krieger, N., Kosheleva, A., Waterman, P., et al. (2011). Racial discrimination, psychological distress and self rated health among US-born and foreign-born Black Americans. *American Journal of Public Health, 101* (9), 1704–1713.

74. Hatzenbuehler, M.L. (2009). How does sexual minority stigma "get under the skin"? A psychological mediation framework. *Psychological Bulletin, 135* (5), 707–730.

75. Meyer, I.H. (2003). Prejudice, social stress and mental health in lesbian, gay and bisexual populations: Conceptual issues and research evidence. *Psychological Bulletin, 129* (5), 674–697.

76. Verkuil, B., Brosschot, J., Korrelboom, K., et al. (2011). Pretreatment of worry enhances the effects of stress management therapy. *Psychotherapy and Psychosomatics, 80,* 189–190.

77. Vaccaro, P. (2000, September). The 80/20 principle of time management. *Family Practice Management, 7* (8), 76.

78. Ornish, D. (1998). *Love and survival: 8 pathways to intimacy and health.* New York: Harper Perennial.

79. Cacioppo, J.T., & Patrick, W. (2008). *Loneliness: Human nature and the need for social connection.* New York: Norton.

80. Christakis, N.A., & Fowler, J.H. (2009). *Connected: The surprising power of social networks and how they shape our lives.* New York: Little Brown.

81. Sacks, M.H. (1993). Exercise for stress control. In D.P. Goleman & J. Gurin (Eds.), *Mind-body medicine: How to use your mind for better health* (pp. 315–327). Yonkers, NY: Consumer Reports Books.

82. Davis, M., McKay, M., & Eshelman, E.R. (2000). *The relaxation and stress reduction workbook* (5th ed.). Oakland, CA: New Harbinger.

83. Geschwind, N., Peeters, F., Drukker, M., et al. (2011). Mindfulness training increases momentary positive emotions and reward experience in adults vulnerable to depression: A randomized control trial. *Journal of Consulting and Clinical Psychology, 79* (5), 618–628.

84. de Vibe, M., Solhaug, I., Tyssen, R., Friborg, O., Rosenvinge, J., Sørlie, T., Bjørndal, A. (2013). Mindfulness training for stress management: a randomized controlled study of medical and psychology students, *BMC Medical Education,* 13 (107).

85. Holzel, B., Lazar, S., Gard, T., et al. (2011). How does mindfulness meditation work? Proposing mechanisms of action from a conceptual neural perspective. *Perspectives on Psychological Science, 6* (6), 537–559.

86. Schwartz, M., & Andrasik, F. (Eds.). (2003). *Biofeedback: A practitioner's guide* (3rd ed.). New York: Guilford.

87. Duckworth, A.L., and Eskreis-Winkler, L. (2013). True Grit, *Association for Psychological Science* Observer, 26(4).

Chapter 3

1. Fowler, J., and Christakis, N. (2010, March 23). Cooperative behavior cascades in human social networks. *PNAS, 107* (12), 5334–5338.

2. Grant, A. (2013). *Give and Take: A Revolutionary Approach to Success,* Viking Press, New York.

3. Fowler, J., & Christakis, N. (2009). The dynamic spread of happiness in a larger social network. *British Medical Journal, 337,* 1–19.

4. Smith-Lovin, L. (2006). Social isolation in America: Changes in core discussion networks over two decades. *American Sociological Review, 71,* 353–375.

5. Christakis, N., & Fowler, J. (2009). *Connected: The surprising power of our social networks and how they shape our lives.* New York: Little, Brown.

6. Preciado, P., Snijders, T., Burk, W., et al. (2012). Does proximity matter? Distance dependence of adolescent friendships. *Social Networks, 34,* 18–31.

7. *Social support: A buffer against life's ills.* (2005). www.mayoclinic.com.

8. Gottman, J., Gottman, J.S., & DeClaire, J. (2006). *10 lessons to transform your marriage.* New York: Three Rivers Press.

9. Pines, A. M. (2005). *Falling in love: Why we choose the lovers we choose.* New York: Routledge Press.

10. Fisher, H. (2004). *Why we love: The nature and chemistry of romantic love.* New York: Henry Holt.

11. Fisher, H. (2009). *Why him? Why her?* New York: Henry Holt.

12. Christakis, N., & Fowler, J. (2009). Love the one you're with. *Scientific American Mind, 20* (6), 48–55.

13. Cacioppo, J., Cacciopo, S., Gonzaga, G., Ogburn, E., Vanderweele, T. (2013). Marital satisfaction and break-ups differ across on-line and off-line meeting venues, *PNAS.* 110 (25) 10135–10140.

14. Hatfield, E., Bensman, L., & Rapson, R. (2012). A brief history of social scientists' attempts to measure passionate love. *Journal of Social and Personal Relationships, 29* (2), 143–164.

15. Fisher, H. (2011). The brain, how we fall in love, and how we stay together: An interview with Helen Fisher. *Family Therapy Magazine, 10* (3), 22–25.

16. Sternberg, R. J. (2006). *The new psychology of love.* New Haven, CT: Yale University Press.

17. Tannen, D. (2010). He said, she said. *Scientific American Mind, 21* (2), 55–59.

18. Gallup Organization. (2000, December). Gallup poll: Traits of males and females.

19. Hill, D., Rozanski, C., & Willoughby, B. (2007). Gender identity disorders in childhood and adolescence: A critical inquiry. *International Journal of Sexual Health, 19,* 57–74.

20. Kinsey, A.C., Pomeroy, W.B., & Martin, C.E. (1948). *Sexual behavior in the human male* (reprint edition, 1998). Bloomington, IN: Indiana University Press.

21. Kinsey, A.C., Pomeroy, W.B., Martin, C.E., & Gebhard, P.H. (1953). *Sexual behavior in the human female* (reprint edition, 1998). Bloomington, IN: Indiana University Press.

22. Copen, C.E., Daniels, K., Vespa, J., & Mosher, W.D. (March 22, 2012). First marriages in the United States: Data from the 2006–2010 National Survey of Family Growth. *National Health Statistics Reports, 49.* www.cdc.gov/nchs/data/nhsr/nhsr049.pdf

23. Aizer, A., Ming-Hui, C., McCarthy, E., Mendu, M., Koo, S., Wilhite, T., Graham, P., Choveiri, T., Hoffman, K., Martin, N.,

Hu, J., Nguyen, P. (2013). Marital status and survival in patients with cancer, *Journal of Clinical Oncology, 31* (31) 3869–3876.

24. Olson, D.H., & Olson, A.K. (2000). *Empowering couples: Building on your strengths.* Minneapolis, MN: Life Innovations.

25. Weaver, J. (2007). Cheating hearts: Who's doing it and why. www.msnbc.msn.com/id/17951664.

26. Bepko, C., & Johnson, T. (2000). Gay and lesbian couples in therapy: Perspectives for the contemporary family therapist. *Journal of Marital and Family Therapy, 26* (4), 409–419.

27. van Wormer, K., Wells, U., & Boes, M. (2000). *Social work with lesbians, gays, and bisexuals: A strengths perspective.* Boston: Allyn & Bacon.

28. Brumbaugh, S.M., Sanchez, L.A., Nock, S.L., & Wright, J.D. (2008). Attitudes toward gay marriage in states undergoing marriage law transformation. *Journal of Marriage and the Family, 70,* 345–359.

29. Willoughby, B., Carroll, J., & Busby, D. (2011, December 28). The different effects of "living together": Determining and comparing types of cohabiting couples. *Journal of Social and Personal Relationships,* 1–23, published online.

30. Kuperberg, A. (2014, April). Age at coresidence, premarital cohabitation, and marriage dissolution: 1985–2009, *Journal of Marriage and Family, 76,* 352–369.

31. Musick, K., & Bumpass, L. (2012, February). Reexamining the case for marriage: Union formation and changes in well-being. *Journal of Marriage and Family, 74,* 1–18.

32. Whitehead, B.D., & Popenoe, D. (2006). The state of our unions: The social health of marriage in America. http://marriage.rutgers.edu/publications/soou/textsoou2006.htm.

33. Olson, D.H., & Defrain, J. (2003). *Marriage and families: Intimacy, diversity, and strength* (4th ed.). New York: McGraw-Hill.

34. Cacioppo, J., & Patrick, W. (2008). *Loneliness: Human nature and the need for social connections.* New York: Norton.

35. Bruhn, J. (2011). *The sociology of community connections* (2nd ed.). New York: Springer.

36. Smith, K., and Christakis, N. (2008). Social networks and health. *Annual Review of Sociology, 34,* 405–429.

37. Fowler, J., & Christakis, N. (2008). Estimating peer effects on health in social networks. *Journal of Health Economics, 27* (5), 1400–1405.

38. Christakis, N., & Fowler, J.H. (2009). *Connected: The surprising power of our social networks and how they shape our lives.* New York: Little, Brown.

39. Ho, D.Y.F., & Ho, R.T.H. (2007). Measuring spirituality and spiritual emptiness: Toward ecumenicity and transcultural applicability. *Review of General Psychology, 11* (1), 274.

40. Gallup Inc. (2009). Religion. www.gallup.com/poll/1690/religion.aspx#1.

41. Aten, J.D., & Schenck, J.E. (2007). Reflections on religion and health research: An interview with Dr. Harold G. Koenig. *Journal of Religion and Health, 46* (2), 183–190.

42. Koening, H.G., Larson, D.B., & Larson, S.S. (2001). Religion and coping with serious medical illness. *Annals of Pharmacotherapy, 35,* 352–359.

43. Rosmarin, D., & Wachholtz, A. (2011). Beyond descriptive research: Advancing the study of spirituality and health. *Journal of Behavioral Medicine, 34,* 409–413.

44. Masters, K. & Hooker, S., (2013). Religiousness/spirituality, cardiovascular disease and cancer: Cultural integration for health research and intervention, *Journal of Consulting and Clinical Psychology, 81* (2) 206-216.

45. Mueller, P.S., Plevak, D.J., & Rummans, T.A. (2001). Religious involvement, spirituality, and medicine: Implications for clinical practice. *Mayo Clinic Proceedings, 76* (12), 1225–1235.

46. Blumenthal, J.A., Babyak, M.A., Ironson, G., et al. (2007). Spirituality, religion and clinical outcomes in patients recovering from an acute myocardial infarction. *Psychosomatic Medicine, 69,* 501–508.

47. Hummer, R.A., Richard, R.G., Charles, N.B., & Christopher, E.G. (1999). Religious participation and U.S. adult mortality. *Demography, 36* (2), 273–285.

48. Strawbridge, W.J., et al. (2001). Religious attendance increases survival by improving and maintaining good health behaviors, mental health, and social relationships. *Annals of Behavioral Medicine, 23,* 68–74.

49. Brady, M.J., et al. (1999). A case for including spirituality in quality of life measurement in oncology. *Psychooncology, 8,* 417–428.

50. Koenig, H.G., McCullough, M.E., & Larson, D.B. (2001). *Handbook of religion and health.* Oxford, UK: Oxford University Press.

51. Larson, D.B., Swyers, J.P., & McCullough, M.E. (1998). *Scientific research on spirituality and health: A report based on the scientific progress in spirituality conferences.* Rockville, MD: National Institute for Healthcare Research.

52. Seybold, K.S., & Hill, P.C. (2001). The role of religion and spirituality in mental and physical health. *Current Directions in Psychological Science, 10,* 21–24.

53. Touissaint, O, & Cheadle, A. (2012). Forgive to live: Forgiveness, health and longevity. *Journal of Behavioral Medicine, 35* (4) 375–386.

54. Chen, Y.Y., & Koenig, H.G. (2006). Do people turn to religion in times of stress? An examination of change in religiousness among elderly, medically ill patients. *Journal of Nervous and Mental Disease, 194,* 114–120.

55. Aaker, J. & Smith, A. (2010). The dragonfly effect: quick, effective and powerful ways to use social media to drive social change. San Francisco: Jossey-Bass.

56. Ruvinsky, J. (2011, Winter). Volunteering for number one. *Stanford Social Innovation Review, 7.*

57. Luks, A. (1988, October). Helper's high. *Psychology Today, 22* (10), 39–42.

58. Farino, L. (n.d.). Do good, feel good. *MSN Health & Fitness.* www.health.msn.com.

59. Hafen, B.Q., et al. (1996). *Mind/body health: The effects of attitudes, emotions and relationships.* Boston: Allyn & Bacon.

60. Luks, A., & Payne, P. (1992). *The healing power of doing good: The health and spiritual benefits of helping others.* New York: Fawcett Columbine.

61. Howe, N., & Strauss, W. (2000). *Millennials rising: The next great generation.* New York: Vintage Books.

62. House, J.S., Landis, K.R., & Umberson, P. (1988). Social relationships and health. *Science, 241,* 540–545.

63. Beckett, W. (1993). *The mystical now: Art and the sacred.* New York: Universe Publishing.

Chapter 4

1. American College Health Association. (2009). National college health assessment—Spring 2008. www.acha-ncha.org/docs/ACHA-NCHA_Reference_Group_ExecutiveSummary_Spring2008.pdf.

2. Forquer, L.M., Camden, A.E., Gavriau, K.M., et al. (2008). Sleep patterns of college students at a public university. *Journal of American College Health, 56* (5), 563–565.

3. National Sleep Foundation. (2010). 2010 Sleep in America poll. www.sleepfoundation.org.

4. National Sleep Foundation. (2009). 2009 Sleep in America poll, executive report. www.sleepfoundation.org.

5. Lockley, S.W. (2012). *Sleep: A very short introduction.* New York: Oxford University Press.

6. Institute of Medicine. (2006). *Sleep disorders and sleep deprivation.* Washington, DC: National Academies Press.

7. American Sleep Association. What is sleep? http://sleepassociation.org/index.php?p=what is sleep.

8. Kryger, M.H., Roth, T., & Dement, W.C. (2011). *Principles and practices of sleep medicine.* New York,: Saunders.

9. Breus, M. (2011). *The sleep doctor's diet plan.* New York: Rodale Press.

10. Bower B., Bysma, L.M., & Morris, B.H., et al. (2010). Poor reported sleep quality predicts low positive affect in daily life among healthy and mood disordered persons. *Journal of Sleep Research, 19* (27), 323–332.

11. Massimiliano, Z., Naima, B., & Tena, D. (2010). Sleep onset and cardiovascular activity in primary insomnia. *Journal of Sleep Research, 20* (2), 318–325.

12. Perlis, M., Aloia, M., & Kuhn, B. (2010). *Behavioral treatments for sleep disorders.* New York: Academic Press.

13. Stickgold, R., & Wehrwein, P. (2009, April 27). Sleep now, remember later. *Newsweek, 153* (17), 56–57.

14. Epstein, L.J. (2007). *A good night's sleep.* New York: McGraw-Hill.

15. Tononi, G., & Cirelli, C. (2013). Perchance to prune. *Scientific American, 309* (2), 34–39.

16. Moore, R.Y. (2011). The neurobiology of sleep-wake regulation. www.medscape.com/viewarticle/491041.

17. National Sleep Foundation. (2011). In your dreams. www.sleepfoundation.org/article/hot-topics/your dreams.

18. Ferrreni, A.F., & Ferreni, R.L. (2008). Health in the later years. New York, NY: McGraw Hill.

19. National Sleep Foundation. (2007). Stressed-out American women have no time for sleep [press release]. www.sleepfoundation.org.

20. National Sleep foundation. (2013). Stress and insomnia. www.sleepfoundation.org/article/ask-the-expert/stress-and-insomnia.

21. National Sleep Foundation. Obstructive sleep apnea and sleep. www.sleepfoundation.org/article/sleep-related-problems/obstructive-sleep-apnea-and-sleep.

22. Lloberes, P., Lourdes, L., Sampol, G., et al. (2010). Obstructive apnea and 24-h blood pressure in patients with resistant hypertension. *Journal of Sleep Research, 19* (4), 577–602.

23. Wang, H., Newton, G.E., Floras, J.S., et al. (2007). Influence of obstructive sleep apnea on mortality in patients with heart failure. *Journal of American Cardiology, 49,* 1625–1631.

24. Lewis, P.A. (2013). *The secret world of sleep.* New York: Palgrave MacMillan.

25. Chokroverty, S. (2009). *Sleep disorder medicine.* Philadelphia: Saunders/Elsevier.

26. Griefahn, B., Brode, P., Marks, A., et al. (2008). Autonomic arousals related to traffic noise during sleep. *Journal of Sleep, 31* (4), 569–577.

27. National Sleep Foundation. (2013). Sleep aids. www.sleepfoundation.org.

28. Surgeon General. (2010). How tobacco smoke causes disease. Atlanta, GA: U.S. Department of Health and Human Services.

29. Boggan, B. (2011). Alcohol, chemistry and you: Ethanol and sleep. www.chemcases.com/alcohol/alc-09.htm.

30. National Sleep Foundation. (2011). *2011 Sleep in America poll: Communications technology in the bedroom.* Washington, DC: National Sleep Foundation.

31. Sleep Care. Electronic screens: How do they affect your sleep. www.sleepcare.com/ondex.php/electronic-screens-how-do-they-affect-your-sleep/.

32. *Huffington Post.* Sleep texting is on the rise. www.huffingtonpost.com/2013/02/14/sleep-testing-on-the-rise_n_2677739.html.

33. National Sleep Foundation. Napping. www.sleepfoundation.org/article/sleep-topics/napping.

34. O'Hanlon, B. (2000). *Overcoming sleep disorders: A natural approach.* Freedom. CA: Crossing Press.

35. Park, M. *CNN Health.* Anti-energy drinks: Relaxation in a can. www.cnn.com/2011/HEALTH/02/04anti-energy.drinks/index.html?eref=rss_health.

36. White House Briefing. *Fox News.* www.foxnews.com/story/2010/08.anti-energy.soda-drinks-to-help-sleep-hit-us-st.

Chapter 5

1. Wardlaw, G.M., & Smith, A.M. (2011). *Contemporary nutrition.* New York: McGraw-Hill.

2. Sizer, F.S., & Whitney E. (2011). *Nutrition: Concepts and controversies.* Belmont, CA: Wadsworth.

3. Schiff, W. (2011). *Nutrition for healthy living.* New York: McGraw-Hill.

4. U.S. Department of Agriculture. (2005). *2005 dietary guidelines for Americans.* www.health.gov/dietaryguidelines.

5. Bao, Y., Nimptsch, K., Wolpin, B.M., et al. (2011). Dietary load, dietary insulin index, and risk of pancreatic cancer. *American Journal of Clinical Nutrition, 24* (3), 862–868.

6. Johnson, R.K., Appel, L.J., Brands, M., et al. on behalf of the American Heart Association Nutrition Committee of the Council on Nutrition, Physical Activity, and Metabolism and the Council on Epidemiology and Prevention. (2009). Dietary sugars intake and cardiovascular health: A scientific statement from the American Heart Association. *Circulation, 120,* 1011–1020.

7. Smolin, L.A., & Grosvenor, M.S. (2010). *Nutrition: Science and education.* Hoboken, NJ: John Wiley & Sons.

8. Vasanti, S.M., & Huh, F.B. (2011). Sugar sweetened beverages and health: Where does the evidence stand? *American Clinical Nutrition, 94* (5), 1161–1162.

9. Liebman, B. (2011, March). Carbo loading: Do you overdo refined grains? *Nutrition Action Health Letter, Center for Science in the Public Interest, 38* (2), 3–6.

10. Dong, J.-Y., Ka, H., Wang, P., et al. (2011). Dietary fiber intake and risk of breast cancer: A meta-analysis of prospective cohort studies. *American Journal of Clinical Nutrition, 94* (3), 900–905.

11. Furtado, J.D., Campos, H., Appel, L.J., et al. (2008, June). Effect of protein, unsaturated fat, and carbohydrate intakes on plasma apolipoprotein B and VLDL and LDL containing apolipoprotein C-III: Results from the Omniheart Trial. *American Journal of Clinical Nutrition, 87* (6), 1623–1630.

12. Klingburg, S., Ellegard, L., Johansson, I., et al. (2008). Inverse relation between dietary intake of naturally occurring plant sterols and serum cholesterol in northern Sweden. *American Journal of Clinical Nutrition, 87* (4), 993–1001.

13. Hallowy, C.J., Cochlin, L.E., Emmanuel, Y., et al. (2011). A high-fat diet impairs cardiac high energy phosphate metabolism and cognitive function in healthy human subjects. *American Journal of Clinical Nutrition, 93* (4), 748–755.

14. Key, T.J., Appleby, P.N., Cairns, B.J., et al. (2011). Dietary fat and breast cancer: Comparison of results from food diaries and food frequency questionnaires. *American Journal of Clinical Nutrition, 94* (4), 1043–1052.

15. Mursu, J., Robien, K., Harnack, L.J., et al. (2011). Dietary supplements and mortality rate in older women: The Iowa women's health study. *American Journal of Clinical Nutrition, 92* (2), 338–347.

16. Ribnicky, D.M., Poulev, A., Schmidt, B., et al. (2008). Evaluation of botanicals for improving human health. *American Journal of Clinical Nutrition, 87* (2), 472S–475S.

17. Hutchinson, C. (2011). Heart disease death rate drops with each added fruit and veggie serving. *ABC News.* http://abcnews.go.com/CleanPrint/cleanprintproxy.aspx?1296051874491.

18. Geleijnse, J.M., & Hollman, P. (2008). Flavanoids and cardiovascular health: Which compounds, which mechanisms. *American Journal of Clinical Nutrition, 87* (7), 12–13.

19. Cassidy, A., O'Reily, E.J., Kay, C., et al. (2011). Habitual intake of flavonoids subclasses and incident hypertension in adults. *American Journal of Clinical Nutrition, 93* (2), 338–347.

20. U.S. Food and Drug Administration. (2007). Final rule promotes safe use

of dietary supplements. www.fda.gov/consumer/updates/dietarysupps062207.html.

21. U.S. Department of Agriculture. (2011). USDA's MyPlate. www.choosemyplate.gov/.

22. Center for Science in the Public Interest. 2013. Six reasons to eat lean red meat. Nutrition Action Health Letter. June, pp. 7.

23. Mayo Clinic. Gluten-free diet: What's allowed, What's not. www.mayoclinic.org/healthy-living/nutrition-and-healthy-eating/in-depth/gluten-free-diet/art-20048530. Accessed September 2013.

24. Nestle, M., & Ludwig, D.S. (2010). Front of package food labels: Push products, not health. *Journal of the American Medical Association, 303* (8), 771–772.

25. Institutes of Medicine. (2011). Examination of front-of-package symbols: Phase I and II reports. National Academy of Sciences. www.nap.edu.

26. Food and Drug Administration. FDA proposes updates to Nutrition Facts label on food packages. www/fda.gov/NewsEvents/Newsroom/PressAnnouncements/ucm387418.htm.

27. Center for Science in the Public Interest. (2010). Health reform to deliver calorie contents to chain restaurant menus nationwide. www.cspinet.org/new/201003211.html.

28. National Center for Chronic Disease Prevention and Health Promotion. (2006, September). Does drinking beverages with added sugars increase the risk of overweight? *Division of Nutrition and Physical Activity. Research to Practice Series,* No. 3.

29. Koning, L., Malik, V.S., Rimm, E.B., et al. (2011). Sugar-sweetened and artificially sweetened beverage consumption and risk of type 2 diabetes in men. *American Journal of Clinical Nutrition, 93* (67), 1321–1327.

30. Malik, V.S., & Hu, F.B. (2011). Sugar-sweetened beverages and health: Where does the evidence stand? *American Journal of Clinical Nutrition, 94* (5), 1161–1162.

31. Oaklander, M. (2012, October 19). Diet soda is doing 7 awful things to your body. *Today Show,* NBC News. www.today.com/health/diet-soda-doing-these-7-awful-things-your-body-1C6558748.

32. Centers for Disease Control and Prevention. Most Americans should consume less sodium (1,500mg/day or less). www.cdc.gov/Features/Sodium/.

33. Institutes of Medicine. (2013, May). Sodium intake in populations.

34. Zinczenko, D. (2008). *Eat this, not that.* New York: Rodale.

35. National Institute of Allergy and Infectious Diseases. (2010). Guidelines for the diagnosis and management of food allergy in the United States. www.jacionline.org/article/S0091-6749(10)01566-6/fulltext.

36. Mayo Clinic. Celiac Disease. www.mayoclinic.com/health/celiac-disease/DS00319. Accessed September 2013.

37. Howland, J., & Rohsenow, D.J. (2013). Risks of energy drinks mixed with alcohol. *Journal of American Medical Association, 309* (3), 245–246.

38. Sepkowitz, K.A. (2013). Energy drinks and caffeine-related adverse effects. *Journal of American Medical Association, 309* (3), 243–244.

39. Medical News Today. (2010). Energy drinks: Is it time to tighten regulations? www.medicalnewstoday.com/articles/206310.php.

40. Freedman, D.H. (2013, July/August). How junk food can end obesity. *The Atlantic,* 68–89. www.theatlantic.com/magazine/archive/2013/07/how-junk-food-can-end-obesity/309396/.

41. Boone-Heinonen J., Gordon-Larsn, P., Kiefe, C.I., et.al. (2011). Fast food restaurants and food stores: Longitudinal associations with diet in young to middle-aged adults: The CARDAA study. *Archives of Internal Medicine 171* (13), 1162–1170.

42. Cook, C. The food divide. (2011). *San Francisco Bay Guardian.* www.sfbg.com/2011/11/29/food.

43. Centers for Disease Control and Prevention. Recipe for food safety. *Vital signs.* www.cdc.gov/vitalsigns/listeria/index.html.

44. Stobbe, M. (2013, January 29). Study says leafy green vegetables top source of food poisoning. Associated Press. http://news.yahoo.com/study-says-leafy-greens-top-food-poisoning-source-150043222.html.

45. Zimmer, C. (2011, June 13 & 20). Rise of the superbug. *Newsweek, 157* (26), 11–12.

46. Centers for Disease Control and Prevention. (2011). CDC and food safety. www.cdc.gov/foodsafety.cdc-and-food-safety.html.

47. Centers for Disease Control and Prevention. (2011). Salmonella from dry pet food and treats. www.cdc.gov/Features/SalmonellaDryPetFood/.

48. Antibiotic Resistance Threats in the United States, 2013 Report. www.cdc.gov/drugresistance/threat-report-2013/.

49. U.S. Department of Agriculture. (2009, January 19). USDA issues final rule on mandatory country-of-origin labeling. www.usda.gov.

Chapter 6

1. Centers for Disease Control and Prevention. Facts About Physical Activity. www/cdc.gov/physicalactivity/data/facts.html.

2. American College Health Association. (2011). *ACHA, National Collegiate Health Assessment.* ACHA-NCHA Reference Group Report. www.acha.org.

3. Sharkey B.J., & Gaskill S.E. (2013). *Fitness & health.* Champaign, IL: Human Kinetics.

4. Bassuk S.S., Church T.C., & Manson J.E. (2013). We all know we should exercise. *Scientific American.* August, 764–779.

5. Bushman, B. (2011). *ACSM's complete guide to fitness and health.* Champaign, IL; Human Kinetics.

6. Morey, M.C., Snyder, D.C., Sloane, R., et al. (2009). Effects of home-based diet and exercise on functional outcomes among older, overweight, long-term cancer survivors. *Journal of the American Medical Association, 310* (18), 1883–1891.

7. Gleason, M., & Bishop N. (2013). *Exercise immunology.* Paterson, NJ: Routledge.

8. Krange, J. (2012). *Nutritional metabolism in sports, exercise, and health.* Paterson, NJ: Routledge.

9. Gamble, P. (2012). *Strength and conditioning for team sports.* Paterson, NJ: Routledge.

10. Smith D.L., & Fernhall B. (2013). *Advanced cardiovascular exercise physiology.* Champaign, IL. Human Kinetics.

11. Eklund, U., Besson, H., Luan, J., et al. (2011). Physical activity and gain in abdominal adiposity and body weight: Prospective cohort study in 288,498 men and women. *American Journal of Clinical Medicine.* www.ajcn.org/content/93/4/826.abstract.

12. Scarmeas, N., Luchsinger, J.A., Schupf, N., et al. (2009). Physical activity, diet, and risk of Alzheimer's disease. *Journal of the American Medical Association, 302* (6), 627–636.

13. Davis, C.L., Tomporowski, P.D., McDowell, J.J., et al. (2011). Exercise improves executive function and achievement and alters brain activation in overweight children. *Health Psychology, 30* (1), 91–98.

14. Church T. (2012). It's your move. *Nutrition Action Health Letter.* December 1–6.

15. Barton, J., Griffin, M., & Pretty, J. (2011). Exercise, nature, and socially interactive based initiatives improve mood and self-esteem in a clinical population. *Perspectives in Public Health.* doi: 10.1021/1757913910393862.

16. Barton, J., & Pretty, J. (2010). What is the best dose of nature and green exercise for improving mental health? A multi-study analysis. *Environmental Science and Technology, 44* (10), 3946–3955.

17. Coon, T., Boddy, K., Stein, K., et al. (2011). Does participating in physical activity in outdoor natural environments have a greater effect on physical and mental wellbeing than physical activity indoors? A systematic review. *Environmental Sciences and Technology.* doi: 110203115102046: 10,1021/es10294t.

18. Department of Health and Human Services. (2008). *2008 physical activity guidelines for Americans.* www.health.gov/paguidelines/.

19. American College of Sports Medicine. (2010). *ACSM's guidelines for exercise testing and prescription.* Baltimore: Lippincott, Williams & Wilkins.

20. Target Heart Rate Calculator. www.racedaynutrition.com/HeartRate.aspx.

21. HIT Training. www.hittraining.net/.
22. American College of Sports Medicine. (2009, March). Position stand: Progression models in resistance training for healthy adults. *Medicine & Science in Sports & Exercise, 41* (3), 687–708.
23. Juris, P.M. (n.d.). The truth on fitness: Should we use unstable surfaces? Cybex Institute. www2.cybexintl.com/education/thetruth.aspx.
24. What are the benefits of a stability ball? www.ehow.com/about_5061285 _benefits—stability-ball.html.
25. Benardot, D. (2010). *Advanced sports nutrition.* Champaign, IL: Human Kinetics.
26. Williams, M. H. (2013). *Nutrition for health, fitness and sport* (7th ed.). New York: McGraw-Hill.
27. Johnson, J. (2012). *Therapeutic stretching.* Champaign, IL: Human Kinetics.
28. Nutrition Action Health Letter. (2008, April). Chair today, gone tomorrow. 1, 3–6.
29. Duvall, J., & De Young, R. (2013). Some strategies for sustaining a walking routine: Insights from experienced walkers. *Journal of Physical Activity & Health, 10,* 10–18.
30. 10,000 Steps Program. (2003). Shape up America. www.shapeup.org.
31. Mestek, M.L., Plaisance, E., & Grandjean, P. (2008). The relationship between pedometer-determined and self-reported physical activity and body composition variables in college-aged men and women. *Journal of American College Health, 57* (1), 39–44.
32. Sisson, S.B., McClainn, J.J., & Tudor-Locke, C. (2008). Campus walkability, pedometer determined steps, and moderate-to-vigorous physical activity: A comparison of 2 university campuses. *Journal of American College Health, 56* (5), 585–592.
33. Levine, J.A., & Yeager, S. (2009). *Move a little, lose a lot.* New York: Three Rivers Press.
34. Bassett D.R., Browning R., Conger S.A., et al. (2013). Architectural design and physical activity: An observational study of staircase and elevator use in different buildings. *Journal of Physical Activity & Health, 10,* 556–562.
35. Garn A.C., Baker B.L., & Beasley E.K., et al. (2012). What are the benefits of a commercial exergaming platform for college students? Examining physical activity, enjoyment, and future intentions. *Journal of Physical Activity & Health, 9,* 311–318.
36. Graf, D.L., Pratt, L.V., Hester, C.N., et al. (2009). Playing active video games increases energy expenditure in children. *Pediatrics, 124* (2), 534–540.
37. Barnett, A., Cerin, E., & Baranowski, T. (2011). Active video games for youth: A systematic review. *Journal of Physical Activity and Health, 8* (5), 724–737.
38. Mark, R.S., and Rhodes R.E. (2013). Testing the effectiveness of exercise videogame bikes among families in the home-setting: A pilot study. *Journal of Physical Activity & Health, 10,* 211–221.
39. Lepp, A., Barkley, J.E., Sanders, G.J., et al. (2013). The relationship between cell phone use, physical and sedentary activity, and cardiorespiratory fitness in a sample of U.S. college students. *International Journal of Behavioral Nutrition and Physical Activity, 10* (79). Published online 2013 June 21, doi: 10.1186/14795868-10-79.
40. Spivock, M., Gauvin, L., Riva, M., et al. (2008). Promoting active living among people with physical disabilities: Evidence for neighborhood-level buoys. *American Journal of Preventive Medicine, 34* (4), 291–298.
41. Frank, L., & Kavage, S. (2009). A national plan for physical activity: The enabling role of the built environment. *Journal of Physical Activity and Health, 6* (suppl 2), S186–S195.
42. Armitage, C.J. (2005). Can the theory of planned behavior predict the maintenance of physical activity? *Health Psychology, 24* (3), 235–245.
43. Floyd, M.F., Crespo, C.J., & Sallis, J.F. (2008). Active living research in diverse and disadvantaged communities: Stimulating dialogue and policy solutions. *American Journal of Preventive Medicine, 34* (4), 271–274.
44. Centers for Disease Control and Prevention. (2005). Creating or improving access to places for physical activity is recommended to increase physical activity. www.thecommunityguide.org/pa/paint-create-access.pdf.
45. Sallis, J.F., Bowles, H.R., Bauman, A., et al. (2009). Neighborhood environments and physical activity among adults in 11 countries. *American Journal of Preventive Medicine, 36* (6), 484–490.
46. Duany, A. (n.d.). Smartcode: A comprehensive form-based planning ordinance. www.smartcodecentral.com.
47. Centers for Disease Control and Prevention. (n.d.). Physical activity resources for health professionals: Active environments. www.cdc.gov/nccdphp/dnpa/physical/health_professionals/active_environments/index.htm.
48. Friederichs, A.A.H., Kremers, A.P.J., Lechner, L., et al. (2013). Neighborhood walkability and walking behavior: the moderating role of action orientation. *Journal of Physical Activity & Health, 10,* 515–522.
49. Duvall J. (2012). A comparison of engagement strategies for encouraging outdoor walking. *Journal of Physical Activity and Health, 9,* 62–70.

Chapter 7
1. Ogden, C.L., Carroll, M.D., Kit, B.K., & Flegal, K.M. (2014). Prevalence of childhood and adult obesity in the United States, 2011–2012. *Journal of the American Medical Association, 311* (8):806–814.
2. Centers for Disease Control and Prevention. (2013). U.S. obesity data. www.cdc.gov.
3. World Health Organization. (n.d.). Global strategy on diet, physical activity and health: Obesity and overweight. www.who.int/dietphysicalactivity/strategy/eb11344/en/index.html.
4. Ogden, C.L., & Carroll, M.D. (2010). Prevalence of obesity among children and adolescents: United States, trends 1963–1965 through 2007–2008. NCHS Health E-Stats. www.cdc.gov.
5. Centers for Disease Control and Prevention (2012). Trends in the prevalence of extreme obesity among US preschool-aged children living in low-income families, 1998–2010. *Journal of the American Medical Association, 308* (24), 2563–2565
6. Gallagher, D., Heymsfield, S.B., Heo, M., et al. (2000). Healthy percentage body fat ranges: An approach for developing guidelines based on body mass index. *American Journal of Clinical Nutrition, 72* (3), 694–701.
7. Bray, G.A. (2003). *An atlas of obesity and weight control.* New York: Parthenon Publishing Group.
8. Loomba, L.A., & Styne, D.M. (2009). Effect of puberty on body composition: Current opinion in endocrinology. *Diabetes and Obesity, 16,* 10–15.
9. Tchernof, A., & Despres, J.P. (2013). Pathophysiology of human visceral obesity: An update. *Physiology Review, 93* (1), 359–404.
10. Aviram, A., Hod, M., & Yogev, Y. (2011). Maternal obesity: Implications for pregnancy outcome and long-term risks a link to maternal nutrition. *International Journal of Gynecology and Obstetrics, 115* (S1), S6–S10.
11. Flegal, K.M., Kit, B.K., Orpana, H., & Graubard, B.I. (2013). Association of all-cause mortality with overweight and obesity using standard body mass index categories: a systematic review and meta-analysis. *Journal of the American Medical Association, 309* (1), 71–82.
12. Masters, R.K., Reighter, E.N., Powers, D.A., et al. (2013). The impact of obesity of U.S. mortality levels: The importance of age and cohort factors in population estimates. *American Journal of Public Health, 103* (10), 1895–1901.
13. Fradkin, J.E. (2012). Confronting the urgent challenge of diabetes: An overview. *Health Affairs, 31* (1), 12–19.
14. Puhl, R., & Brownell, K. D. (2001, December). Bias, discrimination, and obesity. *Obesity Research, 9* (12), 788–805.
15. Dor, A., Ferguson, C., et al. (2011). Gender and race wage gaps attributable to obesity. George Washington University and School of Public Health. www.gwumc.edu/sphhs/departments/healthpolicy/dhp_publications/pub_uploads/dhpPublication_FA85CB 82-5056-9D20-3DBD361E605324F2.pdf.

16. Sutin, A.R., & Terracciano, A. (2013). Perceived weight discrimination and obesity. *PLoS One, 8* (7), e70048.

17. El-Sayed Moustafa, J.S., & Froguel, P. (2013) From obesity genetics to the future of personalized obesity therapy. *Nature Reviews Endocrinology, 9,* 402–413.

18. Neary, M.T., & Batterham, R.L. (2009). Gut hormones: Implications for the treatment of obesity. *Pharmacology and Therapeutics, 124* (1), 44–56.

19. Berthoud, H. (2012). The neurobiology of food intake in an obesogenic environment. *Proceedings of the Nutrition Society, 71,* 478-487.

20. Guyenet, S.J., & Schwartz, M.W. (2012). Regulation of food intake, energy balance, and body fat mass: Implications for the pathogenesis and treatment of obesity. *Journal of Clinical Endocrinology and Metabolism, 97,* 745–755.

21. Youngson, N.A., & Morris, M.J. (2013) What obesity research tells us about epigenetic mechanisms. *Philosophical Transactions of the Royal Society Biological Sciences, 368,* 20110337.

22. Centers for Disease Control and Prevention. (2011). Physical activity levels of high school students—United States, 2010. *MMWR, 60,* 773–777.

23. Kwan, M.Y., Cairney, J., Faulkner, G.E., & Pullenayegum, E.E. (2012). Physical activity and other health related behaviors during the transition to early adulthood. *American Journal of Preventive Medicine, 42* (1), 14–20.

24. Girz, L, Polivy, J., Provencher, V., et al. (2013). The four undergraduate years: Changes in weight, eating attitudes and depression. *Appetite, 69,* 145–150.

25. Drewnowski, A., & Eichelsdoerfer, P. (2009). Can low-income Americans afford a healthy diet? *CPHN Public Health Research Brief.* www.cphn.org/reports/brief1.pdf.

26. Darmon, N., & Drewnowski, A. (2008). Does social class predict diet quality? *American Journal of Clinical Nutrition, 87* (5), 1107–1117.

27. Giskes, K., Lenthe, F., et al. (2011). A systematic review of environmental factors and obesogenic dietary intakes among adults: Are we getting closer to understanding obesogenic environments? *Obesity Reviews, 12,* e95–e106.

28. Crombie, A.P., Ilich, J.Z., Dutton, G.R., et al. (2009). The freshman weight gain phenomenon revisited. *Nutrition Reviews, 67* (2), 83–94.

29. Wang, Y., & Beydom, M.A. (2007). The obesity epidemic in the United States—Gender, age, socioeconomic, racial/ethnic, and geographic characteristics: A systematic review and meta-regression analysis. *Epidemiologic Review, 29* (1), 6–28.

30. Gunderson, E., & Abrams, B. (2000). Epidemiology of gestational weight gain and body weight changes after pregnancy. *Epidemiology Reviews, 22* (2), 261–274.

31. American College Health Association. (2013, Spring). *American college health association—National college health assessment II: Reference group executive summary Spring 2013.* Hanover, MD: American College Health Association.

32. National Center for Chronic Disease Prevention and Health Promotion, Division of Nutrition and Physical Activity. (2006). Do increased portion sizes affect how much we eat? (Research to Practice Series, No. 2.) Centers for Disease Control and Prevention. www.cdc.gov/nccdphp/dnpa/nutrition/pdf/portion_size_research.pdf.

33. New Menu and Vending Machines Labeling Requirements. U.S. Food and Drug Administration. www.fda.gov/Food/LabelingNutrition/ucm217762.htm.

34. Papas, M.A., Alberg, A.J., Ewing, R., et al. (2007). The built environment and obesity. *Epidemiological Reviews, 29,* 129–143.

35. Ding, D., Sallis, J.F., Kerr, J., et al. (2011). Neighborhood environment and physical activity among youth: A review. *American Journal of Preventive Medicine, 41* (4), 442–455.

36. The Nielsen Company. (2011). State of the media trends in TV viewing—2011 TV Upfront. http://blog.nielsen.com/nielsenwire/wp-content/uploads/2011/04/State-of-the-Media-2011-TV-Upfronts.pdf.

37. Zick, C.D., Stevens, R.B., et al. (2011). Time use choices and healthy body weight: A multivariate analysis of data from the American Time Use Survey. *International Journal of Behavior, Nutrition and Physical Activity, 8,* 84.

38. Owen, N., Sugiyama, T., Eakin, E.E., Gardiner, P.A., et al. (2011). Adults' sedentary behavior: Determinants and interventions. *American Journal of Preventive Medicine, 41* (2), 189–196.

39. Nielsen, L.S., Danielsen, K.V., & Sorenson, T.I.A. (2011). Short sleep duration as a possible cause of obesity: A critical analysis of the epidemiological evidence. *Obesity Review, 12* (2), 78–92.

40. Mitchell, J.A., Rodriguez, D., Schmitz, K.H., et al. (2013). Sleep duration and adolescent obesity. *Pediatrics, 131* (5), e1428–e1434.

41. Christakis, N.A., & Fowler, J.H. (2007). The spread of obesity in a large social network over 32 years. *New England Journal of Medicine, 357* (4), 370–379.

42. Leroux, J.S., Moore, S., & Dubé, L. (2013). Beyond the "I" in the obesity epidemic: A review of social relational and network interventions on obesity. *Journal of Obesity, 2013,* Article ID 348249, 10 pages, 2013. doi:10.1155/2013/348249.

43. Market Data Enterprises Inc. (2011). *The U.S. weight loss and diet control market* (11th ed.). Tampa, FL: Author.

44. Sacks, F.M., Bray, G.A., Carey, V.J., Smith, S.R., et al. (2009). Comparison of weight-loss diets with different compositions of fat, protein and carbohydrates. *New England Journal of Medicine, 360* (9), 859–873.

45. Tsai, A.G., & Wadden, T.A. (2005). Systematic review: An evaluation of major commercial weight loss programs in the United States. *Annals of Internal Medicine, 142* (1), 56–67.

46. Colman, E. (2012). Obesity: Food and Drug Administration's obesity drug guidance document. *Circulation, 125,* 2156–2164.

47. Colman, E., Golden, J., Roberts, M., Egan, A., et al. (2012). The FDA's assessment of two drugs for chronic weight management. *New England Journal of Medicine, 367,* 1577–1579.

48. Rueda-Clausen, C.F., Padwal, R.S., & Sharma, A.M. (2013). New pharmacological approaches for obesity management. *Nature Reviews Endocrinology, 9,* 467–478.

49. Neff, K J.H., & le Roux, C.W. (2013). Bariatric surgery: A best practice article. *Journal of Clinical Pathology, 66,* 90–98.

50. Poddar, K., Kolge, S., Bezman, L., et al (2011). Nutraceutical supplements for weight loss: A systematic review. *Nutrition in Clinical Practice, 26* (5), 539–552.

51. International Size Acceptance Association. www.size-acceptance.org.

52. National Association to Advance Fat Acceptance. www.naafaonline.com/dev2/.

53. Spark, A. (2001). Health at any size: The self-acceptance non-diet movement. *Journal of the American Medical Association, 56* (2), 69–72.

Chapter 8

1. Neighbor, L.A., & Sobal, J. (2007). Prevalence and magnitude of body weight and shape dissatisfaction among university students. *Eating Behaviors, 8* (4), 429–439.

2. Cramblitt, B., & Pritchard, M. (2013). Media influence on the drive for muscularity in undergraduates. *Eating Behaviors, 14* (4), 441–446.

3. Morris, A.M., & Katzman, D.K. (2003). The impact of the media on eating disorders in children and adolescents. *Adolescent Medicine, 14* (1), 109–118.

4. Derenne, J.L., & Beresin, E.V. (2006). Body image, media, and eating disorders. *Academic Psychiatry, 30* (3), 181–198.

5. Striegel-Moore, R.H., & Bulik, C.M. (2007). Risk factors for eating disorders. *American Psychologist, 62* (3), 181–198.

6. Hogan, M.J., & Strasburger, V.C. (2008). Body image, eating disorders, and the media. *Adolescent Medicine State of the Art Review, 19* (3), 521–546.

7. Grave, D.R. (2011, April). Eating disorder: Progress and challenges. *European*

Journal of International Medicine, 22 (2), 153–160.

8. Barlett, C.P., Vowels, C.L., & Saucier, D.A. (2008). Meta-analysis of the effects of media images on men's body-image concerns. *Journal of Social and Clinical Psychology, 27* (3), 279–310.

9. Blond, A. (2008). Impacts of exposures to images of ideal bodies on male body dissatisfaction: A review. *Body Image, 5* (3), 244–250.

10. Kanayama, G., & Pope, H. (2011). Gods, men and muscle dysmorphia. *Harvard Review of Psychiatry, 19* (2), 95–98.

11. Hudson, J.I., Hiripi, E., Pope, H.G., & Kessler, R.C. (2007). The prevalence and correlates of eating disorders in the National Comorbidity Survey Replication. *Biological Psychiatry, 61*, 348–358.

12. Hautala, L.A., Junnila, J., Helenius, H., et al. (2008). Towards understanding gender differences in disordered eating among adolescents. *Journal of Clinical Nursing, 17* (3), 1803–1813.

13. American Psychiatric Association. (2013). *Diagnostic and statistical manual of mental disorders* (5th ed., DSM-5). Washington, DC: American Psychiatric Association Press.

14. Quick, V.M., & Byrd-Bredbenner, C. (2014). Disordered eating, socio-cultural media influences, body image and psychological factors among a racially/ethnically diverse population of college women. *Eating Behaviors, 15* (1), 37–41.

15. Webb, J.B., Warren-Findlow, J., et al. (2013). Do you see what I see?: An exploration of inter-ethnic ideal body size comparisons among college women. *Body Image, 10* (3), 369–379.

16. Gillen, M.M., & Lefkowitz, E.S. (2012 January 9). Gender and racial/ethnic differences in body image development among college students. *Body Image, 9* (1), 126–130.

17. Ricciardelli, L.A., McCabe, M.P., Williams, R.J., & Thompson, J.K. (2007). The role of ethnicity and culture in body image and disordered eating among males. *Clinical Psychology Review, 27*, 582–606.

18. Becker, A.E. (2007). Culture and eating disorders classification. *International Journal of Eating Disorders, 40* (Suppl. 3), S111–S116.

19. Sundgot-Borgen, J., & Torstveit, M.K. (2010). Aspects of disordered eating continuum in elite high intensity sports. *Scandinavian Journal of Medicine and Science in Sports, 20* (2), 112–121.

20. Berg, K.C., Frazier, P., & Sherr, L. (2009). Changes in eating disorder attitudes and behavior in college women: Prevalence and predictors. *Eating Behaviors, 10* (3), 137–142.

21. Klump, K.L., Bulik, C.M., Kaye, W.H., et al. (2009). Academy for Eating Disorders position paper: Eating disorders are serious mental illnesses. *International Journal of Eating Disorders, 42* (2), 97–103.

22. Alvy, L. (2013). Do lesbian women have a better body image? Comparisons with heterosexual women and model of lesbian specific factors. *Body Image, 10* (4), 524–534.

23. Smith, A.R., Hawkswood, S.E., Bodell, L.P., & Joiner, T.E. (2011). Muscularity versus leanness: An examination of body ideals and predictors of disordered eating in heterosexual and gay college students. *Body Image, 8* (3), 232–236.

24. Feldman, M.B., & Meyer, I.H. (2007). Eating disorders in diverse lesbian, gay and bisexual populations. *International Journal of Eating Disorders, 40* (3), 218–226.

25. Dingemans, A.E., & van Furth, V.F. (2011). Binge eating disorder psychopathology in normal weight and obese individuals. *International Journal of Eating Disorders, 45* (1), 135–138.

26. Arcelus, J., Mitchell, A.J., Wales, J., & Nielsen, S. (2011). Mortality rates in patients with anorexia nervosa and other eating disorders. *Archives of General Psychiatry, 68* (7), 724–731.

27. Ecklund, K., Vajapeyam, S., Feldman, H.A., et al. (2010). Bone marrow changes in adolescent girls with anorexia nervosa. *Journal of Bone and Mineral Research, 25* (2), 298–304.

28. Steinhausen, H.C., & Weber, S. (2009). The outcome of bulimia nervosa: Findings from one-quarter century of research. *American Journal of Psychiatry, 166* (12), 1331–1341.

29. Steinhausen, H.C. (2009). Outcome of eating disorders. *Child and Adolescent Psychiatric Clinics of North America, 18* (1), 225–242.

30. Walsh, B.T. (2013). The enigmatic persistence of anorexia nervosa. *American Journal of Psychiatry, 170*, 477–484.

31. Sim, L.A., et al. (2010). Identification and treatment of eating disorders in the primary care setting. *Mayo Clinic Proceedings, 85* (8), 746–751.

32. Pavan, C., Simonato, P., Marini, M., et al. (2008). Psychopathologic aspects of body dysmorphic disorder: A literature review. *Aesthetic Plastic Surgery, 32*, 473–484.

33. Tadisina, K.K., Chopra, K., & Singh, D.P. (2013). Body dysmorphic disorder in plastic surgery. *Eplasty, 13*, ic48.

34. National Institute on Drug Abuse. (n.d.). NIDA InfoFacts: Steroids (anabolic-androgenic). National Institute of Health. www.drugabuse.gov/infofacts/steroids.html.

35. American Society for Aesthetic Plastic Surgery (2013). Quick facts: Highlights of the ASAPS 2012 Statistics on Cosmetic Surgery. www.surgery.org/sites/default/files/2012-quickfacts.pdf.

36. Swami, V. (2011). Marked for life? A prospective study of tattoos on appearance anxiety and dissatisfaction, perceptions of uniqueness, and self-esteem. *Body Image, 8* (3). 237–244.

37. Bergstrom, K.G. (2013). Tattoo removal: New laser options. *Journal of Drugs in Dermatology, 12* (4), 492–493.

38. GS Blog. (2013, October 30). Dove and Girl Scouts bring you "Free Being Me." http://blog.girlscouts.org/2013/10/dove-and-girl-scouts-bring-you-free.html

39. Student Bodies Prevention Program. National Association of Anorexia Nervosa and Associated Eating Disorders. www.anad.org/get-help/online-program/.

Chapter 9

1. In the Know Zone. (2011). Prevalence of binge drinking. www.intheknowzone.com/substance-abuse-topics/binge-drinking/statistics.html.

2. Singleton, R.A., & Wolfson, A.R. (2009). Alcohol consumption, sleep, and academic performance among college students. *Journal of Studies of Alcohol, 70* (3), 355–363.

3. Parks, K.A., Hsieh, Y.P., Collins, R.L., et al. (2009). Predictors of risky sexual behavior with new and regular partners in a sample of women bar drinkers. *Journal of Studies of Alcohol, 70* (2), 197–205.

4. Highland K.B., Hersschl L.C., Klanecky A., et al. (2013). Bioppsychosocial pathways to alcohol-related problems. *American Journal on Addictions, 22* (4), 366–372.

5. National Institute on Alcohol Abuse and Alcoholism. (2009). *Rethinking drinking.* NIH Publication No. 09-3770. Washington, DC: U.S. Department of Health and Human Services.

6. National Institute on Alcohol Abuse and Alcoholism; National Institutes of Health. (2000). *Alcohol and health.* Washington, DC: U.S. Department of Health and Human Services.

7. Huff, R.M., & Kline, M.V. (1999). Health promotion in the context of culture. In R.M. Huff & M.V. Kline (Eds.), *Promoting health in multicultural populations.* Thousand Oaks, CA: Sage.

8. Hodge, F.S., & Fredericks, L. (1999). American Indian and Alaska native populations in the United States: An overview. In R.M. Huff & M.V. Kline (Eds.), *Promoting health in multicultural populations.* Thousand Oaks, CA: Sage.

9. American College Health Association. (Spring 2012). *American College Health Association–National College Health Assessment Reference Group data report.* www.acha.org.

10. National Center on Addiction and Substance Abuse. (2007). *Wasting the best and the brightest: Substance abuse at America's colleges and universities.* New York: Columbia University.

11. Wechsler, H. (2000). *Binge drinking on America's college campuses: Findings*

from the Harvard School of Public Health College Alcohol Study. www.hsph.harvard.edu/cas/Documents.monograph_2000cas_mono_2000pdf.

12. Nelson, T.F., Naimi, T.S., Brewer, R.D., et al. (2005). The state sets the rate: The relationship among state-specific college binge drinking rates, and selected state alcohol control policies. *American Journal of Public Health, 95* (3), 441–446.

13. HAMS Harm Reduction Network. (2012). Heavy drinking. *HAMS: Harm reduction for alcohol.* http://hamsnetwork.org/heavy/.

14. Mohler, K., Dowdall, M., Koss, G.W., et al. (2004). Correlates of rape while intoxicated in a national sample of college women. *Journal of Studies on Alcohol, 65* (1), 37–45.

15. Haydocy A. (2011). Pregaming and use of alcoholic energy drinks: Underage and legal age college students. *Proceedings of the National Conference on Undergraduate Research (NCUR).* Ithaca College, New York, March 31–April 2.

16. Hass, A.L., Smith, S.K., and Kagan, K. (2013). Getting "game": Pregaming changes during the first weeks of college. *Journal of American College Health, 61* (2), 95–105

17. Trauma Foundation. Alcohol and spring break. www.traumaaf.org/featured/3-14-02springbreak.shtml.

18. Buddy T. (2013, March 10). Spring break is potentially life threatening. Alcoholism: *About.com.* http://alcoholism.about.com/cs/college/a/aa020318a.htm.

19. Ksir, C., Hart, C.L., & Ray, O. (2006). *Drugs, society, and human behavior* (11th ed.). New York: McGraw-Hill.

20. Centers for Disease Control and Prevention. (2013, October 11). Binge drinking: A serious, under-recognized problem among women. *Vital Signs.* www.cdc.gov/vitalsigns/bingedrinkingfemale/index.html.

21. National Institute on Alcohol Abuse and Alcoholism. (2004). Alcohol's damaging effects on the brain. *Alcohol Alert.* http://pubs.niaaa.nih.gov/publications/aa63/aa63.htm.

22. Wingert, P. (2010, November 22). Why it's so risky. *Newsweek,* p. 14.

23. Breen, S. Would you smoke a beer? People are inhaling alcohol. *Greatist.* http://greatist.com/health/inhaling-alcohol-061213.

24. Health Check Systems. Alcohol—It's effect on your body and health. www.healthchecksystems.com/alcohol.htm.

25. Meekis, L. (2013, Sep 8). Beer and alcohol enemas: A drinker's death-wish. *Yahoo! Voices.* http://voices.yahoo.com/beer-alcohol-enemas-drinkers-deathwish-2489511/html?cat+5/.

26. National Institute on Alcohol Abuse and Alcoholism. (2011). Interactive body content. *College drinking: Changing the culture.* http://collegedrinkingprevention.gov/Collegestudents/anatomy/Body_nonflash.aspx.

27. Nelson, D.E., Jarman, D.W., Rehm, J., et al. (2013). Alcohol-attributable cancer deaths and years of potential. *American Journal of Public Health, 103* (4), 641–648.

28. Chen, W.Y., Rosner, B., & Hankinson, S.E. (2011). Moderate alcohol consumption during adult life, drinking patterns, and breast cancer risk. *Journal of the American Medical Association, 306* (17), 1884–1890.

29. Barry, A.E., & Piazza-Gardner, A.K. (2012). Drunkorexia: Understanding the co-occurrence of alcohol consumption and eating/exercise weight management behaviors. *Journal of American College Health, 60* (3), 236–243.

30. Bryant, J.B., Darkes, J., & Rahal, C. (2012). College students compensatory eating and behaviors in response to alcohol consumption. *Journal of American College Health, 60* (5), 350–356.

31. Cherpitel, C.J., Martin, G., Macdonald, S., et al. (2013). Alcohol and drug use as predictors of intentional injuries in two emergency departments in British Columbia. *American Journal on Addictions, 22* (2), 87–92.

32. Office of Applied Studies. (2006). Alcohol and drug use: 2004–2005. *National survey on drug use and health* (DHHS Publication No. SMA 05-4061). Rockville, MD: U.S. Department of Health and Human Services.

33. Mercken, M., & de Cabo, R. (2010). A toast to your health, one drink at a time. *American Journal of Clinical Nutrition, 92* (1), 1–2. http://ajcn.org/content/92/1/1.full.

34. Greenfield, T.K., & Kerr, W.C. (2011). Tracking alcohol consumption over time. National Institute of Alcohol Abuse and Alcoholism. Pubs.niaanih.gov.

35. Szalavitz, M. (2013, January 23.) Mental health manual changes may turn binge drinkers into mild alcoholics. *Time.* http://healthland.time.com/2013/01/23/revisions-to-mental-health-manual-may-turn-binge-drinkers-into-mild-alcoholics/.

36. Difulvio, G., Linowski, S., Mazzioti, J., et al. (2012). Effectiveness of the brief alcohol and screening intervention for college students (BASICS) program with a mandated population. *Journal of American College Health, 60* (4), 269–280.

37. Paschall, M.J., Antin, T., Ringwalt, C.L., et al. (2011). Evaluation of an Internet-based alcohol misuse prevention course for college freshmen: Findings of a randomized multi-campus trial. *American Journal of Preventive Medicine, 41* (3), 300–308.

38. Weschler, H., & Nelson, T.F. (2010). Will increasing alcohol availability by lowering the minimum legal drinking age decrease drinking and related consequences among youths? *American Journal of Public Health, 100* (6), 986–992.

39. Lo, C.C., Weber, J., & Cheng, T. (2013). A spatial analysis of student binge drinking, alcohol-outlet density, and social disadvantages. *American Journal on Addictions, 22* (4), 391–401.

40. Williams, J., Chaloupka, F.J., & Wechsler, H. (2002, January). Are there differential effects of price and policy on college students' drinking intensity? ImpacTeen Research Paper Series, no. 16. www.impacteen.org/generalarea_PDFs/differentialeffectsJan2002_final.pdf.

41. Harwood, E.M., Erickson, D.J., Fabian, L.E.A., et al. (2003). Effects of communities, neighborhoods and stores on retail pricing and promotion of beer. *Journal of Studies on Alcohol, 64* (5), 720–726.

42. Centers for Disease Control and Prevention. (2012). Current cigarette smoking among adults—United States, 2011. *Journal of American Medical Association, 309* (6), 539–541.

43. Centers for Disease Control and Prevention. (2013, February). Adult smoking: Focusing on people with mental illness. *Vital Signs.* www.cdc.gov/vitalsigns/SmokingAndMentalIllness/.

44. Centers for Disease Control and Prevention. (2011). Adult cigarette smoking in the United States: Current estimate. www.cdc.gov/tobacco/data_statistics/fact_sheets/adult_data/cig_smoking/.

45. U.S. Department of Health and Human Services. (2000). *Tobacco use among U.S. racial/ethnic minority groups—African Americans, American Indians and Alaska Natives, Asian Americans and Pacific Islanders, and Hispanics: A report of the surgeon general.* Atlanta, GA: U.S. Department of Health and Human Services.

46. E-Cigarette Dangers (blog). (2012, April 11). New York Times shed light on E-cigarette dangers. http://e-cigarettedangers.com/

47. Trumbo, C.W., & Harper, R. (2013). Use and perception of electronic cigarettes among college students. *Journal of American College Health, 61* (3), 149–155.

48. American College Health Association. (2011, Spring). *American College Health Association–National College Health Assessment (ACHA-NCHA-II) reference group report.* www.acha-ncha.org/docs/ACHA-NCHA-II_ReferenceGroup_DataReport_Spring2011.pdf.

49. Sharma E., Beck K.H., & Clark P.I. (2013). Social context of smoking hookah among college students: Scale development and validation. *Journal of American College Health, 61* (4), 204–211.

50. Centers for Disease Control and Prevention. (2013, December 17). Hookahs. *Smoking and Tobacco Use.* www.cdc .gov/tobacco/data_statistics/fact_sheets/ tobacco_industry/hookahs/.

51. National Cancer Institute. (n.d.). Smokeless tobacco and cancer. *Fact Sheet.* www.cancer.gov/cancertopics/factsheet/ Tobacco/smokeless.

52. Surgeon General. (2010). *How tobacco smoke causes disease.* Atlanta, GA: U.S. Department of Health and Human Services.

53. National Cancer Institute. (n.d.). Questions and answers about cigar smoking and cancer. *Fact Sheet.* www.cancer.gov/ cancertopics/factsheet/tobacco/cigars.

54. Goren, S.S., & Schnoll, R.A. (2006). Smoking cessation. In S.S. Goren & J. Arnold (Eds.), *Health promotion in practice.* San Francisco: Jossey-Bass.

55. Ulrich, J., Meyer, C., Jurgen, H., et al. (2006). Predictors of increased body mass index following cessation of smoking. *American Journal of Addiction, 15* (2), 192–197.

56. Centers for Disease Control and Prevention. (2011). Inhaling tobacco smoke causes immediate harm. *CDC Features.* www.cdc.gov/Features/smokeExposure.

57. Centers for Disease Control and Prevention. (2011). Health effects of secondhand smoke. *Smoking and Tobacco Use.* www .cdc.gov/tobacco/data_statistics/ fact_sheets/secondhand_smoke/ health_effects/.

58. Centers for Disease Control and Prevention. (2011). Tobacco use, smoking and secondhand smoke. *Vital Signs.* www.cdc.gov/VitalSigns/TobaccoUse/ SecondhandSmoke/.

59. U.S. Department of Health and Human Services. (2006). *The health consequences of involuntary exposure to tobacco smoke: A report of the U.S. surgeon general.* Rockville, MD: U.S. Department of Health and Human Services.

60. National Cancer Institute. (n.d.). Cigarette smoking and cancer. *Fact Sheet.* www .cancer.gov/cancertopics/factsheet/ tobacco/cancer.

61. Kenfield, S.A., Stampfer, M.J., Rosner, B.A., et al. (2008). Smoking and smoking cessation in relation to mortality in women. *American Journal of Preventive Medicine, 299* (17), 2037–2047.

62. Larabee, L. C. (2005). To what extent do smokers plan quit attempts? *Tobacco Control, 14* (6), 425–428.

63. Food and Drug Administration. (2012, December 12). FDA 101: Smoking cessation products. www.fda.gov/ ForConsumers/ConsumerUpdates/ ucm198176.htm.

64. Reinberg, S. (2009). Anti-smoking drugs get FDA "black-box" warning. *HealthDay News.* www.healthday.com/Article .asp?AID=628667.

65. Americans for Nonsmokers' Rights. (2003). Recipe for a smoke free society. www.no-smoke.org.

66. Wikipedia. (2014, February 4). List of smoking bans in the United States. http:// en.wikipedia.org/wiki/List_of_smoking _bans_in_the_United_States.

67. Parascandola, M. (2011). Tobacco harm reduction and the evolution of nicotine dependence. *American Journal of Public Health, 101* (4), 632–641.

68. Centers for Disease Control and Prevention. (2011). Tobacco controls have public health impact. *CDC Features.* www.cdc.gov/Features/ tobaccoControls/.

69. Glantz, S.A. (2003). *Tobacco biology and politics.* Waco, TX: Health Edco.

70. Villant, A.C. (2011). Food and Drug Administration regulation of tobacco: Integrating science, law, policy, and advocacy. *American Journal of Public Health, 101* (7), 1160–1162.

71. Americans for Nonsmokers' Rights. (2014, January 2). Going smokefree: Colleges and universities. www.no-smoke.org/ goingsmokefree.php?id=447.

72. Fennell, R. (2012). Should college campuses become tobacco free without an enforcement plan? *Journal of American College Health, 60* (7), 491–494.

Chapter 10

1. National Center on Addiction and Substance Abuse. (2007). *Wasting the best and the brightest: Substance abuse at America's colleges and universities.* New York: Columbia University Press.

2. Substance Abuse and Mental Health Services Administration. (2013). *Results from the 2012 National survey on drug use and health: Summary of national findings,* NSDUH Series H-46, HHS Publication No. (SMA) 13-4795. Rockville, MD: Substance Abuse and Mental Health Services Administration.

3. American Psychiatric Association. (2013). *Diagnostic and statistical manual of mental disorders* 5. Washington DC: American Psychiatric Association Press.

4. National Institute of Drug Abuse. (2012, December). The science of drug abuse and addiction. *Media guide.* www .drugabuse.gov/publications/media-guide/ science-drug-abuse-addiction.

5. Saal, D., Dong, Y., Bonci, A., & Malenka, R. (2003). Drugs of abuse and stress trigger a common synaptic adaptation in dopamine neurons. *Neuron, 37* (4), 577–582.

6. National Institute on Drug Abuse. (2010, March). InfoFacts: Cocaine. www.nida .nih.gov/Infofacts/cocaine.html.

7. National Institute on Drug Abuse. (2010, March). InfoFacts: Methamphetamine. www.nida.nih.gov/ infofacts/methamphetamine.html.

8. National Institute on Drug Abuse. (2010, December). InfoFacts: MDMA (Ecstasy). www.drugabuse.gov/publications/ infofacts/mdma-ecstasy.

9. National Institute on Drug Abuse. (2010, December). InfoFacts: Synthetic Cathinones ("Bath Salts"). www .drugabuse.gov/publications/drugfacts/ synthetic-cathinones-bath-salts.

10. National Institute on Drug Abuse. (2010, July). InfoFacts: Club drugs (GHB, Ketamine, Rohypnol). www .drugabuse.gov/publications/infofacts/ club-drugs-ghb-ketamine-rohypnol.

11. Hart, C., Ksir, C., & Ray, O. (2009). *Drugs, society and human behavior* (13th ed.). New York: McGraw-Hill.

12. National Institute on Drug Abuse. (2010, March). InfoFacts: Heroin. www.drugabuse .gov/publications/infofacts/heroin.

13. Daubresse, M., Chang, H., Yu, Y., Viswanathan, S., et al. (2013, October). Ambulatory diagnosis and treatment of nonmalignant pain in the United States, 2000–2010. *Medical Care, 51* (10), 870–878.

14. National Institute on Drug Abuse. (2009, June). InfoFacts: Hallucinogens—LSD, Peyote, Psilocybin, & PCP. www.google. com/search?client=safari&rls=en&q= hallucinogens+infofacts&ie=UTF-8 &oe=UTF-8.

15. National Institute on Drug Abuse. (2010, March). InfoFacts: Inhalants. www.drugabuse.gov/publications/ infofacts/inhalants.

16. Johnston, L., O'Malley, P., Miech, R., Bachman J., & Schulenberg, J. (2014). 2013 Overview: Key findings on adolescent drug use. *Monitoring the future: National survey results on drug use, 1975–2013.* Ann Arbor, MI: University of Michigan, Institute for Social Research, NIDA, NIH.

17. National Institute on Drug Abuse. (2010, November). InfoFacts: Marijuana. www.drugabuse.gov/publications/ infofacts/marijuana.

18. National Institute on Drug Abuse. (2011, December). InfoFacts: Spice. www .drugabuse.gov/publications/infofacts/ spice.

19. U.S. Department of Justice. (2011, April). *The impact of illicit drug use on American society.* Washington, DC: National Drug Intelligence Center.

20. The National Center on Addiction and Substance at Columbia University. (2009). *Shoveling it up II: The impact of substance abuse on federal, state and local budgets.* www.casacolumbia.org.

21. National Institute on Drug Abuse. (2011, May). InfoFacts: Drug related hospital emergency room visits. www.drugabuse

.gov/publications/infofacts/drug-related -hospital-emergency-room-visits.

22. National Institute on Drug Abuse. (2011, May). Topics in brief: Treating offenders with drug problems: Integrating public health and public safety. www.drugabuse .gov/publications/topics-in-brief/treating -offenders-drug-problems-integrating -public-health-public-safety.

23. Glaze, S. (1995). Treating addiction. *Congressional Quarterly Researcher, 5* (1), 1–24.

24. Califano, J. (1998). Crime and punishment —and treatment too. National Center of Addiction and Substance Abuse at Columbia University. www.casacolumbia.org.

25. National Institute on Drug Abuse. (2009, September). InfoFacts: Treatment approaches for drug addiction. www .drugabuse.gov/publications/infofacts/ treatment-approaches-drug-addiction.

26. Marlatt, G.A., Larimer, M., & Witkiewitz, K. (Eds.). (2012). *Harm reduction: Pragmatic strategies for managing high-risk behaviors.* New York: Guilford.

27. Drug Policy Alliance. (2010). Reducing drug harm. www.drugpolicy.org/issues/ reducing-drug-harm.

28. Visser, S.N., Danielson, M.L., Bitsko, R.H., Holbrook, J.R., Kogan, M.D., Ghandour, R.M., Perou, R., & Blumberg, S.J. (2013). Trends in the parent-report of health care provider-diagnosed and medicated ADHD disorder: United States, 2003–2011. *Journal of the American Academy of Child and Adolescent Psychiatry*, 53, (1): 34–46.

Chapter 11

1. Hutcherson, H. (2002). *What your mother never told you about sex.* New York: Putnam.

2. Abramson, P.R., & Pinkerton, S.D. (1995). *With pleasure: Thoughts on the nature of sexuality.* New York: Oxford University Press.

3. Yarber, W.L., Sayad, B.W., & Strong, B. (2010). *Human sexuality: Diversity in contemporary America* (7th ed.). New York: McGraw-Hill.

4. Olson, D.H., & Defrain, J. (2003). *Marriage and families: Intimacy, diversity, and strength* (4th ed.). New York: McGraw-Hill.

5. Sanders, S.A. (2006). Issue 3: Is Masters and Johnson's model an accurate description of sexual response? In T. Williams (Ed.), *Taking sides: Clashing views and controversial issues in human sexuality.* New York: McGraw-Hill.

6. Caron, S.L. (2007). *Sex matters for college students.* Upper Saddle River, NJ: Pearson/Prentice Hall.

7. Basson, R. (2000). The female sexual response: A different model. *Journal of Sex and Marital Therapy, 26,* 51–65.

8. Godson, S. (2002). *The sex book.* London: Cassell Illustrated.

9. Wingert, P., & Kantrowitz, B. (2007, January 15). The new prime time. *Newsweek,* 39–50, 53–54.

10. Wald, M. (2005). Male infertility: Causal cures. *Sexuality, Reproduction and Menopause, 3* (2), 83–87.

11. Milsten, R., & Slowinski, J. (1999). *The sexual male: Problems and solutions.* New York: Norton.

12. Hughes, S.M., Harrison, M.A., and Gallup, G.G. (2007). Sex differences in romantic kissing among college students: An evolutionary perspective. *Evolutionary Psychology, 5,* 612–631.

13. Regan, P.C., Shen, W., de la Peña, E., et al. (2007). "Fireworks exploded in my mouth:" Affective responses before, during, and after the very first kiss. *International Journal of Sexual Health, 19* (20), 1–16.

14. Bullough, V.L. (2005). Masturbation: 100 years ago and now. *Journal of Sex Research, 42* (2), 175–176.

15. Silverberg C. Latex versus non-latex condoms. *About.com.* http://sexuality .about.com/od/contraception/a/ latexfreecondom.htm/.

16. Boskey, E. (2014, February 3). The hidden dangers of nonoxynol-9. *About.com.* http://std.about.com/od/prevention/a/ n9increaserisk.htm.

17. Sessions Stepp, L. (2007). *How young women pursue sex, delay love, and lose at both.* New York: Riverhead Books.

18. U.S. Department of Health and Human Services. (2004). The surgeon general's call to action to promote sexual health and responsible sexual behavior. www.ejhs.org/volume4/calltoaction.htm.

19. Urology Channel. (2003). Female sexual dysfunction. www.urologychannel.com/ fsd/index.shtml.

20. Crawford, M., & Popp, D. (2003). Sexual double standards: A review and methodological critique of two decades of research. *The Journal of Sex Research, 40* (1), 13–26.

21. Levin, R.J. (2005). The mechanisms of human ejaculation: A critical analysis. *Sexual and Relationship Therapy, 20* (1), 123–131.

22. American College Health Association. (2011, Spring). *American College Health Association–National College Health Assessment (ACHA-NCHA-II) Reference Group Report.* www.acha-ncha.org/docs/ ACHA-NCHA-II_ReferenceGroup _DataReport_Spring2011.pdf.

23. Heldman, C., & Wade. L. (2010, July.) Hook-up culture: Setting a new research agenda. *Sexual Research and Sexual Policy.* DOI 10.1007/213178-010-0024-z.

24. Nielsen S.L. (2012, March 27). Hook-up culture leaves students wanting. *The Crimson.* www.thecrimson.com/ article/2012/3/27/sex-week-hook-ups/.

25. Kenney, S.R., Thadani V., Ghaidarov T., et al. (2013). First-year college women's motivations for hooking up: A mixed-methods examination of normative peer perceptions and personal hookup participation. *International Journal of Sexual Health. 25* (3), 212–224.

26. Freitas, D. (2013). *The end of sex: How hookup culture is leaving a generation unhappy, sexually unfulfilled, and confused about intimacy.* New York: Basic Books.

27. Epstein, M., Calzo, J.P., Smiler, A.P., et al. (2009). Anything from making out to having sex: Men's negotiations of hooking up and friends with benefits scripts. *Journal of Sex Research, 46* (5), 414–424.

28. Eberstadt, M., & Layden, M.A. (2010). *The social costs of pornography: A statement of findings and recommendations.* Princeton, NJ: The Witherspoon Institute.

29. Carroll, J.S., Padilla-Walker, L.M., Nelson, L.J, et al. (2008). Generation XXX: Pornography acceptance and use among emerging adults. *Journal of Adolescent Research, 23* (1), 6–30.

30. Sukel, K. (2012). *Dirty minds.* New York: Free Press.

31. Lohman, R.C. (2012). The dangers of teen sexting. *Psychology Today.* www.psychology today.com/blog.teen-angst/201207/ the-dangers-teen-sexting.

32. Sankinaaron, A. (2013, June 5). Revenge porn: California legislators go after troubling new trend. *Huffington Post.* www.huffingtonpost. com/2013/06/05/revenge-porn- california_n_3391638.html.

33. Silverberg C. Teledildonics. *About.com.* http://sexuality.about.com/ od/sexandtechnology/a/teledildonics.htm.

34. Crystal meth and sex. www.crystal townhalls.org/methsex.html.

35. Hartney, E. (2010). What is sexual anorexia? *About.com.* http://addictions. about.com/od/sexaddiction/a/what_is_ sexual_anorexia.htm.

36. Counseling Affiliates. Sexual anorexia. www.sexaddictionhelp.com/page. asp?pageID=13&content=Sexual%20 anorexia.

Chapter 12

1. Finer, L.B., & Zolna, M.R. (2014). Shift in intended and unintended pregnancies in the United States, 2001–2008. *American Journal of Public Health,* Feb 104 Suppl 1: S43-8.

2. Hughey, A.B., Neustadt, A.B., et al. (2010). Daily context matters: Predictors of missed oral contraceptive pills among college and graduate students. *American Journal of Obstetrics and Gynecology, 203,* 323.e1–7.

3. Hatcher, R.A., Trussell, J., Nelson, A.L., Cates, W., et al. (2011). *Contraceptive*

technology (20th ed.). New York: Ardent Media.

4. Teichmann, D.A., et al. (2009). Continuous, daily levonorgestrel/ethinyl estradiol vs. 21-day cyclic levonorgestrel/ethinyl estradiol: Efficacy, safety and bleeding in a randomized, open-label trial. *Contraception, 80* (6), 504–511.

5. Bitzer, J., & Simon, J. (2011). Current issues and available options in combined hormonal contraception. *Contraception, 84* (4), 342–356.

6. Winner, B., Peipert, J.F., Zhao, Q. et al. (2012). Effectiveness of long-acting reversible contraception. *New England Journal of Medicine, 366,* 1998–2007.

7. New condoms eyed for men, women. (2011, September 1). *Contraceptive Technology Update.*

8. PATH. (July 2013). SILCS Diaphragm. Technology Updates. www.path.org/publications/detail.php?i=1233

9. Arevalo, M., Jennings, V., Nikula, M., & Sinai, I. (2004). Efficacy of the new Two Day Method of family planning. *Fertility and Sterility 82* (4), 885–892.

10. Jones, R.K., Fennell, J., Higgins, J.A., & Blanchard, K. (2009). Better than nothing or savvy risk-reduction practice? The importance of withdrawal. *Contraception, 79* (6), 407–410.

11. Doherty, I.A., & Stuart, G.S. (2009). Coitus interruptus is not contraception. *Sexually Transmitted Disease, 38* (5), 779–787.

12. Miller, L.M. (2011). Emergency contraceptive pill (ECP) use and experiences at college health centers in the mid-Atlantic United States: Changes since ECP went over-the-counter. *Journal of American College Health, 59* (8), 683–689.

13. Miller, L.M. (2011). College student knowledge and attitudes toward emergency contraception. *Contraception, 83,* 68–73.

14. Glasier A., Cameron S.T., Blithe D., et al. (2011). Can we identify women at risk of pregnancy despite using emergency contraception? Data from randomized trials of ulipristal acetate and levonorgestrel. *Contraception, 84,* 363–367.

15. Peterson, H.B. (2008). Sterilization. *Obstetrics and Gynecology, 111* (1), 189–203.

16. Nagler, H.M., & Jung, H. (2009). Factors predicting successful microsurgical vasectomy reversal. *Urologic Clinics of North America, 3* (3), 383–390.

17. Lino, M. (2013). *Expenditures on children by families, 2012.* U.S. Department of Agriculture, Center for Nutrition and Policy Promotion Publication No. 1528-2012. www.cnpp.usda.gov/Publications/CRC/crc2012.pdf.

18. Unmarried father involvement (info sheet 16). (2008). Minnesota Fathers and Families Network. www.mnfathers.org/Resources/Documents/InfoSheet FragileFamilies%20COLOR.pdf.

19. Guttmacher Institute. (2013). In brief: Facts on induced abortion in the United States. www.guttmacher.org/pubs/fb_induced_abortion.html

20. Pazol, K., Creanga, A.A., Burley, K.D., et al. (2013, November 29). Abortion Surveillance—United States 2010. *Morbidity and Mortality Weekly Report, 62* (8), 1–44.

21. Schlangen, R. (2006). Global illegal abortion: Where there is no "Roe": An examination of the impact of illegal abortion around the world (Issue brief). www.plannedparenthood.org/issues-action/international/global-abortion-6480.htm.

22. Ling, F.W. (2013). Overview of Pregnancy Termination. www.uptodate.com.

23. Devroey, P., Fauser, B.C.J.M., & Diedrich, K. (2009). Approaches to improve the diagnosis and management of infertility. *Human Reproduction Update, 15* (4), 391–408.

24. McGrath, J.J., Petersen, L., Agerbo, E., et al. (2014) A comprehensive assessment of parental age and psychiatric disorders. *Journal of the American Medical Association Psychiatry, 71* (3), 301–309.

25. The American College of Obstetricians and Gynecologists. (2013). Frequently asked questions. Nutrition during pregnancy. www.acog.org/~/media/For%20Patients/faq001.pdf?dmc=1&ts=2013 1211T1232118685.

26. Cunningham, R.G., et al. (2009). *Williams obstetrics* (23rd ed.). New York: McGraw-Hill.

27. The American College of Obstetricians and Gynecologists. (2013). Update on immunization and pregnancy: tetanus, diphtheria and pertussis vaccination. Number 566. www.acog.org/Resources_And_Publications/Committee_Opinions/Committee_on_Obstetric_Practice/Update_on_Immunization_and_Pregnancy_Tetanus_Diphtheria_and_Pertussis_Vaccination.

28. Chasnoff, I J., et al. (2005). The 4P's Plus screen for substance use in pregnancy: Clinical application and outcomes. *Journal of Perinatology, 25,* 368–374.

29. Woolf, S.H., & Aron, L. (2013). *U.S. health in international perspective: Shorter lives, poorer health.* Washington, DC: National Academies Press, Institute of Medicine.

Chapter 13

1. Playfair, J., & Bancroft, G. (2013). *Infection and immunity* (4th ed.). New York: Oxford University Press.

2. Centers for Disease Control and Prevention. (n.d.). Parasitic diseases. www.cdc.gov/ncidod/dpd/index.htm.

3. Centers for Disease Control and Prevention. (1999). Achievements in public health, 1900–1999: Impact of vaccines universally recommended for children—United States, 1990–1998. *Morbidity and Mortality Weekly Report, 48* (12), 243–248.

4. Roush, S.W., Murphy, T.V., et al. (2007). Historical comparisons of morbidity and mortality for vaccine-preventable diseases in the United States. *Journal of the American Medical Association, 298* (18), 2155–2163.

5. Segerstrom, S.C. (2010). Resources, stress and immunity: An ecological perspective on human psychoneuroimmunology. *Annals of Behavioral Medicine, 40,* 114–125.

6. Dragos, D., & Tansescu, M.D. (2010). The effect of stress on the defense systems. *Journal of Medicine and Life, 3* (1), 10–18.

7. Locavore. *Oxford dictionary.* http://oxford-dictionaries.com/definition/locavore.

8. Centers for Disease Control and Prevention. (2013). Investigation update: Multistate outbreak of multidrug-resistant Salmonella Heidelberg infections linked to Foster Farms Brand Chicken. www.cdc.gov/salmonella/heidelberg-10-13/index.html.

9. World Health Organization—Western Pacific Region. (2004). *SARS.* www.wpro.who.

10. World Health Organization. (2012). *Global alert and response,* www.who.int/csr/en/.

11. Panic, M. and Ford, J.D. (2013). A review of national-level adaptation planning with regards to the risks posed by climate change on infectious diseases in 14 OECD nations. *International Journal of Environmental Research and Public Health, 10,* 7083–7109.

12. Center for Disease Control and Prevention (2013). *Climate and health program.* www.cdc.gov/climateandhealth/.

13. Downing-Matibag, T.M., & Geisinger, B. (2009). Hooking up and sexual risk taking among college students: A health belief model perspective. *Qualitative Health Research, 19* (9), 1196–1209.

14. Centers for Disease Control and Prevention. (n.d.). *Hepatitis C FAQs for health professionals.* www.cdc.gov/hepatitis/HCV/HCVfaq.htm#section2.

15. Centers for Disease Control and Prevention. (2011). Transatlantic taskforce on antimicrobial resistance. www.cdc.gov/drugresistance/pdf/tatfar-report.pdf.

16. World Health Organization (2013) Antimicrobial resistance. *Fact Sheet 194.* www.int/mediacentre/factsheets/fs194/en

17. Flaherty, D.K. (2011). The vaccine-autism connection: A public health crisis caused by unethical medical practices and fraudulent science. *Annals of Pharmacotherapy, 45* (10), 1302–1304.

18. Atkinson, W., Hamborsky, J., McIntyre, L., & Wolfe, S. (Eds.). (2007). *Epidemiology and prevention of vaccine-preventable diseases* (10th ed.). Washington, DC: Public Health Foundation.

19. Walker, C.F., Rudan, I., Liu, L., et al. (2013). Global burden of childhood pneumonia and diarrhea. *The Lancet, 381,* 1405–1416.

20. World Health Organization. (2013). The top ten causes of death. *Fact Sheet 310.* www.who.int/mediacentre/factsheets/fs310/en/index.html.

21. Centers for Disease Control and Prevention. (2013). Advisory Committee on Immunization Practices (ACIP) recommended immunization schedule for persons aged 0 through 18 years—United States, 2013. *Morbidity and Mortality Weekly Report, 62* (01), 2–8.

22. World Health Organization. (2013). *Global tuberculosis report 2013.* www.who.int/tb/publications/global_report/en/index.html.

23. Rowland, K. (2012, January 13). Totally drug-resistant TB emerges in India. *Nature, 481* (7380), www.nature.com/news/totally-drug-resistant-tb-emerges-in-india-1.9797.

24. World Health Organization. (2013). World malaria report 2013. www.who.int/malaria/publications/world_malaria_report_2013/report/en/index.html.

25. American College Health Association. (2013). *American College Health Association—National college health assessment: Reference group data report spring 2013.* Baltimore: American College Health Association.

26. Centers for Disease Control and Prevention. (2011). Updated recommendations for use of tetanus toxoid, reduced diphtheria toxoid, and acellular pertussis (TdaP) vaccine from the advisory committee on immunization practices, 2010. *Morbidity and Mortality Weekly Report, 60* (1), 13–15.

27. Centers for Disease Control and Prevention (2013). Guidelines for vaccinating pregnant women. www.cdc.gov/vaccines/pubs/preg-guide.htm.

28. Hansra, N.K., & Shinkai, K. (2011). Cutaneous community acquired and hospital-acquired methicillin-resistant Staphylococcus aureus. *Dermatologic Therapy, 24* (2), 263–272.

29. Colgan, R., & Williams, M. (2011). Diagnosis and treatment of uncomplicated cystitis. *American Family Physician, 84* (7), 771–776.

30. World Health Organization. (2013). *Global report: UNAIDS report on the global AIDS epidemic 2013.* www.unaids.org/en/media/unaids/contentassets/documents/epidemiology/2013/gr2013/UNAIDS_Global_Report_2013_en.pdf.

31. Johnson, A.S., Hall, I., Hu, X. et al (2014). Trends in diagnosis of HIV infection in the United States, 2002–2011. *Journal of the American Medical Association*, 312 (4), 432–434.

32. Centers for Disease Control and Prevention. (2013). Estimates of new HIV infections in the United States, 2007–2010. www.cdc.gov/nchhstp/newsroom/docs/2012/HIV-Infections-2007-2010.pdf.

33. Keele, B.F., Heuverswyn, F.V., Li, Y., et al. (2006). Chimpanzee reservoirs of pandemic and nonpandemic HIV-1. *Science, 313* (5786), 523–526.

34. Occupational Safety and Health Administration. (2011). Bloodborne pathogens and needlestick prevention. www.osha.gov/SLTC/bloodbornepathogens/.

35. Branson, B.M., Handsfield, H.H., Lampe, M.A., et al. (2006). Revised recommendations for HIV testing of adults, adolescents, and pregnant women in health-care settings. *Morbidity and Mortality Recommendations and Reports, 55* (RR14), 1–17.

36. Centers for Disease Control and Prevention (2013). National HIV testing day—June 27, 2013. *Morbidity and Mortality Recommendations and Reports, 62* (24), 489.

37. Centers for Disease Control and Prevention. (n.d.). National HIV and STI testing resources. www.hivtest.org.

38. HIV Vaccines and Microbicides Resource Tracking Working Group. (n.d.). Investing to end the AIDS epidemic: A new era for HIV prevention research and development. www.hivresourcetracking.org/.

39. Centers for Disease Control. Department of Health and Human Services. (2014). 2014 preexposure prophylaxis for the prevention of HIV infection in the United States - 2014. www.cdc.gov/hiv/pdf/prepguidelines2014.pdf.

40. Marrazzo, J.M., & Cates, W. (2011). Interventions to prevent sexually transmitted infections, including HIV infection. *Clinical Infectious Diseases, 53* (3), 64–78.

41. Centers for Disease Control and Prevention. (2012). *Sexually transmitted disease surveillance, 2011.* Atlanta: U.S. Department of Health and Human Services.

42. Centers for Disease Control and Prevention. (n.d.). *Sexually transmitted diseases treatment guidelines 2011.* www.cdc.gov/STI/treatment/default.htm.

43. ACOG Practice Bulletin No. 131: Screening for Cervical Cancer. ACOG Committee on Practice Bulletins—Gynecology. (2012 November). *Obstetrics and Gynecology, 120* (5), 1222–1238. doi: http://10.1097/AOG.0b013e318277c92a.

44. Salit, I.E., et al. (2011). The role of cytology (Pap tests) and human papilloma virus testing in anal cancer screening. *AIDS, 24* (9), 1307–1313.

45. D'Souza, G., Rajan, S.D., Bhatia, R., et al. (2013). Uptake and predictors of anal cancer screening in men who have sex with men. *American Journal of Public Health, 103* (9), 88–95.

46. U.S. Food and Drug Administration. (2009). Gardasil. www.fda.gov/BiologicsBloodVaccines/Vaccines/ApprovedProducts/UCM094042.

47. U.S. Food and Drug Administration. (2009). Cervarix. www.fda.gov/BiologicsBloodVaccines/Vaccines/ApprovedProducts/ucm186957.htm.

48. Bernstein, D.I., Bellamy, A.R., Hook, E.W., et al. (2013). Epidemiology, clinical presentation and antibody response to primary infection with herpes simplex virus type 1 and type 2 in young women. *Clinical Infectious Disease, 56* (3), 344–351.

Chapter 14

1. World Health Organization. (2011). *Global status report on noncommunicable diseases 2010.* www.who.org.

2. World Health Organization. (2011). *Noncommunicable diseases: Country profiles 2011.* www.who.org.

3. American Heart Association. (2013). *Heart disease and stroke statistics—2013 update.* www.americanheart.org.

4. Strong, J.P. (1999). Prevalence and extent of atherosclerosis in adolescents and young adults: Implications for prevention from Pathobiological Determination of Atherosclerosis in Youth Study. *Journal of the American Medical Association, 281* (8), 727–735.

5. Rubini Gimenez, M., Reiter, M., Twerenbold, R., et al. (2014, Feb). Sex specific chest pain characteristics in the early diagnosis of acute myocardial infarction. *Journal of the American Medical Association Internal Medicine, 174*(2): 241–249.

6. Canto, J.G., Goldberg, R.J., Hand, M.M., et al. (2007). Symptom presentation in women with acute coronary syndromes: Myth vs reality. *Archives of Internal Medicine, 167* (22), 2405–2413.

7. Mackay, M.H., Ratner, P.A., Buller, C.E., et al. (2009). Gender differences in reported symptoms of acute coronary syndromes. *Canadian Journal of Cardiology, 25* (Suppl. B), 115b.

8. National Heart, Lung, and Blood Institute. (2011). Congenital heart defects. www.nhlbi.nih.gov/health/health-topics/topics/chd/.

9. Erhardt, L. (2009). Cigarette smoking: An undertreated risk factor for cardiovascular disease. *Atherosclerosis, 205* (1), 23–32.

10. National Heart, Lung, and Blood Institute. (2003). Seventh report of the Joint National Committee on Prevention, Detection, Evaluation and Treatment of High Blood Pressure. www.nhlbi.lnih.gov/guidelines/hypertension/.

11. Holmes, L., Hossain, J., Ward, D., & Opara, F. (2013). Racial/ethnic variability in hypertension prevalence and risk factors

in National Health Interview Survey. *ISRN Hypertension,* Article ID 257842.

12. Stone, N.J., Robinson, J., Lichtenstein, A.H., Merz, N.B., et al. (2013). 2013 ACC/AHA Guideline on the treatment of blood cholesterol to reduce atherosclerotic cardiovascular risk in adults. *Journal of the American College of Cardiology.* doi:10.1016/j.jacc.2013.11.002.

13. Executive summary of the third report of the National Cholesterol Education Program Expert Panel on Detection, Evaluation, and Treatment of High Blood Cholesterol in Adults. (2001). *Journal of the American Medical Association, 285* (19), 2486–2497.

14. Player, M.S., King, D.E., Mainous, A.G., & Geesey, M.E. (2007). Psychosocial factors and progression from prehypertension to hypertension or coronary heart disease. *Annals of Family Medicine, 5,* 403–411.

15. Yusuf, S., Hawken, S., Ounpuu, S., et al. (2004). Effect of potentially modifiable risk factors associated with myocardial infarction in 52 countries (the INTER-HEART study): Case-control study. *Lancet, 364* (9438), 937–952.

16. Cooper, D.C., Mills, P.J., Bardwell, W.A., Ziegler, M.G., & Dimsdale, J.E. (2009). The effects of ethnic discrimination and socioeconomic status on endothelin-1 among Blacks and Whites. *American Journal of Hypertension, 22* (7), 698–704.

17. Kim, D., Kawachi, I., Hoorn, S.V., & Ezzati, M. (2008). Is inequality at the heart of it? Cross-country associations of income inequality with cardiovascular diseases and risk factors. *Social Science and Medicine, 66* (8), 1719–1732.

18. National Research Council and Institute of Medicine. (2013). *U.S. Health in International Perspective: Shorter Lives, Poorer Health. Panel on Understanding Cross-National Health Differences Among High-Income Countries,* S.H. Woolf & L. Aron (Eds.), Committee on Population, Division of Behavioral and Social Sciences and Education and Board on Population Health and Public Health Practice, Institute of Medicine. Washington, DC: The National Academies Press.

19. O'Keefe, J.H., et al. (2004). Psychosocial stress and cardiovascular disease: How to heal a broken heart. *Comprehensive Therapy, 30* (1), 37–43.

20. Cross, B.J., Estes, M., & Link, M. (2011). Sudden cardiac death in athletes and nonathletes. *Current Opinion in Critical Care, 17* (4), 328–334.

21. Office of Minority Health and Health Disparities (OMHD). (n.d.). Eliminate disparities in cardiovascular disease. www.cdc.gov/omhd/AMH/factsheets/cardio.htm.

22. Rossouw, J.E., et al. (2002). Risks and benefits of estrogen plus progestin in healthy postmenopausal women. *Journal of the American Medical Association, 288* (3), 321–333.

23. Temmerman, J.C. (2011). Vitamin D and cardiovascular disease. *Journal of American College Nutrition, 30* (3), 167–170.

24. Helfand, M., Buckley, D.I., Freeman, M., et al. (2009). Emerging risk factors for coronary heart disease: A summary of systemic reviews conducted for the U.S. Preventive Services Task Force. *Annals of Internal Medicine, 151* (7), 496–507.

25. Warren-Gash, C., Smeeth, L., & Hayward, A.C. (2009). Influenza as a trigger for acute myocardial infarction or death from cardiovascular disease: A systematic review. *Lancet Infectious Diseases, 9* (10), 601–610.

26. Harding, R. (2005). Fetal origins of postnatal health and disease. *Early Human Development, 81* (9), 721–722.

27. Fradkin, J.E. (2012). Confronting the urgent challenge of diabetes: An overview. *Health Affairs, 31* (1), 12–19.

28. Centers for Disease Control and Prevention. (2011). *National diabetes fact sheet, 2011.* Atlanta, GA: U.S. Department of Health and Human Services. www.cdc.gov/diabetes/pubs/pdf/ndfs_2011.pdf.

29. DeFronzo, R.A., & Abdul-Ghani, M.A. (2011). Preservation of beta-cell function: The key to diabetes prevention. *Journal of Clinical Endocrinology and Metabolism, 96* (8), 2354–2366.

30. Leroith, D. (2012). Pathophysiology of the metabolic syndrome: Implications for the cardiometabolic risks associated with type 2 diabetes. *American Journal of the Medical Sciences, 343* (1), 13–16.

31. Villarivera, C., Wolcott, J., et al. (2012). The US Preventive Task Force should consider a broader evidence base in updating its diabetes screening guidelines. *Health Affairs, 31* (1), 35–42.

32. Oostdam, N., van Poppel, M.N., et al. (2011). Interventions for preventing gestational diabetes mellitus: A systemic review and meta-analysis. *Journal of Women's Health, 20* (10), 1551–1563.

33. National Heart, Lung, and Blood Institute. (2012). What is asthma? U.S. Department of Health and Human Services. www.nhlbi.nih.gov/health/health-topics/topics/asthma/.

34. Zhang, Y., Moffatt, M.F., & Cookson, W.O.C. (2012). Genetic and genomic approaches to asthma: New insights for the origins. *Current Opinion in Pulmonary Medicine, 18,* 6–13.

35. Fanta, C.H., & Fletcher S.W. (2012). An overview of asthma management. *UpToDate.* www.uptodate.com/contents/an-overview-of-asthma-management?view=print.

36. Centers for Disease Control and Prevention. (2012). Asthma action plan. www.cdc.gov/asthma/actionplan.html.

37. Lloyd-Jones, D.M., Hong, Y., Labarthe, D., et al. (2010). Defining and setting national goals for cardiovascular health promotion and disease reduction. *Circulation, 121,* 586–613.

Chapter 15

1. American Cancer Society. (2013). Cancer facts and figures 2013. www.cancer.org.

2. American College Health Association. (2013). *American College Health Association—National College Health Assessment II: Reference group executive summary spring 2013.* Baltimore: American College Health Association.

3. Produce for Better Health Foundation. (n.d.). Fruits and veggies—more matters. www.fruitsandveggiesmorematters.org/.

4. Kushi, L.H., Doyle, C., et al. (2012). American Cancer Society guidelines on nutrition and physical activity for cancer prevention: Reducing the risk of cancer with healthy food choices and physical activity. *CA: A Cancer Journal for Clinicians, 62* (1), 30–67.

5. World Cancer Research Fund/American Institute for Cancer Research. (2007). *Food, nutrition, physical activity, and the prevention of cancer: A global perspective.* Washington, DC: World Cancer Research Fund.

6. Lomas, A., Leonardi-Bee, J., & Bath-Hextall, F. (2012, January 17). A systematic review of worldwide incidence of non-melanoma skin cancer. *British Journal of Dermatology, 166* (5), 913–915.

7. The Cancer Council Australia. (n.d.). SunSmart. www.cancer.org.au/preventing-cancer/sun-protection/.

8. United Nations. (2010). Report of the United Nations Scientific Committee on the Effects of Atomic Radiation 2010. Summary of low-dose radiation effects on health. Accessed February 7, 2014, at www.unscear.org/docs/reports/2010/UNSCEAR_2010_Report_M.pdf.

9. Gilbert, E.S. (2009). Ionizing radiation and cancer risks: What have we learned from epidemiology? *International Journal of Radiation Biology, 85* (6), 467–482.

10. International Agency on Research for Cancer. World Health Organization. (2011). Press release No 208. IARC classifies radiofrequency electromagnetic fields as possibly carcinogenic to humans. www.iarc.fr/en/media-centre/pr/2011/pdfs/pr208_E.pdf.

11. Szmigielski, S. (2013). Cancer risks related to low-level RF/MW exposures, including cell phones. *Electromagnetic Biology and Medicine, 32* (3), 273–280.

12. Davis, D.L., Kesari, S., Soskolne, C.L., et al. (2013). Swedish review strengthens grounds for concluding that radiation from cellular and cordless phones is a probable human carcinogen. *Pathophysiology, 20* (2), 123–129.

13. Young, G.S., Fox, M.A., Trush, M., et al. (2012) Differential exposure to hazardous air pollution in the United States: A multilevel analysis of urbanization and neighborhood socioeconomic deprivation. *International Journal of Environmental Research and Public Health, 9* (6), 2204–2225.

14. Fontham, E.T.H., Thun, M.J., Ward, E., Balch, A.J., et al. (2009). American Cancer Society perspectives on environmental factors and cancer. *CA: A Cancer Journal for Clinicians, 59* (6), 343–351.

15. Clapp, R.W., Howe, G.K., & Jacobs, M.M. (2007). Environmental and occupational causes of cancer: A call to act on what we know. *Biomedicine and Pharmacotherapy, 61* (10), 631–639.

16. Ruttkay-Nedecky, B., Jimenez, A.M., Nejdl, L., et al. (2013). Relevance of infection with human papillomavirus: The role of the p53 tumor suppressor protein and E6/E7 zinc finger proteins. *International Journal of Oncology, 43* (6), 1754–1762.

17. Hasegawa, Y., Ando, M., Kubo, A., et al. (2014). Human papilloma virus in non-small cell lung cancer in never smokers: A systematic review of the literature. *Lung Cancer ,83* (1), 8–13.

18. Tolstov, Y., Kadaschik, B., Pahernik, S., et al. (2014) Human papillomaviruses in urologic malignancies: a critical assessment. *Urology Oncology, 32* (1), 46e19–27.

19. Shah, K.M., & Young, L.S. (2009). Epstein-Barr virus and carcinogenesis: Beyond Burkitt's lymphoma. *Clinical Microbiology and Infection, 15* (11), 982–988.

20. Higgs, M.R., Chouteau, P., & Lerat, H. (2014). Liver let die: oxidative DNA damage and hepatotropic viruses. *Journal of General Virology, 10,* 1099/vir.o.o59485-0

21. Hsu, W., Lin, C., Lin, C., et al. (2014) The relationship between Helicobacter pylori and cancer risk. *European Journal of Internal Medicine, S0953-6205* (14), 00010–00017.

22. Deng, B., Li, Y., Zhang, Y., Bai, L., & Yang, P. (2013). Helicobacter pylori infection and lung cancer: A review of an emerging hypothesis. *Carcinogenesis, 34* (6), 1189–1195.

23. Wojas-Krawczyk, K., Krawczyk, P., Biernacka, B., et al. (2012). The polymorphism of the CHRNA5 gene and the strength of nicotine addiction in lung cancer and COPD patients. *European Journal of Cancer Prevention, 21* (2), 111–117.

24. Suqimura, H., Tao, H., Suzuki, M., et al. (2011). Genetic susceptibility to lung cancer. *Frontiers in Bioscience, 1* (3), 1463–1477.

25. Humphrey, L., Deffebach, M., Pappas, M., Baumann, C., et al. (2013). Screening for lung cancer: Systematic review to update the U.S. Preventive Services Task Force Recommendation. July Report No. 13-05188-EF-1. Rockville, MD: Agency for Healthcare Research and Quality.

26. American Cancer Society. (2011). Colorectal cancer facts and figures 2011–2013. www.cancer.org/acs/groups/content/@epidemiologysurveillance/documents/document/acspc-028323.pdf.

27. Centers for Disease Control and Prevention. (2013). National breast and cervical cancer early detection program. www.cdc.gov/cancer/nbccedp/index.htm.

28. U.S. Preventive Task Force. (2009, November). Screening for breast cancer. www.ahrq.gov/clinic/uspstf/uspsbrca.htm.

29. American Cancer Society. (2013, December). Mammograms and other breast imaging procedures. www.cancer.org/acs/groups/cid/documents/webcontent/003178-pdf.pdf.

30. National Cancer Institute. (201, December 5). Breast cancer screening (PDQ®)–Health professional. www.cancer.gov/cancertopics/pdq/screening/breast/HealthProfessional.

31. Berry, D.A. (2013). Breast cancer screening: controversy of impact. *The Breast, 22* (2), S73–S76.

32. American Cancer Society (January 2014). Breast awareness and self exam. www.cancer.org/cancer/breastcancer/moreinformation/breastcancerearly-detection/breast-cancer-early-detection-acs-recs-bse.

33. U.S. Food and Drug Administration. (2010). Provenge. vaccines, bloods and biologics. www.fda.gov/Biologics BloodVaccines/CellularGeneTherapy Products/ApprovedProducts/ucm210012.htm.

34. National Cancer Institute. (n.d.). Ovarian cancer. www.cancer.gov/cancertopics/types/ovarian/.

35. U.S. Preventive Services Task Force. (2012). Screening for ovarian cancer. Accessed February 9, 2014, at www.uspreventiveservicestaskforce.org/uspstf12/ovarian/ovarcancersum.htm.

36. Runger, T. M., & Kappes, U. P. (2008). Mechanisms of mutation formation with long-wave ultraviolet light (UVA). *Photodermatology, Photoimmunology, and Photomedicine, 24* (1), 2–10.

37. National Cancer Institute. (n.d.). SEER stats fact sheet: Testis. http://seer.cancer.gov/statfacts/html/testis.html#risk.

38. Hayes-Lattin, B., & Nichols, C.R. (2009). Testicular cancer: A prototypic tumor of young adults. *Seminars in Oncology, 36* (5), 432–438.

39. Dunne, E.F., Markowitz, L.E., Saraiya, M., et al. (2014). CDC grand rounds: Reducing the burden of HPV-associated cancer and disease. *Morbidity and Mortality Weekly Report, 63* (4), 69–72.

40. National Cancer Institute. (n.d.). Types of treatment. www.cancer.gov/cancertopics/treatment/types-of-treatment.

41. National Center for Complementary and Alternative Medicine. (n.d.). Cancer and CAM at a glance. http://nccam.nih.gov/health/cancer/camcancer.htm.

42. Cramer, H., Cohen, L., Gustav, D., & Witt, C.M. (2013). Integrative oncology: Best of both worlds—theoretical, practical and research ideas. *Evidence-based Complementary and Alternative Medicine, 2013,* 383142.

Chapter 16

1. Centers for Disease Control and Prevention, National Center for Injury Prevention and Control. (2009). CDC injury fact book. www.cdc.gov/injury/publications/factbook/.

2. Centers for Disease Control and Prevention. (2011). Injuries among American Indians/Alaska Natives (AI/AN): Fact sheet. www.cdc.gov/motorvehiclesafety/native/factsheet.html.

3. National Highway Traffic Safety Administration. (2013). *Early estimates of motor vehicle traffic fatalities 2012* (Publication No. DOT HS 811 741). Washington, DC: U.S. Department of Transportation.

4. Centers for Disease Control and Prevention. (April 19, 2013). Motor Vehicle traffic-related pedestrian deaths—United States, 2001–2010. *Morbidity and Mortality Weekly Report, 62* (15), 277–282.

5. Centers for Disease Control and Prevention. Distracted driving in the United States and Europe. www.cdc.gov/motorvehiclesafety/distracted_driving/.

6. Coben, J.H. (2013). Keeping an eye on distracted driving. *Journal of American Medical Association, 309* (9), 877–878.

7. Centers for Disease Control and Prevention. (January 4, 2013). Drowsy driving—19 states and the District of Columbia, 2009–2010. *Morbidity and Mortality Weekly Report, 61* (51), 1033–1037.

8. National Highway Traffic Safety Administration. (2006). *The impact of driver-inattention on near crash/crash risk: An analysis using the 100-Car Naturalistic Driving Study data* (Publication No. DOT HS 810594). Washington, DC: U.S. Department of Transportation.

9. Road Ragers. (2011). What is road rage. www.roadragers.complaint-is-road-rage.htm.

10. National Highway Traffic Safety Administration. (2009). *Alcohol-impaired drivers involved in fatal crashes, by gender and state: 2007–2008* (Publication No. DOT HS 811195). Washington, DC: U.S. Department of Transportation.

11. Centers for Disease Control and Prevention. (2012). Preventing injuries in America: Public health in action. www.cdc.gov.

12. NHTSA Federal Motor. (2011). Test procedures. www.nhsta.gov/vehicle+safety/testprocedures.

13. Centers for Disease Control and Prevention. (2011). Vital signs: Adult seat belt use in the US. www.cdc.gov/vitalsigns/SeatBeltUse/index.html.

14. Centers for Disease Control and Prevention. (2011). Still, 1 in 7 adults do not wear a seat belt on every trip. www.cdc.gov/media/releases/2011/p0104_vitalsigns.html.

15. Decker, M.D., Rice, T.M., & Anderson, C.L. (2009). The use and efficacy of child restraint devices. *American Journal of Public Health, 99* (7), 1161–1162.

16. Homer, J., & French, M. (2009). Motorcycle helmet laws in the United States from 1990 to 2005: Politics and public health. *American Journal of Public Health, 99* (3), 408–415.

17. Insurance Institute for Highway Safety, Highway Loss Data Institute. (2008). Current U.S. motorcycle and bicycle helmet laws. www.iihs.org/laws/helmetusecurrent.aspx.

18. American College Health Association. (Spring, 2012). *National College Health Assessment II.* www.acha-ncha.org/reports_ACHA-NCHAII.html.

19. Centers for Disease Control and Prevention. Walk this way! Taking steps for pedestrian safety. www.cdc.gov/Features/PedestrianSafety/.

20. Centers for Disease Control and Prevention. (2011). Pedestrian safety: Fact sheet. www-nrd.nhtsa.gov/Pubs/811888.pdf.

21. Jaffe, E. (2013). Distracted walking puts 1,500 people into the hospital a year. *The Atlantic.* www.theatlanticcities.com/arts-and-lifestyle/2013/07/distracted-walking-puts-1500-people-into-the-hospital-a-year.

22. Main E. Distracted driving addressed by politicians, scientists, and advocates. www.rodale.com/print/2239.

23. Lowy, J. The big story: Drunk walking leads to pedestrian fatalities. Associated Press. http://bigstory.ap.org/article/drunk-walking-leads-pedestrian-fatalities.

24. Praderelli, M. (2005). As ATV usage soars, safety needs to take a front seat. *Midwest Injury Prevention Control, 7* (1), 1.

25. Crispi, K. (n.d.). Pocket bikes. *FindLaw.* http://injury.findlaw.com/personal-injury-a-z/pocket-bikes.html.

26. Saluja, G., Brenner, R.A., Trumble, A., et al. (2006). Swimming pool drownings among U.S. residents aged 5–24 years: Understanding racial/ethnic disparities. *American Journal of Public Health, 96* (4), 778–783.

27. Centers for Disease Control and Prevention. (2008). Water-related injury: Fact sheet. www.cdc.gov/ncipc/factsheets/drown.htm.

28. Fiore, K. (2009). Rock climbing injuries going up. *ABC News.* http://abcnews.go.com/print?id=8165004.

29. Centers for Disease Control and Prevention. (2009). Fire deaths and injuries: Fact sheet. www.cdc.gov/ncipc/factsheets/fire.htm.

30. National Fire Protection Agency. (2006). *Fire in your home.* Washington, DC: National Fire Protection Agency.

31. Centers for Disease Control and Prevention. (2008). Poisoning in the United States: Fact sheet. www.cdc.gov/ncipc/factsheets/poisoning.htm.

32. Centers for Disease Control and Prevention. (2008). Tips to prevent poisoning. www.cdc.gov/ncipc/factsheets/poisonprevention.htm.

33. Centers for Disease Control and Prevention. (2011). Lead hazards in some holiday toys. www.cdc.gov/Features/LeadInToys/.

34. Centers for Disease Control and Prevention. (2014). Carbon monoxide (CO) poisoning prevention. www.cdc.gov/features/copoisoning/.

35. Centers for Disease Control and Prevention. (2011). Unintentional poisoning—Keep yourself and others safe. www.cdc.gov/Features/PoisonPrevention/.

36. Aleccia, J. (2013, June 4). Deaths in hot cars claim 8 children so far this spring. *NBC News: Vitals.* http://vitals.nbcnews.com/_news/2013/06/04/18732520-deaths-9n-hot-xars-claim-8-children-so-far-this-spring.

37. Park, A. (2009). iPod safety: Preventing hearing loss in teens. *Time.* http://time.com/time/printout/0,8816,1881130,00.html.

38. Centers for Disease Control and Prevention, National Center for Injury Prevention and Control. (2013, July 23). Concussion in sport. *Traumatic Brain Injury.* www/cdc.gov/concussion/sports/index.html.

39. Mitka, M. (2013). Guideline: Tailor appraisal of concussion during sports. *Journal of the American Medical Association, 309* (15), 3980.

40. University of Washington School of Medicine. (2014). Survive cardiac arrest. http://depts.washington.edu/survive/cardiac/arrest.

41. Wilson, J. (2012, September 20). Your smartphone is a pain in the neck. *CNN: Our Mobile Society.* www.cnn.com/2012/09/20/health/mobile-society-neck-pain/.

42. Mozaffarian, D., Hemenway, D., & Ludwig, D. (2013). Curbing gun violence: Lessons from public health success. *Journal of the American Medical Association. 309* (6), 551–552.

43. Kellermann, A.L., & Rivers, F.P. (2013). Silencing the science on gun research. *Journal of the American Medical Association, 309* (6), 549–550.

44. Frieden, T. (2011, September 19). FBI: 2010 sees further decline in violent crime. *CNN News: Justice.* www.cnn.com/2011/09/19/justice/fbi-crime-report/.

45. Aronwitz, T. (2013). How safe are college campuses? *Journal of the American Medical Association, 61* (2), 57–58.

46. Hazing Prevention Organization. (n.d.). Hazing facts. *Hazing Information.* www.hazingprevention.org/hazing-information.html.

47. Couch, C. (n.d.). The lowdown on college hazing. College Bound Network. www.collegebound.net/content/article/the-,lowdown-onpcollege0hazing/19224.

48. Hudson, D.L. (2007). Hate speech and campus speech codes. www.firstamendmentcenter.org/speech/pubcollege/topic.aspx?topic=campus_speech_codes.

49. Centers for Disease Control and Prevention. (November 2011). *The national intimate partner and sexual violence survey.* Atlanta, GA: National Center for Injury Prevention and Control.

50. Carr, J. L. (2005). *Campus violence white paper.* Baltimore, MD: American College Health Association.

51. Bureau of Justice Statistics. (2012). *National crime victimization survey, 2012.* www.ojp.usdoj.gov/bjs.

52. U.S. Department of Education. (2011). Dear colleague letter: Sexual violence background, summary, and fast facts. www2.ed.gov/about/offices/list/ocr/docs/dcl-factsheet-201104.html.

53. Flack, W.F., Coran, M.L., Seinen, S.J., et al. (2008). The red zone: Temporal risk for unwanted sex among college students. *Journal of Interpersonal Violence, 23* (9), 1177–1196.

54. Rape Abuse and Incest National Network. (2009). RAINN's back-to-school tips for students. www.rain.org/news-room/sexual-assault news/2009-back-to-school-tips.20.

55. Rapoza, K.A., & Drake, J.E. (2009). Relationships of hazardous alcohol use, alcohol expectancies, and emotional commitments to male sexual coercion and aggression in dating. *Journal of*

the Study of Alcohol and Drugs, 70 (1), 55–63.

56. Center for Public Integrity. (2009). Sexual assault on campus shrouded in secrecy. www.publicintegrity.org/investigations/campus_assault/articles/entry/1838/.

57. Center for Public Integrity. (2009). Campus sexual assault statistics don't add up. www.publicintegrity.org/investigations/campus_assault/articles/entry/1841/.

58. Center for Public Integrity. (2009). Barriers curb reporting on campus sexual assault. www.publicintegrity.org/investigations/campus_assault/articles/entry/1822/.

59. Finkelhor, D., Turner, H., Ormond, R., et al. (2009). Violence, abuse, and crime exposure in a national sample of children and youth. Pediatrics, 124, 1411–1423.

60. Wallace, H. (2005). Family violence: Legal, medical and social perspectives. Boston: Allyn & Bacon.

61. McCarty, C. (2007). New Jersey attorney general subpoenas Facebook over sex offender data. http://news.cnet.com/8301-13577_3-9790064-36.html.

62. U.S. Equal Employment Opportunity Commission. (2008). Sexual harassment. www.eeoc.gov/types/sexual_harassment.html.

63. Rospenda, K.M., Richman, J.A., & Shannon, C.A. (2009). Prevalence and mental health correlates of harassment and discrimination in the workplace. Journal of Interpersonal Violence, 24 (50), 819–843.

64. National Center for Victims of Crime. (n.d.). Stalking. www.ncvc.org.

65. Crime Library. (n.d.). Cyber-stalking: Risk management. www.crimelibrary.com/criminal_mind/psychology/cyberstalking/6.html.

66. U.S. Department of Health and Human Services. (2007). Child maltreatment. Washington, DC: Administration for Children and Families.

67. Love Is Not Abuse. http://loveisnotabuse.com/web/guest/home/journal_content/56/10123/193872/155832.

68. Cornelius, T.L., Sullivan, K.T., Wyngarden, N., et al. (2009). Participation in prevention programs for dating violence. Journal of Interpersonal Violence, 24 (6), 1057–1078.

69. McPhail, B.A., & Dinitto, D.M. (2006). Prosecutorial perspectives on gender bias and hate crimes. Violence Against Women, 11 (19), 1162–1185.

70. Mitka, M. (2013). Search for ways to reduce gun violence spurred by toll of recent shootings. Journal of the American Medical Association, 309 (8), 755–756.

71. Record K.L., & Gostin L.O. (2013). A systematic plan for firearms law reform. Journal of the American Medical Association, 309 (12), 1231–1232.

72. Institute of Medicine and National Research Council. Firearm-related violence. Washington, DC: National Academies Press.

73. Students for Concealed Carry on Campus. (2011). http://concealedcampus.org; GunFacts; www.GunFacts.info.

74. Lewiecki E.M., & Miller S.A. (2013). Suicide, guns, and public policy. American Journal pf Public Health, 103 (1), 27–31.

75. Minnebo, J. (2006). The relation between psychological distress, television exposure, and television-viewing motives in crime victims. Media Psychology, 8 (2), 61–63.

76. Murray, C. (2002). The physical environment. In J.Q. Wilson & J. Petersilia (Eds.), Crime: Public policies for crime control (pp. 349–361). San Francisco: ICS Press.

77. Samson, R.J. (2002). The community. In J.Q. Wilson & J. Petersilia (Eds.), Crime: Public policies for crime control (pp. 225–252). San Francisco: ICS Press.

78. Stephens, K.A. (2009). Rape prevention with college men. Journal of Interpersonal Violence, 24 (6), 996–1013.

79. Furedi, F. (2005). The culture of fear: Why Americans are afraid of the wrong things. New York: Continuum Intermediate Publishing Group.

About the Authors

Photos courtesy of Michael Teague, Sara Mackenzie, David Rosenthal.

Table of Contents

Page iv(yoga) © Imagemore/Getty Images; Page v(Asian man): © Creative/Getty Images; Page vi(girl friends): © Susanne Walstrom/Getty Images; Page vii(soccer player): © Stockbyte/PunchStock; Page viii(two women): © FredFroese/E+/Getty Images; Page ix(cannabis plant): Courtesy of U.S. Drug Enforcement Agency; Page x(Gardasil vaccine): © AP Images/John Amis; Page xi(almonds): © Image Source/PunchStock; Page xii(headphones): © Image Source/Getty Images; Page xiii(recycling): © E+/Getty Images.

Design Elements

Speech Bubbles icon: © lushik/iStock Vectors/Getty Images; Checkmark icon: © funnybank/iStock Vectors/Getty Images; Warning Symbol icon: © Imagotres/Getty Images; Clipboard icon: © Stockbyte/PunchStock; Athlete shoes icon: © McGraw-Hill Education. Ken Karp, photographer; Whistle icon: © iStock/Getty Images; People icon: © McGraw-Hill Education.

Chapter 1

Opener: © Stockbyte/Getty Images; 1.2a © Brand X Pictures/PunchStock; p.3: Stockbyte/PictureQuest; 1.3a: © Creative/Getty Images; 1.5a(left)© Beyond/SuperStock; 1.5b(right): © Custom Medical Stock Photo/Alamy; p.12: © McGraw-Hill Education. Mark Dierker, photographer; p.13: © Peter Dazely/Iconica/Getty Images; p.14(top): © Comstock/PunchStock; p.14(woman): © Barbara Penoyar/Getty Images; p.14(man): © Stockbyte/PunchStock; p.14(couple): © John Henley/Getty Images; p.14(baby): © Purestock/Superstock; p.15: © Mehdi Taamallah/AFP/Getty Images; p.17: © McGraw-Hill Education. Andrew Resek, photographer; p.19: © 2012 NBAE Photo by Rocky Widner/NBAE via Getty Images; p.19: © Rachel Epstein /The Image Works; 1.9a: © Angelo Cavalli/Getty Images.

Chapter 2

Opener: © Yellow Dog Productions/Digital Vision/Getty Images; p.24: © MXA/Getty Images; 2.2: © Tinette Reed/Brand X Pictures/JupiterImages; 2.3: © Fuse/Getty images; p.33: © Michael Reynolds/EPA/Corbis; p.34: Stockdisc/Stockbyte/Getty Images; 2.4(beer): © Burke/Triolo Productions/Getty Images; 2.4(bong): Courtesy of U.S. Drug Enforcement Agency; 2.4(ashtray): © Photodisc Collection/Getty Images; 2.4(coffee): © Ingram Publishing/Fotosearch; 2.4(donuts): © Comstock/PunchStock; 2.4(cards): © RF/Corbis; 2.4(hangers): © Janis Christie/Getty Images; 2.4(sign): © RF/Corbis; 2.4(woman): © RF/Corbis; p.7: © Photodisc Collection/Getty Images; 2.5: © Galen Rowell/Corbis; p.42: © Peter Parks/AFP/Getty Images; p.43: © Ariel Skelley/Blend Images/Corbis; p.45: © C Squared Studios/Getty Images; p.48: © Maskot/Getty Images; p.49: © Brand X Pictures/JupiterImages/Getty Images; p.50: © Trinette Reed/Blend Images LLC; p.51: © Dougal Waters/Digital Vision/Getty Images.

Chapter 3

Opener: © Amy Eckert/Taxi/Getty Images; p.55: © Susanne Walstrom/Getty Images; p.56: © Steve Cohen/Getty Images; p.58(Burt): © Ingram Publishing; p.58(Savannah): © Onoky/SuperStock; p.58(Peter, Sara): © Image Source/Getty Images; p.58(Nick): © Stockbyte/Getty Images; p.58(Leslie): © Jose Luis Pelaez Inc./Blend Images LLC ; p.58: © Image Source/Getty Images; p.58: © Ronnie Kaufman/Larry Hirshowitz/Blend Images LLC; p.60: © Monica Lau/Photodisc/Getty Images; p.62: © Ben Sklar/Dallas Morning News/Corbis; p.64(top): © Stephane Lehr/Corbis; p.64(bottom): © Juanmonino/E+/Getty Images; p.67(top): © Banana-Stock/Alamy; p.67(bottom): © Steve Debenport/E+/Getty Images; p.70: © SW Productions/Brand X/Corbis; p.71: Corporation for National & Community Service; p.73: © James Marshall/The Image Works.

Chapter 4

Opener: © rubberball/Getty Images; 4.1a: © Stockbyte/Getty Images; p.79: © FilmMagic/Getty Images; p.85: © Russ Elliot/AdMedia/AdMedia/Corbis; 4.2a: © PhotoAlto/PunchStock; p.82: © Buena Vista Images/Stockbyte/Getty Images; p.83: © Design Pics/Pete Stec/Getty Images; p.86: © Photodisc; p.87: © Stuart O'Sullivan/The Image Bank/Getty Images; p.90: © PhotoAlto Agency/Getty Images; p.91: © Koichi Kamoshida/Getty Images; p.92: McGraw-Hill Education.

Chapter 5

Opener: © Andersen Ross/Blend Images/Getty Images; p.96: © Colin Hawkins/cultura/Corbis; p.97: © JupiterImages/Getty Images; p.100: © Tooga/Getty Images; p.102: © Jonelle Weaver/Getty Images; 5.2: MyPlate, 2010, U.S. Department of Agriculture, Center for Nutrition Policy and Promotion; p.5.3: © McGraw-Hill Education. Jill Braaten, photographer; p.5.4(left): © McGraw-Hill Education; p.5.4(right): © McGraw-Hill Education. Mark Steinmetz, photographer; p.115: © McGraw-Hill Education. Jill Braaten, photographer; p.117: © C Squared Studios/Getty Images; p.120: © Dave & Les Jacobs/Blend Images/Getty Images; p.120: © Tarek El Sombati/E+/Getty Images; p.120: © Alex Cao/Photodisc/Getty Images; p.120: © Inmagine.

Chapter 6

Opener: © Hero Images/Getty Images; 6.1: © Ingram Publishing/Alamy; p.128: © Photodisc/Getty Images; p.127© : Stockbyte/PunchStock; p.130: © Lisa Noble/flickr Editorial/Getty Images; p.131: © Norma Jean Gargasz/Alamy; p.133: © Ingram Publishing/Alamy; p.134: © Tobias Titz/Getty Images; p.136: © Ryan McVay/Getty Images; p.136: © Mark Hamel/Getty Images; p.138: © CB2/ZOB/WENN/Newscom; p.139: © keepics/Alamy; p.140: © Rick Bowmer/AP Images; p.140: © Howard Lipin/ZUMA Press/Newscom; p.141: © Adam Pretty/Getty Images; p.141: © mlorenzphotography/Flickr/Getty Images; p.143: © Barry Lewis/In Pictures/Corbis.

Chapter 7

Opener: © Adam Crowley/Blend Images/Getty Images; p.148: © Brand X Pictures/PunchStock; p.150: © NBAE 2010 Photo by Issac Baldizon/NBAE via Getty Images; p.152: © Hero Images/Vetta/Getty Images; p.155: © Scott Olson/Getty Images; 7.1(fist): © Photodisc/Getty Images; 7.1(ball): © Pixtal/ Superstock; 7.1(cards): © McGraw-Hill Education. Richard Hutchings, photographer; 7.1(mouse): © Brand X Pictures; 7.1(ping pong): © Image Source/PunchStock; 7.1(dice): C Squared Studios/Getty Images; p.157: Stockbyte; p.159: iStockphoto.com/luoman; p.161: Ed Andrieski/AP Images; p.163: Paul Burns/Getty Images.

Chapter 8

Opener: © Michael Rowe/DK Stock/Getty Images; p.166: © Evan Agostini/AP Images; p.167(left): © McGraw-Hill Education; p.167(right): © Bloomberg via Getty Images; p.168(top): © David J. Green-Lifestyle/Alamy; p.168(bottom): © Luca Bruno/AP Images; p.169(top): © JG Photography/Alamy; p.169(bottom): © Jonathan Kantor Studio/Photodisc/Getty Images; p.172: © Jeff Kravitz/FilmMagic/Getty Images; 8.2: © photosindia/Getty Images; 8.3: © BananaStock/PunchStock; p.175: © Simon Lees/Tap Magazine/Getty Images; p.177: © Anatoly Repin/E+/Getty Images; p.178: © Hero Images/Getty Images; p.180: © FredFroese/E+/Getty Images.

Chapter 9

Opener: © Stockbyte/Getty Images; 9.1(beer): © iStockphoto.com/Bjorn Heller; 9.1(wine): © iStockphoto.com; 9.1(shot): © C Squared Studios/Getty Images; 9.1(drink): © Comstock Images/Alamy; p.185: © Rudi Von Briel/PhotoEdit; p.186: © Image Source/Getty Images; 9.2a: © George Doyle/Getty Images; 9.4a: © Getty Images; p.193: Courtesy of National

Institute on Alcohol Abuse and Alcoholism of the National Institutes of Health; p.195: © Victor R. Caivano/AP Images; p.195: © Janine Wiedel/Photolibrary/Alamy; p.197: © Blend Images/Alamy; p.199: Photo by Bob Nichols, USDA Natural Resources Conservation Service; p.200: © Simon de Glanville/Alamy; p.201(top): Aleksandar Jocic/iStockphoto.com; p.201(bottom): © Vehbi Koca/Alamy; 9.6: © Tim Large–Youth Social Issues/Alamy; p.203: © Newscom; p.205: California Department of Health Services and CDC/Office on Smoking and Health (OSH) Media Campaign Resource Center (MCRC); p.208: © Newscom; p.208: © Brooks Kraft/Corbis.

Chapter 10

Opener: © Seth McConnell/The Denver Post via Getty Images; p.219(top): © James Carman/Blend Images/Getty Images; p.219(bottom): © RF/Corbis; 10.4: © ER Productions/Getty Images; p.225(top): © Michael Loccisano/Getty Images for Sundance Film Festival; p.225(bottom): Multnomah County Sheriff's Office/Barcroft USA/Getty Images; p.226: © Mills, Andy/Star Ledger/Corbis; p.228: © AP Images; p.229: © Darren McCollester/Getty Images; p.230: Courtesy of U.S. Drug Enforcement Agency; p.234: © Albert Mollon/Moment/Getty Images.

Chapter 11

Opener: © Vstock LLC/Getty Images; p.238: © Don Emmert/AFP/Getty Images; p.244: © Steve Granitz/WireImage/Getty Images; p.245: © Blend Images/Ariel Skelley/Getty Images; p.246: © Radius Images/Alamy; p.250, 256: © McGraw-Hill Education.

Chapter 12

Opener: © Tom Merton/OJO Images/Getty Images; p.260: © Juanmonino/E+/Getty Images; 12.1: © Image Source/Getty Images; p.263: © Photodisc/Getty Images; p.266: © McGraw-Hill Education. Jill Braaten, photographer; p.268: © Justin Sullivan/Getty Images; p.271: © Jacopo Raule/FilmMagic/Getty; p.273: © LWA/The Image Bank/Getty Images; p.274: © Andy Levin/Photo Researchers, Inc.; p.277: © Kevin Brofsky/Getty Images; p.280: © Francisco Cruz/Purestock/SuperStock.

Chapter 13

Opener: © Nina Shannon/E+/Getty Images; p.286: Courtesy of the Center for Disease Control; 13.4: © JupiterImages/Getty Images; p.289:

© Ale Ventura/PhotoAlto Agency/PhotoLibrary; p.290: © moodboard/Corbis; p.292: © Anna Yu/Alamy; p.294: © Glowimages/Getty Images; p.298(left): © McGraw-Hill Education. Barry Barker, photographer; p.298(right): © Scott Camazine/Alamy; p.302: © browndogstudios/iStock-photos.com; p.304: © Mario Tama/Getty Images; p.305: © McGraw-Hill Education. Christopher Kerrigan, photographer; p.309: © AP Images/John Amis.

Chapter 14

Opener: © Michael Krinke/iStock/360/Getty Images; p.317: © McGraw-Hill Education. Jill Braaten, photographer; p.318: © McGraw-Hill Education. Rick Brady, photographer; p.319: © Jason LaVeris/FilmMagic/Getty Images; p.323: © Blend Images; p.324: © Moodboard/360/Getty Images; p.325: © Image Source/PunchStock; p.326: © Lawrence Sawyer/E+/Getty Images; p.328: © Jonathan Fredin/AP Images; p.331: © Jon Kopaloff/FilmMagic/Getty Images; p.335: © Rubber ball/Nicole Hill/Getty Images.

Chapter 15

Opener: © Comstock/Alamy; p.338: Holly Anissa Photography/Moment/Getty Images; 15.1: Rubberball/Getty Images; p.342: Jason Merritt/Getty Images; p.343: © Sean Sprague/The Image Works; p.348: Charles Norfleet/FilmMagic/Getty Images; p.350: PhotoDisc/Getty Images; p.353: Jose Luis Magana/AP Images; p.356: Valerie Macon/AFP/Getty Images.

Chapter 16

Opener: © Bloomberg via Getty Images; p.362: © Gene Chutka/E+/Getty Images; p.363: © McGraw-Hill Education. Rick Brady, photographer; 16.1(driver): © iStockphoto.com; 16.1(stadium): © David Madison/Corbis; p.364: © Insurance Institute for Highway Safety/AP Images; p.366: © S. Solum/PhotoLink/Getty Images; p.367: © RF/Corbis; p.367: © Cultura/Alamy; p.368: © Comstock/Alamy; p.368, 369: © Photodisc/Getty Images; p.371: © Tetra Images/Getty Images; p.371: © Image Source/Getty Images; p.373: © Ted S. Warren-Pool/Getty Images; p.377: © Steve Shepard/iStock/360/Getty Images; p.378: Courtesy MenCan-StopRape.org; 16.5: © Monica Lau/Getty Images; p.383: © Shawn Baldwin/AP Images; p.384: © Brian Branch-Price/AP Images; p.384: © Comstock/JupiterImages/Getty Images; p.386: © S. Meltzer/PhotoLink/Getty Images.